HEALTH UNIT COORDINATING

Expanding the Scope of Practice

MADELINE A. CLARK, RN, BGS, CHUC

VIRGINIA S. MAZZA, RN, CHUC

W.B. SAUNDERS COMPANY
A Division of Harcourt Brace & Company
Philadelphia London Toronto Montreal Sydney Tokyo

W.B. SAUNDERS COMPANY
A Division of Harcourt Brace & Company

The Curtis Center
Independence Square West
Philadelphia, Pennsylvania 19106

Library of Congress Cataloging-in-Publication Data

Health unit coordinating : expanding the scope of practice / [edited by] Madeline A. Clark, Virginia S. Mazza.—1st ed.

p. cm.

Includes index.

ISBN 0–7216–7036–9

1. Hospital ward clerks—Miscellanea. I. Clark, Madeline A. II. Mazza, Virginia S. [DNLM: 1. Personnel, Hospital. 2. Medical Records. 3. Health Facilities—organization & administration. WX 159 bH4344 1999]

RA972.55.H43 1999 651.5′04261—dc21

DNLM/DLC 98-24850

HEALTH UNIT COORDINATING
Expanding the Scope of Practice ISBN 0–7216–7036–9

Printed in the United States of America

Last digit is the print number: 9 8 7 6 5 4 3 2 1

To Mickey Sperry and the late Judy Graham, whose devotion to furthering the cause of the health unit coordinator inspired me to try to do the same; and to my friend Betty, who provided patience and support through this long and arduous project.

Madeline Clark

To my students, who taught me more than I could ever teach them; and to my beloved husband, Joe, whose love and understanding have endured through all my efforts.

Virginia Mazza

Contributors

Section Editors

E. Anne Mason, RN
Director, Clinical Services,
Mercy Home Care of Western New York,
Lockport, New York
Home-Based Care

Cynthia Nault, CHUC
Information Systems Specialist,
Surgical Services,
St. Joseph Health Center,
Kansas City, Missouri
The Emergency Department
The Operating Room

Sandy Ayres, CHUC, BBA
Unit Secretary Coordinator/Educator,
Luther Midelfort, Eau Claire, Wisconsin
Special Care Units: Overview

Donna Baker, CHUC
Madonna Rehabilitation Hospital,
Lincoln, Nebraska
Rehabilitation Facility

Lynda Black, BSED, ASN
Registered Nurse in Open Heart Recovery Unit,
Certified Health Unit Coordinator,
Charleston Area Medical Center,
Charleston, West Virginia
Special Care Units: Open Heart Recovery

Wendy Bollinger, CHUC, HUC II
University of Wisconsin Hospitals & Clinics,
Madison, Wisconsin
Transplant Unit

Beth C. Brace, CHUC
Health Unit Coordinator Instructor,
University of Wisconsin Hospitals & Clinics,
Madison, Wisconsin
Introduction

Jan Bumgarner, CHUC
Staffing Coordinator,
Osteopathic Medical Center,
Fort Worth, Texas
Centralized Staffing/Scheduling Coordinator

Louise A. Butterfield, CHUC
Gundersen/Lutheran Hospital,
La Crosse, Wisconsin
Same Day Admission Unit

Kathryn Bymers, CHUC
St. Joseph's Hospital,
Marshfield, Wisconsin
Special Care Units: Coronary Care

Nancy Charley, BA, CHUC
Application Analyst,
Appalachian Regional Healthcare,
Lexington, Kentucky
Computer Specialist

Madeline A. Clark, RN, BGS, CHUC
Health Unit Coordinator AD Program;
Professor, Adjunct Faculty (Retired),
New Hampshire Technical College,
Manchester, New Hampshire
Home Health Nurse,
Alternative Care Medical Services,
Salem, New Hampshire

Dialysis Unit
The Geriatric Unit
Community Relations
Long-Term Care/Skilled Nursing Facility

Gloria Cornelius, HUC
Clinical Research Coordinator
Marshfield Medical Research Foundation,
Marshfield, Wisconsin
Research Facility

Nancy Fuerstenau Cutler, HUC
Health Care Applications Analyst,
Rockford Health System,
Rockford, Illinois
The Health Unit Coordinator Supervisor

Karen DiFrancesco, CHUC
Adjunct Instructor, Medical Terminology,
Somerset County Vocational & Technical College,
Bridgewater, New Jersey
Agency Staffing Services

Diane Faulkner, CHUC
Library Coordinator, Memorial Hospital & Medical Center Health Science Library,
Memorial Hospital & Medical Center,
Midland, Texas
Medical (Health Sciences) Library Assistant

Sandy Fisher, CHUC
Deaconess Medical Center,
Spokane, Washington
Special Care Units: The Postanesthesia Care Unit

M. Mairata Frankwick, BA, CHUC
Health Unit Coordinator Instructor,
Mid-State Technical College,
St. Joseph's Hospital,
Marshfield, Wisconsin
The Hematology/Oncology Unit

Roylene Galbraith, CHUC
Program Assistant 2,
University of Wisconsin Hospital & Clinics,
Madison, Wisconsin
Administrative Assistant to Nurse Manager

Winona Hardy, MBA
Associate Professor, Adjutant Faculty,
New Hampshire Technical Institute,
Concord, New Hampshire
Residential Assisted Living Home

Patricia A. Hassan Ibrahim, AS, CHUC
Health Unit Coordinator Supervisor,
Naval Medical Center, San Diego, California
Special Care Units: Neonatal Intensive Care

Joi Heierling, CHUC
Founder/Director,
What-Ev-Er!,
Chicago, Illinois
Private Medical Transcription Company

Diane Helms, CHUC
Patient Appointment Counselor,
Marshfield Clinic, Marshfield, Wisconsin
Multispecialty Clinics

Elizabeth A. Howe, CHUC
Franklin Medical Center,
Greenfield, Massachusetts
Hospice Organization

Donna Knecht, CHUC
Office Manager,
Clyde Knecht, MD,
Libby, Montana
Private Medical Office

Betty Lamb, CHUC
Program Coordinator, Valley Children's Hospital,
Madera, California
The Pediatric Unit

Audrey Langhorne, CHUC
Human Services, Inc.,
Downingtown, Pennsylvania
Community Mental Health Services

Lois Lawton, CHUC
Ortho/Neuro/Joint Replacement Center,
Henrico Doctor's Hospital,
Richmond, Virginia
The Orthopedic Unit

Gayle Levi-McLouden, CHUC
Fairviews University Medical Center,
Adult Chemical Dependency,
Minneapolis, Minnesota
Mental Health Unit

Charles S. Leyer, CHUC
Health Services Unit,
Milwaukee County Sheriff's Department
and Milwaukee House of Corrections,
Milwaukee, Wisconsin
Criminal Justice Facilities

Monica L. Lowe, CHUC
Adjunct Faculty/Clinical Preceptor for HUC Program,
New Hampshire Technical College,
Manchester, New Hampshire
Early Intervention Program

Nancy Mania, HUC
Northern Michigan Hospital,
Petoskey, Michigan
Special Care Units: The Surgical Intensive Care Unit

Virginia S. Mazza, RN, CHUC
HUC Instructor (Retired),
Midstate Technical College,
Marshfield, Wisconsin
The Pharmacy Assistant

Jackie Perkins, HUC
Clinic Clerk,
University Medical Associates,
Larista, Nebraska
Diagnostic Laboratory

Patricia Noonan Rice, CHUC, AAS, BA
Instructor,
Rock Valley College
Rockford, Illinois
Educator in Hospital-Based Training Program

Linda Sanford Face, HUC
HUC/Cardiac Monitor Technician,
Memorial Hospital and Medical Center
Midland, Texas
Monitor Technician

Lou Ann Schraffenberger, MBA, RRA, CCS
Clinical Assistant Professor, Health Information Management,
The University of Illinois at Chicago;
Clinical Data Consultant,
Advocate Health Care,
Oak Brook, Illinois
Overview of Clinical Coding
The Coding Process
The Clinical Coder

Jessie Shelby, CHUC
Pharmacy Assistant/Buyer,
Central Baptist Hospital,
Lexington, Kentucky
The Pharmacy Assistant

Nancy Shepherd, CHUC
Operations Assistant,
St. John's Mercy Medical Center,
St. Louis, Missouri
The Burn Unit

Gloria Smith
Administrator,
Inn at Deerfield, Inc.,
Deerfield, New Hampshire
The Geropsychiatric Unit

Patty Sopko, RN
Staff RN,
Nursing Information Specialist,
St. Vincent Mercy Medical Center,
Toledo, Ohio
Health Unit Coordinator Preceptor

Mary Andrew Stirrup, HUC
Pediatric Intensive Care Unit,
Children's Hospital of Wisconsin,
Milwaukee, Wisconsin
Special Care Units: Pediatric Intensive Care Unit (PICU)

Nadine Stratford, CHUC
Adjunct Instructor,
Salt Lake Community College;
Unit Clerk Supervisor,

Primary Children's Medical Center, Salt Lake City, Utah
Community/Vocational/Technical Colleges

Dawne Pfile Thomas, CHUC
Maternity Center Coordinator,
Mercy Maternity Center,
Charlotte, North Carolina
Birth Center

Christina Washington, CHUC
Open Heart Recovery Unit,
Charleston Area Medical Center,
Charleston, West Virginia
Special Care Units: Open Heart Recovery

Jo-Ann Polis Wilkins, CHUC
Receptionist, Home Care Department,
Temple/Lower Bucks Hospital,
Bristol, Pennsylvania
Hospital-Based Home Care

Linda Winslow, BS
Educator,
Marquette General Health System,
Marquette, Michigan
Neurology/Rehabilitation

Janice Wyse, CHUC
Northern Michigan Hospital,
Petoskey, Michigan
Special Care Units: The Surgical Intensive Care Unit

Preface

The idea for this book was conceived at a meeting of educators, officers of NAHUC, and representatives of the W.B. Saunders Company, who were all in Salt Lake City for the NAHUC Convention in July 1995. Myrna LaFleur, author of the basic textbook *Health Unit Coordinating*, had suggested such a meeting to explore what might be done to broaden the professional knowledge of health unit coordinators. Many ideas were considered. Among them was a suggestion that there was a need for a book that looked beyond the basic information available to students. Such a book could detail the opportunities that exist for the experienced practitioner as well as graduating students. It seemed as though it was an idea whose time had come. With that in mind we began to delve into the possibility of writing such a book. It quickly became obvious to us that the scope of such a book was vast. As we began to research the topic, using, in part, information gathered by the Health Care Reform Committee of NAHUC, we discovered many different situations in which health unit coordinator practitioners could be involved in work opportunities outside the typical hospital nursing unit. After considering many possible approaches we felt that the best way to present the information to the reader was to go to the practitioners themselves. Our experience on the NAHUC Education Board and the Continuing Education Committee had acquainted us with many people throughout the country who were already working in such situations. It became an easy decision to ask them to write about the environment in which they worked and to describe the actual work that they did. This is the result. Consequently, the information contained in this volume has great validity because, for the most part, it is a book for health unit coordinators written by health unit coordinators. We know that you will find it helpful.

This book is intended to reach students and practitioners of health unit coordinating as well as institutions that provide education and health care. Therefore, it can be used for the following:

- Students of health unit coordinating will find it helpful in examining all the possibilities that may exist for the entry-level employee as well as the experienced practitioner. Its focus is the exploration of opportunities and situations for the health unit coordinator throughout the health care industry. Although it is not meant to be a skills-oriented manual, it is a textbook that can be used as the basis for courses in the diploma or associate's degree programs. It does explain in detail many of the alternative positions that health unit coordinators may pursue, some with little or no further education. Some of the situations will require more extensive educational pursuits; however, graduates of a health unit coordinator program or experienced practitioners will find that their background makes them "naturals" to acquire this education and move into these positions.
- Practitioners who desire to build upon their current knowledge base or move into a different facet of health care will find many situations in this text that can help them analyze their skills and fortify them in their pursuit of new endeavors.
- For providers of health care the book can serve as a resource to explore how best to use current employees and also aid in recruiting employees into available positions. In the rapidly changing health care environment having a multiskilled employee is very advantageous.
- Providers of continuing education, in both health care institutions and colleges, will find the book a useful tool in developing programs in career exploration. It could be used for semi-

nars and workshops to provide some of the credits necessary for recertification.

There are several things that make this book unique, in addition to the fact that it is written by your contemporaries. The book is divided into four sections, each of which concentrates on a specific health care environment. It is set up in such a way that whether you are reading one chapter, all of a section, or the entire book, you will be able to find the information you are seeking easily and in a uniform manner. Every chapter contains a vocabulary list, and most contain an abbreviation list for the terms used in that chapter. In each chapter the vocabulary is printed in boldface type and the word itself is boldfaced the first time it is used in the text. Many chapters contain an additional listing of medical terms that are important to that particular area of interest but are not used in the text. When that is the case the terms are listed separately. The abbreviations are included in a single list, but only those used in the text appear in boldface type, and these are also boldfaced when they are used for the first time in the text. This should allow for easy reference to the list for the meaning.

In addition, most chapters contain a bibliography. This should be considered as a list of recommended reading as well as a reference for information contained in the chapter. Where no bibliography is listed it can be assumed that none is available. That is because these are situations that have been created without precedent, and nothing has been published that would be appropriate to the chapter. Consider that these are the pathfinders for your profession. We have found this experience to be most educational and rewarding. It is astonishing to discover the talents and creativity of the people who responded to the call. Perhaps this effort will uncover many more who are doing things of which we are not yet aware. It is our hope that reading of the endeavors of others in your profession will stimulate you to explore and create your own opportunities as well as pursue some of the opportunities that the contributors have described.

Health care is a dynamic field. It will only continue to be so in the future. The opportunities will be ever-expanding and the challenges even more exciting. Continue to broaden your horizons.

MADELINE A. CLARK
VIRGINIA S. MAZZA

Acknowledgments

Any effort of this magnitude requires the assistance of many people. We are grateful to all the contributors who worked so hard to meet deadlines and provide us with the information contained in this volume. In many cases it was their first effort at writing, and their dedication to the task is commendable.

We are especially grateful to Myrna LaFleur-Brooks and Lisa Biello for their confidence in us and their encouragement to undertake the project. Without them this book would never have become a reality.

We would also like to acknowledge Velma Kerschner and the Health Care Reform Committee of NAHUC, who did a tremendous job in identifying so many of the areas in which the skills of health unit coordinators could be utilized. Our thanks also go to Rosemary Boiselle, NAHUC President, for her assistance in providing us with the information on the organization found in the appendix.

Lynda Bernier was most helpful in providing her expertise in the areas dealing with cardiology and cardiovascular surgery.

Our section editors, Anne Mason and Cynthia Nault, spent countless hours editing the outlines and original manuscripts. They provided us with encouragement when we needed it and a shoulder to cry on when we were discouraged. We can never thank them enough. Cecil Powell also was very helpful in the early stages of the book, and we thank him for that effort.

We wish to express our gratitude to Bill Armstrong, Chicago, Illinois, for his expertise and patience in taking most of the pictures that appear in this text. His attention to detail and his willingness to go to any lengths to get the best photograph are sincerely appreciated. St. Joseph's Hospital, Marshfield Clinc, and Midstate Technical College, all in Marshfield, Wisconsin, were most cooperative in allowing us the use of their facilities for the photographs. A special thank you goes to Marcella Reigel of Marshfield, who allowed us to come into her home to take the photographs for residential living.

Northern Michigan Hospital in Petoskey, Michigan, deserves a special note of thanks for allowing their employees work time to write the section on surgical intensive care.

To the staff of W.B. Saunders Company, especially Scott Weaver, we owe a very special thank you. Scott never tired of answering our questions and providing us with the information that we needed. He was our solid rock through several staffing changes, and we could not have managed without him.

In addition, many persons contributed to the efforts of each individual chapter; they are listed below, with thanks for their assistance in whatever manner.

Agency Staffing
Joan Gorman

Birth Center
C. Dian Blades
Rita Ciarla
Deborah Johnson
Beth Rickenbaugh
Cheryl Sarna
Sue Uhryk
Mercy Maternity Staff
D. O'Brien
B. Mast
M. Janvrin
M. Hamilton
Georgia Duncan (deceased)

Community Mental Health Services
Cheryl Flanagan
Anjum Irfan

Home-Based Care
Tom Briody
Molly Facho
Donna Peters
Brian Egan

Long-Term Care Facility
Sister M. Elias Foley
Carol Boilard
Marsha Lancaster

Mental Health Unit
Lenore McLouden
Nancy Klug
Christine Maghrak-Sherve
Barb Bartkowiak

Monitor Technician
Wanda Brewer

Multispecialty Clinic
M. Mairata Frankwick

Pharmacy Assistant
James Adler
Tom Urbanek
Sue Johnson
Barb Blanchard
Kathy Stini
Jane Anderson
Patty Rindfleisch

Postanesthesia Care Unit
Judy Demand

Contents

Introduction

Beth C. Brace

Congratulations! By making the decision to purchase this book, you have opened a window. The window that I am referring to is the window of opportunity. As a health unit coordinator, you are in a perfect position to explore the many rewarding and satisfying careers in health care. This book will help you recognize and understand career opportunities that can evolve directly from your role as a health unit coordinator. If you are exploring ways to move forward in your career, you will find chapters filled with excellent first-hand examples of how other health unit coordinators have advanced their practice. For those of you who may not believe that it is possible to transform your job as a health unit coordinator into an exciting and rewarding career, I would like to share my personal journey into professional development.

In 1986, I accepted a position as a float unit clerk at a large teaching hospital. With a nursing assistant background, I completed the required 6-week training program. I was overwhelmed by the amount of responsibility required in my new role, but I accepted the challenge. Within 6 months I was confident of my ability to float to any unit. After 2 years as a float HUC, I had become a walking, talking resource. I still know phone numbers that I memorized as a HUC! I never really planned the changes in my career. Most were dictated by basic needs, such as a schedule that would accommodate child care. I needed a job that allowed me to work a set schedule, so I started looking for a new job.

My experience as a health unit coordinator provided an excellent background for a position in the information systems department. As the department secretary, my knowledge of the computer system and customer service skills were assets. I learned how to use a word processor and began to feel more comfortable using computers. After a year, I was promoted to a position in the outpatient clinic setting. My experience as a health unit coordinator provided the perfect background for this job. I used many of the skills that I learned as a health unit coordinator to coordinate admissions and schedule diagnostic tests and procedures. Two years later, I applied for a position as health unit coordinator instructor, a position I have held for the past 6 years. During that time our hospital has made the following strides to promote the professional development of health unit coordinators:

- It officially changed the working title from unit clerk to health unit coordinator.
- It provides resources and support for certification and recertification for HUCs.
- It has taken a leadership role in the development of a citywide consortium to provide educational offerings specifically for health unit coordinators.
- It encourages and supports HUC participation in total quality improvement activities.
- It has become an educational provider of contact hours for HUC recertification.

In addition, I have had the opportunity to become involved in nationwide efforts to promote health unit coordinator education and certification. And it all started with that job as a float unit clerk.

Although my transformation from health unit coordinator to health unit coordinator instructor took place over several years, there are some basic strategies to consider that will help you along the way. I offer these suggestions:

1. Talk to the people you work with every day.

Creating networks is a natural part of the role of health unit coordinator. There are opportunities daily to meet and work with people in all aspects of health care: nursing staff, physicians, pharmacy, respiratory therapy, PT, OT, medical records, business office, admissions, information systems, outpatient clinics, radiology. If you list all the people you know and who know you, it would undoubtedly be a cross section of people from every department in the hospital. When making a move down a different career path, these networks can work for you.

2. Volunteer for committees and work groups.

Getting involved in the decision-making process is an important step toward employee empowerment. Become part of the solution. Talk to your manager about team training or classes related to total quality improvement. Volunteer to help review and revise procedure manuals. Help develop training materials. Look for ways to become involved in the changes that are happening around you.

3. Take advantage of classes and training opportunities.

If you have access to tuition reimbursement or scholarship funds, take a class! I don't have my degree yet; I'm on the 14-year plan. Start with an easy class, something you enjoy. The benefits will reach far beyond your grade report. I firmly believe that you must be willing to learn new things if you want to grow professionally. If taking an evening class at a tech school seems like a big step, start with classes offered by your employer. Computer training of any kind is especially valuable. Computer systems are an integral part of the health unit coordinator role; learn more. Hospital information systems departments will only continue to grow.

4. Become involved in teaching.

After you get through the initial "shock" of the role and have gained some experience as a health unit coordinator, share your knowledge. Volunteer to be a preceptor for a new health unit coordinator. Ask to participate in unit training for new nurses, residents, and students.

5. Don't get bogged down in the mire.

The position of health unit coordinator puts you in the role of "information central." It is a burdensome task to become the personal advisor for an entire staff. Take on responsibilities that help promote you as a professional. It is difficult but worthwhile to rise above the daily grind and grouching in order to champion change!

Employing these strategies in your current position will increase your marketability for future employment opportunities. Take advantage of the skills and knowledge that you have gained as a health unit coordinator to maximize your potential!

When I accepted that position as a float unit clerk, I had no idea where it would lead. I took advantage of the many opportunities around me to enhance my career. I am still involved in health unit coordinator education, but my role has continued to evolve and expand. I am working on several total quality improvement project teams and have recently been assigned responsibilities for the implementation of a new information system for our home health agency. As I continue to learn and grow, I expect my career options will too! I believe that the health unit coordinators who have contributed to this book would agree; the window of opportunity is just waiting to be opened.

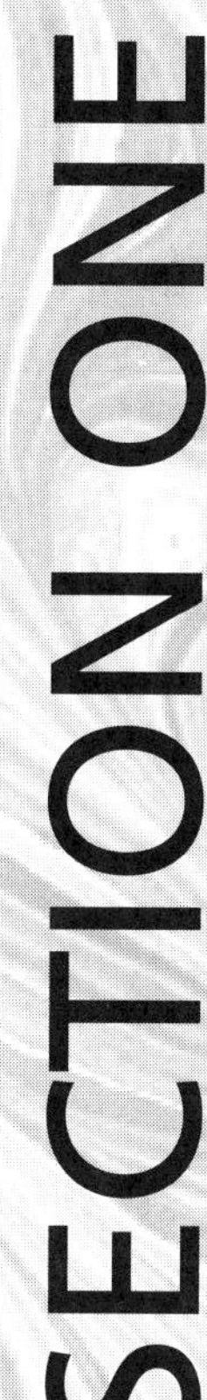

THE HEALTH UNIT COORDINATOR IN HOSPITAL SPECIALTY UNITS

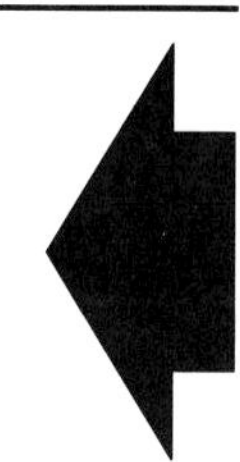

1

Birth Center

Dawne Pfile Thomas

Objectives

Upon completion of this chapter the reader will be able to:

1. Explain the LDRP model of care in obstetrics.
2. Identify the four stages of labor.
3. List three diagnostic tests performed in the birth center.
4. List five treatments or procedures performed on the mother or infant.

Vocabulary

Nägele's rule: A system to estimate the date of the onset of labor

Ripening: Hormonal effects that soften the cervix at the end stages of pregnancy, making it ready for labor

Effacement: The thinning of the cervix

Cardinal movements: Positional changes of the fetus during passage through the birth canal

Descent: Coming down

Flexion: The act of bending or a condition of being bent, in contrast to extension

Internal rotation: Rotating within the body

Extension restitution: The turning of a fetal head to the right or the left after it has completely emerged through the vagina

External rotation: Twisting of the fetal head as it follows the curves of the birth canal downward

Expulsion: Delivery of the child and subsequently the placenta and membranes from the mother

Primigravida: A woman during her first pregnancy

Multigravida: A woman who has been pregnant two or more times

Tocolytic therapy: Inhibition of uterine contractions. Drugs used for this include adrenergic antagonists, such as magnesium sulfate.

Continued

Vocabulary *Continued*

Lamaze: A method of psychoprophylaxis for childbirth in which the mother is instructed in breathing techniques that permit her to facilitate delivery by relaxing at the proper time with respect to the involuntary contractions of abdominal and uterine musculature. Those who are able to use the method effectively require little if any anesthesia during delivery.

Bradley: A specific approach to delivery that is partner-coached and uses no medications or drugs

Common Abbreviations

Accel	Acceleration of fetal heart rate
ACOG	American College of Obstetrics and Gynecology
AWHONN	Association of Women's Health, Obstetrics and Neonatal Nurses
AORN	Association of Operating Room Nurses
BOW	Bag of waters
CNM	Certified Nurse Midwife
C/S	Cesarean section, C-section
D&C	Dilatation and curettage
Decel	Deceleration of fetal heart rate
DHEC	Department of Health Environmental Control
EPIS	Episiotomy
FHT	Fetal heart tone
IUFD	Intrauterine fetal death
IUGR	Intrauterine growth retardation
JCAHO	Joint Commission on Accreditation of Health Care Organizations
LBW	Low birth weight
LDRP	Labor, delivery, recovery, post-partum
LFD	Low forceps delivery
LGA	Large for gestational age
Mec	Meconium
NNP	Neonatal nurse practitioner
NSVD	Normal spontaneous vaginal delivery
OCT	Oxytocin challenge test
PGE^2	Prostaglandin
Pit	Pitocin
PKU	Phenylketonuria
RDS	Respiratory distress syndrome
ROM	Rupture of membranes
SGA	Small for gestational age
STD	Sexually transmitted disease
VAD	Vacuum-assisted delivery

History of the LDRP

In the past, the model of care in obstetrics was the multitransfer system. A patient was admitted to one area, transferred to a labor area, and then, as she progressed in labor, brought to a delivery room. When the infant was delivered, the mother was taken to a recovery area until she was stabilized. Once stabilized, she was transferred to the post-partum unit.

The possibility of a smoother transition was being discussed as early as the late 1970s. Several factors determined the need for the **LDRP** (labor, delivery, recovery, post-partum) model of care that was instituted in the early 1980s. These were (1) cross training of nurses to increase cost efficiency and decrease staffing needs; (2) greater continuity of care, facilitating mother and infant bonding, especially in the first hours after delivery; (3) the fact that LDRP units are methodically

The abbreviations listed for this chapter are those that a HUC working in this area would be expected to know. Only those in **boldface** type are used in the text and appear in boldface when they are used for the first time.

designed for efficiency and maximum utilization of space in a most productive manner; and (4) most importantly, a recognized need for a more intimate setting for the birth process. Once the need to modify the traditional obstetrics unit was recognized, the advantages soon became clear. Those advantages were patient satisfaction, safety, increased marketability, and cost efficiency. During the early 1980s the first alternative birthing centers were opened on the West Coast.

A productive LDRP considers the following: (1) the philosophy, or mission statement, of the institution in which it is located; (2) the clinical care needs of the patient base; (3) the importance of structural design as it affects clinical care: (4) the needs of the consumer for education both before and after the birth process; and (5) the importance of marketing to remaining competitive in the health care market.

The Birthing Center

The Birthing Center consists of (1) LDRP suites (Fig. 1–1), which are designed to provide a homelike atmosphere while containing state-of-the-art equipment for a vaginal delivery; (2) high-tech surgical suites (Fig. 1–2), which enable the patient to remain on the unit in the event of a scheduled or emergent cesarean section; (3) the newborn nursery (Fig. 1–3), which is complete with necessary equipment for the newborn, e.g., scales, infant warmer, and bathing area; (4) a level II nursery, which provides stabilization and continuing intensive care for the premature or ill newborn (in some hospitals this may be a separate neonatal intensive care unit [NICU]; see Chapter 14, Part 3); and (5) a triage area, which allows the patient to be treated comfortably in the maternity area. It is designed for the special needs of the

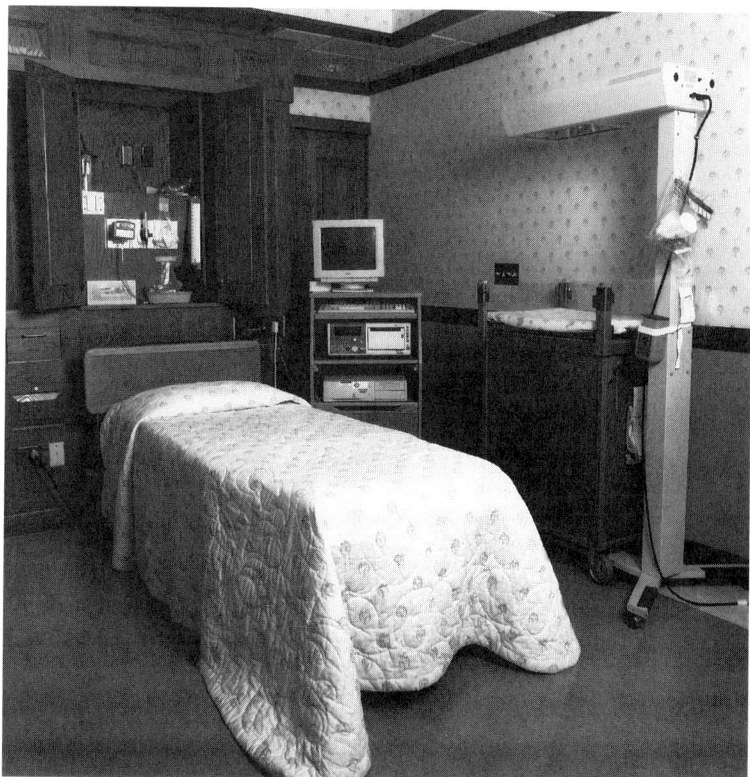

Figure 1–1
LDRP suite.

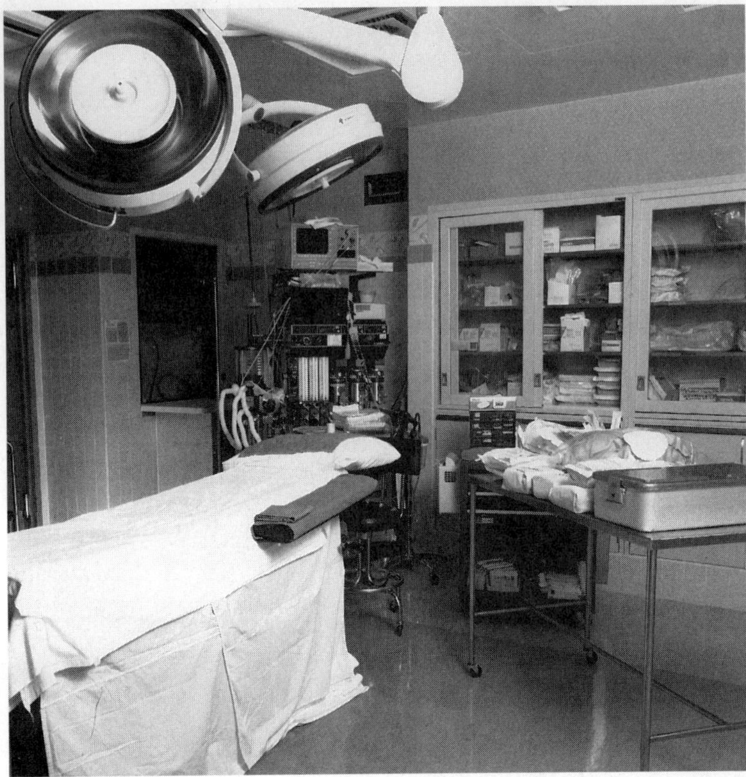

Figure 1–2
Birth center surgical suite.

antepartum patient and diagnostic procedures as well as examination/evaluation of labor (Fig. 1–4).

Some facilities continue to operate on the LDR model of care, with post-partum care administered apart from the delivery area, and some obstetric units may have both models.

Also important for the center are educational classes provided by the perinatal educator and his or her assistants. It is important for the health unit coordinator (HUC) to assist in marketing and directing the needs of patients through the perinatal educator. The HUC may assist with scheduling tours of the unit and classes for the ante-partum and post-partum patients.

Lactation consultants facilitate the work of the maternity center with regard to breast feeding of infants, with classes prior to delivery and on-site teaching post partum.

The HUC must know the assignments of the staff in order to guide the coverage for each designated area. He or she oversees the centrally located nurses' station, which is the originating point for patients as they arrive. The HUC facilitates a smooth transition from one area to another.

Anatomy and Physiology of the Reproductive System

The female reproductive system is composed of internal and external pelvic organs as well as the breasts. The female pelvis is instrumental in childbearing. The external genitalia include the mons pubis, vagina, labia majora, labia minora, clitoris, urethral meatus, vaginal orifice, and perineal body. Internal genitalia consist of the vagina,

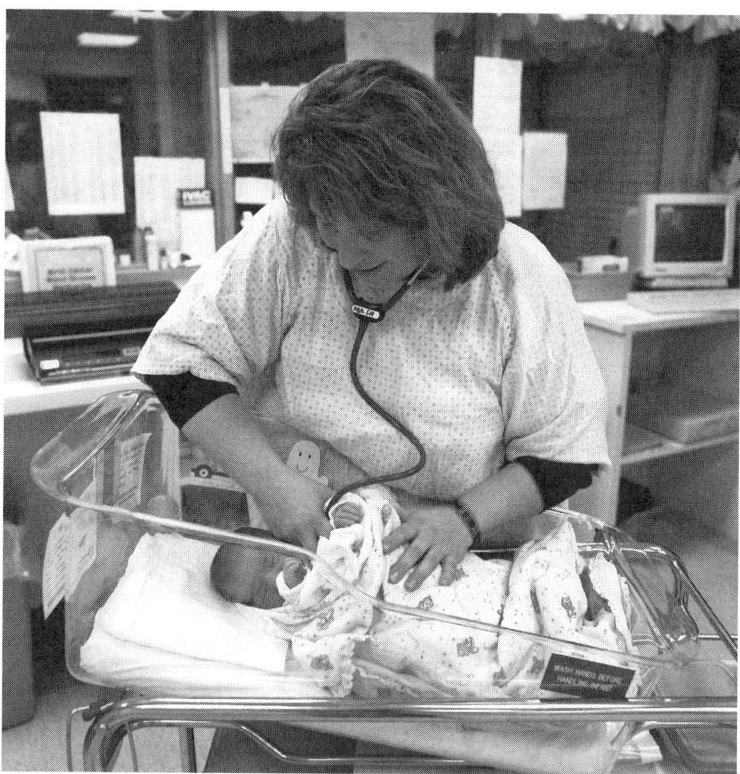

Figure 1–3
Pediatrician examining baby in newborn nursery.

uterus, fallopian tubes, and ovaries. The pelvis is made up of four bones: two innominate bones, the sacrum, and the coccyx.

Conception occurs when a sperm from the male unites with the ovum of the female. The fertilized ovum is where all human life begins. This single cell then undergoes several cell divisions. Implantation in the uterus occurs between 7 and 10 days after fertilization. Embryonic membranes begin to form at the time of implantation. Development of the fetus takes 38 to 40 weeks in a normal pregnancy cycle. Nägele's rule is used to determine the estimated date of confinement.

It is very important for the HUC to understand the progression of the birth process.

Factors relating to the birth process include **effacement** of the cervix, **dilatation** of the cervix, and station of the fetus within the pelvis. The fetus must go through many positional changes during the birth process. These changes are called **cardinal movements.** Listed in order of occurrence, they are **descent, flexion, internal rotation, extension restitution, external rotation,** and, finally, **expulsion.** Effacement of the cervix occurs with dilatation. The thinning and dilatation of the cervix is known as **ripening** and is influenced by hormones. Cervical dilatation during labor generally begins at 2 cm and is considered complete at 10 cm (Fig. 1–5).

Labor is defined as the process by which the fetus is expelled from the mother's uterus. It is divided into four stages. The first stage of labor begins with the onset of regular uterine contractions (rhythmic tightening of the uterus). Dilatation and effacement of the cervix occur during this time. As the cervix dilates, a patient is progressing

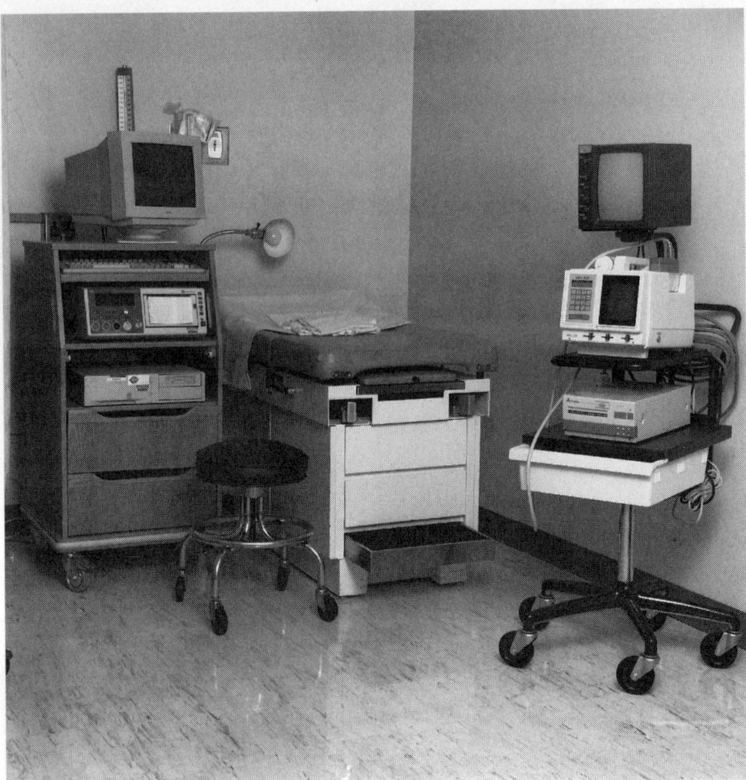

Figure 1–4
Triage area.

from labor to delivery. Transition to birth ends the first stage of labor, when cervical dilatation is usually from 8 to 10 cm. The transitional phase usually is no longer than 3 hours for **primigravidas** and 1 hour for **multigravidas**. Contractions are more frequent, longer, and more intense. The second stage of labor begins when the cervix is completely dilated at 10 cm and ends with birth (Fig. 1–6). The third stage, also known as placental separation, normally occurs minutes after the infant is born. However, sometimes the placenta is retained, and further intervention is needed. The fourth stage occurs 1 to 4 hours after birth. It is important bonding time for mother, infant, and family (Fig. 1–7).

Health care providers in the birth center may include technicians, registered nurses, midwives, and physicians. Anesthesia staff may become involved for pain management or if a crisis develops.

Medications Specific to the Birthing Process

Medications specific to the birthing process are included in the orders, which are often computer-generated standing orders. These orders are specific for the various groups of health care providers. The HUC pulls the specific orders and gives them to the assigned nurse. It is the registered nurse's responsibility to assess the patient's pain medication needs and administer the drugs as necessary.

Ante-partum medications can include prenatal vitamins prescribed by the physician or nurse midwife. Other ante-partum medications that may be ordered are drugs that are given in the event of premature labor (contractions). Prophylactic antimicrobial medications may also be given to reduce the risk of infection to the infant or if

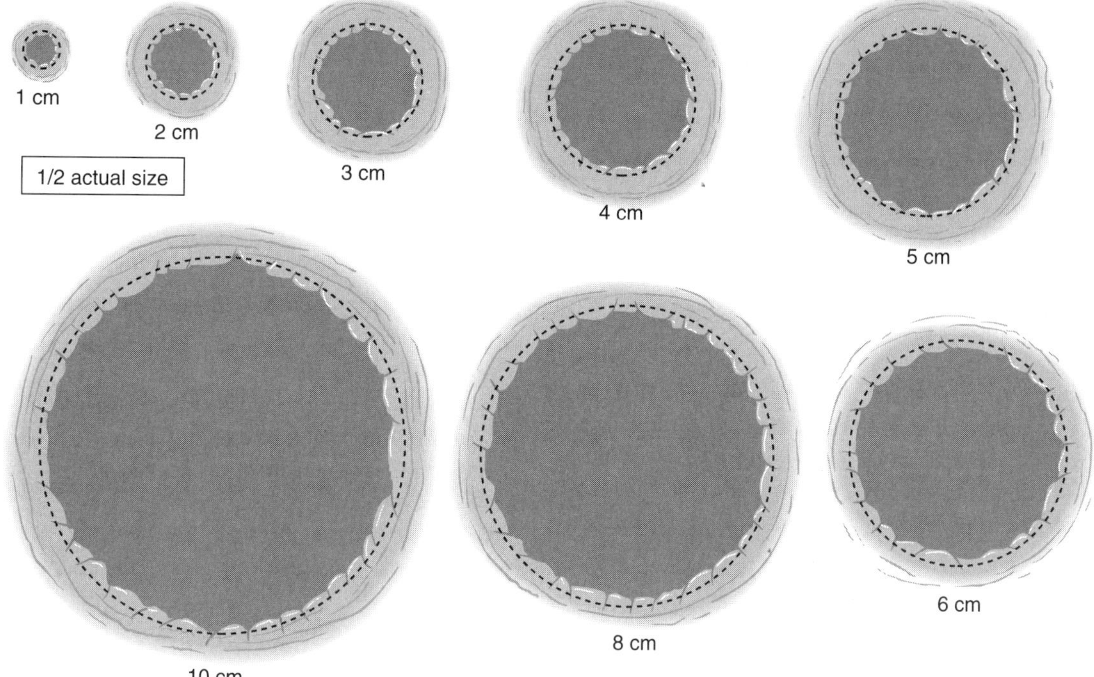

Figure 1–5
Cervical dilatation.

the mother is a group B strep carrier. There are several medications that may be given to induce labor. These include Pitocin (**Pit**) and prostaglandin gel.

During labor the mother may have a difficult time with pain control. She may choose pain-relieving drugs such as Nubain or Stadol or opt for epidural anesthesia. This form of anesthesia is given by an anesthesiologist, who inserts a catheter into the patient's spinal column in the epidural space in order to initiate pain management. This allows the patient to be awake and alert. She will continue to have contractions but will feel them without pain. The anesthesia is discontinued immediately after birth, enabling the patient to ambulate.

Post-partum medications given after birth, if necessary, include Pitocin, to prevent uterine atony, and Hemabate or Methergine, which may be given to a patient who has excessive bleeding. Analgesics are also ordered to help the new mother with discomfort immediately after delivery.

Normal newborn medications include vitamin K, which facilitates the blood clotting factor in the infant; erythromycin eyedrops, which are given to prevent infection from the delivery; and hepatitis B vaccine, which is now required for newborns. Topical lidocaine may also be used after circumcision. Tylenol elixir is a p.r.n. medication offered by some physicians for infant discomfort after circumcision. Injectable lidocaine may be used prior to circumcision as an anesthetic agent at the physician's discretion or the parents' request.

Medications are given in cases of maternal high risk, e.g., when premature labor has begun and there is a risk of premature delivery. Betamethasone, a steroid, benefits the infant by improving fetal lung maturity. Magnesium sulfate and terbutaline may be given in an attempt to reduce con-

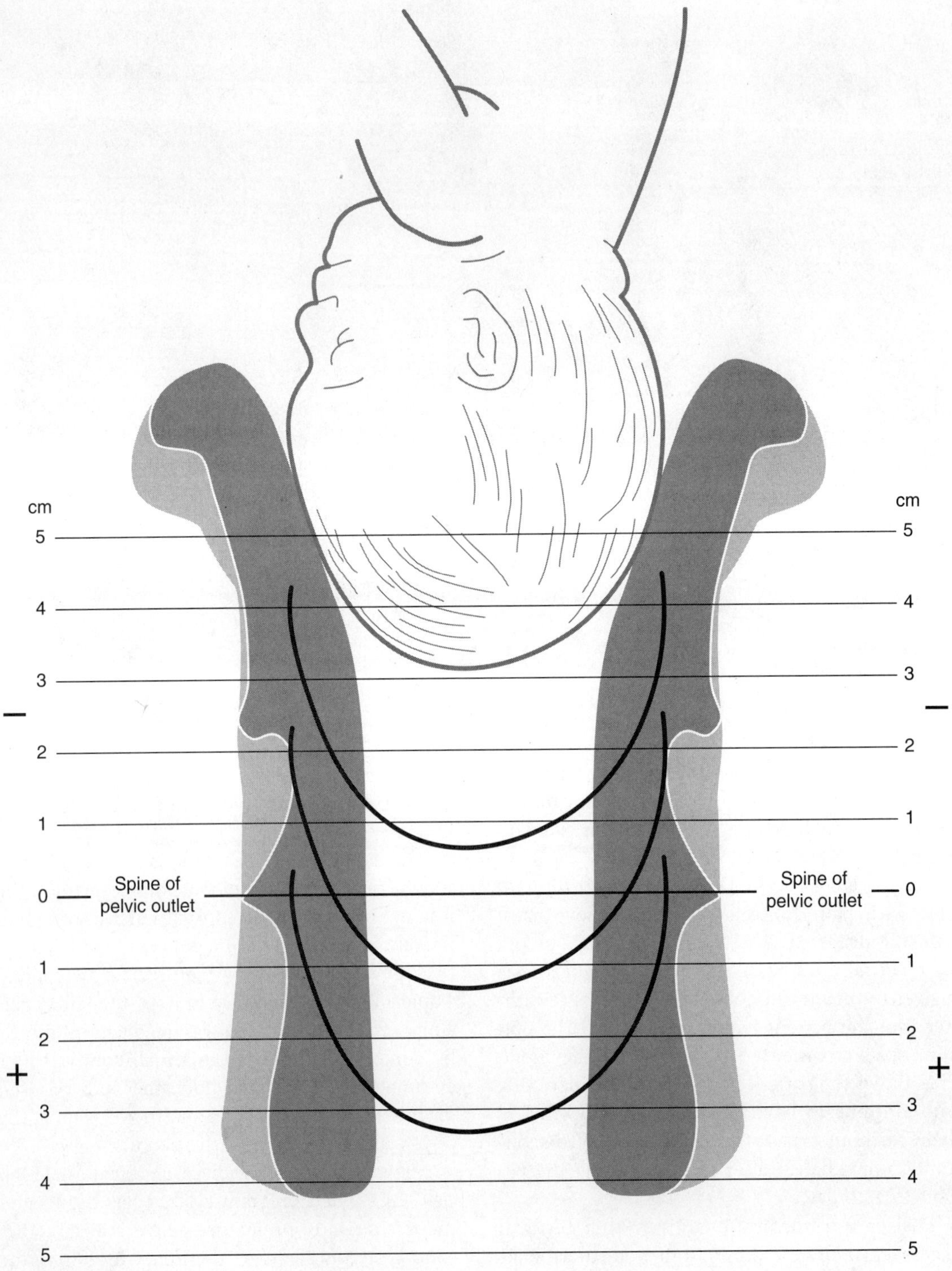

Figure 1–6
Second stage of labor.

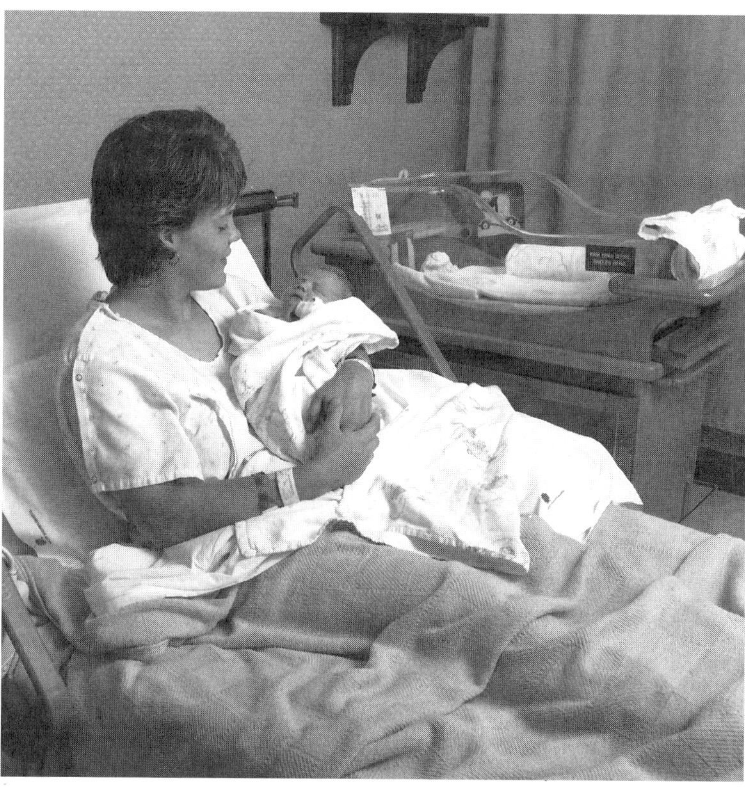

Figure 1–7
Mother with newborn infant.

tractions and stop labor. This is referred to as **tocolytic therapy**. Antibiotic coverage is given also for premature rupture of membranes, maternal fever, or if the patient has been in labor for more than 24 hours.

Diagnostic Testing

Diagnostic testing in the maternity center consists of several tests to check the welfare of the infant and mother. They may be performed in a triage area on an outpatient or an observation basis. Once the patient has been greeted, has registered, and has signed the necessary consents, the nurse or physician will conduct the appropriate tests. These may include the following:

NST—non-stress test

Fetal monitoring—auscultation of the fetal heart rate

Speculum examination—use of an instrument called a speculum, which is inserted in the vagina in order to view internal organs

Contraction stress test—nipple stimulation causing contraction to occur

Oxytocin challenge test (OCT)—administration of oxytocin to stimulate contractions

Nitrozine test—evaluation for ruptured membranes

Amniocentesis—the removal of amniotic fluid through the abdomen; the fluid is tested to determine fetal lung maturity. This procedure is performed by the doctor.

External version—external manipulation of fetus from breech to vertex presentation.

The HUC is responsible for registering the patient, gathering appropriate documents for charting, and transcription of the orders. After-discharge duties may include charging patient accounts accurately, disassembling the chart, and making a follow-up appointment with the patient's physician or midwife.

Equipment

The Birthing Room

Equipment in the birthing center room may consist of, but is not limited to, the following:

- Fetal monitor—allows the health care provider to listen to the infant's heart rate
- Fetascope—uses bone conduction to determine the infant heart rate
- Doppler—allows the health care provider to listen to the infant's heart rate while the patient is ambulatory
- Delivery cart—table that contains instruments and supplies for the health care provider during a vaginal delivery
- Infant care station—provides a flat surface for the infant to be examined immediately after delivery and contains items necessary for an emergency
- Epidural cart—contains all the necessary supplies and equipment in the event that the patient requires epidural anesthesia

Supplies

Sterile supplies that are used in the birth center are often prepared as packs in the central supply or services area. They are generally cleaned and sterilized immediately after use and returned to the birth center. These may include such supplies as a vaginal pack, a C-section pack, and a circumcision pack. These packs would include all the items necessary for the procedure being carried out. It is important that supplies always be readily available.

The Newborn Nursery

Equipment in the newborn nursery may consist of the following:

Infant cribs/bassinets
Otoscope
Portable lights
Ophthalmoscope
Circumcision table
Baby linens
Infant warmer
Suction
Stethoscope
Oxygen

Treatments and Procedures

Maternal child treatments and procedures that are invasive to the mother or child are as follows:

Cerclage insertion/removal—This procedure reinforces the weakened cervix by encircling it at the level of the internal os. Removal is clipping the suture.

Vaginal delivery—This term refers to the delivery of the infant through the vaginal opening.

Cesarean section—This is a surgical procedure that involves the removal of the infant through an incision in the abdomen.

Circumcision—This is the surgical removal of the foreskin of the penis on male infants.

PKU testing—The phenylketonuria test is carried out on the infant prior to discharge. It is a simple blood test using drops of blood from the infant's heel that are placed on a special filter paper.

Digit tie-off—This is the removal of an extra digit with a string tied tightly at the base of the extra digit, which eventually falls off.

Communication With and About Patients

During the second trimester the patient may schedule a tour with the HUC so that she can visit the birth center, where she wants to deliver. Several forms may be made available to her during this time. One of these forms is the birth plan. Using this plan the patient states her preferences as well as her dislikes. She reviews this with her health care provider, who sends it to the hospital at 36 weeks together with the patient's prenatal record. This may not be done formally in all parts of the country.

The prenatal records, containing the patient's personal history and physical data, are sent to the hospital anywhere from 32 weeks, for high-risk patients, to 36 weeks, for the normal OB patient. Vital information about the patient that is extremely confidential is in the prenatal records: prior menstrual history, previous surgeries, pregnancies, **STDs**, and general medical information.

During the course of prenatal care, the patient is given a brochure on prenatal classes. This assists her in preparing for and having a better understanding of the birth process. **Lamaze**, **Bradley**, breast feeding, infant care, and siblings at birth are just some of the information discussed. The HUC assists the perinatal educator in scheduling tours and classes and in providing information about the hospital system.

Post-partum communication with the new parents begins with the birth certificate. The HUC will ascertain that all information is correct and answer any questions that the parents may have in regard to the registration of the birth. Some hospitals provide a computer-generated birth certificate, and this can be used to check the information with the parents before the document is sent to the state.

It may be a responsibility of the HUC to act as a notary public in the event that the new parents are not married or if the infant is being placed for adoption.

The HUC can handle scheduling, insurance, and preregistration and answer billing questions. Training is offered by the admissions office, which also provides updates on changes in insurance. All admitting is done in the maternity center upon arrival. Basic billing questions can be handled in the maternity center, although inquiries about general costs are normally transferred to a billing officer.

Post-partum teaching with regard to caring for the mother and infant is done by the nurse. Videos are available for the patient to view as well as visits by the lactation consultants. The patient is encouraged to call her, or the infant's, health care provider if she has any questions once she is at home.

Quality/Risk Management

JCAHO and **DHEC** require a process of ongoing patient care improvement. Quality or problems improvement is another area in which the HUC plays a vital part. The ability to oversee the entire operation of the unit allows the HUC to identify problems in registration, flow through the hospital system, and family responses to care. To ensure a high standard of care, staff are given extensive training. In addition to JCAHO standards, many hospitals will use the standards set by **AWHONN**, **AORN**, and **ACOG**. The HUC may be responsible for tabulating data from monthly audits of certain areas within the unit. A patient satisfaction survey might also be used to allow the families to critique the care that was provided to them.

Risk management issues are primarily those of security and safety. With the danger of infant abductions, birth centers instruct families on how to identify staff. Many hospitals use specially designed badges. Each family unit may be identified with bands issued by the hospital. The staff should identify themselves and stress the importance of infant security in the rooming-in circumstance and also the extreme importance of NEVER leaving the infant unattended. The nurses and the HUC also protect the security of the nursery with locks on the doors.

Closing Thoughts

A Day in My Life

I feel blessed to have been trained in the manner that I was. The first role of a good HUC is to set the tone for the unit. The pace may change several times throughout your shift, but you set the tone as well as the atmosphere in helping it all come together with the staff, various departments, and visitors.

As the day begins and each nurse is given his or her particular assignment, your job is to (1) be aware of what is happening with all of them, (2) have ongoing updates with the charge nurse, and (3) manage what comes in your door.

The dynamics of the position require you to be flexible and highly organized, owing to the fact that patients and staff are at various stages throughout the day. Several activities are generally going on at once. As my day begins, I have the usual list of duties to be performed for the unit to run smoothly: being aware of the list of incoming patients for various procedures, tests, or inductions; filing lab reports; checking charts to add any necessary forms; making sure that charts are in order for health care provider rounds; and having my nurses' assignment lists close at hand. This does not include the patients who come in unexpectedly or the patient who progresses quickly and has a rapid delivery. Once the laboring patient arrives, it is very important to note what her comfort level is. Ideally, she will have preregistered. If not, a clipboard will be taken to the room so that she or a family member can fill out the registration form. The standard questions are asked, and the HUC then enters the patient data into the computer. As stated earlier, both mother and infant have computer-generated orders that the HUC transcribes.

After delivery and family bonding, teaching and the birth certificate process are initiated. During this process of documenting the birth with the state, the HUC must be aware of the additional information that may be needed in those special circumstances that were discussed earlier.

The HUC must handle the activity on the unit smoothly as well as dealing with the phone and the patient intercom system. Also important in terms of telephone skills is the ability to forward calls in the right direction.

The work of the HUC is critical in assisting the patient, health care providers, and visitors. He or she is a vital part of the team. The ultimate goal is for the family unit to experience a happy and natural birth process.

Review Questions

1. Explain what is meant by the LDRP model of care in obstetrics.
2. Identify the four stages of labor.
3. List three diagnostic tests that would be performed in the birth center.
4. List five treatments or procedures that would be performed on the mother or infant.

Bibliography

McKay S, Phillips CR: Family Centered Maternity Care. Rockville, MD, Aspen Publications, 1984.

2

The Burn Unit

Nancy Shepard

Objectives

At the completion of this chapter the reader should be able to:

1. Describe the four classifications of burns.
2. List the six burn categories.
3. Explain the "rule of nines" for measuring the extent of burns.
4. List the other hospital departments that would be involved with the care of a burn patient.
5. Identify three special pieces of equipment used for burn patients.

Vocabulary

1st Degree: Superficial burn of top of skin

2nd Degree: Burn extends through top layer of skin

3rd Degree: Burn damages underlying tissue

Alloderm: Human skin that has been processed aseptically from the donor site

Debride: To remove damaged tissue

Dermis: Inner layers of skin (below the epidermis)

Donor site: Area that skin graft is taken from

Easyderm: Fine pigskin that is placed over burn area to protect it from infection

Epidermis: Outer (top) layers of skin

Eschar: A dry scab that results from a burn

Frostbite: Freezing part of the body

Graft: To move healthy skin to the area of damaged tissue

Hypovolemia: Diminished blood volume

Hypovolemic shock: A condition occurring when there is an insufficient amount of blood in the circulatory system

Sepsis: A condition that results from the presence of microorganisms or their poisonous products in the bloodstream

Continued

Vocabulary *Continued*

Slough: To shed or cast off

Skin graft: A piece of skin transplanted to replace a lost portion of the body skin surface

Xeroflo: Coating of Xeroform dressing that allows drainage

Common Abbreviations

ADA	Americans With Disabilities Act
B	Blister
C	Crust
CEA	Culture epidermal autograft
$CeNo_3$	Cerous nitrate
COBH	Carboxyhemoglobin
D	Dry
Dnr	Donor
E	Eschar
EP	Epithelization
ES	Escharotomy
EX	Excised
FL	Flaky
FS	Fasciotomy
G	Granulation
I	Intact
Ivy	Ivory
LE	Leathery eschar
M	Margins
MT	Mottled
P	Pink
PL	Pale
R	Red
S	Separating
Scr	Scar
STSG	Split-thickness skin graft
TBSA	Total body surface area
TE	Tacky eschar
V	Vascular
W	Wet
WH	White

Related Terminology

The following terms do not appear in the text of the chapter; however, they are terms that someone who works on a burn unit would be expected to know.

Coalescence: The process of putting two pieces of growing skin together so they overlap

Indolent: Inactive or not developing

Description of the Burn Unit

Patient Rooms

The burn unit may look more like an ICU or other specialty unit because of the uniqueness of the supplies and equipment needed to care for the special patients with burns. The Americans With Disabilities Act (**ADA**) has provided guidelines to ensure that the physical environment is appropriate for this type of patient. The rooms must be large enough to handle lifters, wheelchairs, and special dressing or burn carts. There should be enough clear space for a wheelchair to make a 180 degree turn. All doors should be wide,

The abbreviations listed for this chapter are those that a HUC working in this area would be expected to know. Only those in **boldface** type are used in the text and appear in boldface when they are used for the first time.

at least 32 inches for easy wheelchair access. The doors should have special handles that make it easy to open and close them with one hand, giving a patient with healing burns the opportunity to move about without pulling or twisting to open the door. All burn unit rooms should be equipped with a wall panel that contains vacuum, air, and oxygen. The patient call light system may be a modification of that used in the rest of the hospital. Burn patients are often confined by heavy bandages and dressings, and the call lights should be large enough to activate under these conditions. The same is true for TV/radio/bed controls; they should be easy to push, despite a heavy wound dressing.

All patient rooms should have an area for sterile and nonsterile supplies, a separate container to dispose of any blood-soiled dressings, and the proper hand washing area with supplies. All unused dressings should be kept in a cabinet to prevent contamination when not in use. Infection is the major enemy of any burn patient, and extra precautions must be taken with these patients.

Bathrooms and Showers

The patient bathrooms must be large enough for wheelchair access and have the appropriate grab bars, making transfers safe and easy for the patient. If the patient bathroom contains a shower it also must have the safety grab bars and either be equipped with a safety seat or be large enough to accommodate a special rolling chair. Showers should be equipped with both a fixed showerhead and a hand-held unit. Some burn units may have shower or tub rooms that are large enough to accommodate a special lift chair for transferring patients in and out of the tub (Fig. 2–1). These rooms should be equipped with the same emergency wall panel of vacuum, air, and oxygen. All showers and tubs should be cleaned and disinfected prior to use.

Isolation Rooms

The burn unit may have special isolation rooms with a positive airflow system and double doors going into the patient room. The positive airflow system allows air to recirculate without pulling in air from the outside. This protects the patient from airborne infections. The outer room contains the garments and supplies needed by the health care worker before entering the patient room.

Acute Care Rooms

Some rooms for the acute care burn patient may have additional heating and cardiac monitoring. Patients with large areas of severe burns have trouble maintaining normal body temperature, and during dressing changes they need to be in a very warm environment. The special heating system may be utilized during dressing changes or whenever the patient needs to be kept warm. Because acutely ill burn patients may also need kidney dialysis, the rooms must be designed to handle the special equipment and supplies for these treatments.

Classification of Burns

First-Degree Burns

First-degree burns are characteristically painful, red, and dry and blanch with pressure (Fig. 2–2). First-degree burns typically occur secondary to prolonged exposure to low-intensity heat (as in the sun) or a short-duration flash exposure to a heat source (stove, iron). Only a superficial layer of epidermal cells is destroyed, and they **slough** (peel away from healthy underlying tissue) without scarring. Medical attention may be required if symptoms such as nausea, vomiting, or fever occur. If the burned area becomes cracked or appears infected, a local antibiotic ointment may be applied to the affected area. Antihistamines and analgesics may be prescribed for swelling and pain. These burns usually heal within 2 to 3 days.

Second-Degree Burns

Second-degree burns may be divided into two groups: superficial partial-thickness and deep partial-thickness wounds. Superficial partial-

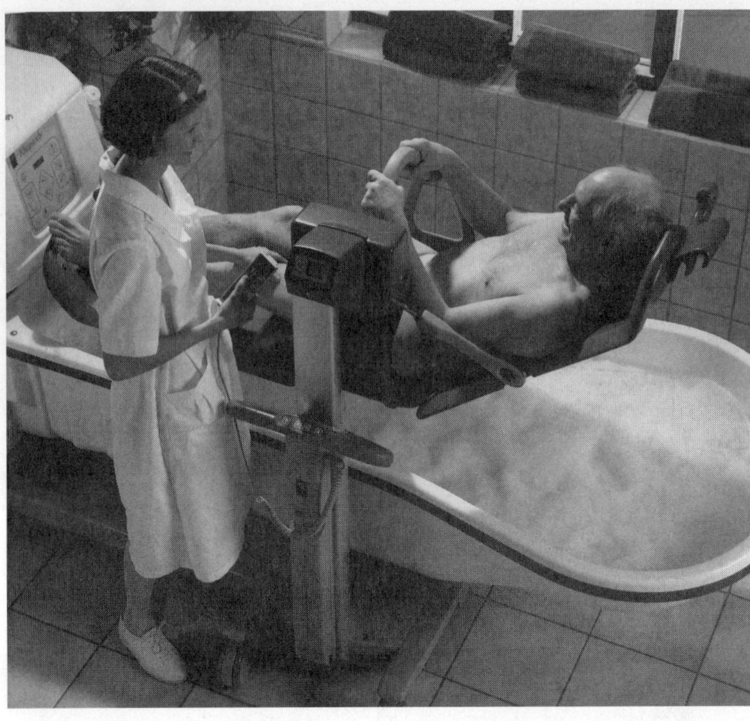

Figure 2–1
Patient using special lift to transfer to tub. (Courtesy of Arjo, Morton Grove, IL.)

			WOUND APPEARANCE	WOUND SENSATION	COURSE OF HEALING
EPIDERMIS Sweat duct Capillary	PARTIAL-THICKNESS BURN	1st-degree	Epidermis remains intact and without blisters. Erythema; skin blanches with pressure.	Painful	Discomfort lasts 48—72 hours. Desquamation in 3—7 days
Sebaceous gland Nerve endings DERMIS Hair follicle	PARTIAL-THICKNESS BURN	2nd-degree	Wet, shiny, weeping surface Blisters Wound blanches with pressure.	Painful Very sensitive to touch, air currents	Superficial partial-thickness burn heals in < 21 days. Deep partial-thickness burn requires > 21 days for healing. Healing rates vary with burn depth and presence/absence of infection.
Sweat gland Fat Blood vessels	FULL-THICKNESS BURN	3rd-degree	Color variable (i.e., deep red, white, black, brown) Surface dry Thrombosed vessels visible No blanching	Insensate (↓ pinprick sensation)	Autografting required for healing
Bone	FULL-THICKNESS BURN	4th-degree	Color variable Charring visible in deepest areas Extremity movement limited	Insensate	Amputation of extremities likely Autografting required for healing

Figure 2–2
Classification of burns. (From Black JM, Matassarin-Jacobs E (eds): Medical-Surgical Nursing: Clinical Management for Continuity of Care, 5th ed. Philadelphia, WB Saunders, 1997.)

thickness burns are characterized by blisters (**B**) and are commonly caused by contact with hot (not boiling) liquids, hot grease, flame, and explosions producing flash burns. The injury goes through the outer layer of skin (**epidermis**) to the inner layers (**dermis**) but does not destroy the basal layers of the skin; new skin is regenerated within a few days to a week. Second-degree burns produce blisters, which provide a seal that protects the wound from infection and excessive fluid loss. The injured area is usually red, wet, and painful and may blanch with pressure. In the absence of infection, these wounds heal without scarring, usually within 14 days.

If the depth of the burn involves the basal layer of the dermis, it is considered a deep partial-thickness burn. Sensation in and around the wound may be diminished because of the destruction of basal layer nerve endings. The injury may appear red and wet or white and dry, depending on the degree of vascular injury. Wound infection, **sepsis**, and fluid loss are major complications of these injuries. Uncomplicated, deep partial-thickness burns will heal within 3 to 4 weeks. In some cases, skin grafting may be necessary to speed the healing process or to minimize the formation of thick scar tissue that may restrict movement and cause pain and disfigurement. Physical therapy is started the day after admission on all joints, using active and passive range of motion to help prevent contractures.

Third-Degree Burns

Third-degree burns are serious and may be life threatening. Both the inner and the outer layers of skin and tissue are destroyed. The wound appears pearly white, charred, or leathery. A definitive sign of third-degree burn is a translucent surface in the depths of which thrombosed veins are visible. Because the burn has destroyed the small blood vessels and nerve endings, pain may be minimal or absent in these patients, while blood and fluid loss may be severe. Loss of fluid and blood may lead to infection and sepsis. Third-degree burns must be treated with **skin grafts** to close the full-thickness wounds, to minimize complications, and to allow for full range of motion.

Fourth-Degree Burns

Some burn classifications describe a fourth-degree burn as a full-thickness injury that penetrates both the inner and the outer layers of skin, muscle, and bone. These burns usually result from incineration type exposure and electrical burns in which heat is sufficient to destroy tissues below the skin.

Burn Categories

Smoke Inhalation

Smoke inhalation most often occurs when the victim is in a closed environment, such as a building, automobile, or airplane, and is caused by the accumulation of toxic by-products of combustion. It is also possible to suffer a smoke inhalation injury in an open area where the smoke may be intense or toxic, such as a forest or the site of a chemical fire. All burn patients should be evaluated for this injury. The dangers are caused by the fact that the fire consumes the available oxygen while producing carbon monoxide and other toxic gases.

Patients with smoke inhalation may also have severe burns to the respiratory system. Respiratory burns are very serious and often require a tracheotomy and ventilator breathing assistance.

Chemical Burns

Chemical burns occur when a chemical agent comes into contact with the skin. Spilling a strong cleaning agent on a bare hand may cause the hand to become red and irritated. This is a minor chemical burn and should be treated by quickly washing the chemical off the affected area. Most chemical burns are minor and require no further treatment. Major chemical burns generally occur in an industrial environment where the chemicals may be moderately to extremely toxic and are stored in vast containers. The initial treatment for an industrial chemical burn is the same as for the household burn—huge amounts of water. Chemical burns, like any other burn, may require surgical intervention and hospitalization.

Electrical Burns

Electrical burns occur from direct and indirect contact with electricity. The degree of voltage may determine the severity of the injury. The circumstances of the accident may also play an important role. Touching a lamp with a short in the cord may result in a minor electrical shock; touching the same lamp with wet hands or while standing in water could result in a major electrical injury. Under normal conditions, household 110 current will not cause death—but add water to the situation and death could occur because water acts as a conductor for electricity.

High-voltage electrical burns are often life threatening, and many of these are in the fourth-degree category. In addition to the burns, the electricity interferes with the cardiac and respiratory systems. This could result in cardiac or respiratory arrest, irregular heart rate, or any other system failure. Once the electricity enters the body it can bounce around before it finds an exit. The exit area skin may be more severely burned than the initial area of contact. The internal organs are the greatest cause for concern. It is necessary to assess the internal damage immediately. The pathway of the current will give a clue about which anatomic structures may have been damaged.

Thermal Injury

Thermal injury occurs when there is contact with flame, no matter what the source of the flame. Severity will depend on the length of contact as well as the amount of body surface exposed.

Scald Injury

Scald injuries result from contact with hot liquids or steam.

Lightning Strike

Burns resulting from a lightning strike produce tissue injuries that differ from those seen in an electrical injury. Because the duration of the lightning is short, skin burns are less severe than those from high-voltage current, and third-degree burns are rare. Patients with minor lightning injuries are usually conscious, but they are frequently confused and exhibit memory loss. Lightning injuries commonly occur on golf courses. Patients with moderate to severe injury have the same potential for internal damage and complications as victims of electrical burn injury. Careful evaluation is critical in all patients with a lightning strike injury.

Medications

Medications for burn patients include those used for pain relief as well as antibiotics to prevent infection. Only a few of the more common medications are mentioned here.

Thrombin is used to control bleeding when grafts are being taken. It can also be used postoperatively and during dressing changes when there is danger of heavy bleeding.

Oxandrin is a steroid that is used to help in the healing process. Vitamins such as C, folate, and thiamine are often ordered to assist in the healing process as well.

Polysporin, Thermazene, and Sulfamylon cream are used directly on the burn to promote healing.

Norcuron, ketamine, morphine, Demerol, Versed, and Percocet are analgesics used to help control pain. In addition, many patients may receive Valium, which is a tranquilizer.

Eucerin and Nivea are used on the healing skin to protect it from cracking, to prevent breakdown, and to decrease itching.

Patients with extensive burns will receive IV therapy as well to replace fluid loss, prevent dehydration, and provide additional nutrition. Vitamins and antibiotics will often be a part of the IV therapy.

Treatments

Measuring the Extent of the Burn

Just as important as determining the degree and type of burn is knowing the extent of body area that the injury covers. A third-degree burn in a small area is not as serious as a second-degree burn that covers a large area. The method commonly used is called the rule of nines (Fig. 2–3). This is a measurement that divides the total body surface area (**TBSA**) into segments that are multiples of 9 percent. This method provides a rough estimate of burn injury size and is most accurate for adults and children over the age of 10 years. The measurement is as follows: head and neck, 9%; each arm, 9%; each leg, 9%; anterior trunk, 18%; posterior trunk, 18%. When there is an irregular burn pattern the rule is, the size of your palm equals 1%. Using this scale on a patient who was burned on the right arm and right side of chest, the extent of the burn might be reported as 11% body involvement.

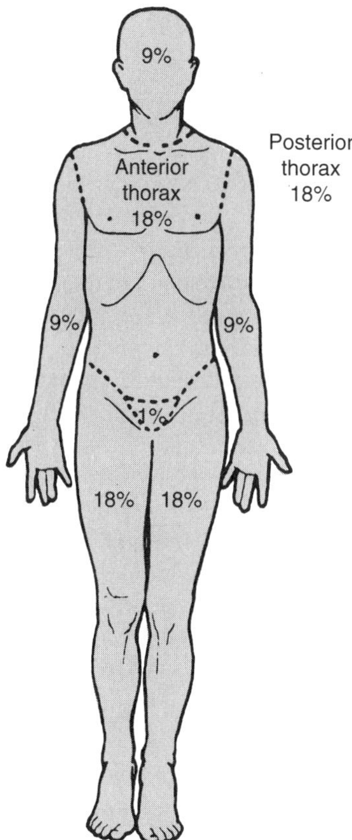

Figure 2–3
Rule of nines. (From Black JM, Matassarin-Jacobs E (eds): Medical-Surgical Nursing: Clinical Management for Continuity of Care, 5th ed. Philadelphia, WB Saunders, 1997.)

Body Response to Injury

The human body is programmed to take care of itself whenever possible. If one part of it is sick or injured, it sends help from other areas, and the whole body goes on alert during the crisis. This state of crisis along with the burn injury causes added stress on the system, which may compromise a positive outcome. Many severe burn patients lose a lot of blood and fluid at the onset of the burn. Since, because of the injury, they are unable to maintain a good fluid level, they go into **hypovolemic** (low fluid volume) **shock.** This, in turn, causes the heart to decrease output, beginning a chain of events as the body tries to adjust to the injury and maintain normal function. Major body functions may be affected by the burn and its complications—the lungs, the kidneys, and the GI system are of primary concern.

In addition to the physical complications of severe burns, there is the emotional and psychological stress suffered by burn patients and their families. The patient must go through a long and often painful recovery, sometimes involving multiple surgical procedures. He or she is frequently isolated from family and friends to protect them from infection. These patients are concerned about disfigurement, deformities, disability, altered self-image, and depression. They may also have the worry of financing the prolonged and expensive treatments. Treating the patient's emotional injury is as important as the skin grafting for the tissue injuries.

Burn Shock

Shock after a burn injury results from swelling and fluid accumulation in the tissues in the area of injury. The loss of blood and fluid begin immediately following the burn and may continue for 24 to 36 hours. Burn shock may be complicated by damage to internal body organs (such as the lungs if hot gases are inhaled) and by secondary infection. Patients suffering burn shock may have a weak, thready pulse; cold, clammy extremities; and pale skin color. They may be anxious, restless, and confused and may have increased respirations. Fluid and pain therapy should be administered immediately.

Escharotomy

Removal of the **eschar** formed on the skin and underlying tissue of severely burned areas is known as escharotomy (ES). This procedure is particularly helpful in restoring circulation to the extremities when the eschar forms a thick band around a limb.

Debridement

Debridement is removal of dead or damaged tissue so that the healing process can begin. Burn patients may undergo debridement procedures many times during the course of healing. For severe burns the patient will go to surgery and be given general anesthesia. Minor debridement may be done at the bedside or sometimes in the whirlpool bath after the tissue has been softened by water. Debridement is generally painful and difficult to endure over and over. Frequently the patient will be given pain medication before the procedure to minimize the discomfort.

Skin Grafting

Placing healthy skin over damaged tissue to promote healing is a common treatment for burn patients. Three different types of skin are used to cover burns to aid in the healing process.

Alloderm is human skin that has been processed aseptically from human donor **(Dnr)** skin. The skin is processed to remove any cells that may be targets of immune response without altering the proteins and collagen of the dermis. Any-time that Alloderm is used there is the possibility of tissue rejection.

Xeroflo is a coating of Xeroform dressing that allows drainage. It has bacteriostatic action, which aids in the prevention of infections.

Culture epidermal autograft **(CEA)** is skin that is grown in the laboratory under sterile conditions from cells of the patient's healthy skin.

Easyderm is a roll of very fine pigskin that is placed over the damaged area to help protect the burn from outside infection.

Dressings

The average burn patient has some sort of dressing that covers the injury. These dressings may be changed several times a day depending on the severity of the injury, the level of infection, or the amount of drainage. Although each dressing change is different depending on the size, location, and type of injury, there are some basic dressing supplies that almost all burn patients require. The most important thing to remember during a dressing change is that infection is the downfall of any burn injury, so supplies should be stored carefully when not in use. Gloves should be worn during the process. The basic burn dressing change includes gauze bandages, 4 × 4s, tube gauze, and various sizes of gauze rolls. Also needed are tweezers, scissors, safety pins, sterile basin, saline or water, and stockinette for the outside covering.

The first step is to carefully remove the old dressing and clean the wounds, removing the residue from the previous dressing. If the dressing is adherent to the wounds, either saline or water may be used to soak the material until it can be lifted off without damage to the tissue. When the burn area is extensive and involves the trunk, a special whirlpool tub (Fig. 2–4) may be used to soften the eschar. If there are small areas of dead tissue or scabbing, the tweezers are used to debride the wound. Once the area is clean and free of all dead tissue, medicated ointment or cream may be applied. The area is then loosely covered and wrapped with gauze bandage; 4-inch gauze is used on arms and lower legs, and 9-inch gauze

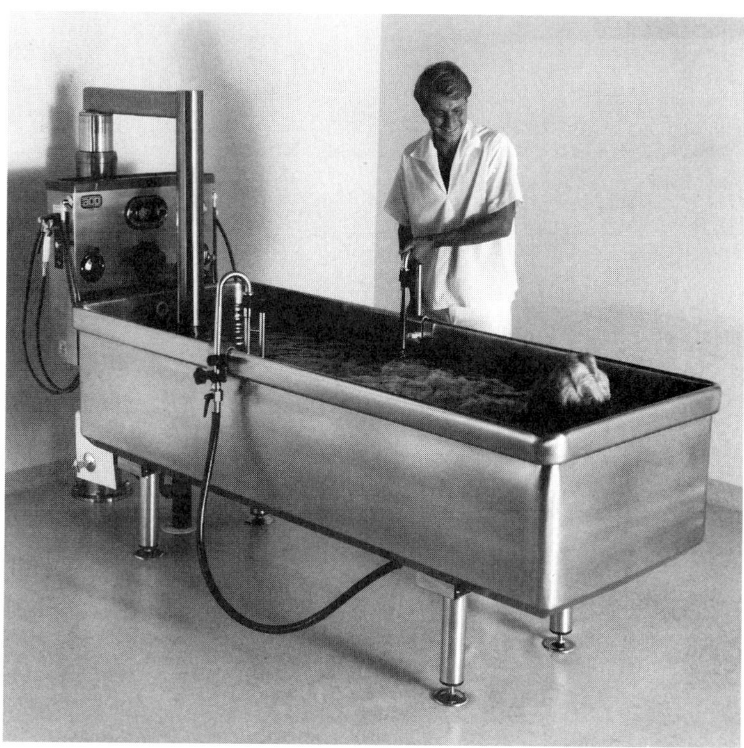

Figure 2–4
Hydro whirlpool tub. (Courtesy of Arjo, Morton Grove, IL.)

for the thighs and torso. This dressing may be secured by safety pins or an outer covering of stockinette. An Ace bandage may be applied for added protection. Dressing changes may be very painful to the patient, and pain medication may be administered prior to beginning the procedure. The idea is to get through the entire process as quickly and smoothly as possible; this cuts down on the possibility of infection and discomfort to the patient. Patients with large area burns may lose body temperature during dressing changes, and care should be taken to increase the room temperature if necessary.

Equipment and Supplies

Specialized Dressings

In addition to the normal types of dressings that the burn patient may have, there are some specialized dressings and skin coverings. Extremity splints are used postoperatively to stabilize the extremity in order to allow the **skin grafts** time to start adhering. An elasticized tubular stocking or sleeve (Tubi-Grip) to minimize hypertrophic scarring is generally used after the skin has begun the healing process. Once the patient is ready to go home, special custom-made pressure covers (Jobskin) (Fig. 2–5) may be applied to minimize the burn scar. Isotoner gloves may also be used as a compression garment that will initiate scar management and decrease swelling of the hand.

Electrocautery

The Bovie is an electrocautery machine (Fig. 2–6) used to make incisions through the full depth of the skin, allowing the eschar to separate with a minimum of bleeding.

Lifts, Chairs, and Beds

Most hospitals have lifts, chairs, and beds for the special patient, but in a burn unit all the patients

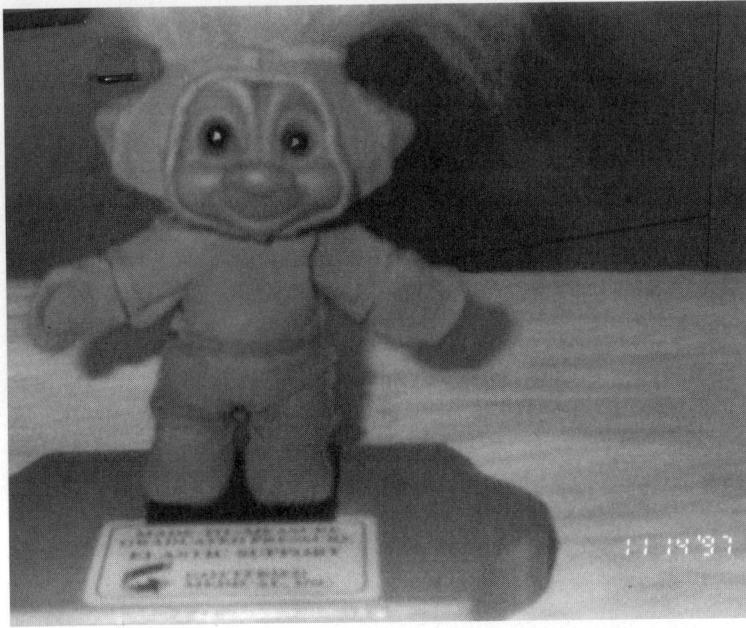

Figure 2–5
Teaching doll used to explain Jobskin to patients. (Courtesy of Jobskin, Clayton, MO.)

are special. Because of the delicate condition of burned or newly formed skin, extra care must be taken not to damage it further when moving the patient. Also, some patients may be so heavily bandaged that mobility is difficult to accomplish without the aid of special equipment. Lifts are used to transfer patients from bed (Fig. 2–7) to tub or transport cart (Fig. 2–8). Because of the large fluid loss most burn patients require an accurate record of their weight. Lifts may be used to place the patient on a special scale, or bed scales may be utilized for the acutely ill.

Special tilt tables are used to assist long-term bedridden patients. Allowing patients to remain flat in the supine position may cause the lower extremities to weaken from lack of exercise and decrease of blood supply. By placing the patient on a tilt table the body is allowed to maintain some of its normal positions.

Air beds are used to help prevent further breakdown of the skin and bone. Many different companies manufacture these specialty beds. They may be leased on a patient-by-patient basis, or the hospital may own a few for the special patient. The expense of purchasing and maintaining this type of equipment generally forces hospitals into the rental arrangement.

Communication With and About Burn Patients

Health Unit Coordinator

Health unit coordinators may not be involved in the clinical care of the burn patient, but they have a role in communicating with the patient. Burn patients are often on the unit for an extended period and may spend some of that time in a state of isolation. The HUC may have the opportunity to get to know both the patient and the family on a far more personal level than is the case with the typical hospital patient. Burns are among the most devastating of traumatic injuries because of the loss of body image, low self-esteem, disability, disfigurement, and long rehabilitation process. Because the burn victim experiences anxiety, depression, and loneliness there may be a decrease of motivation and a reduction in the patient's compliance with treatment. There are many

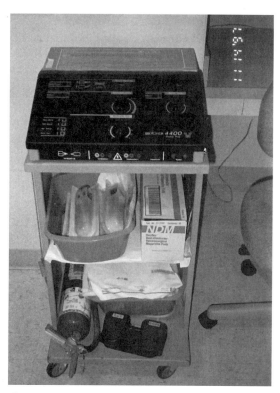

Figure 2–6
Electrocautery machine.

things that the HUC can do to help both the patient and family members and at the same time maintain patient confidentiality. Answering the call light quickly gives the patient the feeling that someone is out there who cares. Listening to patients talk when they need a friendly ear is one of the easiest services that the HUC can perform. When patients feel frustrated or lonely they often just need a few minutes for someone to listen to them. The HUC in this special unit will also recognize that a burn patient or family member may take out their anger or frustration on the next person they see. So a simple, "Hi, how are you?" could be met with a lot more than was expected. People need to vent, and sometimes the HUC is nearby when this occurs. The HUC will know how to evaluate the situation and decide if just listening with interest will help or if it might be necessary to call in a social service worker, a chaplain, or the nurse. The HUC may choose to ask, "Who can I call for you?" Maybe another family member or a close personal friend would put the problem in a different perspective. Whatever course the HUC takes, the first step is to realize not to take it personally and that it is the situation that is upsetting the person.

In addition to communicating with patients

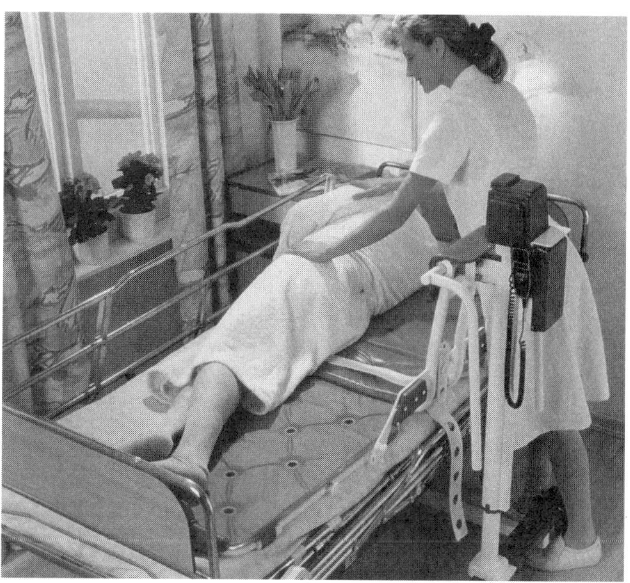

Figure 2–7
Transfer lift. (Courtesy of Arjo, Morton Grove, IL.)

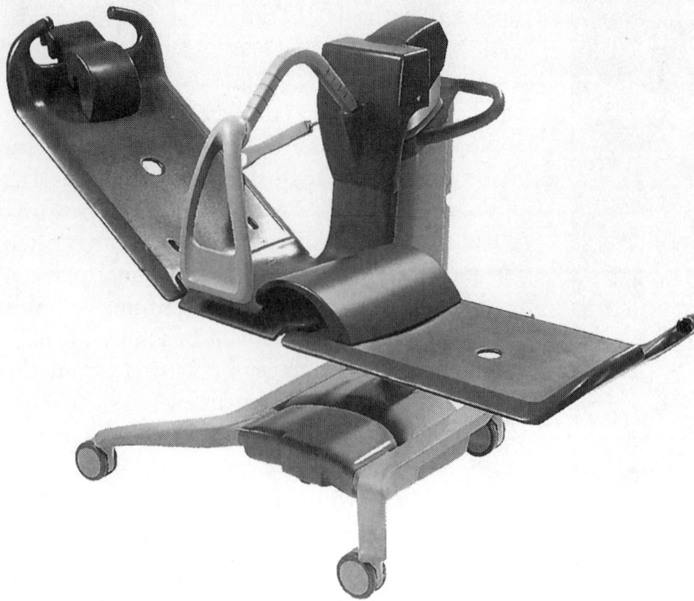

Figure 2–8
Transport chair. (Courtesy of Arjo, Morton Grove, IL.)

and families, the HUC will be communicating with many other departments within the hospital in order to carry out the orders for patient care.

Since the needs of many burn patients may be similar, standard orders are often written to assist the staff in implementing care. This system allows the HUC to begin the process of order transcription in an effective manner. Figure 2–9 shows a sample of some of the standard orders that might be written. Although most of these orders are ones with which an experienced HUC might be familiar, it is helpful to see how they apply to a patient with burns.

Spiritual Services

Chaplains are generally involved in the teamwork of caring for the burn patient. As with any traumatic injury that causes a possible deformity or long-term recuperation it is important to treat all aspects of the patient. Chaplains may offer the needed link to a church or religion or just be a willing ear. Pastoral care is as important to the healing process as medical care. Family members are encouraged to ask for support and to verbalize their fears in a setting apart from the patient. By assisting the family, the pastoral care worker will promote healing for the patient.

Social Services

Social Services may become involved with the patient and family shortly after admission. They may be able to assist with medical insurance questions or concerns. Patients without medical insurance may qualify for special assistance and the Social Services office will know what is available and how to obtain the help that is needed for both the patient and the family. The family may need assistance with temporary housing if they are from out of town. As soon as possible a discharge plan will be developed for the patient and Social Services will play a major role. Some patients go from the hospital to a rehabilitation center for continued care and treatments. Other patients may be able to go home from the hospital but will require special equipment for home recovery. These are all situations that the social service worker will handle for the patient and family.

STANDARD ADMISSION ORDERS		
Order	Major Burns	Minor Burns
Admit to Burn Center with ____ %TBSA ____ %2nd ____ %3rd	X	X
Continuous Cardiac Monitor (if indicated circle)	X	X
I & O	X	X
Vital Signs	X	X
Consults: Ophthalmology	X	X
Infectious Disease	X	X
Pulmonary	X	X
Psychiatry		X
Insert # ____NG/Salem Sump	X	
Insert # ____Foley Catheter	X	
Chest X-Ray	X	X
Oxygen via ____@ ____ L/min	X	
Admit labs: CBC, Chem-6, Chem-12, UA	X	X
ABG's, Mg, Ca, Phos	X	
Carboxyhemoglobin, PT/PTT, Toxicology	X	
Screen-Ethanol Level		
Type and Crossmatch for ____ units PRBC	X	
Wound Culture on admission and then every Mon.	X	
Photograph wounds on admission and discharge	X	X
Dressing changes with ____________ OD, BID (circle choice)	X	X
Elevate burned extremities	X	X
PT/OT Indicate frequency	X	X
Start IV of ________ in non-burned area with # ____ Angiocath Infuse at _____ ml/h	X	
Calorie Count x 3 days	X	
Hi Cal Hi Pro diet		X
Tetanus toxoid 0.5 ml IM		X

Figure 2–9
Standard admission orders.

Physical and Occupational Therapy

Both physical and occupational therapy are begun for most burn patients shortly after admission. Physical therapy focuses on active and passive range-of-motion exercise to prevent contractures. Occupational therapy assists the patient in activities that will promote a return to as normal a life as possible.

Dietitian

Nutrition is an essential part of any healing process, and this is especially true for the patient with a burn injury. Regardless of the method of caloric intake—oral feeding, tube feeding, or parenteral nutrition—a professional dietitian is needed to manage this part of the patient's recovery. In addition to providing the number of calories that the body needs for healing, it is important to ensure that vitamins, minerals, protein, and fat levels are balanced so that the patient can achieve maximum results from food or IV intake.

Family and Friends

Family and friends are very important to the burn patient. In addition to giving emotional support and comfort, it is important to show the patient that he or she is loved regardless of physical appearance. Family and friends will need extra support from the staff in several areas. Whenever one member of a family is injured the whole family unit is damaged and will need the same emotional support that the injured person receives. After the initial shock of the injury has set in, the anxiety of caring for the patient begins. In the case of many burn patients the recovery journey may take months or years before the individual can return to a normal lifestyle. Friends and family will need help adjusting to these facts as well as assistance in coping during this adjustment stage.

Support Groups

Burn support groups are one of the best forms of therapy for burn victims. These groups offer emotional and practical support to both the patient and the family. Support group involvement may begin by meeting with other patients and families while the patient is still in the hospital. Sometimes just hearing about others in a similar situation is a great relief. Many support groups maintain long-term involvement by sending members to meet with new hospital patients. This gives the patient and family the reassurance that the support will be ongoing and not end after a few short meetings. It is often difficult for health care workers to understand everything that the patient may be dealing with; the support group members will not encounter this barrier. Past burn victims and their families have been there and will have practical answers to many questions.

Support groups are especially important when the burn victim is a child. Children may have many years of skin grafting (every time they grow), and dealing with disfigurement is difficult. They need to understand how to handle teasing from other children when they return to school. Some support groups may send members to the school to give a talk on burns and and suggest ways for the children to help their classmate. Parents of burns victims will benefit from talking with other parents to know where to go for special assistance.

The support group is an invaluable network of people who have been there and can help show the way. The only requirement is to pass that service along to the next person who needs help.

Closing Thoughts

The survival rates in burns provide witness to significant improvements each year in overall care and prognosis. This is due, in part, to the increased number of surgical techniques, advances in the different types of skin available, and the public knowledge of burns. Patients are treated by a specialized team of caregivers who dedicate their time to the treatment of burns. The team is able to recog-

nize the special problems and complications associated with the burn victim and to deal with them effectively.

The HUC can help make the unit run like a well-greased wheel. By checking daily to make sure that all supplies are available and up to date, by returning equipment promptly, by being prepared to handle the next admission, and in a hundred other ways the HUC helps ensure that the burn patient will receive the best possible care.

Review Questions

1. Describe the four classifications of burns.
2. List the six burn categories.
3. Explain the "rule of nines" for measuring the extent of burns.
4. List the other hospital departments that would be involved with the care of a burn patient.
5. Identify three special pieces of equipment used for burn patients.

Bibliography

Baker R, Jones S, Sanders C, et al: Degree of burn, location of burn and length of hospital stay as predictors of psychosocial status and physical functioning. J Burn Care Rehabil. July/August, 1996; 2:327–333.

Gottschlich: Nutrition Forum. J Burn Care Rehabil. May/June, 1996; 17:263.

Kirby D, O'Keefe S, Neal J, et al: Does the architectural design of burn centers comply with The Americans With Disabilities Act? J Burn Care Rehabil. March/April, 1996; 17:156–160.

Monafo W: Early Care: The Treatment of Burns Principles and Practice, 1st ed. St. Louis, 1971.

Sanders M, Lewis M, Quick G, et al: Mosby's Paramedic Textbook, 1st ed. St. Louis, CV Mosby, 1994.

Thomas C (ed): Taber's Cyclopedic Medical Dictionary, 14th ed. Philadelphia, FA Davis, 1981.

Dialysis Unit

3

Madeline Clark

Objectives

Upon completion of this chapter, the reader will be able to:

1. List the diagnostic tests most often done in renal dialysis cases.
2. Explain the roles of team members in the "predialysis" phase.
3. Identify and describe various dialysis techniques.
4. List the factors that account for the differences in what is expected of the HUC in the dialysis unit.

Vocabulary

Biocompatible: Being harmless to living systems

Dialysate: A fluid used to remove or deliver compounds or electrolytes that the failing kidney cannot excrete or retain in proper concentrations

Dialysis: The passage of a solute through a membrane

Dialyzer: The apparatus used in performing dialysis

Diffusion: The tendency of molecules of a substance to move from a region of high concentration to one of lower concentration

Nephrotoxic: Destructive to the tissue of the kidney

Reticulocyte: The last immature stage of a red blood cell

Rhabdomyolysis: An acute, often fatal disease characterized by the destruction of skeletal muscle

Scleroderma: A chronic progressive disease characterized by systemic sclerosis, in which the skin becomes taut, firm, and edematous, limiting motion

Tenckhoff catheter: A special catheter that is placed for use in peritoneal dialysis

Common Abbreviations

A-V	Arteriovenous
BUN	Blood urea nitrogen
CAPD	Continuous ambulatory peritoneal dialysis
CCPD	Continuous cycle peritoneal dialysis
Cr	Creatinine
EPO	Erythropoietin
ESRD	End-stage renal disease
IPD	Intermittent peritoneal dialysis
K(subd)	Dialyzer clearance (used in dosage calculations)
kcal	One thousand calories
NIDDKD	National Institute for Diabetes and Digestive and Kidney Diseases
NKUDIC	National Kidney and Urologic Diseases Information Clearinghouse
PCR	Protein catabolism rate
r	residual renal urea clearance (used in calculations)
t	treatment time (used in calculation formula)
URR	Urea reduction ratio
V	Total body urea distribution volume (used in calculations)

History

As early as the 1930s and 1940s, work was being done in selected facilities to develop renal dialysis centers. The equipment was cumbersome, and the procedures used for dialysis were often accompanied by complications and a high morbidity and mortality rate. The procedure was reserved in most instances for the treatment of acute renal failure.

Prior to 1960, end-stage renal disease (**ESRD**) was nearly uniformly fatal. A new era in dialysis was launched with the development of the **A-V** shunt by Brian Scribner and Wayne Quinton. The shunt provided a relatively safe method for repeated vascular access and, coupled with other improvements in the technology, provided a method for chronic intermittent hemodialysis. The development and application of peritoneal dialysis followed soon thereafter.

Much of the progress that followed has been in the area of financing the treatment. In the 1970s legislation was passed to provide Medicare coverage for the treatment of ESRD to individuals regardless of age. This made it possible for hundreds of thousands of patients to receive life-sustaining renal replacement therapy.

The incidence of ESRD patients treated in the United States is over 180 million and rises at a rate of approximately 7.8 percent per year. Of the individuals being treated, 43% are over 64 years of age and less than 2 percent are under 20 years of age. The Health Care Financing Administration (HICFA) estimates that by the year 2000 there will be 300,000 patients enrolled in the ESRD program. The amount of this increase reflects an increase in the diabetic population as well as the increasing life span.

Despite the improvements in technology and in the procedure itself, the mortality in the ESRD population remains high. For example, an average person at age 49 years would be expected to live another 30 years, but the same person with treated ESRD has a life expectancy of only 7 more years. **Biocompatible** membranes have been developed that appear to be positively influencing the mortality rates.

Introduction

Two thirds of **dialysis** patients suffer from either or both of two diseases: diabetes mellitus and hypertension. Patients with kidney failure often have anemia as well, requiring special medication and transfusions. Children with renal disease to

The abbreviations listed for this chapter are those that a HUC working in this area would be expected to know. Only those in boldface type are used in the text and appear in boldface when they are used for the first time.

the extent that dialysis is required are usually dialyzed on a temporary basis, until a suitable organ for transplantation can be procured.

Payment sources for these expensive procedures are as follows:

- Medicare pays 80 percent of the cost of dialysis for ESRD. To qualify, a person must have worked under Social Security or be the child of someone who has. The person must be receiving Social Security benefits and must have applied for Medicare.
- Private insurance often pays for the entire cost of treatment. In some instances it will pay for the 20 percent that Medicare does not cover. Private insurance may also pay for the prescription drugs.
- Medicaid is administered by the states. Some states will pay for the 20 percent not covered by Medicare. If the person's income is below a certain level, Medicaid will pay for the treatments if the patient is ineligible for Medicare.
- VA benefits can help pay for the treatment for veterans. Information for this program is available from local VA offices.

The cost of treatment alone, not including necessary drugs, supplies, or disability payments, was 7.26 billion dollars in 1990. This figure does include covered physician services such as direct patient care services, medical direction of the staff providing care, procedures such as insertion of access catheters, and medically appropriate pre- and postdialysis medical examinations.

Dialysis was originally provided in hospital-based areas, but now there are dedicated outpatient facilities. Private investors have set up companies that specialize in dialysis and can provide the equipment and even the manpower to hospitals. These companies often have several units in ever-expanding territories. All these options make the treatment more readily available to those who need it.

Design of the Unit

Dialysis can actually be done in several units. The intensive care units may have specially equipped rooms to perform dialysis on acutely ill patients. In some facilities there is an area dedicated to inpatient dialysis and a separate area for outpatient dialysis; in others the two are combined.

Many dialysis units have a triage area, which is compared by some patients to the traffic control center. The patients are assessed on arrival; the information is reported to the nephrologist; and the patients are directed for further testing or to their dialysis area, which is referred to as a treatment station.

The areas for each treatment station must be large enough to accommodate the equipment and a recliner or bed (Fig. 3–1). The fact that several staff members may have to be around a patient in an emergency has to be considered as well. Each area is supplied with the equipment needed to monitor the patient's vital signs.

Many of the patients read, watch TV, or engage in some other activity while they are receiving treatment, so adequate nonglare lighting is a must. If children are dialyzed in the unit, education and play facilities should be provided.

There a technical department within the unit and space for equipment as well as an area dedicated to storage and preparation of medication

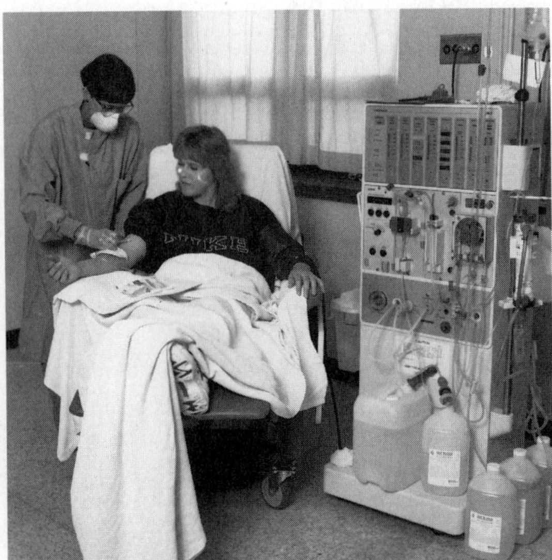

Figure 3–1
Dialysis station.

that is administered during treatment. A central desk area for the nurses and the HUC is the seat of communication in the unit, and most of the nonclinical activities take place here.

Staffing of the Unit

The leader of the dialysis team is the nephrologist. Other team members include trained dialysis technicians, registered nurses, renal dietitian, mental health professional, social worker, and health unit coordinator.

The nephrologist examines the patient, studies the test results to develop a medical care plan unique to that individual, and orders whatever is necessary for the plan to be carried out. The actual dialysis orders are calculated based on a formula for each patient; the goal is to achieve a urea reduction ratio (**URR**) of approximately 60 percent. URR is calculated as predialysis blood urea nitrogen (**BUN**) minus postdialysis BUN divided by predialysis BUN expressed as a percentage.

If children are routinely treated in the unit, a pediatric nephrologist should be available as well.

The dialysis technicians handle the dialysis equipment according to manufacturer's guidelines and institute the dialysis by facility policy. They are usually responsible for scheduling any maintenance and repairs that need to be done. They must use strict aseptic technique and observe OSHA guidelines for the handling of body fluids.

The nursing staff monitor the patients, administer medications as needed, and see to the comfort of the patient during the procedure. They are in constant communication with the nephrologist to report progress as well as the slightest sign of a potential problem. Vital signs, including temperature, are taken every 30 minutes during treatment. The patient has to be weighed during treatment and blood samples taken. The lines of the dialyzer must be checked regularly. Intake and output are recorded. After the procedure, the access site is monitored for bleeding. The nurses provide ongoing education to the patients and families, particularly to those who are candidates for home dialysis. They are also involved in the teaching if the patient is a candidate for transplantation.

A dietitian with special training in renal dietetics is preferred in the dialysis unit because of the complexities of nutritional interventions required by these patients. The renal dietitian develops food plans based on the physician's orders and educates patients in food choices that comply with their special needs. Before beginning dialysis treatment, the patient is on a limited protein diet that is based on the protein catabolism rate (**PCR**) and is adequate in calories. Once dialysis therapy is initiated, protein intake can be liberalized. Most of the patients on dialysis have special dietary needs because of other disorders. Constant monitoring of many parameters must be done and adjustments made accordingly.

The mental health professional is critical to the success of the dialysis program. Because the patients and their families must adjust to a new lifestyle, it is important to have assessed their coping skills and prepared appropriate plans for interventions. The range of responses by individuals facing a lifetime of dialysis extends from full rehabilitation to suicide. Often the course of treatment is a mix of "honeymoon periods," such as initially, when a sudden improvement in general condition occurs, and periods of disillusionment and discouragement from the realization that the treatment is for the long term.

This is one occasion when denial becomes a useful coping mechanism. If patents remain less than fully aware of the realities of the life-threatening situation and dependence on a machine, they are less likely to be overwhelmed and more likely to resume normal activities. Too much denial, however, can lead to noncompliance and rejection of treatment. The mental health professional is available to assist and support the patient dealing with these and other behaviors that occur as a result of dialysis.

The social worker is available to assess family function and coping mechanisms. Based upon the evaluation, additional services may be arranged. He or she can help the family find sources of funding and fill out the necessary paperwork to apply to various programs. Social workers have access to and can provide the family with information from the National Kidney Foundation, **NKUDIC**, American Association of Kidney Patients, **NIDDKD**, and the American Kidney Fund. As the mental health professional is cast in the role of patient advocate, the social worker becomes the family advocate.

The HUC is the nerve center and heart of the unit. In order to make the best use of the equipment, scheduling must be precise. Each patient will have individualized orders as well as standing orders to be processed. The tests must be carried out efficiently. Medications have to be given on schedule. Equipment and supplies need to be ordered. Amid all this ativity, the HUC must know where all the team members and patients are located and at what stage of treatment the patients are.

The most critical team member is not a staff member, but the patient. Patient participation as an integral member of the renal team is absolutely necessary for the success of the program and the achievement of its goals.

Anatomy and Physiology Related to the Dialysis Unit

The kidneys are two bean-shaped organs located in the posterior of the abdomen. They lie one on each side of the vertebral column and are generally located between the twelfth thoracic and third lumbar vertebrae. The left kidney is often positioned up to an inch higher than the right one. Each kidney weighs from 4 to 6 ounces and is 4 to 5 inches long and 2 inches thick. The high degree of vascularity in the kidneys is responsible for their reddish brown color.

Facing the midline of the body in each kidney is a concavity known as the hilus. The renal artery, renal vein, renal nerve, and the ureter are admitted at the hilus. Within the kidney is the renal sinus or cavity. The functional groups called nephrons are contained within the renal sinus (Fig. 3–2). There are more than 1 million nephrons in each kidney. The nephron is made up of a cluster of small blood vessels called a glomerulus. The glomerulus is attached to a tubule. If both kidneys were combined, there would be about 140 miles of these tubes and filters.

The kidneys are responsible for filtering ingested water, toxins, mineral salts, and wastes out of the bloodstream. The filtration process that separates the waste products from the blood takes place in the glomerulus. The entire blood supply is processed in this way every 2 minutes. The wastes are eliminated in the urine.

The kidneys maintain body fluid levels by excreting fluid and sodium when there is an overabundance of fluid in the body and, in dehydration, conserving fluid. The kidneys contribute to the regulation of blood pressure through this fluid balancing and play a role in the regulation of acid-base balance by excreting alkaline salts when called upon to do so.

Kidney Disease

Human beings are "blessed" with the capacity for sufficient kidney function such that symptoms of renal failure will not start until 90 percent of the total kidney function is lost. At this point the waste products that are not cleansed from the system become toxic to the body. Kidney disease is a broad term to describe a large number of disease processes that directly or indirectly affect the kidneys. It is often the indirect processes, such as the effects of long-standing diabetes, autoimmune disease, or hypertension, that destroy the kidney over a period of years. The condition that results is known as chronic renal failure and can progress to ESRD. A condition that acutely compromises kidney blood flow can precipitate renal failure. If it results in a sudden onset of decline in renal function, it is referred to as acute renal failure. Table 3–1 lists the various causes of kidney failure and whether they are likely to cause acute or chronic failure.

The symptoms of renal failure are:

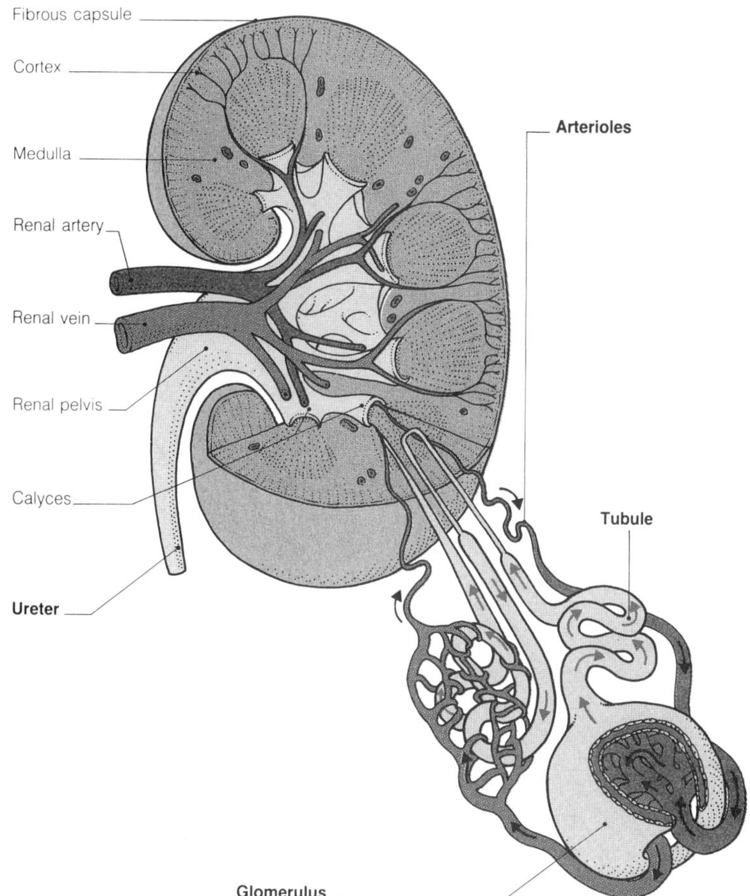

Figure 3–2
Kidney and nephron. (From Clayman CB [ed]: AMA Encyclopedia of Medicine. New York, Random House, 1989.)

- Decreased urine output
- Weakness and lack of energy and endurance
- Dry and itchy skin
- Peculiar odor to breath (urine-like)
- Smoky or cocoa-colored urine
- Net weight gain from fluid accumulation but with loss of muscle and fat
- Pallor from anemia
- Shortness of breath on minor exertion (from anemia)
- Total body edema, worse in lower extremities
- Confusion, lethargy, dementia, delirium
- Memory loss
- Coma in late stages
- Tremors
- Seizures in later stages
- Vomiting
- Lack of sensation in hands and feet
- Anorexia
- Hiccups

Evaluation of kidney disease begins with a detailed history and thorough physical examination. Testing, including testing of blood and urine, is done to evaluate kidney function. Additional tests are done as indicated in an attempt to identify the precipitating factors, which often can be corrected. If, with all this testing, the answer is not clear, a kidney biopsy may be required. Treatment is prescribed based upon the conclusions that the nephrologist draws from all the test results.

Table 3–1 CAUSES OF RENAL FAILURE

Kidney infection	A	Kidney stones	A
Severe dehydration	A	Drug toxicity	A
Kidney cancer	B	Sepsis	A
Chronic diabetes	C	Chronic hypertension	C
Chronic drug abuse (heroin)	C	Inherited kidney disease	B
Lupus	C	Post-"strep" glomerulonephritis	B
Polycystic kidney	C	Scleroderma	C
Malignant hypertension	A	Shock	A
Burns	A	Acute tubular necrosis	B
Rhabdomyolysis	A	Obstructive uropathy	A
Acute glomerulonephritis	A	Interstitial nephritis	B
Transfusion reaction	A	Post-partum renal failure	A

A, Acute renal failure; C, chronic renal failure; B, both.

Laboratory Testing

The types of laboratory testing done in both the predialysis and the dialysis phases are as follows:

- BUN (blood urea nitrogen) is produced in the liver as a by-product of protein metabolism. The normal range is 8 to 23 gm/dl (may vary with institutions and laboratories). Elevations are seen not only in kidney disease and renal failure but also in dehydration, starvation, congestive heart failure (CHF), increased protein ingestion, severe burns, shock, and gastrointestinal bleeding as well as with the use of several medications. Lower than normal values are seen in liver failure, diets low in protein, and overhydration as well as with the use of chloramphenicol and streptomycin.
- Cr (creatinine) is a by-product of muscle metabolism. The normal range is 0.6 to 1.2 mg/dl (may vary with institutions and laboratories). Elevated values may occur in kidney disease, renal failure, acromegaly, muscular dystrophy, preeclampsia, shock, CHF, and **rhabdomyolysis.** Cimetidine, cisplatin, and the antibiotics gentamicin, tobramycin, and amikacin may all cause elevations in creatinine. Lower than normal results may be seen in myasthenia gravis and late-stage muscular dystrophy.
- Arterial blood gas to check for acidosis or alkalosis
- Electrolytes to check for problems with sodium or potassium
- CBC (complete blood count) to check for anemia and infection
- **Reticulocyte** count to monitor erythropoietin (**EPO**) effects
- Serum EPO level
- PTT (partial thromboplastin time) to monitor the results of the use of heparin
- Urinalysis to check for specific gravity, protein, and infection
- Urine Cr requires a 24-hour specimen to be collected; must be accompanied by a serum creatine for evaluation.

Predialysis Phase

Studies have shown that this phase may offer the best opportunity to positively influence the outcomes of dialysis. Many of the patients who enter dialysis are at risk for a cardiovascular event such as stroke or myocardial infarction; such events account for 50 percent of the mortality in dialysis patients. The rising mean age of dialysis candidates will undoubtedly influence these numbers in an upward direction. Many believe that predialysis intervention in the patients with chronic renal failure will reduce the morbidity and mortality rates.

An individual who is considered to be a potential candidate for dialysis is referred to the dialysis team by a primary care physician or specialist. The team meets with the individual and family or significant other to establish a rapport as well as to establish the clinical condition of the patient. The predialysis phase is also the time to get the potential patient interested in support groups of people with similar problems.

Teaching begins with the predialysis visits.

Disease and Dialysis-Specific Education. The nephrologist and the RN explain the procedures and testing that need to be done and advise the patient on some lifestyle changes that may improve his or her condition. Of primary interest are hypertension and smoking. Nearly all dialysis patients who have achieved 20-year survival rates no longer smoked and were compliant with treatments to keep their blood pressure in a normal range. Perhaps the most important learning that will be done is that dialysis is an acceptable replacement for failed kidneys but that it is *not* a cure.

Psychosocial Considerations. Early predialysis evaluation and intervention by the mental health professional and social worker have been found much more effective than intervention after treatment has been established. The assessment by these two team members produces measurements of the individual's quality of life, social and family role functions, mental acuity, economic status, and the presence or absence of depression. This time offers a unique opportunity to ensure the patient's understanding and positive participation in a care plan and its implementation. It is also an opportunity to optimize the relationship between the patient and other team members. The earlier the assessments are carried out and proper interventions are initiated, the greater will be the impact on physical and social rehabilitation.

If the patient is a child with chronic renal failure, a cycle of depression, anxiety, and lowered self-esteem is typically encountered. The difficulties often result in family stress as evidenced by a higher divorce rate in families with chronically ill children. As with adults, early and continuous assessment and intervention by the mental health professional and social worker are essential for the program to succeed.

Nutritional Factors. The nutritional status is a major consideration in the predialysis phase because it is imperative to avoid malnutrition. Based upon the results of testing, the renal dietitian can recommend diets to maintain nutrition or correct malnutrition. Malnutrition will be evidenced by decreases in serum albumin below 3.5 gm/dl and loss of body weight. Ordinarily, in the predialysis phase calories in the range of 35 **kcal**/kg/day are needed, with restricted protein in the range of 0.7 to 0.8 gm/kg/day. The renal dietitian will have the opportunity to work with patients and families to develop appropriate meal plans that take individual preferences into account.

Exercise Planning. A physical therapist can do an assessment of the patient's current status and develop a home exercise program to optimize his or her physical capabilities. Physical training can add to general well-being and best results when it is started early and continued throughout therapy.

Care Planning. Throughout the predialysis period, the results of the ongoing assessments will help determine which type of treatment will be best and where it will be provided. At every stage patients are kept aware of both their status and their options.

When the determination is made that dialysis is imminent, either an A-V shunt (for hemodialysis) or a **Tenckhoff** or other type of catheter (for peritoneal dialysis) will be placed in advance and allowed to mature.

In the A-V shunt, a fistula is created surgically between an artery and a vein in the forearm to provide multiple vascular access (Fig. 3–3). The recommendation is that the fistula be created at least a month before the first hemodialysis treatment is planned. If there is not time for the shunt to mature before dialysis is initiated, a tunneled subcutaneous femoral catheter may be placed that can be used temporarily. In those patients for whom a shunt is not feasible, a synthetic graft is placed. This is used only when absolutely necessary because studies have shown that 60 percent of these grafts fail each year owing to thrombosis.

The peritoneal dialysis catheter is inserted under sterile techniques by a trained practitioner. It, too, should be placed a month before the planned initiation of dialysis. In some centers, the catheters are placed very early in the planning phase. The distal end of the catheter is buried subcutaneously and brought out to the exterior at a later date to avoid contamination and infection.

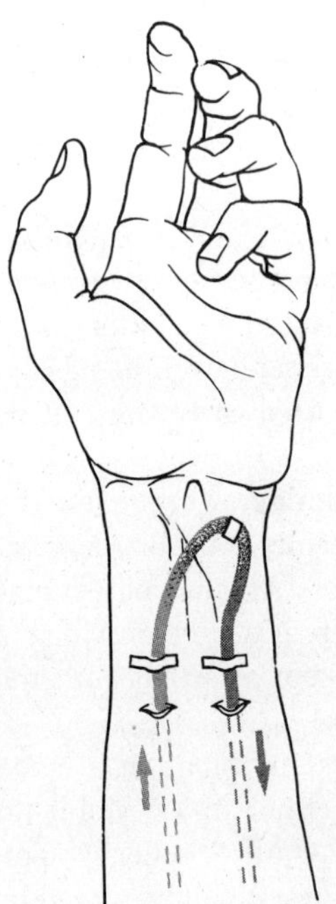

Figure 3–3
AV shunt. (From Ignatavicius DD, Workman ML, Mishler MA [eds]: Medical-Surgical Nursing. Philadelphia, WB Saunders, 1995.)

Procedures on the Dialysis Unit

The goal of dialysis procedures is to remove toxic materials and to maintain blood pressure, fluid electrolyte and acid-base balance in a person whose kidneys are unable to do so.

Hemodialysis

Hemodialysis is the method for providing kidney function by circulating blood through a machine called a dialyzer. Tubes take the patient's blood to the dialyzer and through the hemodialyzer, an apparatus consisting of semipermeable membranes, where filtering takes place, in one of the following forms: (1) hollow fibers the size of hairs; (2) coils of cellophane tubing separated by mesh spacers; or (3) parallel sheets of cellophane sealed at edges between grooved membrane supports.

The dialyzing membranes are continually bathed in **dialysate,** a solution that selectively removes unwanted materials. The machine is set up before each procedure according to the manufacturer's guidelines. The dialysate is added according to the prescription developed by the nephrologist.

Before the treatment is started, any ordered lab studies are done. The shunt is accessed with two needles, one to direct the blood to the dialyzer and one to return the blood to the patient's body (Fig. 3–4). Vital signs and weight are taken and recorded before the treatment starts. Vital signs are repeated every half hour during the treatment. Any ordered medications are given.

Hemodialysis treatments are typically done three times a week and generally last 3 to 4 hours. Hemodialysis may be done in a hospital dialysis unit, a freestanding kidney center, or at home. Home dialysis is sometimes referred to as self-care dialysis. If the dialysis is to be done at home, a partner is trained to do the procedure.

When deciding which option to take, the patient will want to weigh the following pros and cons.

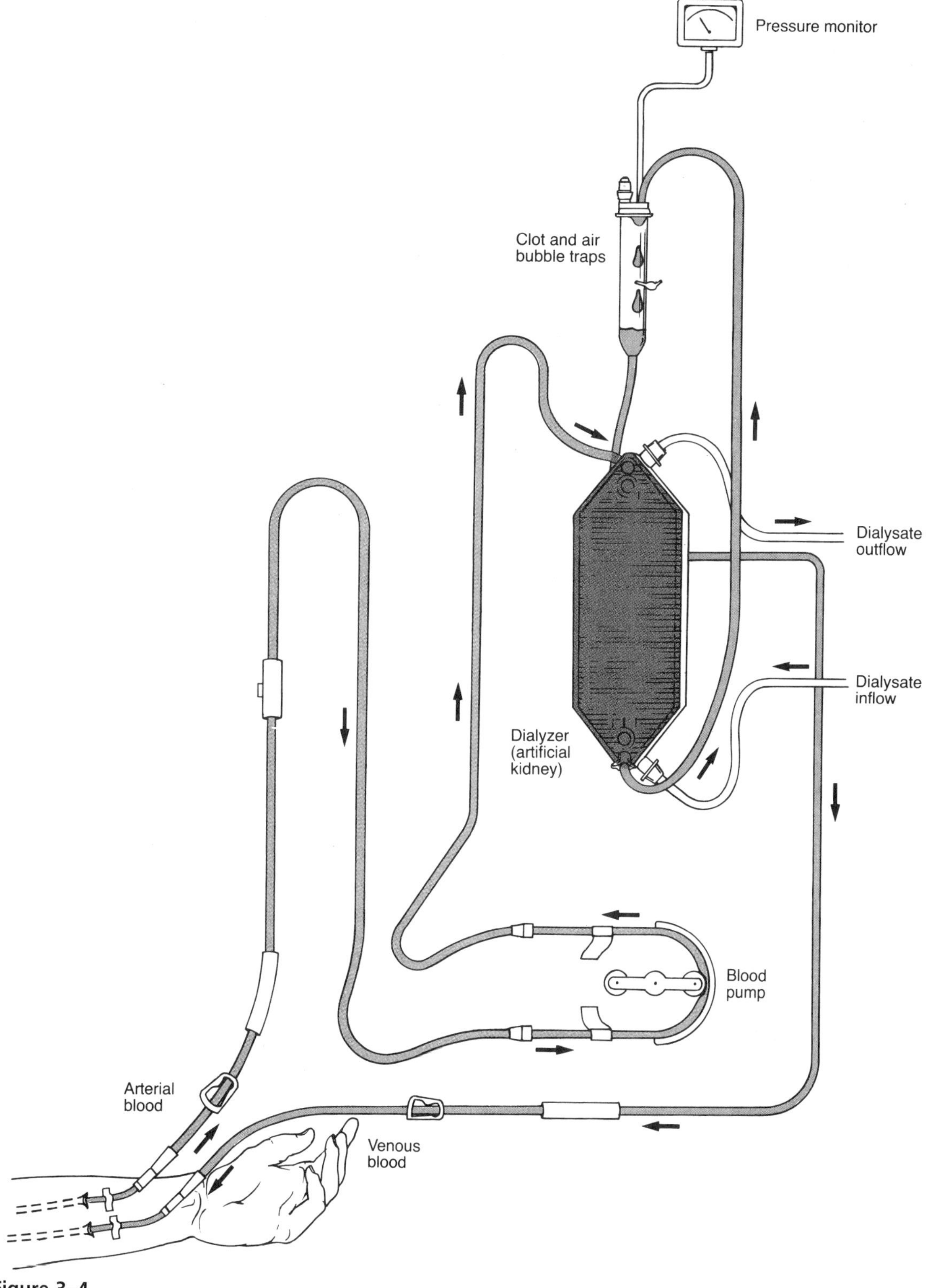

Figure 3–4
Hemodialysis. (From Ignatavicius DD, Workman ML, Mishler MA [eds]: Medical-Surgical Nursing. Philadelphia, WB Saunders, 1995.)

In-Unit Hemodialysis

Pro

Constant availability and attention of trained professionals
Opportunity to get to know others with common problems.

Con

Treatments are scheduled by the unit
Necessary to travel to the unit for each treatment.

Home Hemodialysis

Pro

Patient can choose time of day (within framework of doctor's orders)
No need to travel to unit on a routine basis
Patient gains a sense of independence and control of his or her life.

Con

Helping with treatments may become stressful for partner and family
Special training needed
Designated space needed at home to store the machine, equipment, and supplies.

Complications of Hemodialysis

Infection is an ever-present possibility in a person who is on a hemodialysis schedule; it is usually heralded by fever. Side effects can be caused by rapid changes in the body's fluid and electrolyte balance during treatment. Muscle cramps are common. Sudden hypotension can cause weakness, dizziness, and nausea. Some of these symptoms lessen as the patient adjusts to hemodialysis.

Problems can develop with the shunt. The patient may bleed from the heparin that is added to prevent the blood from clotting as it goes through the dialyzer. Disorders of calcium, phosphorus, vitamin D, and parathyroid hormone may occur and become disabling.

Peritoneal Dialysis

Peritoneal dialysis is the procedure in which the lining of the body's peritoneal cavity is used as the dialyzing membrane. This is possible because the peritoneum contains vast networks of blood vessels that are capable of mimicking the action of the fibers in the hemodialyzer. The warm sterile dialysate is introduced into the abdominal cavity by way of a catheter and is left for a period of time and then drained, in the process known as exchange. The procedure is carried out under sterile technique. This procedure is usually used in renal failure. It can also be used to clear the body of certain ingested drugs, chemicals, and other **nephrotoxic** substances. In some facilities the same principle is used to treat heat stroke, with chilled isotonic saline solution replacing the dialysate (Fig. 3–5). Peritoneal dialysis can be accomplished in three ways.

Continuous Ambulatory Peritoneal Dialysis (CAPD)

This is the most common type of peritoneal dialysis. The dialysate passes from a plastic bag through the catheter into the abdomen. The solution remains in the abdomen for the length of time prescribed by the physician, is drained, and then is replaced.

Continuous Cyclic Peritoneal Dialysis (CCPD)

CCPD differs from CAPD in that it is accomplished overnight, utilizing a machine that automatically fills and drains the dialysate from the abdomen. The time ranges from 10 to 12 hours every night.

Intermittent Peritoneal Dialysis (IPD)

IPD uses the same type of machine as CCPD to add and drain the dialysate. The treatment is generally performed in the kidney unit. IPD takes longer than CCPD, being done several times a week for a total of 36 to 42 hours. In some conditions, sessions may last up to 24 hours.

In determining which type of peritoneal dialysis is most suitable, the following should be considered:

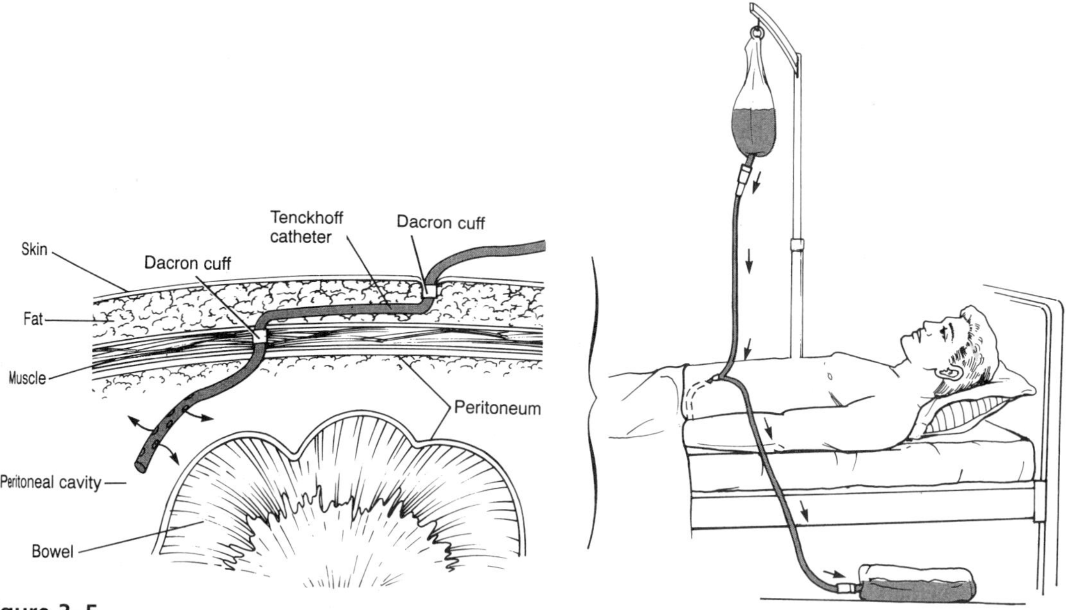

Figure 3–5
Peritoneal dialysis. (From Ignatavicius DD, Workman ML, Mishler MA [eds]: Medical-Surgical Nursing. Philadelphia, WB Saunders, 1995.)

CAPD

Pro

Treatment can be performed alone
Treatment can be done at times chosen by the patient
Treatment can be done in many locations
No need for a machine
Relatively inexpensive.

Con

Disruption of daily schedule.

CCPD

Pro

Can be done at night, mainly while patient is sleeping.

Con

Requires a machine and a storage place for it
Requires help from a partner.

IPD

Pro

Health professionals usually perform the treatment.

Con

Usually done in dialysis unit, requiring scheduling and travel.

Complications

Peritonitis can occur if the entry site or catheter becomes infected. Peritonitis will cause fever, nausea and vomiting, and abdominal pain and distention. If the dialysate looks cloudy when it is emptied from the abdominal cavity, this should be reported to the doctor immediately.

Patients are taught to seal the catheter entry site before bathing, showering, or swimming to prevent infection. They must also report any redness or drainage from the catheter entry site.

About 85 percent of people on dialysis use

hemodialysis, while the remainder use peritoneal dialysis. Generally speaking, there isn't one optimal method. It is a decision to be made by the patient and renal team. The factors that the patient must consider are:

How involved they want to be with their care
Whether a reliable helper is available
How difficult it is to arrange transportation to the dialysis unit
What kind of lifestyle restrictions they can be comfortable with.

Hemoperfusion

Hemoperfusion involves perfusing the blood through substances such as activated charcoal or ion exchange resins to remove toxic materials. The blood is then returned to the body. The procedure differs from dialysis in that the blood is not separated from the chemicals or solutions by a semipermeable membrane.

Hemofiltration

This technique differs from dialysis in that it is not accomplished by **diffusion.** It provides a more effective means to remove larger and heavier substances from the blood. The greatest advantage to the technique is that it is less disturbing to the blood pressure.

The tradeoff for this is that the treatment time is longer because removal of small molecules, such as urea and creatinine, is less effective. Hemofiltration is often the treatment of choice in the critically ill pediatric patient. It is more expensive than traditional hemodialysis.

Communication in the Dialysis Unit

The members of the renal dialysis unit team have to be in constant communication. The HUC is often at the center of this communication because he or she is the only person to know the location of everyone else. In some units, bulletin boards are used to list where each team member is. In others, everyone reports verbally to the HUC.

The HUC is called upon to convey the urgency of the calls he or she is making and give the messages concisely. Communication with parties outside the facility is often necessary. Some will be to families to confirm scheduling or to tell them that the patient will be delayed or even admitted to the hospital from outpatient dialysis. A patient may need a taxi for a ride home.

In the hospital-based dialysis unit, there is a need for communication with the other hospital departments, especially the laboratory. In some facilities, communication and order transfer can be done by computer; in others, it is done by phone. The pharmacy must be notified of urgent medication needs and medication changes. The unit that houses the in-patient dialysis area must be kept aware of when the patient will be returning and of any special orders that must be carried out. If the patient is being treated through mealtime, snacks or light meals may have to be arranged.

Communication with the patients on a dialysis unit requires sensitivity because their moods may range from near-euphoria when they notice a positive change in their condition to the agitation that accompanies loss of control and to periods of depression when they will barely communicate at all. Often, all they need is a compassionate "ear" with good listening skills.

When the course of treatment is initiated, the family, particularly if the patient is a child, will be concerned and have many questions that must be directed to the appropriate staff.

In cases of poisoning or acute failure, lives may be in the balance. The predialysis teaching will have been forgone, which increases the stress for the patient (if alert) and family. The HUC is in a position to provide support and calm and to arrange for the assistance of pastoral counselors and social workers as the need arises.

Medications Used in the Dialysis Unit

Some of the medications used in the dialysis unit are much the same as in other units. Some that are frequently used include:

Erythropoietin (EPO). EPO (epoetin alfa, Epogen, Procrit) is the most often used hematocrit stimulator. Technically it is classified as a hormone. It plays a role in the rate of red blood cell production. It is given subcutaneously three times a week, usually at the dialysis treatment visit. The results of its use are monitored by performing reticulocyte counts.

Iron. In some individuals, iron deficiency anemia may be so profound that the IV form of the drug is needed. The injectable form of iron is known as iron dextran, Imferon, or InFeD. The drug is classified as a hematinic. A test dose is given initially to check for allergy. Iron can cause shivering, nausea, vomiting, and cramps, which are also symptoms of complications of dialysis.

Heparin. Heparin is added to the dialysate to prevent the blood from clotting when it is passing through the dialyzer. Since the blood from the dialyzer is returned to the body, the patient must be watched for signs of bleeding. A PTT is done to check for the effects of heparin.

Insulin. Insulin is kept on the unit because so many dialysis patients are insulin-dependent diabetics. If their blood sugars are found to be high, they can be given insulin on the unit.

Other Medications. If a dialysis patient is found to have an acute infective process, he or she will receiving a loading dose of an IV antibiotic on the unit. Other medications used are those for nausea and pain.

The Role of the HUC in the Dialysis Unit

In the dialysis unit, an individual treatment may last as little as 3 hours. Then another patient will be present to use that station. The support of the HUC to facilitate the turnover of the chart and completion of orders in a timely fashion is essential.

In the dialysis unit, the HUC must be:

Flexible—hours start early in the morning and go into the evening.

Accurate—orders for the same patient will not necessarily be the same for two treatments in a row.

Able to self-motivate—much of the time the other staff members will be busy with their assigned tasks.

Capable in the role of customer service representative—the HUC may be the first person to be approached by families, who are often stressed and distraught.

Organized and able to prioritize.

It is also helpful if the HUC who applies to the dialysis unit has experience with scheduling and extracting data.

Risk Management and Quality Assurance

Few units in the hospital offer as much ongoing exposure to blood and body fluids as the dialysis unit. Strict adherence to OSHA guidelines is mandatory. Those guidelines must be kept accessible for the staff to refer to. Any splashes and exposures must be reported and followed up.

An outline of OSHA Standards is as follows:

I. Who is Covered?
II. The Exposure Control Plan
III. Who Has Occupational Exposure?
IV. Communicating Hazards to Employees
V. Preventative Measures
VI. Methods of Control
VII. What to do if an Exposure Incident Occurs

All the manufacturers' guidelines for the use of equipment as well as policies and procedures must be organized and available on a moment's notice to the staff. The HUC will always be the one asked to locate them.

Quality assurance monitors are usually based on potential and real complications. The studies accumulated and shared by the dialysis centers have been responsible for many of the advances in the field. The HUC can provide a valuable service by accessing the data for the studies and collating the information. Similar information can be gathered for the morbidity and mortality committee that reviews all serious complications and deaths of dialysis patients.

Closing Thoughts

The dialysis unit may not be for everyone. The team, including the HUC, gets intensely involved with patients whom they will see gradually deteriorate rather than get well. In this respect, strong emotional attachments are likely to happen. Some staff counter this by being unwilling to accept the seriousness of the patient's illness, and this may lead to unrealistic expectations and early burnout. The person who will succeed in this unit is the one who can promote the patients' desires to live in ways that are uniquely theirs.

If you have this foundation, a wonderful career can be built in this ever-changing and exciting field. There are opportunities for flexible HUCs with good organizational skills not only in hospital dialysis units but also in freestanding units.

Review Questions

1. Name and describe the two lab tests most frequently done on the dialysis unit patients.
2. Describe the roles of two of the team members in the "predialysis" phase.
3. List three differences between hemodialysis and hemofiltration and hemodialysis and peritoneal dialysis.
4. Describe one advantage and one disadvantage for an HUC working in a dialysis unit.

Bibliography

Home Medical Advisor, Dr. Schueler's Health Informatics. TLC Properties, A Subsidiary of The Learning Company, 1997.

http://www.nhibi.nih.gov/nhibi.nhibi.htm

http://www.niddk.nih.gov/EndStageRenalDisease/EndStageRenalDisease.html

http://www.healthtouch.com/level1/leaflets/kidne/kidne023.htm

http://www.medicinenet.com/mainmenu/encyclop/ARTICLE/ART/dialyis.htm

http://www.kidney.org

http://cybermart.com/aakpaz/aakp.html

http://intellihealth.com/JohnsHopkinsHealthInformation

http://MayoHealthO@sis

Taber's Cyclopedic Medical Dictionary, 18th ed. Philadelphia, FA Davis, 1997.

The Merck Manual, 14th ed. Rahway, NJ, Merck, Sharp and Dohme Research Laboratories, 1982.

4

The Emergency Department

Cynthia Nault

Common Abbreviations

DNR	Do not resuscitate
ED	Emergency department
EMT	Emergency medical technician
HIR	Health information records
HMO	Health maintenance organization
ME	Medical examiner
PPO	Preferred Provider Organization
SOB	Shortness of breath

Objectives

At the completion of this chapter the reader will be able to:

1. List the various patient care rooms in the emergency department.
2. Explain the purpose for each of the patient care rooms.
3. Discuss the other departments in the hospital that might be called to the emergency department and how they would serve the ED patient.
4. Discuss the importance of good communication skills in the emergency department.
5. Describe the role of the health unit coordinator as a "detective" in the emergency department.

Vocabulary

Triage: A system of assigning priorities of medical treatment based on urgency and chance for survival

Conscious sedation: Sedation that allows the patient to sleep but not to the point of needing airway assistance

Code blue: Term used to signify that a person has stopped breathing and has no heart rate

History

The origins of emergency medicine can be traced to the first time a person was injured by a human or by nature. Emergency care was given for injuries suffered in battle, encounters with wild animals, and accidents caused by natural disasters. History tells us that most societies utilized the services of a medicine man of some type to deal with illnesses, injuries, and strange behaviors.

The use of guns during battle became more widespread during the 14th century, thereby advancing the art of surgery in the field. This early form of emergency care often resulted in amputations, since most people with wound infections died.

Emergency medicine as a formal speciality did not emerge until the early 1960s. Medical schools began offering courses in emergency medicine, and the emergency room expanded into departments providing more than just immediate lifesaving services. Today we expect more than a "room" for emergency care. We expect the same expertise from the emergency department physician that we get from a surgeon, oncologist, or other medical specialist.

Current Emergency Departments

The emergency department (**ED**) of any hospital is both connected and disconnected to the activities of the organization in which it is located. Although the ED is housed in the same building and the staff is governed by the same policy and procedures, it is often so completely different from other patient care areas that it is easy to view it as another world. Patient census is either feast or famine. Patient acuity goes from the walking wounded to the worst trauma case. At any given moment and without warning, the people who work in this area must be prepared for everything and surprised by nothing. The ED HUC is a vital member of the emergency team and can handle the diverse activities with calm efficiency.

Description of the Emergency Department

Physical layout will vary depending on the size and age of the building and also will be determined by the intent of the organization. A large urban hospital that takes major trauma cases will be laid out much differently from a smaller community hospital. This discussion will cover aspects of both the great and the small.

Triage areas have become common and necessary to the ED not only to make it possible to give better patient care but also to expedite diagnosis and treatment. Triage areas are staffed by a nurse, **EMT**, paramedic, intern, or resident. This is the first person that the patient will come in contact with, and this person will make the first decision regarding the acuity of the patient's needs. Vital signs and a brief history are obtained; in many cases initial blood work may be done, and the patient may be sent to the x-ray department for routine films. By the time the patient is placed into an exam room, all the doctor may have to do is examine and interview the patient, making treatment efficient and timely. Triage areas are usually located close to the waiting room and registration area.

Registration of the patient is often like the chicken and the egg. Which comes first? Should the patient register before or after going to triage? Should ambulance patients go through the registration process before being seen by the doctor? There is no answer that will fit all patients. Ambulatory patients are best served by going to triage first to determine if they are well enough to go though the registration process. If warranted, a very ill patient might be taken directly into the treatment area, leaving a relative to relay the proper information for registration. Ambulance patients or lone patients can bypass the registration desk and have the staff member ask the necessary questions at the bedside.

With managed care, **HMOs**, and **PPOs**, the registration process can be vital to the type of treatment that a patient receives in the ED. Although any life-threatening case will be attended to without question of payment, all other cases will be handled according to the rules and regulations set by the patient's insurance. Some plans call for the patient to obtain permission prior to arrival in the ED. If this has not been done, the HUC can either call to inquire if the visit can be approved or inform the patient of the possibility that the insurance company will not pay for treatment. Either way, it is important for both the hospital and the patient to understand that emergency care is expensive and responsibility for the payments must be determined. If the patient is responsible for payment, it is not unusual for partial payment to be collected in advance of treatment.

The registration staff often consists of HUCs with special training and understanding of the insurance plans and rules. Registration staff might report to ED, admitting, ambulatory services, nursing, or other departments in the hospital. Registration staff may cross train with HUCs from these other departments or have extensive specialized training that would necessitate keeping them in the registration area full time. Special qualifications required for this position are very good interpersonal skills, computer knowledge, medical terminology, advanced insurance knowledge, math skills, general office skills (typing, spelling, office machines), and telephone skills. Interpersonal skills are especially important because it is necessary to deal with people who are sick, injured, afraid, grieving, worried, angry, and generally not at their best—it takes someone with a good HUC background and a lot of patience.

The HUC working desk is the heart and hub of the emergency department (Fig. 4–1). The HUC who sits in this chair is often the one person in the department who knows where every staff member can be found, what each patient is waiting for, who has been called, and who has not been to lunch. This is a HUC with very special organizational skills. To the outsider the entire department may look like a whirlwind of people running every which way, but in reality, if the HUC is organized, the department will be running smoothly and with purpose.

The patient charts are usually located close to the HUC desk along with telephones, computer, fax, and copy machines. If the area is shared with the nursing staff, cardiac monitors and ambulance radios are also present (Fig. 4–2). The HUC is in constant motion between the patient chart, the computer, and the telephones. Since the goal in the ED is to treat patients in the quickest and most effective manner, this is not the place to spend a lot of time reading the chart. Many times the HUC will enter the orders before they are written on the chart; patients who come in with chest pain cannot wait for paperwork. The HUC will begin ordering tests as soon as the information reaches the desk, even if only making the necessary STAT calls. It is common for EDs to have standing orders for certain patient complaints (Fig. 4–3): chest pain, shortness of breath (**SOB**), trauma, asthma, and other common problems seen in the ED. The nursing staff may begin these orders and pass along this information to the HUC to continue orders even before the patient is seen by a physician.

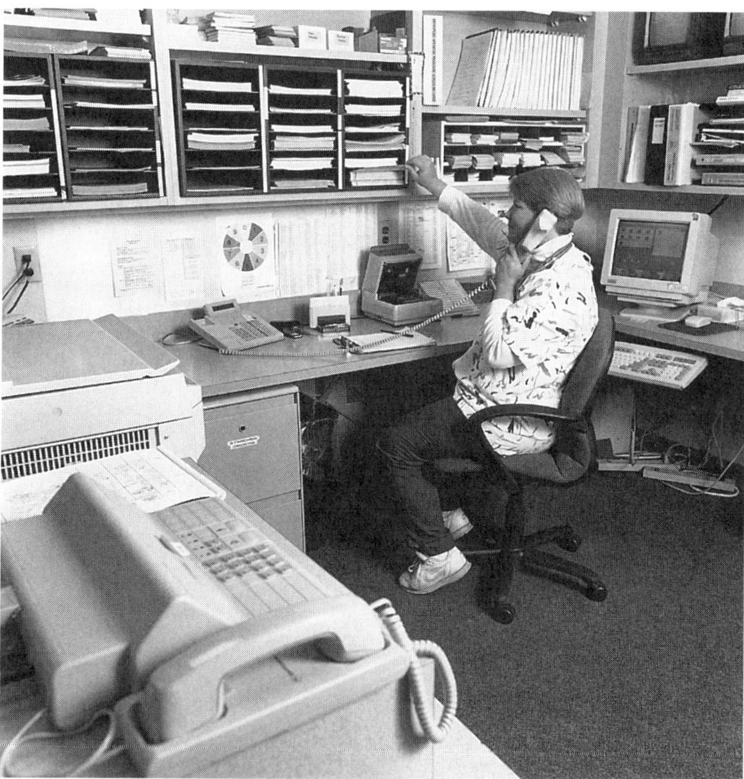

Figure 4–1
The emergency department HUC.

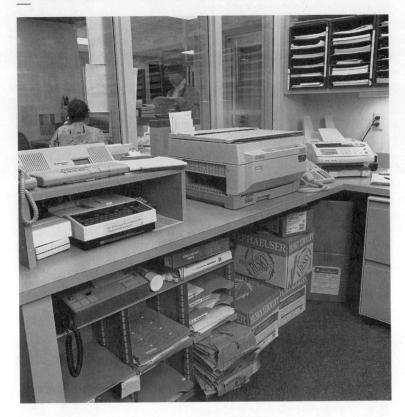

Figure 4–2
Emergency department equipment (ambulance radio, copy machine, fax machine).

HUCs in the ED must also be on top of the various stages of test results: Which patients are waiting for which tests, and how long have they been waiting? At what point should the lab be called to see if there is a problem? How much time should pass before a second call is placed to the attending physician for admitting orders? Who is taking pediatric call, and how long before the bed is ready upstairs? The ED HUC is the encyclopedia of information for the department. It is important to work closely with the nursing staff and keep them informed regarding their patients.

The **medication area** is one place where the HUC does not usually spend a lot of time working,

STANDING ORDERS; EMERGENCY DEPARTMENT
CHEST PAIN

1. Cardiac monitor
2. STAT EKG
3. IV, D5W @ 125 ml/H
4. 2 liters Oxygen, nasal cannula
5. STAT LAB: CBC, Lytes, Glucose, Cardiac enzymes
6. Pulse Ox., if level is below 90%; STAT ABGs
7. STAT portable chest x-ray

Figure 4–3
Example of standing orders.

yet someone working in ED should know it well. Some hospitals now have computer-generated medication dispensers (Fig. 4–4); the nurse signs in, types in the patient ID number, chooses the medication from a screen, and the correct drawer or door opens so the medication can be removed. At the same time the computer sends the charge to the billing office. One step dispenses, counts, bills the patient, and keeps a record of who dispensed that medication. If this advanced method is not present, there will be locked narcotic cabinets or carts. Cabinets and refrigerators with medications, IVs, and supplies will also be a part of the medication area. All additional medications will be obtained through the hospital pharmacy, for example, IV antibiotic piggybacks and other medications prepared specially for a patient.

Supplies for patient care can be located throughout the department or in specially designed areas. Most supplies for patient use are disposable and considered patient charge items. The HUC may be responsible for keeping track of these supplies and entering these charges on the patient record or in the computer. Supplies can be dressings, disposable treatment trays, suture, casting supplies, crutches and walkers, syringes, tubing, and even reusable instruments. The ED HUC should have a working knowledge of the supplies common in the area and be able to locate them in a crisis. The HUC may be the

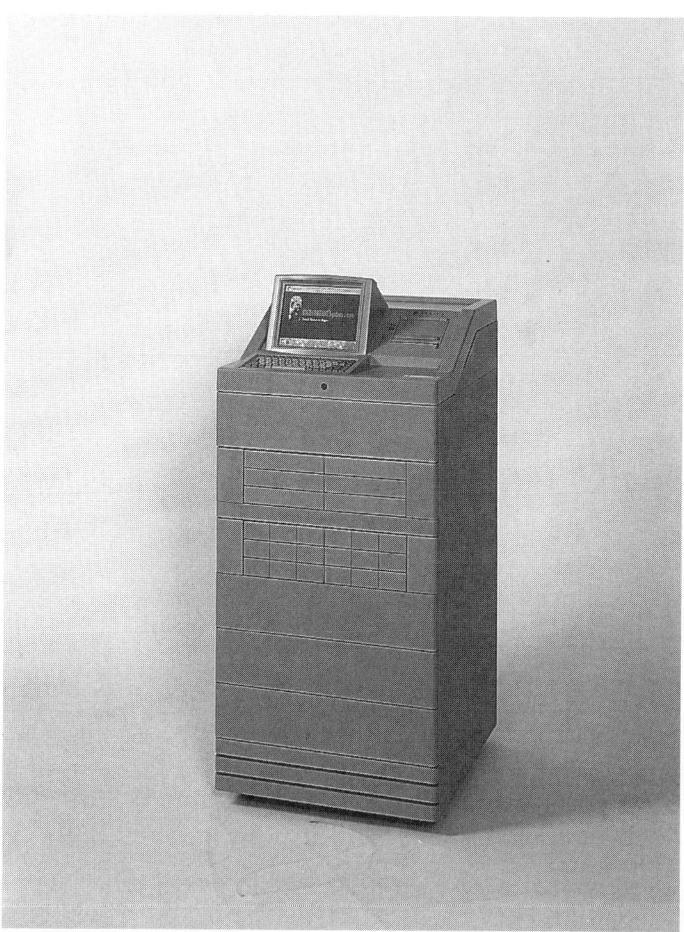

Figure 4–4
Automated medication dispenser. (Photo courtesy of Pyxis Corporation.)

only person not giving direct patient care when a supply item is needed.

Linen is a staple in the ED and needs to be replaced frequently depending on the acuity of patients and census. During the winter months it is hard to keep enough blankets on hand; if there is a blanket warmer, it should be kept filled with fresh blankets. Sometimes a warm blanket for sick or injured patients is the nicest thing anyone can do for them; fear is a cold feeling. An internal laundry department is a blessing when the hospital linen supply runs low; the HUC orders additional supplies. If the hospital uses an outside linen service, advance planning is needed to ensure adequate supplies. During high-census days or times when it seems that every patient uses several sets of sheets, linen can be just as precious as IV fluids to the department. When the HUC is responsible for the linen supply, another spoke is added to the wheel of responsibility.

It is often the responsibility of the HUC to maintain order and organization in the doctors' desk/dictation area (Fig. 4–5). At the time of discharge it is usually the responsibility of the doctor to dictate the discharge notes and the take-home instructions. In large teaching hospitals, interns or residents often perform these duties, and they may choose to dictate at another time or another place. If dictation and take-home instruction are the responsibility of the ED staff physician, the HUC can facilitate this process by having the necessary records organized for the doctor in the dictation area and making sure that all Dictaphones are in working order. If there are old charts from past patients to be reviewed, these can be located in the same area, and the HUC will be responsible for seeing that these charts are returned to the **HIR** department as soon as they are completed.

The administrative assistant/records secretary/department secretary is often located in an office next to or close by the head nurse or manager of the department. This is another HUC position found in some EDs. Job duties will be as varied as the titles, but in most cases this is a person who functions as the right-hand assistant to the manager. This HUC may make out the staff working schedule, order nonclinical supplies, take the minutes at a meeting, type policy and procedures, maintain the manuals for the department, function on committees, or any number of other activities. HUCs with duties unrelated to patient care are often a vital link between management and staff. It is important that persons with this responsibility maintain the same skills and knowledge as HUCs in patient care areas. They should attend seminars and workshops and maintain a high level of continuing education. It is wise for all ED HUCs to attend as many education sessions as possible and to remain current with emergency medical trends as well as with managed care, insurance reimbursements, and anything else related to the ED. Being prepared for new circumstances makes it much easier to deal with them when they occur.

Minor procedure rooms may be located in one area or spread throughout in several areas of the ED. In some cases there are special rooms set up for certain circumstances. Minor care and eye rooms may be set up without a bed or cart, since these patients are often treated in an upright position. Patients assigned to these rooms will have complaints such as minor lacerations not requiring sutures, colds, sore throats, earaches, foreign body in eyes or ears, and minor injury to eyes or ears; they may also be there for suture removal or another cause for a return visit. These rooms may be stocked with supplies that are commonly used for minor or eye care. The patients utilizing minor care and eye rooms can be treated quickly and efficiently.

Cardiac care rooms will be equipped with cardiac monitors, pulse oxymetry, and EKG equipment (Fig. 4–6). IV supplies and equipment will be either in the room or close by for quick access. In many cases these rooms will be larger than other treatment rooms to accommodate additional equipment and personnel to care for a cardiac emergency. The HUC will be observant of patients entering these areas and be prepared to order the standard cardiac tests, and for the possibility of an ICU admission. Chest pain, SOB, irregular heart rate, syncope, neck or shoulder pain, and code blue are just a few of the reasons patients may be treated in the cardiac care room.

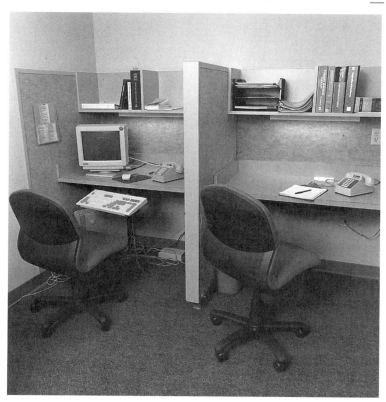

Figure 4–5
Doctors' dictation area.

Orthopedic rooms are very common in EDs, since the supplies and equipment used to treat orthopedic injuries are often specialized (Fig. 4–7). People with sprained, strained, and broken bones generally require ice, elevation, and x-rays. Depending on the results they may leave the ED with splints, casts, crutches, canes, or walkers. Casting and splinting procedures are wet, messy, and sometimes noisy, when the cast saw is used. Patients with back injuries or dislocated joints may also use these rooms, depending on the space available. In many situations orthopedic cases will require surgical intervention. It is the responsibility of the HUC to notify Surgery of a pending case and to determine if the patient will be dismissed after surgery or will be admitted post surgery. The HUC will prepare the patient chart for surgery, ensuring that all the required papers are collected: lab results, radiology films, order sheet, signed permit, nurse's notes, old records, and anything else that has been accumulated during the ED visit.

The trauma room may be reserved for certain types of trauma patients, or it might be used for any ambulance trauma case. If the ED is located in a designated trauma center, the trauma room will be set up following state-approved guidelines. Major trauma centers have trauma teams designated at all times; these teams may include ED personnel in addition to staff from other areas of the hospital: surgery, ICU, pulmonary, radiology, clergy, and social service. The trauma team is called as soon as the ED is notified; by the time the patient arrives the team is in place and assumes full care of the individual, thereby allowing uninterrupted care of the other ED patients. The HUC may be the only staff member focusing total attention on the trauma patient. During this time it might be necessary for other orders to wait until trauma orders are complete. Nursing staff may

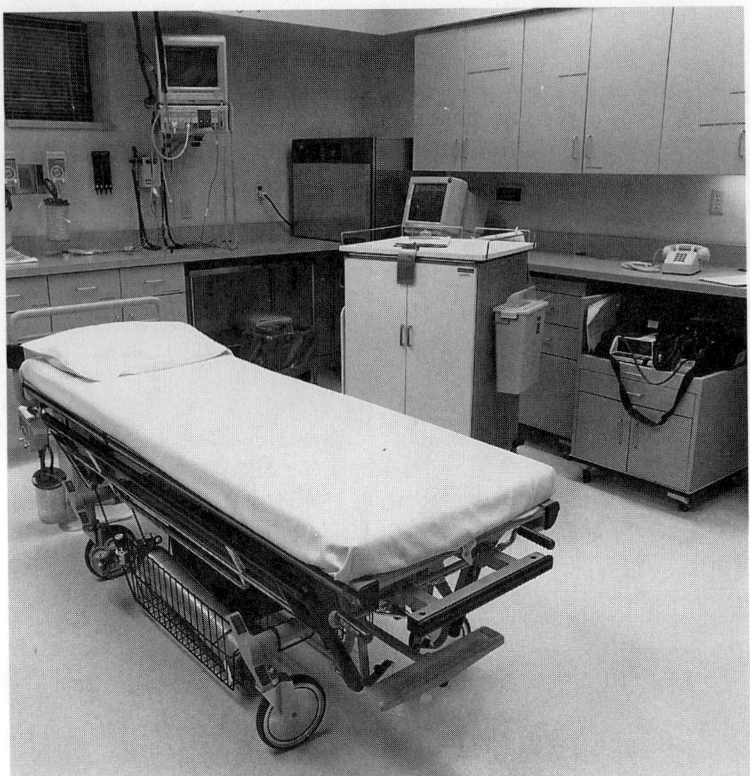

Figure 4–6
Cardiac room.

assist the HUC by ordering tests for their patients if the HUC is involved in a trauma case. It may also be the duty of the HUC to locate relatives of trauma or ambulance patients.

Frequently Used Medications

IV fluids are very common in most emergency departments, since this treatment can be used with a multitude of diagnoses. Patients with the flu often receive IV fluids to combat dehydration. IV fluids are routinely administered for any patient whose condition is critical or may become critical. IV intervention is necessary to administer medication in life-threatening situations. IV piggyback medication is often given to patients in the ED. This could be a one-dose only of antibiotics with the patient being sent home with additional oral antibiotics, or it might be the first dose of many for patients being admitted to the hospital.

Anesthetic agents are frequently administered in the ED for a variety of treatments. Anyone receiving sutures is given a local anesthetic to the affected area. Minor fractures or dislocations may be treated with Bier block or some other form of regional anesthesia. Some patients may receive a form of anesthesia referred to as **conscious sedation.** The patient may actually sleep during the procedure but is able to breathe without artificial assistance and is easily aroused. Some form of conscious sedation may be given to small children requiring multiple sutures, since this may be less traumatic then being held down by three or four people. Also, patients with dislocations may be given this type of medication so that they are able to relax sufficiently to have the joint relocated; shoulders and hips are prime examples. In cases

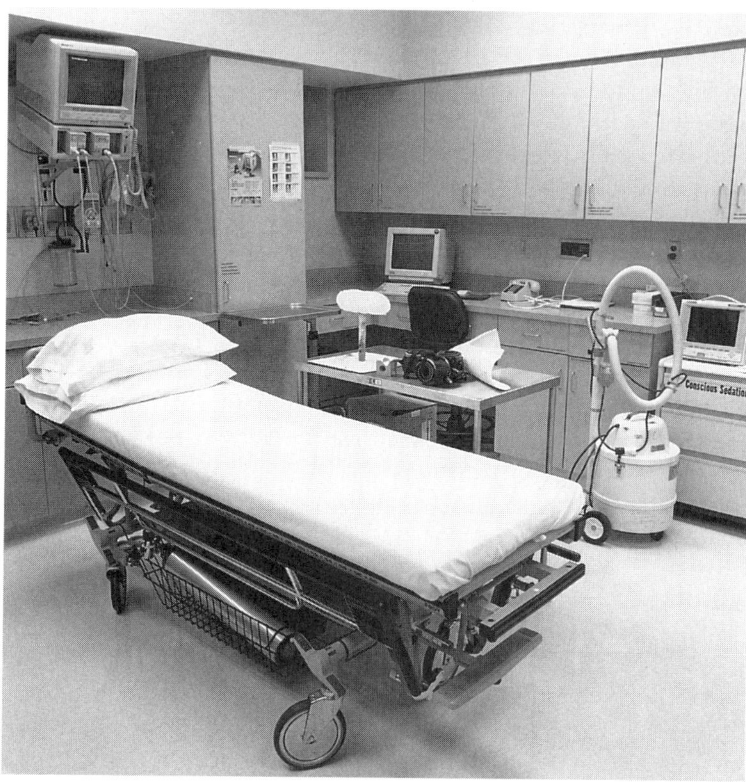

Figure 4–7
Orthopedic room.

of extreme emergency it may become necessary to paralyze a patient and put him or her on an artificial respirator. This type of treatment might be given to someone with acute respiratory distress or in trauma cases. These patients are considered critical and will require an ICU bed.

There are many different types of medications given to ED patients. This may be the one area of a hospital that prescribes and administers the largest variety of medications. Immunizations are routinely given to all patients with lacerations who are not current for tetanus and diphtheria. Other common medications administered in the ED are antibiotics: oral, IM, IV, and/or prescription to take home. Pain medications are given very cautiously. The ED attracts many drug-seeking people, and personnel must be careful with all narcotic medications. It once was common to treat someone in severe pain first and look for the cause second, as in back pain or kidney stones. Today, however, unless the injury can be seen, most ED doctors will not order narcotic medications until test results confirm the source of pain. The patient might be offered an injection of a non-narcotic prior to x-ray or lab studies. Most drug seekers will refuse this by saying that they are allergic and then demand a narcotic. For this reason some EDs keep a list of known drug seekers, and in some areas this list is shared with other EDs in the vicinity. This task is usually one of the duties of the HUC, who may work in conjunction with security staff.

Diagnostic Procedures

Fast result testing is the goal of most emergency departments. It is always in the best interest of both the patients and the staff to "treat 'um & street 'um." Because the ED must always be ready for major trauma or crisis (busload of hemophiliacs) the staff will try to treat existing patients with any timesaving methods available. One timesaver is lab results that can be obtained in the department. If the doctor wants a CBC on a patient, someone is needed to draw the blood and either take or tube the blood to the lab; depending on the turnaround time, this could take from 30 minutes to over an hour. Some EDs now have equipment in the department that will run uncomplicated blood or urine tests in just a few minutes. This equipment is expensive but pays for itself in emergency situations.

Radiology is another area that can be very time consuming depending on the type of films ordered. CT scans, MRIs, ultrasounds, and multiple bone films can all take the patient and the staff out of the department for long periods. Trauma or other critical patients usually require a nurse to go with them for these studies. If possible, the ED doctor may order some initial films as portable until the patient can be stabilized; for example, a patient with severe chest pain or SOB will have a portable chest x-ray. This produces faster results and allows the patient to stay in the area where the appropriate treatment can be administered.

Other testing that can be done from the patient's bedside are EKGs, ABGs, respiratory treatments, and echocardiograms. Some of these tests are run by ED personnel, and some require calling or paging personnel from the specialty area.

Long-term testing is a necessary process, since many patients cannot be diagnosed completely during their stay in the ED. Lab tests may be ordered and the specimen sent to the lab from the ED, but if the results are not going to be available for more than a few hours it will be necessary to treat the patient from home or as an in-patient. Some examples are cultures, drug levels, and drug screening. Hospitals that do not have a laboratory on site or have limited facilities will send a large number of specimens out to be processed. If that is the case, many times the patient will not have a final diagnosis confirmed in the ED. For example, a patient with a wound that is red and swollen would probably have a culture done prior to leaving the ED. Rather than waiting several days to get the results the physician will probably prescribe an antibiotic until the results of the culture are available. This is also true with laboratory tests; sometimes it is better to treat the patient for a positive result than to wait for the actual positive reading. Baseline studies may be ordered from the ED from radiology, neurodiagnostic, cardiovascular, or pathology if the patient shows signs of abnormalities.

Treatments and Procedures Specific to Emergency

Immediate improvement in the patient's condition is the rule in emergency care. As mentioned earlier, the faster patients can be treated, the better chance the staff will have to be ready for a crisis. Also, the faster patients can be treated, the faster they will improve. Immediate results can be seen with asthma patients who receive a respiratory breathing treatment and some IV medication. Insulin-dependent patients with abnormally high or low blood sugar get better very quickly with drug therapy. Patients with congestive heart failure feel immediate results with one dose of Lasix. Once patients have passed the crisis stage, further evaluation can take place without the fear and pain associated with most injury and illness. Patients are able to give the doctor a better history and description of what is currently happening. Whenever possible, the ED staff will work to give some immediate care to all patients.

Lacerations may be the most common complaint in any ED. Lacerations come in all sizes and shapes and happen for a variety of reasons, but the majority can be repaired in the ED. Sometimes it may be necessary to take patients to surgery for the repair of extensive nerve or tendon damage and for multiple or deep lacerations. A plastic surgeon will prefer to work under sterile conditions, and thus these patients may be taken to surgery.

Orthopedic procedures are as common as lacerations. Since none of us can tell if a bone is broken (unless it is an open fracture), it is necessary to investigate, and many people will go the ED. The injured area is x-rayed, and the patient referred back to ED for proper treatment. Treatment is dictated by the severity of the injury. A badly swollen arm or leg may not be casted the same day even if it is broken, because when the swelling goes down the cast will not fit properly. These injuries can be splinted and have a cast applied in a few days. If the bone is not in proper alignment it will be necessary to perform a closed reduction, which consists of pulling on the bone (usually the radius/ulna or the tibia/fibula) until it lines up correctly and then applying a cast. Many closed reductions can be performed in the ED. It may also be necessary to cast a bone that is not broken; a very painful sprain will heal faster if it can rest properly.

Patients with bone injuries often require crutches, canes, or walkers and the necessary training to use these tools. They can usually be treated and released. Patients with more serious fractures may need to go to surgery to have the bone repaired, which sometimes requires the application of plates or screws to assist with alignment. Surgical patients may require overnight or extended hospitalization.

Trauma patients arrive in the ED with or without warning. Many times trauma patients arrive by private car, brought in by someone who could not wait for an ambulance. Surprise trauma patients are difficult because they have not had any advance treatment and are often in shock. Ambulance services are equipped with radios or cell phones and will call ahead to notify the ED of a pending patient. The EMT or paramedic will give the doctor or nurse a brief history of the patient's injuries, a review of the current condition, and the type of treatment administered. He or she will often request further instructions or approval for other treatments. If the hospital has a trauma protocol, this is the time when the trauma surgeon and/or trauma team is alerted to the ED *STAT*. The people on this team must be in house or very close by and should report within a very short time. Ideally, the team will be gowned and ready when the patient is wheeled into the ED. Trauma patients have what is called a "golden hour," meaning that the best survival rate occurs when treatment is instituted within an hour of injury. For this reason trauma patients must be assessed and treated as quickly as possible, transporting them to the OR immediately if necessary. Some hospitals take trauma patients directly into the OR, and all assessment is done there. Trauma patients are very time consuming for the HUC; many, many orders are standard and routine for all trauma patients, including drug screens, alcohol levels, HIV, and type and screening, in addition to other blood work and multiple x-rays. Along with trauma patients are telephone calls, both incoming and outgoing. The trauma team may be calling for additional physicians, specialists, for example; at the same time, as friends, family, and the media hear of the trauma, they begin to call. The HUC will be ordering tests, arranging for surgery, calling ICU or Admitting for bed assignment, placing calls to other physicians or the patient's family, and fielding the incoming calls. Somewhere there is an unwritten rule that says whenever you get a trauma patient you will also get an influx of nonemergency patients who demand to be seen immediately and do not understand why they should have to wait. Often comments such as "I hope I don't die waiting for a doctor" are coming from the person needing care the least. These are the times when a HUC must call on all the past training and patience to get through the shift.

Any person who has ever worked in health care has been through some kind of confidentiality training. This becomes particularly important in the ED. It is very easy to talk about the really bad trauma patient in the ED on your shift; some of them are very sensational and make the TV news and newspapers. The HUC may not, at any time, give out any information that is not public record. This is equally true whether the patient is a famous person or a next-door neighbor. What you see and hear cannot go out of the department. In situations of assault or rape, patients may be given an alias, and incoming calls either will be forwarded to the hospital media department or the HUC will refuse to confirm admission. This may also occur when celebrities are involved. Confidentiality applies to all ED patients, not just the trauma cases. This is difficult if the patient involved is known personally to the staff, but, unless the patient gives permission, the staff may not discuss the case with anyone not directly related to the care of that individual.

Code blue patients are similar to trauma patients, since there is usually very little warning and the patients require immediate treatment. The difference in these two groups is that the majority of code blue patients are elderly and many do not survive. In the past few years the popularity of **DNR** (do not resuscitate) in senior citizens has cut back on many incoming codes. It is very sad when a patient is brought to the ED as a code, only to have the family arrive and report that the patient would not have wanted to be resuscitated. Regardless of a patient's age or circumstances the family members will grieve at their loss, and the staff must give them additional time and assistance to cope with their ordeal.

Grief is a very stressful emotion, whether it is grief on the part of the staff in the department or the grief of a family. It is impossible to be unaffected by tragedy and death. It is not unusual for a staff member to cry at the death of a baby, young child, teenager, adult, or elderly person. It is human to feel sadness over someone's loss of a loved one, and although it is not desirable for the family to see sobbing from the staff, a few tears shed are often very meaningful for them.

Some people deal with their grief in ways other than sadness; sometimes it is anger. Anger is often displayed in a very violent outburst, such as yelling, screaming, hitting a wall, kicking a chair, or throwing objects on the floor. Although this is a recognized form of dealing with tragedy or death, it warrants close monitoring to ensure that these people do not harm themselves or others. Security can be called to assist when these situations arise. Often these individuals are calm and embarrassed after the initial outburst, but sometimes they require medical intervention in the form of a sedative.

The HUC is a key player in these situations, calling additional family or clergy and ensuring that the family has the use of a telephone, phone books, coffee, or whatever they need to get through this life-altering event. The HUC is the person the family may go to for questions and assistance, sometimes only because they do not want to bother the nurses and doctors with nonmedical requests. The HUC may also assist the family with calling a funeral home, although many hospitals will make that initial call when the body is ready to be released.

The HUC must be familiar with the rules and laws pertaining to the disposition of the body. Some cases must go to the county medical examiner, and others can be released to the funeral home. There are also cases in which the **ME** may not require an autopsy but the family will request one. It is now customary to ask families about organ donation if the patient is eligible. There are permits to be signed and calls to be made in these situations, and the HUC will know the correct protocol for each case.

Communication Within the Hospital

The HUC's best skills should probably be in communication. This is one of the biggest and most important duties in the ED. The ED HUC is in constant communication with the clinical staff within the department. While each patient will be in a different stage of treatment, the HUC will know where the patients are in this process and be able to communicate their progress to the clinical staff. This does not stop at the doors of the ED; this level of communication continues throughout the hospital. The telephone is the most commonly used piece of equipment for the ED HUC. All HUCs should have excellent telephone skills, including knowing the proper way to answer each call, even if it rings 1000 times. Most hospitals have guidelines for answering the telephone that include the department, name, and title. It is natural to use shortcuts when it is very busy and say, "ER . . ." or "ER, Mary. . . ." When this happens it immediately gives the wrong impression to the caller; they think that the person does not know how to answer the phone or is too busy to speak clearly. This causes mistrust and anxiety in the caller, and in the ED the caller could be someone in a crisis situation. The HUC must be calm and in control.

Placing calls to other departments within the hospital is routine for HUCs of all units, but in the ED the quantity and variety may be on a larger scale. In some facilities it is routine to call critical care units for a bed assignment prior to calling Admitting. In other facilities the routine is to call Admitting before receiving a bed assignment, and in yet other places all bed assignments are made from Admitting or an assignment office (which may be staffed by a HUC). Whatever the routine, getting a bed for a patient can require several phone calls.

Calling ancillary departments is also routine: if nothing else, to give them information on the patient's current location. A patient with multiple STAT orders for lab, x-ray, EKG, and ultrasound cannot be in more than one place at a time, so the HUC must communicate the progress to each waiting department. Generally EKG and Lab will be first; they can work at the same time in the ED while the doctors and nurses assess and treat the patient. If the orders include x-rays and ultrasound, which must be done outside the ED, they must wait until lab and EKG are finished. The last thing that anyone needs is to hurry to the ED for a STAT order and have to wait in line for the patient. The HUC will see that STAT orders are planned in a timely manner for both patient and staff.

Security, Social Services, and Pastoral Care or Chaplain are called by the ED many times in a day. Disorderly patients or family members may require attention from Security. On-duty police officers who come to ED with patients often check their weapons with hospital security for safety reasons. Police who accompany patients in custody may ask for assistance from hospital security. Social Services can offer assistance for a variety of patients, from arranging placement in extended care facilities to applying for financial assistance or assisting families in crisis. An active social services department is an asset to any ED. The astute HUC will recognize such situations and request a consult from the physician. Some of the same services may also be offered by the Pastoral Care or Chaplain's office. They can be called for critical patients, death or impending death, and patients or families in need of emotional or spiritual support. All of these groups offer services to patients and families that make it possible for the ED staff to concentrate on providing medical care for the patients.

Communication Within the Community

When the ED HUC makes an outside call, the same skills are needed as making a call to an ancillary department inside the hospital, except that now the HUC must put on a public relations hat. The relationship that a hospital creates and maintains in the community is vital to its success. Hospitals need ties to the community, and the community needs the services of the hospital; therefore, a two-way relationship is formed. Without this relationship a hospital may have a difficult time keeping its doors open. HUCs in the ED have a unique opportunity to maintain the good name of the hospital just by using good communication techniques. Many contacts are made in the community on a daily basis.

Patients coming into ED from a mugging, car accident, rape, dog bite, or any other emergency often do not take time to call the police. They arrive frightened and hurt; their first concern is for medical attention and the safety of people. When this happens, the HUC may make the first call to notify the authorities. Emergency departments are also required by law to report anyone with a gunshot or stabbing injury, even if the victim has a good explanation for the injury. The ED staff is not in a position of judgment; their job is to treat the injury and let the police make the judgment calls regarding how or why. When children are brought in for treatment with injuries that are suspect for child abuse, it may be necessary to notify the police if the injuries are severe or if the parent demonstrates or verbalizes threatening behavior to the child. ED personnel are mandated to report ANY injury that they suspect is child abuse or neglect. This can be done on the phone or by filling out a child abuse form.

Ambulance and fire rescue units are often on a first-name basis with people in emergency departments. These units call with patient information prior to arrival. After arriving and turning over care of the patient to ED, they may remain to finish their paperwork. They often call back later in the shift to check on the patient's condition. Ambulance EMTs, paramedics, firemen, and policemen often are able to provide valuable information about an accident that will affect the type of medical care that the patient receives. Sometimes the condition of the car may change the extent of investigation into possible injuries. For example, the patient may state that he or she feels fine. However, firemen state that the patient broke the steering wheel in half. This would alert the doctor to look for internal chest injuries. A patient with a small pneumothorax could go for hours before showing distress from the injury. The same is true of many internal injuries; patients are often so shocked by being injured that they are not in a position to know what is important and what is not.

Placing calls to locate physicians can require real detective work on the part of the HUC. Calling the office or answering service is always first. This may result in leaving a message and waiting for the doctor to call back. Most HUCs have learned that it is smart to know the routine of the doctors most frequently called: Dr. Smith always plays golf on Thursday afternoon at the country club, and if you call George, the pro, he will find Dr. Smith; Dr. Jones volunteers at the free clinic from 6 P.M. to 10 P.M. every Sunday; Dr. Doe won't answer a page inside the building, but if you call the beeper he calls back immediately. This may sound above and beyond, but if you need to find a doctor, it helps if you know where to look. These tips should be written on the card file with the other phone numbers for each physician. The HUC who can locate physicians is a valuable person in the ED.

On the special occasions when a patient in the ED is a celebrity, a new set of callers may be ringing the phone off the hook. A celebrity does not have to be the mayor or a movie star; it could be a fireman, policeman, local politician, or just a citizen who happened to be involved in an event that made the news. In any of these situations you will have local (and possibly national) television, radio, newspapers, and magazines calling to get any information that they can. Most hospitals have a plan for these types of situations, and it usually involves a designated spokesperson. While the HUC may answer all the calls, it is important to know what to say to whom.

Documentation

Documentation is at the center of all patient care. There is a very old saying: "If you didn't document it, it didn't happen." There are several reasons for this; the most common is thought to be for legal reasons. Hospitals and doctors, nurses, and other health care providers are sued every day for a variety of reasons both valid and invalid. Liability in a lawsuit will be determined by the documentation presented to the court. Although the nurse may remember giving an antibiotic to the patient, if it is not written down, the patient did not get it, in the eyes of the court. Who can and who cannot write in a patient's chart has changed a lot in the past few years. In the past, only the nurse or doctor could write anything pertaining to the care and treatment of a patient. HUCs could chart on the vital sign form and put a signature on the order sheet, but that was all. The thought was that only someone with a license should document in the chart.

Today the thoughts and theories have changed, and in most hospitals the person giving the care makes the notations in the chart. HUCs are taking orders from physicians and writing those orders in the chart. These are usually orders for routine tests and not for medications, but soon it may be common for all orders to be taken by the HUC. Other people are also making notations in the patient chart: the nursing assistant on care given; the food service worker for percentage of meal eaten; the volunteer for how the patient was transported off the unit.

While the legal reasons for good documentation are the first to come to mind, another reason is to ensure a complete patient history. It is routine for a patient's old record to be requested at the time of admission. This gives all the caregivers an idea of how the patient responded to treatment during previous hospitalizations. The reason for admission may be completely unrelated, but there will be significant information in the old chart: allergies to medication, family history, psychological reaction to hospitalization, and many other valuable pieces of information that can be helpful in emergencies when the patient may be unable to communicate.

Methods of documentation have also changed over the years, and computers are now a common and routine part of the nursing unit. Endless hours of handwriting in a patient's chart have been replaced with timesaving computer charting. There may be as many different methods as there are hospitals, but the one common thread is speed and efficiency. It might be a checkoff form that replaces narrative charting. It might be a printed set of standards, and the narrative will be only on the exceptions.

OLD: Narrative charting (handwritten):
"The patient is oriented to date, time, place, and person."
NEW: Exception charting: on a preprinted chart
"The patient is oriented to date, time, place, person?" Y/N ___

However the chart is set up, it will be refined over and over in the coming years. Changes in health care reimbursement have forced hospitals to look into the amount of time that documentation takes and how it can be improved and shortened at the same time.

Quality and Risk Management

Quality, risk management, and health care are all interchangeable. It is impossible to have one without the other two. If you are not providing health care with quality and risk management you will not be providing health care for very long. Patients expect quality care with minimal risk to safety or exposure to disease. This has been demonstrated by the drop in available blood at blood banks across the country. People fear becoming infected from donating blood, and blood banks have improved their screening process. These are both quality and risk management issues.

The same issues are true in EDs. It would be rare today to find a staff member in the ED treating a patient with open lacerations without first donning gloves. In some situations gowns and goggles or face shields are automatically added to the list of precautions to be carried out prior to patient care. This is true for trauma patients, GI bleed patients, code blue patients, and any other patient who may expose the staff to blood or other body fluids. Not too many years ago it was routine for a nurse to bring blood tubes, urine specimens, and everything else to the HUC to be labeled and sent to the lab. Today, this is considered an unnecessary risk. If these items are brought to the HUC, they are labeled and put in a plastic bag for transport to the lab. This is also a quality issue. When several unlabeled specimens are brought to the desk at the same time, they could be labeled incorrectly, opening the door for many complications, both risk and quality related.

Statistics are an important quality issue and have begun to play a very important role in health care. Statistics are being used for infection control trends, patient population trends, staff risk trends (for example, needle sticks, lift injuries), and many other quality and risk issues. The HUC may be the data collector for these statistics either by computer outcomes or, the old standby, a tally sheet. Since important decisions are being based on these numbers, gathering and reporting data are becoming a common duty for ED HUCs.

Signatures can sometimes be a roadblock in the care of a patient with minor injuries or illness. In life-threatening situations, emergency care is given first and signatures are taken care of when the time is appropriate. The problems arise when a minor child comes in with an older sibling or neighbor and needs minor care. Care of a minor requires the written or verbal consent of a parent or other designated adult. The HUC may be asked to find the parent. Once again, some detective work may be required: paging a shopping mall; calling shore to cruise ship; asking the beauty shop if Mom mentioned where she was going next. At the same time the HUC must be careful not to release confidential information or cause unnecessary alarm.

Code blue patients and unconscious patients sometimes arrive in the ED without friends or family. While the doctors and nurses tend to the immediate medical care the HUC tries to locate some family member. This usually requires looking through the patient's purse or wallet for forms of identification and recording the valuables and turning them over to Security or locking them in the hospital safe. In some hospitals this requires a witness and two signatures on the valuables sheet. The patient may have personal identification but nothing noting next of kin or whom to call in emergencies. The detective HUC will use every resource available to find some family for this patient. The telephone book is a good place to start; the next step is to use the clues found in the patient's belongings: business cards, appointment book or notes, the name of a doctor or dentist (they may have family data on file)—anything that might lead to someone who knows this patient and can offer some assistance. The patient needs family support, and families need to be with the patient; this is part of the healing process.

Dealing with patients and families who do not speak English can be a tricky situation. For hospitals located in a part of the country that is bilingual this may not be an issue, since someone on the staff is likely to know the language or to know someone who does. If the patient speaks a language unknown to anyone in the ED, the HUC may need to locate someone who can assist with communication. Several issues are involved, including the medical care of the patient and ensuring that the patient understands his or her rights to treatment. Some hospitals maintain a list of employees who speak other languages, so all the HUC would do is consult the list and ask that person to come to ED. Sometimes the doctors, nurses, and patient just have to use whatever method they can to communicate with each other. In these situations, good documentation will reduce the chances of legal risk to the hospital while at the same time record the quality issues with the patient's medical care.

Closing Thoughts

Working in an emergency department is very exciting and boring at the same time. There will be days when you don't eat or go to the bathroom and other days when you wish the phone would ring (hard to believe, but true). The teamwork attitude is stronger in ED than in other departments where I have worked, as is the level of trust in your coworkers. I spent 14 years in the same ED; I knew what to expect from each person, and they knew what to expect from me.

I think that groups of people who experience the same critical events day after day must lean on each other in order to get through the bad times. It is hard when there is a death in the department; it is usually unexpected, and the family is overwhelmed. The staff in many ways goes through a form of grieving along with the family; you are with them, and you feel sad for them. The younger the patient, the harder it is for the staff; the more traumatic the death or the longer the staff was involved with the lifesaving efforts, the harder it is for the staff. I'll always remember the father's face when he ran into the ED after his 5-year-old son fell under the tires of the school bus. There was not a dry eye in the department; those of us with small children called home just to hear their little voices. It was not our child, but we grieved for the loss of this man's child. No one said it, but we all thought it . . . this could be me. This is the hardest part of ED work; you must be able deal with these issues, and you must have very good coping skills.

The rewards override the sad times and make coming to work a different adventure each day. Most patients are frightened when they come to the ED, and the smallest things may make them relax and feel more comfortable. My favorite thing to do was to take new patients, especially ambulance patients, a warm blanket if I had a minute and the nurse couldn't get there immediately. Coming in by ambulance was very stressful, but the warmth of that blanket was like magic; I could almost see them relax. Maybe it is just the fact that someone cared about them, but also the HUC is nonthreatening as far as causing any physical discomfort (no needles). When some people are nervous they like to talk, and just giving them a minute of your time is often appreciated more than the physical care they receive. The rewards sometimes came days, weeks, or months later, when a letter might arrive with thanks to everyone. Some patients will return after they recover to say thanks in person. It is amazing how different they usually look—maybe because they are standing up and dressed!

None of us plan to have emergencies, so when they happen we are usually unprepared to deal with them. I have seen patients and families arrive in nightgowns and bathrobes, swimming suits, tuxedos and wedding gowns; women with half their hair in curlers, without shoes, and covered with mud from working in the garden; kids in full football uniform; Halloween costumes in May, shorts in December. We had a man who said his finger was bitten off by a tiger (his story and he stuck to it!); a woman who came in to see if we would admit her so she would not have to cook for her husband; a 2-year-old with a crayon in her nose. I have seen a doctor pull a live moth out of a man's ear and it flew away! I have seen babies delivered from women who swore that they could not be pregnant and women in labor who were not pregnant. I have seen patients with foreign objects in all body cavities, for all kinds of reasons. After 14 years I doubt that there is much I have not seen or heard in the emergency department, but for all of that time I loved going to work and looked forward to each shift.

Unfortunately, burnout is high in emergency care. The smart ones will move on when it happens, but others are too fearful of change and stay where they are comfortable. Working with burned-out coworkers is very difficult; they don't want to be there, so they really do not give it their best efforts, and others end up covering for them for the good of the patients. Health care is in a rapid stage of change, and soon technology will be the benchmark of the people who staff EDs.

Education and technological skills will be the tools used to determine who works in emergency care. If you are interested in the fast and changing pace of emergency care, you will get as much education as you can: terminology, computers, and statistical data collection are all important skills to have for a future in an emergency department.

Review Questions

1. List four different types of patient care rooms that would be found in an emergency department.
2. Explain how each of the above rooms functions.
3. There are many other departments in the hospital that the ED health unit coordinator might need to contact. Name four of those departments and how they would serve the patient's needs.
4. Discuss the role of the ED HUC in communicating information regarding patients who have been involved in traumatic situations such as rape or accidents.
5. Describe how the HUC may have to act as "detective" to gather information regarding a patient or to locate a physician.

Bibliography

Frenay A, Mahoney RM: Understanding Medical Terminology, 7th ed. St. Louis, Catholic Health Association, 1984.

Merck Index, 12th ed. Rahway, NJ, Merck & Co, 1996.

Stedman's Medical Dictionary, 24th ed. Baltimore, Williams & Wilkins, 1982.

Taber's Cyclopedic Medical Dictionary, 17th ed. Philadelphia, FA Davis, 1993.

5 The Geriatric Unit

Madeline Clark

Objectives

At the completion of this chapter the reader should be able to:

1. Explain the importance of the physical layout of a geriatric unit.
2. List five considerations in planning a geriatric unit that will reduce the risks of falls.
3. Explain what is meant by "polypharmacy" and the impact that this can have on the elderly.
4. Identify the most common cause of emergency admissions in the elderly.
5. Explain how hearing impairment affects the ability to communicate with the elderly.

Vocabulary

Abuse: Improper, injurious action

Frail elderly: Those who are unable to function at anticipated levels for their age owing to disorders of one or more of the body systems. These are the elderly most likely to require one or more hospital admissions.

Geriatrics: The medical specialty involved in the diagnosis and treatment of disease and disorders of the aged

Gerontology: The study of the biologic, psychological, and sociological phenomena associated with old age and aging

Neglect: Culpable omission resulting in lack of proper care

Polypharmacy: The concomitant use of several medications, both prescription and over the counter

Presbycusis: Hearing deficit of old age

Common Abbreviations

ADLs	Activities of daily living
ARDS	Adult respiratory distress syndrome
BPH	Benign prostatic hypertrophy
CHF	Congestive heart failure
COPD	Chronic obstructive pulmonary disease
DJD	Degenerative joint disease
DRG	Diagnosis related group
EPS	Extrapyramidal symptoms
FUO	Fever of unknown origin
HMO	Health maintenance organization
IADL	Instrumental activities of daily living
IDDM	Insulin-dependent diabetes mellitus
NIA	National Institute on Aging
NIDDM	Non–insulin dependent diabetes mellitus
SDAT	Senile dementia, Alzheimer type
THR	Total hip replacement
TIA	Transient ischemic attack
TKR	Total knee replacement
TURP	Transurethral resection of the prostate
URI	Upper respiratory infection
UTI	Urinary tract infection
WDHA	Watery diarrhea, hypokalemia, achlorhydria syndrome

History

Social and medical changes in the United States since 1940 have influenced the average life span of the population in a positive manner. The average life expectancy in 1940 was 47 years. In 1990 it was 75.6 years. This has created an increased interest in **geriatrics**, the medical specialty dealing with the diseases and treatment of the older person.

The 1990 census revealed that there were approximately 31 million residents over the age of 65 years in the United States. This represents a near-doubling of the figures for 1960. It has been projected that 50 million individuals will make up this age group by the year 2020 (Fig. 5–1). The geriatric age group known as the "oldest old" consists of those over the age of 85 years. This group represented 10 percent of the population older than 65 years in 1990 and is expected to represent 17 percent by 2040.

From 1981 to 1987 the inception of **DRGs** influenced the average length of a hospital stay by a geriatric patient. Since 1987, the average has been 7.3 days per admission. It is estimated that persons 65 years of age and older account for 40 percent of all physician visits and 33 percent of all hospitalizations (Fig. 5–2). This percentage represents more than 90 million hospital days per year. Advances in technology and the inception of **HMOs** and managed care have resulted in declining in-patient days in all other age groups. This, coupled with the statistics mentioned above, has dramatically increased the competition among hospitals to gain favor with the aging population.

In 1975 the United States Congress established the National Institute on Aging (**NIA**). In 1978 a report was published recommending the integration of knowledge on geriatrics and aging into the medical school curriculum. A specialization examination in geriatrics was established in 1988. Many physicians who became involved in this specialty have advocated the establishment of special geriatric units in hospitals. It was the philosophy of Robert Butler, the first director of NIA, that influenced many of these efforts. He understood that traditional medical thinking and process are about cure but that these concepts are not always applicable in geriatric practice, in which treatment is aimed at improving function and quality of life.

Description of the Unit

In the past, geriatric patients were placed in the mixed medical-surgical population. Today we see an effort to design units that will meet their

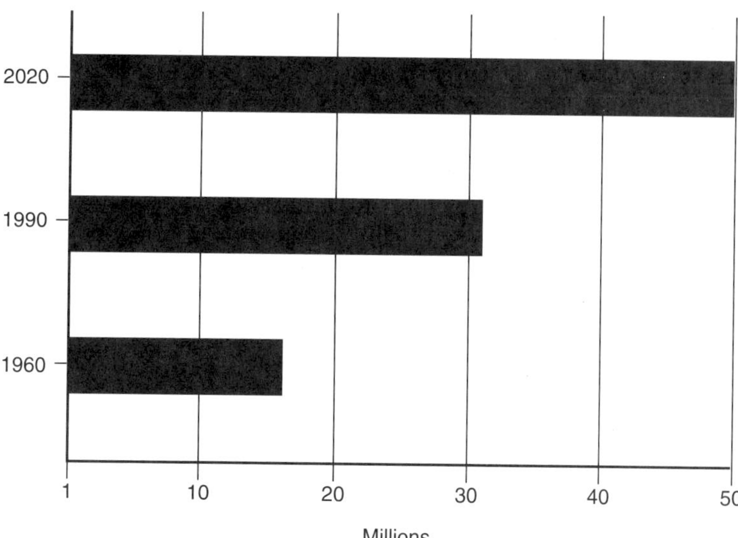

Figure 5–1
U.S. population over age 65.

unique needs. The unit must be devoted to patients with multiple communication, ambulation, orientation, and elimination problems. The unit should be created in such a way as to subdue symptoms and allow for a holistic approach to treatment.

A properly designed patient room in a geriatric unit is spacious enough to accommodate assistive devices for ambulation and medical devices and equipment. Planners should pay particular attention to the following, which will reduce the risk of falls in the elderly:

Ample, glare-reducing indirect lighting
Night-lights in the main room and bathroom
Tile floors treated with nonskid wax
Easily accessible light switches
Nonskid tubs and showers
Grab bars in bathrooms (Fig. 5–3)

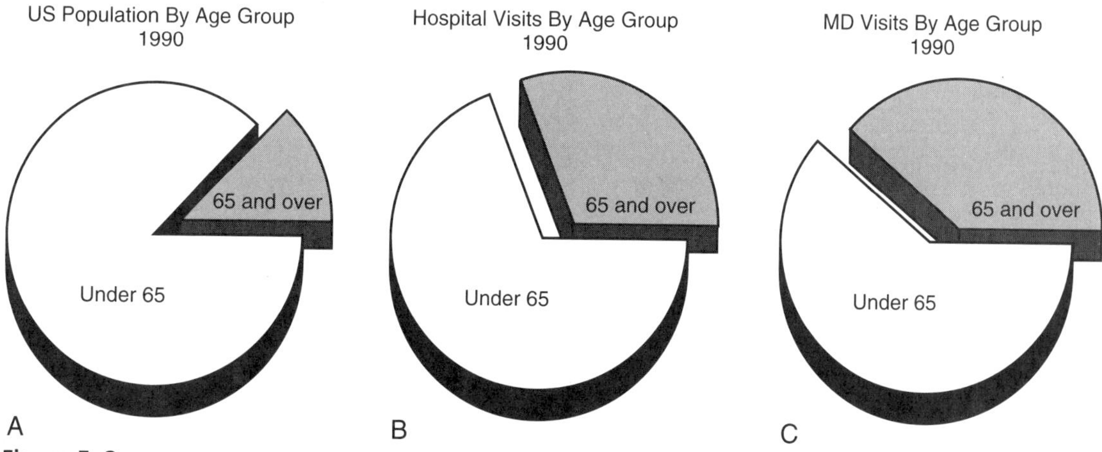

Figure 5–2
A, U.S. population by age group. *B*, Hospital visits by age group. *C*, M.D. visits by age group.

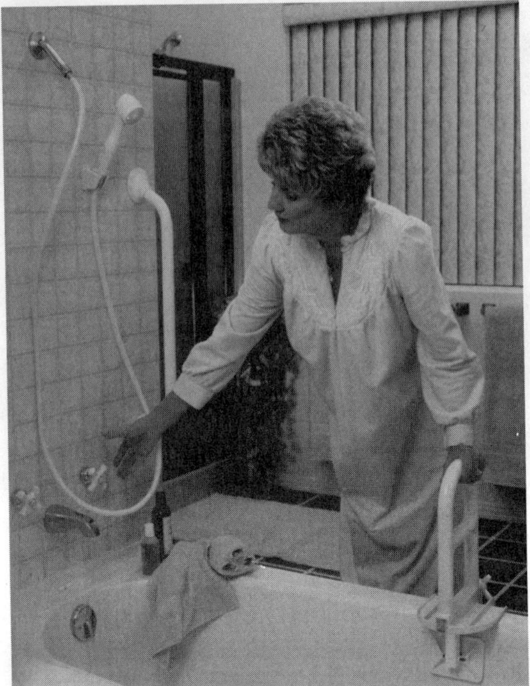

Figure 5–3
Bathroom outfitted with grab bars.

Elevated toilet seats
Bathroom rugs with nonskid backing
Furniture arrangement to maintain clear pathways.

The environment should be designed around the functional status of the aged. A clear color demarcation should be made between walls and floors. Knobs, buttons, and handles that cannot be easily seen should be brightly colored. Chairs should be chosen with sturdy, nonskid legs and firmly padded high seats. The chairs should also have arms to grip. The bed should be adjustable from a low point of 18 inches to a height that is comfortable for the caregivers. Side rails should be attached to the bed. The split side rails are preferable for the independently ambulating patient. Contoured furniture is preferable to that with sharp edges.

Much discussion has been centered on the choice of color for the geriatric room. Some feel that bright, cheery colors are best to prevent and alleviate depression. Others feel that the cool blues and greens will prevent overstimulation in the aggressive individual. A group in Canada has found that pastel shades of pink, peach, green, and muted yellow seem to alleviate both agitation and depression.

Elderly people are very protective about their privacy. Some object to sharing their room with another to the extent that having to do so is viewed as an invasion of territory. This often results in anxiety and forced dependence. Others want the company of a roommate and find that it is an opportunity to make new friends, provided boundaries are respected. Unfortunately, reimbursement and medical issues rather than patient choice usually determine the accommodations.

Families of the elderly are usually active in the workforce, so visiting hours should be set accordingly. A large common area should be available for patients to interact with and enjoy their visitors. In lieu of this, a sufficient number of chairs should be available for visits in patients' rooms.

Terminology

Some new terms were created within this specialty that might be heard around the unit but do not appear elsewhere in the text.

Geriatrician or *geriatrist* is the physician who specializes in the medical care of the elderly.

Gerodontics is the branch of dentistry that deals with the diagnosis, prevention, and treatment of diseases and problems specific to the aged.

Gerontic is a term used to relate to the last phase of life.

Anatomic Changes and Physiology of Aging

A goal of the NIA was to sponsor research into the aging process. Since 1975 several theories have been advanced, based on genetic, cellular, and physiologic studies. A prominent genetics theory, known as the *error theory*, assumes that the deficits of aging are the result of the accumulation of random genetic damage, which causes small errors in the flow of genetic information. These errors prevent or reduce proper cell function.

The best-known theory in cellular research was proposed by an American biologist named Leonard Hayflick. The *Hayflick phenomenon* is based on a study that showed that in tissue cultures, certain human cells are capable of only a certain number of divisions before they die. This finding suggests that aging is programmed into cells. Many experts believe that aging represents many phenomena working in concert.

It is widely believed in **gerontology** circles that 90 to 100 years is the limit for the human life span, but only a few hardy persons attain this age. There may be a familial tendency for aging to begin later and progress more slowly in some individuals. Questions continue to be asked about how changes in smoking, exercise, dietary habits, medical advances, and new technology will affect the aging process in the future.

Anatomic changes in the integumentary system include thinning of the skin, causing bruising to occur more easily. The elasticity is lost, causing wrinkles. Receptor sites become less responsive to stimuli, resulting in a higher pain threshold and diminished capacity in thermal regulation.

In the nervous system, cells atrophy and die, causing some loss of capacity for learning and memorization. The reflexes diminish from a slower response to stimuli. The senses become duller. The loss of smell and taste can affect the appetite and nutritional status of the aged.

The joints deteriorate from constant use. Cartilage disappears, causing "old age shrinking." The muscles lose bulk and strength, which, accompanied by lessening of lean body mass and increase in body fat, change the body's shape and contour. Loss of bone mass occurs, which increases the risk of fractures. The loss of bone mass around the teeth makes the teeth loosen, causing difficulty in chewing. This frequently results in reduced consumption of fresh fruits and vegetables high in dietary fiber.

In the circulatory system, the heart may gain in size but pumps less efficiently, reducing exercise tolerance. The elasticity in the arterial network decreases and plaque accumulates, causing changes in blood pressure. The heart valves often become calcified, interfering with the conduction system.

The gastrointestinal (GI) system loses motility, leading to many functional problems such as altered digestion and bowel habit. The elderly do not absorb the by-products of digestion well. The changes in the GI tract alter the absorption of vitamins and minerals.

In the respiratory system, the thorax becomes more rigid, making it more difficult to breathe deeply. The alveoli and bronchial muscles become less elastic, making it harder to clear the airway. In stressful situations there is less oxygen available to the tissues.

The urinary system is compromised at the renal level by a reduction in the size of the kidneys, accompanied by a decrease in the number of glomeruli, causing less effective filtration. The bladder loses the muscular and nervous ability necessary for control of urination. The prostate in the elderly male usually becomes enlarged, further complicating the problem of incontinence.

A disturbance in response to levels of sodium occurs with the aging of the adrenal cortex in the endocrine system. The pancreas secretes less insulin, creating problems in the metabolism of glucose. The decreased activity of the thyroid gland can cause listlessness, apathy, and confusion in the aged.

The immune system gradually loses its capacity to fight off infections and invaders as an individual ages. Consequently, antibodies are produced that are unable to distinguish between friendly and enemy cells in the host.

Pharmacology and Geriatrics

The majority of the elderly regularly take more than one prescription drug a day as well as several over-the-counter medications. Any of these can interact, causing severe side effects. Some of the elderly go from physician to physician, sometimes expecting miracles, and do not share information about the medications they have at home. This results in "**polypharmacy**," with drugs often being taken to counteract the reactions to others. The approach to pharmacology in this age group is more complex than in any other except newborns. The response to drugs seems to be much more individualized.

In general, the same medications are common to all age groups, but the elderly absorb, distribute, metabolize, and excrete medications less efficiently. Conservative doses of about one-third to one-half the usual dose should be the starting point for drugs that have a low ratio of therapeutic to toxic dose (low therapeutic index). Drugs that have a high therapeutic index, such as antibiotics, do not require dose adjustments. Generally speaking, the elderly require lower doses of:

narcotic analgesics
anticoagulants
diltiazem
naproxen
diazepam
temazepam
levodopa.

They require higher doses of:

tolbutamide
haloperidol
furosemide
prazosin
isoproterenol.

There are more elders taking vitamins and mineral supplements, thyroid hormone, oral hypoglycemics, and eyedrops than any other age group. Unfortunately, the least used drugs in this population are the antidepressants and drugs that positively affect incontinence, such as flavoxate and oxybutynin. It is hoped that, with more physicians specializing in geriatrics and more research and courses available, this will soon change.

Reasons for Hospital Admissions

Presentation of symptoms and syndromes is often different in the elderly and can be complicated by memory deficit and problems with comprehension. For these reasons, differential diagnosis can be difficult.

Emergency Admissions

Because elderly patients frequently arrive in the emergency department (ED) with their complaints, many admissions to the geriatric unit come by way of the ED. The most frequent complaint is chest pain.

Chest Pain

Chest pain, in particular, can be due to many causes. It is important to identify the specific cause, because some chest pains are life-threatening.

Coronary Artery Disease. Chest pain accompanies less than 50 percent of myocardial infarctions in the elderly. Dyspnea, confusion, syncope, or numbness may be the only way that a myocardial infarction is manifested. These symptoms also accompany many other problems, both benign and serious.

Herpes Zoster (Shingles). This condition can cause chest pain, chills, fever, and malaise before the typical skin eruptions appear.

Musculoskeletal Disorders. The chest pain in these disorders is usually chronic but at times can become acute. The tenderness noted on examination is usually generalized.

Pericarditis. A stabbing sensation is typically present in this condition. The pain decreases when the subject is in a sitting position while posturing forward. The pain is also worse on inspiration.

Pneumonia. The elderly patient with pneumonia presents with sharp pleuritic pain. Pneumonia is the fifth leading cause of death in people over 65 years of age. Fever patterns in this group are misleading. The cough is often atypical and is easily mistaken for an upper respiratory infection (URI) with bronchitis.

Pneumothorax. A spontaneous rupture of the pleura is more common in emphysematous patients. Pneumothorax usually causes acute chest pain, dyspnea, and air hunger.

Pulmonary Embolus. This disorder is most

often seen in individuals who have been bedridden or otherwise immobile, particularly in those with varicosities. It is characterized by acute dyspnea and intense pleuritic pain.

Thoracic Aorta Dissection. This is an immediately life-threatening emergency and is usually seen in patients who have hypertension. It is associated with sudden severe, tearing chest pain.

Upper Abdominal Disorders. Acute cholecystitis, peptic ulcer, and esophagitis can all cause referred chest pain. The differential diagnosis can often be suggested by the patient's history.

Other Causes for Evaluation and Admission

Acute Confusional State. This is described as a radical change in the baseline mental status, behavior, and cognition. It is characterized by acute onset, clouding of sensorium, wakefulness, decreased mentation, and increased meaningless motor activity (picking and plucking). There is often impaired memory and orientation, anxiety, transient delusions, hallucinations, and speech abnormalities. The most common cause of this state is medications, some of which also can cause extrapyramidal symptoms (EPS). Also implicated are electrolyte imbalance, TIA, URI, UTI, kidney or liver failure, and hypoxia. Treatment is aimed at eliminating the cause.

Gastrointestinal Bleeding. In the elderly this disorder has a mortality rate approaching 10 percent. If an elderly patient presents with frank rectal bleeding or is vomiting blood, rapid assessment of shock is absolutely necessary in order to start stabilizing measures before the fragile systems fail. After initial stabilization, a cause can be searched for; the most likely are diverticulosis and ulcers.

Syncope. Syncope is a transient loss of consciousness, many causes of which may be a medical emergency (Table 5–1). Syncope usually arises from acutely diminished blood flow to the brain. It can be brought about by several causes ranging from orthostatic hypotension to myocardial infarction. Drugs such as antiarrhythmics, diuretics, nitrates, calcium channel blockers, antipsychotics, β blockers (including ophthalmics) antihypertensives, digoxin, and antidepressants have been implicated in syncopal episodes.

Trauma. Fractures are the most frequent outcome of trauma in the elderly. Fractures occur more easily in this age group because of osteoporosis. In individuals over 85 years of age, one of three women and one of six men will sustain hip fractures. Falls account for 90 percent of geriatric fractures. Initial treatment is immobilization of the fracture to stabilize it and limit the pain associated with it. Time can then be taken to evaluate the whole patient before more definitive procedures and reductions requiring anesthesia are undertaken. Traction, once a popular way to avoid the risks of surgery, has proved to be riskier in the **frail elderly** owing to the complications resulting from being immobile.

Heat Stroke. Heat stroke differs in the elderly in that it occurs without exertion. It usually occurs in the frail elderly, especially those taking drugs that alter fluid balance or temperature regulation. The mortality rate reaches 50 percent in those 65 years and over. The diagnosis is established if during a heat wave an elder presents with a temperature of 100 to 106°F (37.8 to 41°C), altered mental status, hyperventilation, vomiting, poor skin turgor, fatigue, and possibly seizures.

Hypothermia. Hypothermia is defined as a core temperature of less than 94°F (34°C). In the aged it may occur with only modest exposure to temperatures below 50°F. A history of exposure accompanied by confusion, slurred speech, sleepiness, and dilated pupils is diagnostic. Rewarming must be done with particular care in this age group.

Urinary Tract Infections. Emergency evaluation is often indicated in this situation because it presents atypically. It is estimated that bacteremia occurs in up to one third of cases of urinary tract infections (UTIs) in the elderly. Geriatric patients have frequency and dysuria much as their younger counterparts do. Incontinence in a usually continent patient is a clue, especially if accompanied by increased confusion. It is important to have UTI diagnosed early and treatment started before bacteremia can occur.

Table 5–1 DIFFERENTIATION OF SYNCOPAL EPISODES

Onset	Associated Activities	Symptoms	Cause	Recovery
No warning	Nothing out of ordinary; perhaps exertion	Sudden collapse	Arrhythmia	Prolonged
Quick	Coughing, full bladder or bowel, eating big meal	Nausea, pallor, sweating, bradycardia, hypotension	Vasovagal reflex	Rapid
Slower	Exertion, activity, stress	Substernal chest pain, cold, clammy, diaphoretic, anxious	Myocardial infarction	Prolonged
Rapid	Increased activity, stress, change in insulin or oral hypoglycemic dose, loss of appetite	Hunger, sweating, pallor, headache	Hypoglycemia	Fast
Rapid	Changing position from sitting or lying to upright	Dizziness, black spots, lack of balance	Orthostatic hypotension	Quick
Aura first	Flashing lights, certain sounds	Eyes roll back in head; possible twitching	Seizure	Slow

Direct Admissions

Patients can also be admitted directly to the geriatric unit when circumstances do not require a visit to the emergency department first. Often they arrive on the unit after being seen in the physician's office, where hospitalization was determined to be necessary. Direct admissions occur with diagnoses such as:

Acute **CHF** with fluid retention not responsive to usual oral diuretics.

Benign prostatic hypertrophy (**BPH**) requiring **TURP** surgery.

Cancer that requires surgery, complicated chemotherapy, or pain control.

Diabetes and related complications (**IDDM, NIDDM**) with sugar levels below 70 or over 300 and the condition unable to be controlled at home by medication and diet adjustments. The complications may be related to peripheral vascular disease or renal problems.

Fever of unknown origin (**FUO**) with continuous readings of 103°F or higher, that requires a work-up to determine the cause.

Intestinal obstruction, which is often the result of adhesions from prior surgery and frequently requires surgery to alleviate the problem.

Joint replacements (**THR, TKR**) as a result of **DJD**.

Parkinson's disease and its sequelae, which can result in severe motor dysfunction and problems with swallowing, in addition to falls.

Respiratory disorders such as **ARDS** and severe pneumonia in an individual whose respiratory system is already compromised by other problems, such as **COPD**.

Renal failure, which may be severe enough to require dialysis.

Severe gastrointestinal problems such as **WDHA**, for which intravenous hydration and electrolyte replacement are needed.

Stroke that causes severe neurologic deficits. Often this is a "stabilize only" situation, with the patient being hospitalized for a few days before being transferred to a rehabilitation unit or facility.

During the hospital stay, measures must be taken to avoid skin problems from incontinence, which is so prevalent in this age group. Incontinence is further complicated by stress and occasionally occurs in a hospitalized patient who has had no such previous problems.

Diagnostic Testing

Essentially the same diagnostic testing is done for the geriatric patient as for any other patient. There is a tendency to limit the exams, at least initially, to the least invasive procedures. It is of the utmost importance that the HUC bear in mind that many of the elderly have disabilities that will affect their ability to cooperate with the technicians performing the tests. If an individual is hard of hearing, blind, or unable to verbalize or has severe contractures or **SDAT**, it will interfere with his or her participation in the procedure. The HUC should list these types of limitations on the request for testing so that more time can be allowed or other steps taken, if necessary.

Equipment and Supplies

Canes are used to help with balance. They reduce the weight-bearing forces across the hips. Canes come in two basic types: the single-point cane and the quad cane. Each of these comes with a variety of handgrips. The quad canes provide more stability but require the user to move at a slower pace (Fig. 5–4).

Walkers provide a movable stable platform designed to protect the patient from falls. They are not constructed to support weight. The user must ambulate with a slow gait and will encounter difficulty with thresholds and stairs. Walkers can be folded to become more portable. The styles range from those with a simple frame to those with wheels and those that allow the patient to sit (Fig. 5–5).

Geri-Chair is designed to accommodate various positions, with the head and feet moving in a similar fashion to a recliner. The chairs have locking casters. They are covered in a well-padded washable material. A tray is usually attached so that it comes across the front from one side or the other.

Reachers are designed for the elderly person who has problems bending or grasping items. The squeeze grip handle makes it easy to use (Fig. 5–6).

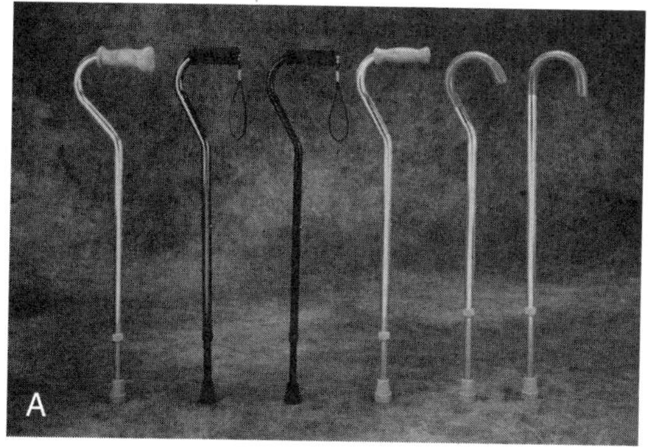

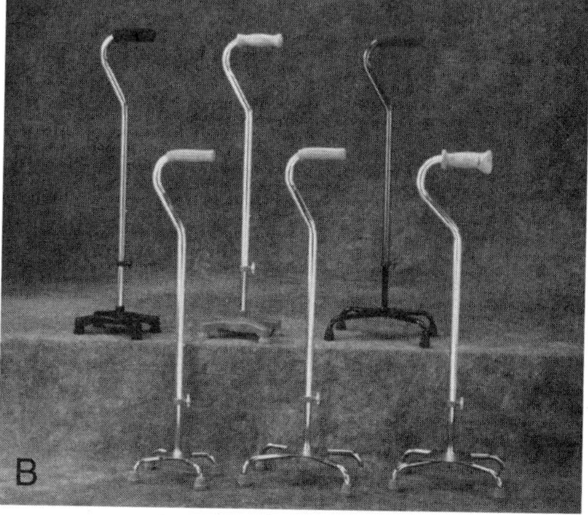

Figure 5–4
A, Single-point canes. *B*, Quad canes.

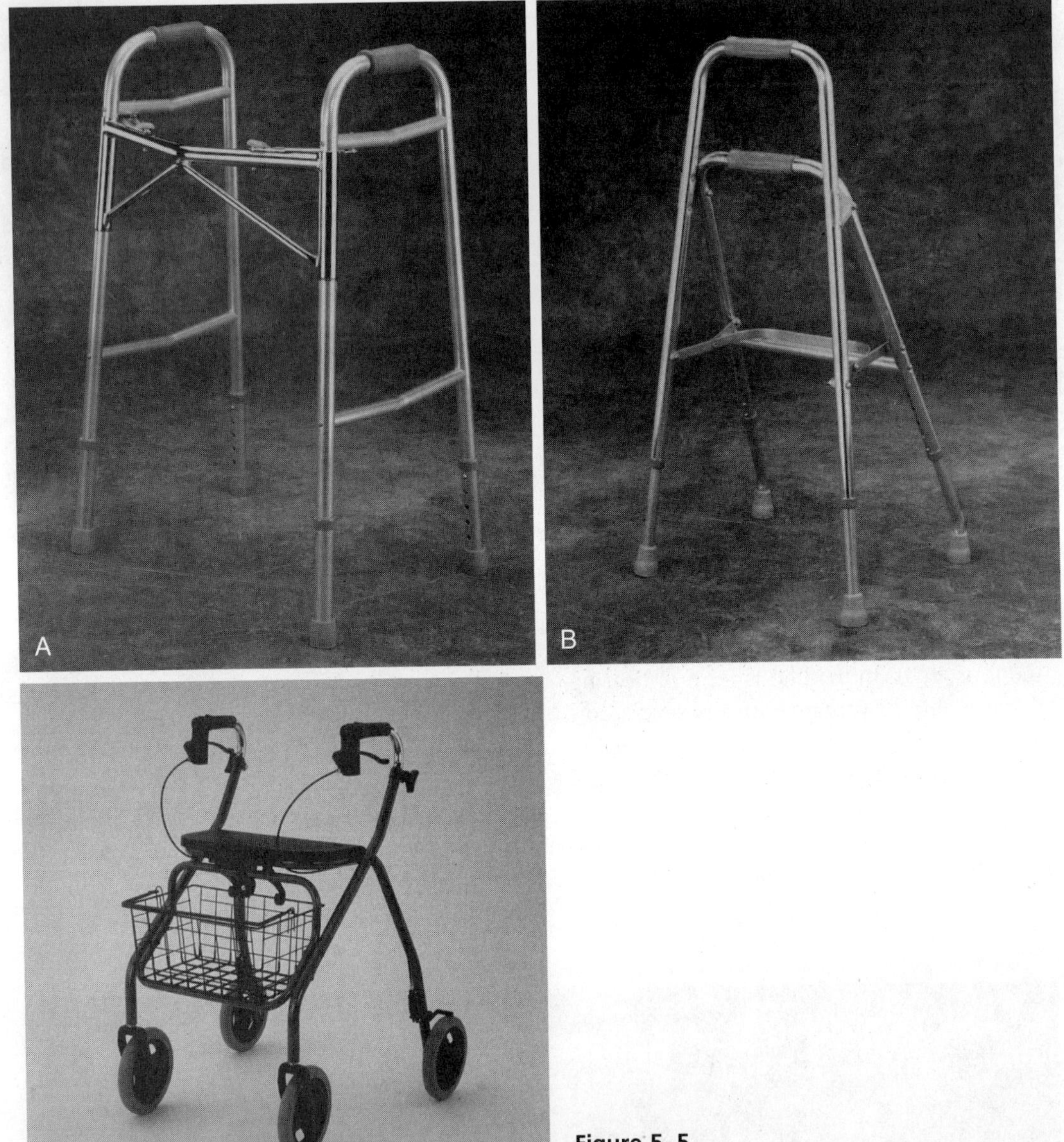

Figure 5–5
A, 7755 Standard walker. *B*, 7770 Hemi walker. *C*, Rolling walker.

Incontinence supplies include bed savers made of plastic or disposable pads. Absorbent pads that can be worn in the undergarments are used for individuals who lose small amounts of urine. Men's shorts that can accommodate the incontinence pads have been designed in jockey and boxer styles. The diapers, which are disposable, may be in an abbreviated style or the full diaper. The diapers are typically used in individuals who have totally lost control of their urine or who go

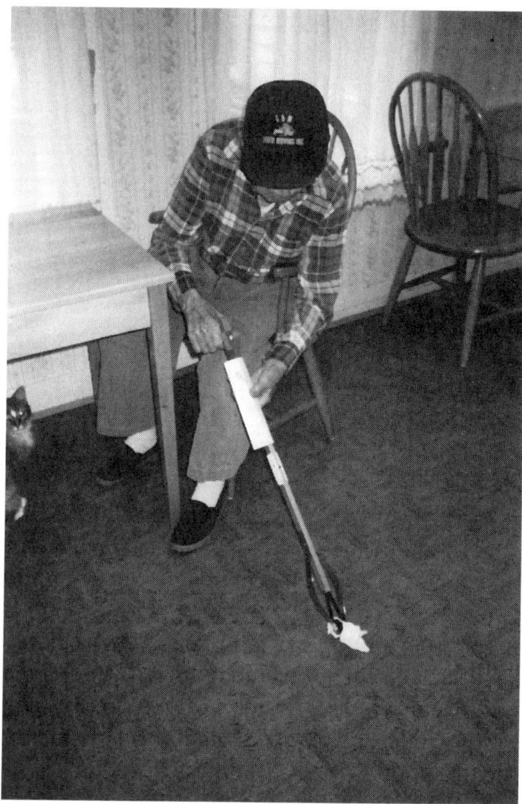

Figure 5–6
A reacher.

to the bathroom only when reminded. Many of the elderly prefer the pads because they are not as noticeable.

Spray deodorants are available to counteract the odor of the urine. Peri-wash solution or moist wipes similar to those for infants are used to cleanse the perineal area when the undergarments are changed.

Communication

Communication with the Elderly

In communicating verbally with geriatric patients, the manner in which they are addressed is of primary importance. The fact that these individuals are old does not necessarily mean that they want to be called by their first name or by the endearing terms that health care workers often use. The person should be asked initially how he or she prefers to be known. If the response is a terse "Mr. (or Mrs.) So and So," that is what should be used until the individual decides differently.

It was mentioned earlier that the senses dull with age. It is estimated that one third of the population between the ages of 65 and 74 years have significant hearing loss. That figure rises to one half in the 75- to 79-year group. Hearing loss in the elderly is most often conductive, in which the transmission of sound from the environment is distorted. A second kind is caused by problems in neurosensory structures. Individuals may have one type or the other or, in some cases, a mixed hearing loss. The most common hearing loss in the elderly is **presbycusis**, the term used to describe "the hearing loss of the aged," the exact cause of which is unknown.

Any type of hearing loss is a detriment to verbal communication. People who are hearing-impaired respond to what they hear, whether the message is accurate or not. If it makes sense in the context of the conversation, the message that they receive is clear to them. Take the example of the elderly grandmother who wished to please a young grandson with a birthday gift. She engaged him in a conversation about his interests and what he wanted for a gift. Imagine her disappointment when he wasn't pleased with her gift of a baseball hat. He had asked for a baseball bat. It is absolutely important to ask for feedback when conversing with the hearing-impaired elderly to be sure that the message sent is the message received.

For unknown reasons, people do not object to wearing glasses to assist their vision but are reluctant to purchase hearing aids when they need them. In some cases, it is reported to be an issue of vanity, but with the availability of small hidden devices, that should no longer be a problem. Another factor is cost, which is over 1000 dollars, not including the cost of batteries, which must be changed about every 2 weeks. In most instances the cost is not reimbursed by insurance carriers.

Hearing aids can help those individuals with conductive or neural hearing loss. A hearing aid contains a miniature microphone that receives the sound and transforms it into electrical energy. The electrical energy is sent to an amplifier to increase the energy output. This has a positive effect on the acoustical quality of the signal that is delivered. The hearing aids are programmed to match the characteristics shown to be needed by the hearing evaluation.

Assisted listening devices are available for use with telephones, televisions, and radios. They are available in portable and fixed models. These are configured so that the hearing-impaired person can enjoy TV or radio without changing the volume for others who are listening.

Amplification can be provided by anyone conversing with a hearing-impaired person. The speaker should face the listener at a distance of about 3 feet, in a well-lighted environment. Extraneous noise should be minimized. The speaker should use facial expressions to convey meaning or emotion and enunciate slowly and clearly. It is important *not to shout,* as this makes it more difficult to discriminate sounds. When feedback is requested or if it obvious that the listener did not understand, the message should be paraphrased rather than repeated word for word. The speaker should not become agitated when having to repeat because it will cause the already embarrassed listener to close down.

The HUC, by location and availability, is in a perfect setting to practice the good principles of communication needed for this often misunderstood group of people.

Legal and Ethical Issues

The rights and responsibilities afforded every other individual in the health care setting are the same for the geriatric patient. Among the patient's rights is the right to refuse care, and this must be allowed. The issue becomes clouded when it comes to competency. The definition is a combined social, ethical, and legal one. Legally, an individual who has not been declared incompetent and assigned a guardian is considered competent. In many states, guardianship is a long and tedious process.

The providers of health care understand short-term memory loss and other signs of early dementia. It is often ethically difficult for them to accept that the understanding required for "informed consent" is present in these elderly patients. An acceptable way to deal with the issue is to have an informed consent form signed not only by the patient but also by the patient's next of kin. One must look for the windows of lucidity when asking the patient to sign. Unless there is an assigned legal guardian, the geriatric patient should be encouraged to participate in the plan of care.

Advanced directives, which include a living will and durable power of attorney for health care (health care proxy), should be explained to all patients, and they should be encouraged to execute them. Those who already have these documents in place should make them available to their physicians and to the facility where they receive medical care. These are legal documents identifying the patient's wishes, and they must be followed by the health care team.

Patients also have rights concerning death. They should have the opportunity to state whether or not they want CPR. This does not suggest that they have a right to euthanasia. Most people understand the request of a competent person who is suffering greatly without hope for cure to have life ended prematurely, but this is not allowable by law in most states. The ethical, legal, and policy debate on this issue will surely continue. The sensitivity required of the HUC and the rest of the health care team in dealing with the families of patients involved in this process is the key to success.

It is unfortunate that each year a large number of older people are injured physically, psychologically, and financially by partners, family, and others. The elderly are particularly vulnerable to mistreatment. The problem may involve physically hitting and slapping or verbally threatening and insulting. **Neglect** is present when a person is deprived of something needed for daily living. Neglect and **abuse** have no socioeconomic barriers and are prevalent in all classes and ethnic groups.

Physical mistreatment is noted by the health care team by observing and reporting unexplained:

Bruising
Burns
Welts
Lacerations
Punctures
Fractures
Dislocations
Unusual genital infections
Dehydration
Missing dentures, glasses, or prostheses.

Psychological mistreatment is evidenced by a combination of any of the following:

Insomnia
Unusual weight gain or loss
Tearfulness
Low self-esteem
Excessive fears
Resignation
A need for excessive sleep.

Indicators of financial mistreatment include:

Sudden inability to pay bills
Unexplained withdrawals of money from accounts
Disproportion between assets and living conditions.

If mistreatment is suspected, it should be reported to the elder protective services agency in the locality, as mandated by law. If mistreatment is identified, appropriate interventions will be put into place.

Discharge Planning

Discharge planning for the geriatric patient is complex because the needs are often multiple. The plans may be as simple as returning home to the care of the family, with the assistance of a home health agency for **ADL** and **IADL** support. Or, plans may be as complex as a complete relocation. Many geriatric patients may have to be transferred to rehabilitation facilities, geropsychiatric units, nursing homes, congregate housing, or residential assisted living homes. They often need additional community services, such as hospice, respite care, community mental health support, adult day care, senior centers, nutrition programs such as Meals On Wheels, and monitoring services such as Lifeline. The discharge plan is based on an individual assessment of each patient's needs and then matching those needs to the appropriate services. A further barrier to discharge planning is that there are not as many nursing home and residential assisted living home beds available as there were in the past.

Quality Assurance Issues

The team can be made up of any number of professionals working on the unit. It is becoming commonplace for the HUC to have a place on the team. The HUC has access to most of the data needed in the studies and can bring an objective perspective to the evaluation of the data. The data are typically collected from chart review survey tools and interviews. They are then collated and a raw analysis is done for interpretation. The team can study the results and make recommendations and communicate them to other involved parties.

A useful tool for any quality assurance team when studying most topics relevant to the care of the geriatric patient is shown in Table 5–2.

Closing Thoughts

Many people do not want to associate with the aged. For some it is the fear of what is to

Table 5–2 QUALITY ASSURANCE TOOL

Category	Basic Question(s)	Findings (Data)
Efficacy	Is/are procedure(s) useful?	
Appropriateness	Is it right for the client?	
Accessibility	If it is right, can the client get it?	
Acceptable	Is it what the client wants?	
Effectiveness	Is it carried out well?	
Efficient	Is it done cost effectively?	
Continuity	Did it progress without interruption, with proper follow-up and referral?	
Compassion	Is there evidence that the staff cares deeply about work with clients?	
Timeliness	Is it made available when needed?	
Privacy	Can client control information relative to care?	
Confidentiality	Is there assurance that privileged information is not discussed without permission?	
Participation	Are client and family included in all decision making regarding care?	
Safety	Is environment free from hazards/ danger?	
Supportiveness	Are materials adequate to meet client needs?	

happen to them. For others, it is considered boring. In truth, our elders have a wealth of experience that they are willing to share with us, and they can do nothing but enrich our lives. It is very rewarding to see a grandparent get well and go home to enjoy the grandchildren.

The geriatric unit presents a unique kind of confusion and stress for the HUC that differs from the high-tech areas, such as the special care units. Managing and coordinating issues concerning individuals with memory deficits and other special needs can be challenging as well. Participating on committees that deal with real issues surrounding the geriatric population, such as the quality assurance committee or the ethics committee, can make a HUC a part of forming the future of this specialty.

Review Questions

1. Explain the importance of the physical layout of a geriatric unit.
2. List five considerations in planning a geriatric unit that will reduce the risks of falls.
3. Explain what is meant by "polypharmacy" and the impact this can have on the elderly.
4. Identify the most common cause of emergency admissions in the elderly.
5. Explain how hearing impairment affects the ability to communicate with the elderly.

Bibliography

Rakel RE: Saunders Manual of Medical Practice. Philadelphia, WB Saunders, 1996.

Merck Manual of Geriatrics. Rahway, NJ, Merck, Sharp & Dohme Research Laboratories, 1996.

Home Medical Advisor, The Learning Company http://www.learningco.com

NIH Library of Medicine, http://www.nih.gov/

Health Care Reform Bookshelf, gopher gopher.counter-point.com

Gerontology. Microsoft Encarta 96 Encyclopedia Microsoft and Funk and Wagnalls, 1996.

The Geropsychiatric Unit

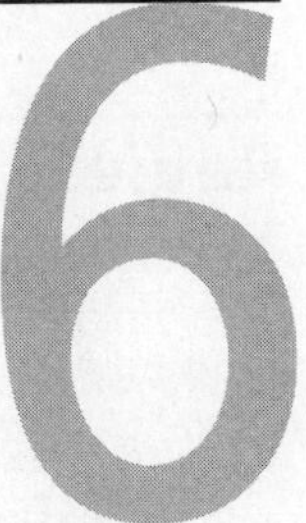

Gloria Smith

Common Abbreviations

AD	Alzheimer's disease
ADRD	Alzheimer's disease and related dementia
CJD	Creutzfeldt-Jakob disease
MAO-B	Monoamine oxidase B
MMSE	Mini-Mental State Exam
MID	Multi-infarct dementia
PET	Positron emission tomography
PSMS	Physical Self-Maintenance Scale
SDAT	Senile dementia of the Alzheimer type
SSRI	Selective serotonin reuptake inhibitor

Objectives

At the completion of this chapter the reader should be able to:

1. List three other names by which geropsychiatric units might be known.
2. Name three diseases seen in patients admitted to a geropsychiatric unit.
3. Explain what is meant by "polypharmacy" and state its impact on the geropsychiatric patient.
4. Describe six types of therapy that may be used to treat the geropsychiatric patient.
5. Discuss the role of the health unit coordinator in communicating with the geropsychiatric patient.

Vocabulary

Acetylcholine: A neurotransmitter that appears to be involved in learning and memory

Aggression: A threatening behavior

Agitation: Disruptive vocal or motor behavior

Apathy: General lack of feeling or emotion; indifference

Behavioral symptoms: Those that relate to emotion and action

Catastrophic reaction: Emotionally violent response to a seemingly trivial occurrence

Cognitive symptoms: Those that relate to thought processes, such as learning, comprehension, memory, reasoning, and judgment

Confabulation: Making up information to fill voids caused by memory deficit

Delirium: Extreme excitement or confusion accompanied by impaired memory, illusions, or hallucinations

Delusion: A fixed, false belief

Dementia: A group of symptoms that accompany certain diseases and conditions. It involves loss of intellectual functioning (thinking, remembering, and reasoning).

Continued

Vocabulary *Continued*

Depression: Emotional dejection greater and more prolonged than that warranted by any objective reason

Dopamine: A neurotransmitter that is essential for normal motor function

Gene: The basic unit of heredity

Hallucination: False sensory experiences. These are heightened in sensory impaired individuals.

Memory: A general term referring to a person's recollection of those things taught or learned; a person's mental storage of information

Monamine oxidase B: An enzyme that breaks down certain neurotransmitters, i.e., dopamine, serotonin, and noradrenaline

Neuritic plaque: An abnormal cluster of dead and dying nerve cells and protein. Also called senile plaque.

Neurofibrillary tangle: An abnormal accumulation of twisted protein fragments inside nerve cells

Neurotransmitter: A specialized chemical messenger, produced and secreted by nerve cells

Noradrenaline (norepinephrine): A neurotransmitter that plays a role in mood, pain, and possibly learning and memory

Paranoid behavior: Behavior characterized by unreasonable suspicion of actions of others

Phosphorylated: Mixed with or bound to phosphorus

Polypharmacy: The use of multiple medications

Prion: A small protein-containing infectious particle that is resistant to the usual methods of inactivation and degradation

Psychosis: A general term for a state of mind in which thinking becomes irrational and/or disturbed

Serotonin: A compound occurring in the brain, intestines, and platelets that induces vasoconstriction

Sleep disturbances: Real or perceived disruption in the normal sleep-wake cycle

Sundowning: An acceleration of behavioral symptoms late in the day (at dusk or after dark). May be a result of fatigue or reduced sensory stimulation by light.

Wandering: A behavioral symptom characterized by the individual's engaging in aimless motor activity.

Related Terminology

The following terms do not appear in the text; however, they are terms that someone working on a geropsychiatric unit would be expected to know.

Neurotransmission: The passage of signals from one nerve cell to another via chemical substances or electrical signals

Neuropathology: Changes in the brain produced by a disease

Serotonergic: The system of nerve cells that uses serotonin to play a role in mood, sleep, and pain

History

Standard psychiatric units within the medical community have traditionally addressed the needs of the mentally ill of various ages. In the past 10 to 20 years the trend has been toward deinstitutionalization. This created a need for environments that could provide care to these individuals when a crisis arose that required immediate medical support and intervention.

The elderly population has grown, as has research into the diseases specific to this age group. As new diagnostic tests have been developed and new treatments discovered, an increasing number of elderly individuals have been recognized with psychiatric disorders. It has become evident that mixing the young, middle-aged, and elderly in a single unit is not a good idea. The result of this thinking created the concept of the geropsychiatric unit. These units are variously known as elder care, senior care, and senior mental health units. It is interesting to note that the word "psychiatric" is often avoided. This is because this population has an aversion to that term. To them it means that they are "crazy."

The mission of the geropsychiatric unit is to provide a supportive environment for those in this population (usually 55 years of age and older) with behavioral problems caused by organic neurologic impairment. The impairment may be exacerbated by a functional neurosis that has existed over a lifetime or may simply result from an existing disease process. The goal is to find the most appropriate form of intervention to calm the patient and to provide the best possible quality of life.

Description of the Unit

There are many types of geropsychiatric units nationwide. Some are freestanding, which means that they are independent of other medical care services and care models. Others are segregated, which means that they are attached to and housed with other medical care services and care models. The segregated units are typically found in hospitals, but they are often operated and maintained separately for treatment purposes. The majority of hospitals have been turning to a continuum of care service model, integrating the service needs of the geropsychiatric unit with other units.

Many units are located in former general patient care areas that were closed as a result of dramatically reduced in-patient days. These units are redecorated in less stimulating colors, have clearly marked areas, and are free of clutter. The unit is preferably located in a quieter area of the facility and ideally will have no overhead paging system. The confused elder has no understanding of the public address system, and its use often starts a **catastrophic reaction.** Radios and television sets are usually kept at low volume.

The latest models of the freestanding units are being built without sharp corners, using open concepts wherever possible and eliminating confusing corridors. The patient rooms are self-contained and have a private bath visible from the bed. The main desk/nurses' station is best located off to one side and enclosed in a transparent shatterproof material to prevent **wandering** or disruptive patients from intruding on staff. This provides for general visibility of activities. It is recommended that a monitoring system be kept active between all patient care areas and the desk so that verbally disruptive behaviors can be noted and defused before becoming full-blown **agitation** or **aggression.** It is important that these behaviors be controlled early on to avoid injuries to the individual or to others.

The geropsychiatric unit must be a secure environment with a locking or alarm system to prevent patients from eloping. It can be an elaborate system of alarms on all doors and windows that exit to the outside or a system whereby patients wear a bracelet or anklet that triggers an alarm when they approach certain off-limits areas.

Staffing

All the patient care staff working on the geropsychiatric unit have special training in the challenges presented by the psychiatric elder patient. The staff is often cross trained in the specialties of geriatrics and psychiatry. This is a specialized field with unique requirements, including the ability to work with agitation, various **psychoses, depression,** mania, anxiety, and **sleep disturbances.**

The medical director is a geropsychiatrist who in many facilities heads a staff of other similarly trained physicians and frequently psychiatric nurse practitioners. The rest of the team working directly with the patient and the family usually consists of geropsychiatric nurses, discharge planners, social workers, and geropsychiatric technicians. The unique psychosocial needs of this unit's population dictates a patient-to-staff ratio of no greater than 3 to 1.

The other departments of the hospital participate on an as-needed basis. An admission physical exam is done by a family practitioner or internist. Consultations with medical specialists, spiritual care staff, nutritionists, and physical and occupational therapists are common. There are usually personnel assigned to contact the patient and family after discharge for follow-up information.

The HUC plays a vital role on this unit, seeing to it that the information from the various aspects of the treatment plan is transcribed in a timely manner and that information is flowing smoothly between all the different direct care professionals. A HUC is in a position to keep the unit running efficiently, enabling the medical and social professionals to do their jobs without losing time in searching out information and constantly backtracking. This one position is the indispensable "glue" to establishing an effective care plan delivery system.

Anatomy and Physiology

The cortex of the brain is the seat of functioning that becomes disturbed in such a way that an individual must be admitted to the geropsychiatric unit. The frontal lobe deals with personality and social conduct. The hippocampus is important in learning and **memory.** Problems in this area cause **cognitive symptoms.** If some of the pathology seen in cortical disturbances affects motor areas of the brain, Parkinson-like symptoms may be seen.

Neurotransmitters are chemicals that mediate the transmission of messages along nerves and across the synapses, which are the junctions between two nerve cells. They are produced and secreted by the nerve cells. Neurotransmitters play complex roles in the body, many of which are still the subject of research. **Acetylcholine** is a neurotransmitter that appears to be involved in learning and memory. **Dopamine** is a neurotransmitter that is essential for motor functions. **Norepinephrine,** also known as **noradrenaline,** plays a role in mood, pain, and possibly learning and memory. **Serotonin** is a neurotransmitter that influences sleep, mood, pleasure, and pain. **Monamine oxidase B (MAO-B)** is an enzyme that breaks down certain neurotransmitters.

Diseases Seen on the Unit

Most of the admissions to the geropsychiatric unit are for control of behaviors seen with **dementia.** Some affected individuals may have had previous psychiatric diagnoses, and many of the dementias have psychiatric symptoms associated with them.

Alzheimer's Disease

Alzheimer's disease (AD) is a progressive neurodegenerative disease characterized by loss of function and death of areas of the brain, leading to loss of mental functions such as learning and memory. There is evidence that acetylcholine levels are severely diminished in the brains of individuals with **ADRD** and **SDAT**.

The following are examples of typical **behavioral symptoms** and changes that come about during the progression of the disease:

- A social facade or a capacity to look and behave well in brief social encounters
- Shadowing or following a family member into the bathroom or around the house
- New demands, irritability, or obsessive-compulsive traits with low frustration tolerance
- **Apathy**, withdrawal, lack of interest, lack of motivation; doesn't start anything or will not do anything new or different; depression, tearfulness
- Hiding things, losing things, accusing others of theft
- Constant packing, pacing, rummaging, searching, moving things about
- Loss of ability to understand or care about the feelings of others
- Taking things belonging to others; hoarding things of value
- Resistant or stubborn refusals in response to changes in routine or being rushed; poor response to strange places; won't bathe or change clothes
- Wandering, getting lost, agitation, excessive worrying, suspiciousness of those closest to them
- Confusing present family members with those from the past; misidentification, **confabulation**
- **Delusions**, or fixed false beliefs; especially suspicious about infidelity or theft
- Nonrecognition of self in mirror; belief that television plots involve self
- **Hallucinations**; hearing, feeling, seeing things that aren't there
- Catastrophic reactions: blowing events out of proportion, usually in response to overstimulation, frustration, fatigue, or failure
- Repetitive statements, questions, telephone calls or movements; ideas seem to get stuck in the person's head
- Bizarre changes in food and activity preferences
- **Sundowning**; increased restlessness in the late afternoon
- Uncharacteristic anger, hitting, biting, screaming, pinching, kicking
- Changes in sexual desires and behaviors
- Inappropriate social behaviors, childishness, silliness
- Safety risks from poor judgment, neglect, abuse, exploitation, falls, exposure, poisoning.

It is easily seen that Alzheimer's dementia resembles human development in reverse.

Disruptive behavior is brought on by fear, frustration, and the feeling of being overwhelmed by a situation. The loss of the sense of time and place and control of impulses goes along with forgetting what is appropriate. If complicated demands are being made there is physical discomfort or difficulty in communicating, resulting in frustration that will bring on disruptive behavior.

There is a form of the disorder known as early-onset Alzheimer's disease. The diagnosis is made before the age of 65 years. This form of the disease has been associated with mutations in **genes** located on chromosome 14 and chromosome 21. Approximately 1 to 10% of AD patients are diagnosed as early onset.

Creutzfeldt-Jakob Disease

Creutzfeldt-Jakob disease (**CJD**) is a rare fatal disorder caused by a transmissible infectious organism called a **prion**. Early symptoms include failing memory, behavioral changes, lack of coordination, and seizures. The disease progresses quickly, with rapidly deteriorating mentation and pronounced involuntary movements. The patient may develop blindness, experience weakness in the extremities, and ultimately lapse into a coma.

Frontal Lobe Dementia

In this type of dementia the frontal lobe is primarily affected. Individuals are usually diagnosed following a fast and dramatic change in personality and social conduct. Memory loss and language impairment vary from patient to patient.

Lewy Body Dementia

Lewy body dementia occurs when Lewy bodies appear in the cortex of the brain. Individuals with this diagnosis have episodes of confusion and memory loss followed by periods of clear thinking and lucidity. Eventually, deterioration causes visual and auditory hallucinations, **paranoid behavior**, and delusions.

Multi-infarct Dementia

Multi-infarct dementia (**MID**) is known as vascular dementia. It is caused by a series of strokes. The cumulative damage from the strokes is impairment of intellectual and motor abilities, including the ability to walk. The damage can cause the individual to experience hallucinations, delusions, or **depression.** The onset of MID is usually abrupt and seems to progress in a stepwise fashion. Treatment is aimed at prevention of the strokes, since the nerve cells that die as a result of the stroke cannot regenerate. Dealing with the risk factors of high blood pressure, stress, cardiac disease, and diabetes will avoid further damage.

Pick's Disease

Pick's disease is a type of dementia diagnosed in individuals suffering from dramatic alterations in personality and social behavior, with memory preserved until late in the course of the disease. There is mostly frontal lobe damage or shrinkage. MMSE results can be in a normal range. The onset of Pick's disease is seen in people between 45 and 65 years of age.

Wernicke-Korsakoff Syndrome

A two-stage neurologic condition, Wernicke-Korsakoff syndrome is a result of malnutrition associated primarily with alcoholism. It is directly caused by a vitamin B_1 deficiency. The first stage is known as Wernicke's encephalopathy and consists of overall confusion and slowness. On a motor level, there is a problem with walking as well as uncoordinated movements. The level of consciousness may decrease to coma. The second stage is known as Korsakoff's syndrome and occurs if treatment is not promptly initiated to correct the vitamin B_1 deficiency. Individuals at the later stage experience permanent memory loss, apathy, and disorientation.

Diagnostic Testing

Medical issues generally are addressed at the outset. Often medical problems in the elderly affect emotional expression. This complicates the mental health evaluation, so every attempt is made to diagnose and deal with medical illnesses. The process is complicated by the fact that there is usually memory deficit involved and problems with verbal expression. The information for history taking must come from family or close friends.

Laboratory Testing

Complete blood count (CBC) is obtained to detect anemia or evidence of infection, either of which can cause symptoms of dementia in the elderly. Blood chemistry panels are used primarily to check for diabetes. Hyper- and hypoglycemia can cause neurologic symptoms and behavior changes. Liver and kidney function are also determined. Thyroid studies are performed to ascertain the presence or absence of hypothyroidism, which manifests itself in lethargy and may be mistaken for depression. Vitamin B_{12} and folate levels are obtained to check for vitamin deficiencies, which are suspected of contributing to dementia.

Diagnostic Imaging

It is not unusual for a baseline CT scan or MRI to be ordered as soon as possible after disturbing symptoms arise. One reason for this is that subsequent imaging studies can be compared with the initial one to track the stages of disease. Another reason is that this may be the only chance to perform these tests; that is, the disease may progress to the point that the client cannot tolerate being quiet long enough to accomplish the tests.

Positron emission tomography (PET) is an imaging scan that measures the activity or functional level of the brain by measuring its uptake of glucose.

Other Diagnostic Testing

Electroencephalogram records electrical activity present in the brain. In the elderly, it is usually attempted in an awake state to gather as much information as possible. If agitation or severe anxiety is a problem, the patient can be sedated.

Global Deterioration Scale provides a tool to objectively measure age-associated cognitive decline and AD (Table 6–1).

Autopsy, unfortunately, is the only mechanism of gathering certain pieces of diagnostic information. Among them are:

The presence of prions in CJD.

The presence of Lewy bodies, which are the abnormal deposits of a filament-like substance on nerve cells, associated with dementia and Parkinson's disease.

The presence of **neuritic plaques**, also known as senile plaques. These consist of an abnormal cluster of dead and dying nerve cells, other brain cells, and protein. They are a characteristic structural abnormality seen in AD.

The presence of **neurofibrillary tangles**, which are an accumulation of twisted protein fragments inside nerve cells. Neurofibrillary tangles are also found in the brain of AD patients in the post-mortem exam.

The presence of the Tau protein in neurofibrillary tangles. Tau is normally involved in maintaining the internal structure of nerve cells. In AD, this protein is abnormally **phosphorylated**.

Evaluation and Care in the Geropsychiatric Unit

The first priority during the admission process is to obtain as much information as possible so that a treatment plan can be developed and initiated. In addition to the diagnostic testing mentioned earlier, the patient is given a physical and neurologic examination. Much of the history is contributed by the family. The occupational therapy staff may be asked to evaluate the patient's abilities with respect to activities of daily living.

A brief baseline mental status examination, such as Mini Mental State Exam (**MMSE**), is done as soon after admission as the patient is found cooperative. The evaluation done during admission can be repeated during follow-up to help ascertain the level of functioning. The Physical Self-Maintenance Scale (**PSMS**) is applied in conjunction with the baseline mental status examination (Figs. 6–1 and 6–2).

At this time, based on the collective information, hopefully a treatment plan can be developed. The term hopefully is used because most of the time excessive behavioral symptoms are the reason for admission, and the patient can be stabilized only through psychopharmacology.

All clinical and historical information gathered enables the psychiatrist to determine which medications are best suited for the individual and the behavior being exhibited. Many changes of medications may be required before the most effective agent or group of agents can be found. Effects and side effects are constantly monitored, and changes are made in response to the findings.

During simultaneous work with families and caregivers, it is important to differentiate between challenging behavior or psychiatric symptoms of a brain disorder and poor family support and communication. The onset of disease is often subtle, and family members must understand that they did not in any way contribute to it and are not to blame for failing to anticipate it.

In detailing a care plan, the behaviors must be considered. Most people with ADRD are very sensitive to nonverbal communication. Care must be taken with body language and tone, especially if the caregiver is upset, angry, or frustrated. The patient will respond to nonverbal cues much more readily than to what is said. People with dementia are sensitive to the environment and to demands. They are less likely to be disruptive in calm, familiar settings with predictable routines. Requests

Text continued on page 89

Table 6–1 GLOBAL DETERIORATION SCALE

GDS #	GDS Stage	Clinical Phase	Clinical Characteristics	Diagnosis
1	No cognitive decline	Normal	No subjective complaints of memory deficit. No memory deficit evident on interview.	Normal
2	Very mild cognitive decline	Forgetfulness	Subjective complaints of memory deficit, most frequently in the following areas: (1) forgetting where one has placed familiar objects; (2) forgetting names one formerly knew well. Objective evidence of memory deficit on interview. No objective deficits in employment or social situations. Appropriate concern over situation.	Normal for age
3	Mild cognitive decline	Early confusional	Earliest clear-cut deficits. Manifestations in more than one of the following areas: (1) gets lost when traveling to an unfamiliar location; (2) coworkers aware of relatively poor performance; (3) word and name finding difficulties evident to people close to patient; (4) very little retention from reading a short passage; (5) decreased facility on remembering names of new people; (6) loses or misplaces articles of value; (7) concentration deficit. Objective evidence on intensive interview. Decreased performance in demanding employment and social settings. Mild to moderate anxiety accompanies symptoms.	Compatible with incipient Alzheimer's disease
4	Moderate cognitive decline	Late confusional	Clear-cut deficit on careful clinical interview. Deficit manifests in following areas; (1) decreased knowledge of current and recent events; (2) may exhibit some deficit in memory of one's personal history; (3) concentration deficit elicited on serial subtraction; (4). decreased ability to travel, handle finances. Frequently no deficit in: (1) orientation to time and person; (2) recognition of familiar persons and faces; (3) ability to travel to familiar places. Denial is dominant defense mechanism. Flattening of affect and withdrawal from challenging situations occur.	Mild Alzheimer's disease

Table continued on following page

Table 6–1 GLOBAL DETERIORATION SCALE *Continued*

GDS #	GDS Stage	Clinical Phase	Clinical Characteristics	Diagnosis
5	Moderately severe decline	Early dementia	Patient can no longer survive without some assistance. On interview, patients are unable to recall a major relevant aspect of their current lives, e.g., address, telephone number, names of grandchildren, high school classmates. Frequently some disorientation to time (day of week, date, season) or to place. May have trouble counting back from 20 by 2's. Retain many facts regarding themselves and others. Need no assistance with toileting or eating but may have difficulty choosing proper clothing to wear.	Moderate Alzheimer's disease
6	Severe cognitive decline	Middle dementia	May occasionally forget the name of spouse upon whom they are entirely dependant for survival. Will be largely unaware of all recent events and experiences of their lives. Retain some knowledge of their life in the past but it is sketchy. Generally unaware of surroundings, the year, season, etc. Difficulty counting to or from 10. Require assistance with ADLs. Ultimately will become incontinent without reminders. May recognize familiar locations when traveling. Diurnal rhythm disturbed. Almost always recall their own name. Can distinguish familiar from unfamiliar persons in their environment. Personality and emotional changes occur: (1) delusional behavior, accusing spouse of being an imposter, talking to imaginary figures in their environment or to themselves in a mirror; (2) obsessive symptoms, repeating simple activities; (3) anxiety and agitation, up to violent behavior. (4) cognitive abulia, i.e., loss of willpower because the person cannot carry a thought long enough to determine a purposeful action.	Moderately severe Alzheimer's disease
7	Very severe cognitive decline	Late dementia	All verbal abilities are lost. Frequently there is no speech at all—only grunting. Incontinent of urine; requires assistance toileting and feeding. Loss of basic psychomotor skills, including the ability to walk. The brain appears no longer able to tell the body what to do. Generalized cortical neurologic signs and symptoms frequently present.	Severe Alzheimer's disease

Components of the Mental Status Exam

Appearance	Age, clothing, personal hygiene, unusual physical characteristics
Activity	Recent change in activity level, hyperactivity, agitation
Mood & Affect	Happiness, sadness, worry; intensity, appropriateness, constricted or expanded feelings
Speech & Language	Mutism, pressured speech, blocking, loose associations, word salad
Thought Content	Obsessions, compulsions, phobias, delusions
Perceptual Disturbances	Illusions, hallucinations
Memory & Attention	Attention; calculation; remote and recent memory
General Intellectual Level	Vocabulary; knowledge of current events, abstract thinking

Figure 6–1
Mental status examination. (From Linton AD, Matteson MA, Maebius NK (eds): Introductory Nursing Care of Adults. Philadelphia, WB Saunders, 1995.)

Physical Self-Maintenance Scale (PSMS)
Activities of Daily Living

Patient's Name ______________________________ **Date** ____________
Rated by ______________________________

Numbers one through five in each category represent worsening states of function. Choose the number that best describes the patient's functional status. Scores in all six categories should then be totaled. The higher the final score, the greater the degree of impairment:

Score

A. Toileting
1. Cares for self at toilet completely, no incontinence.
2. Needs to be reminded or needs help in cleaning self, or has rare (weekly at most) accidents.
3. Soiling or wetting while asleep more than once a week.
4. Soiling or wetting while awake more than once a week.
5. No control of bowels or bladder. ______

B. Feeding
1. Eats without assistance.
2. Eats with minor assistance at mealtimes and/or with special preparation of food, or help in cleaning up after meals.
3. Feeds self with moderate assistance and is untidy.
4. Requires extensive assistance for all meals.
5. Does not feed self at all and resists efforts of others to feed him/her. ______

C. Dressing
1. Dresses, undresses, and selects clothes from own wardrobe.
2. Dresses and undresses self with minor assistance.
3. Needs moderate assistance in dressing or selection of clothes.
4. Needs major assistance in dressing, but cooperates with efforts of others to help.
5. Completely unable to dress self and resists efforts of others to help. ______

D. Grooming (neatness, hair, nails, hands, face, clothing)
1. Always neatly dressed, well groomed, without assistance.
2. Grooms self adequately with occasional minor assistance, eg, shaving.
3. Needs moderate and regular assistance or supervision in grooming.
4. Needs total grooming care, but can remain well groomed after help from others.
5. Actively negates all efforts of others to maintain grooming. ______

E. Physical Ambulation
1. Goes about grounds or city.
2. Ambulates within residence or about one block distance.
3. Ambulates with assistance of (check one)
   a ( ) another person b ( ) railing c ( ) cane d ( ) walker
   e ( ) wheelchair–gets in and out without help
   f ( ) wheelchair–needs help in getting in, out.
4. Sits unsupported in chair or wheelchair, but cannot propel self without help.
5. Bedridden more than half the time. ______

F. Bathing
1. Bathes self (tub, shower, sponge bath) without help.
2. Bathes self with help in getting in and out of tub.
3. Washes face and hands only, but cannot bathe rest of body.
4. Does not wash self but is cooperative with those who bathe him/her.
5. Does not try to wash self, and resists efforts to keep him/her clean. ______

Total Score

To track patient cognitive and functional status, record the base and follow-up scores of the MMSE and PSMS in the chart provided:

	MMSE	PSMS	DATE
Baseline			
Follow-up			
Follow-up			
Follow-up			
Follow-up			
Follow-up			

Figure 6–2
Physical self-maintenance scale. (Adapted from Lawton MP, Brody EM: Gerontologist 1969;9:179.)

should be tailored to their capacity, remaining strengths, and energy levels. The presence of hearing or visual deficits will alter the approach to the care plan as well.

The professional staff has to be sensitive to the fact that there are some situations in which families do not or cannot participate in care or care planning. This situation must be respected. Obviously, the scenario in which the family participates in a partnership to benefit their loved one is the preferred one. Good geropsychiatric programs encourage family involvement. Social services usually coordinate this aspect of care. In AD, it has been found that many families benefit from attending a support group. Meeting with others who have had the same experience gives them the opportunity to gain insights and share their feelings.

Medications

One of the goals of selecting medication regimens for the behavioral and psychotic problems of the elderly is to avoid **polypharmacy**, the use of an inordinate number of medications. This results from prescribing one medication to counteract the side effects of another medication, only to create different side effects. Further medication is added to counteract these side effects, and the cycle continues.

Neuroleptics

Neuroleptics are psychotropic drugs indicated in the treatment of severe agitation, wandering, screaming, assaultiveness, and psychotic or paranoid thinking. The following list gives the generic and trade names of some common neuroleptics:

Generic Name	Trade Name
chloropromazine	Thorazine
clozapine	Clozaril
fluphenazine	Prolixin
haloperidol	Haldol
loxapine	Loxitane
mesoridazine	Serentil
molindone	Moban
perphenazine	Trilafon
risperidone	Risperdal
thioridazine	Mellaril
thiothixene	Navane
trifluoperazine	Stelazine

Neuroleptics have consistent, reliable, and therapeutic effects in controlling agitation and psychosis. They play a role in containing the behaviors that arise from organic mental disorders such as dementia and **delirium**. They are effective in late-life psychoses and major affective disorders. A gradual decline in the therapeutic efficiency is seen in long-term administration of any neuroleptic.

Three types of side effects attributed to neuroleptics are frequent and troublesome:

Sedation is an unwanted side effect in the elderly because it often leads to more confusion and agitation. It can also play a role in sleep disturbances.

Orthostatic hypotension is demonstrated by a drop in systolic blood pressure of 20 mm of mercury or more when the patient changes from a recumbent to a sitting position or from sitting to standing. This is dangerous in the frail elderly, because they either do not understand or forget the instruction that they received to change positions slowly. There is an increased likelihood of falls and resulting fractures.

Extrapyramidal symptoms (EPS) may have a slow or sudden onset. There are meaningless movements of the head and face. There may be pelvic rocking. The gait is shuffling, and there may be leaning to one side or the other. Chewing motions are frequently seen. There seems to be a relationship between age and the severity of the EPS seen. This fact has led to a reduction in the use of the more potent neuroleptics (Haldol, Prolixin) as first-line treatment in the elderly patient.

Antidepressants

For the treatment of a depressive disorder in the elderly patient whose depression is not immediately life-threatening and who is not delusional, cyclic antidepressants are the treatment of choice:

Generic Name	Trade Name
amitriptyline	Elavil
doxepin	Sinequan
imipramine	Tofranil
nortriptyline	Aventyl, Pamelor
desipramine	Norpramin
clomipramine	Anafranil
trimipramine	Surmontil
amoxapine	Asendin

Selective Serotonin Reuptake Inhibitors (SSRIs)

In recent years, **SSRIs** have been added to the list of weapons against depression. It has been noted that the response to these drugs in the elderly has been less predictable than in younger patients:

Generic Name	Trade Name
fluoxetine	Prozac
fluvoxamine	Luvox
paroxetine	Paxil
sertraline	Zoloft

There has been some success using Luvox for obsessive-compulsive disorders or behaviors.

Novel Antidepressants

These agents have had varying levels of success. Often the dose that is needed is not well tolerated by the elderly.

Generic Name	Trade Name
bupropion	Wellbutrin
venlafaxine	Effexor
nefazodone	Serzone
trazodone	Desyrel

The new non-neuroleptics have shown some effectiveness in the treatment of agitation, psychosis, and disruptive behavior. This is an exciting area of geriatric pharmacology.

Drugs such as beta blockers, anticonvulsants, trazodone, lithium, and buspirone (BuSpar) have shown indications of therapeutic effectiveness (Table 6–2). Aricept, a drug to help the memory, was developed and released in 1996. A new psychotropic drug, Zyprexa, which seems to have fewer undesirable side effects, was also released.

One consideration in ordering the drugs for the elderly, particularly those who will be returned to the community, is the cost of the medication. It does no good to stabilize patients on medication on the geropsychiatric unit only to have them be noncompliant at home because they cannot afford the drug.

Another consideration in choosing drugs is the patient's liver, kidney, and cholinergic function. Older patients are more sensitive, more easily sedated, and more likely to become disoriented and lose coordination. Medication is the last resort for sleep disturbances. A short-acting benzodiazepine might have to be given for a limited time for day/night reversal. The goal is to discontinue the drug as soon as possible.

Many patients on the geropsychiatric unit take

Table 6–2 PHARMACOLOGIC STRATEGIES

Target Symptoms	Agents Likely to Be Effective
Depression, persistent sadness	SSRIs Tricyclic antidepressants
Hopelessness, self-deprecation	Novel antidepressants
Hallucinations	Neuroleptics
Delusions	Neuroleptics
Physical aggression	Neuroleptics carbamazepine (Tegretol) valproic acid (Depakote)
Anxiety	buspirone (BuSpar) Benzodiazepines Antidepressants
Apathy	methylphenidate (Ritalin)
Disinhibition	Dopamine agents amantadine (Symmetrel) bupropion (Wellbutrin) bromocriptine (Parlodel) estrogen (for males)

medication for arthritis, cardiovascular disease, GI upsets, constipation, and respiratory disease. The elderly often self-treat with vitamins as well. It is easy to see how the geriatric patient gets into the situation of polypharmacy. Close monitoring of medications is a necessity.

The HUC will process the medication orders, checking for STAT orders, and notifying the pharmacy of the needs of the unit. Many patients will have p.r.n. orders, particularly until their behaviors have stabilized. If the HUC observes any bizarre or accelerated behavior in a patient, it should be reported to the nurse immediately.

Therapies

Spiritual care or therapy is a significant need for most of our elderly, who have grown through a lifetime of religious beliefs and practices that are a very important part of their lives. This need is filled by the Pastoral Care Department, if the hospital has one, or by local clergy.

Color therapy employs color as a therapeutic activity designed to enhance a specific emotional response. Since emotion contributes to behavior, it stands to reason that color therapy can be used in a passive manner to enhance the overall treatment plan.

Music therapy is an older, well-known technique. It has been proved repeatedly to enhance other treatments and provide a calming environment.

Reminiscing therapy is another well-known and widely used technique. The patient is encouraged and allowed to retreat into much-loved memories. Many dementia patients live in the past either by choice or by disease process, and bringing forth pleasant memories helps in modifying behavior.

Validation therapy is a tool that creates reassurance of emotions and feelings. This has significance to the elderly demented patient, who lives in a world of emotion and feelings. Reality is a state of mind. Each of us sees a different reality, based on our lives and experiences. If we should become demented in old age, a totally new version of "reality" is introduced. It is no less real but definitely harder for others to understand. Validation encourages and allows that feeling and does not make judgments of reality.

Exercise therapy can be done individually or in a group. It is a channel for the expulsion of excess energy and excess feelings. It is good for us, body and soul. Often the elderly, who could benefit most from exercise therapy, are overlooked.

Light therapy is the use of a special box light to help treat seasonal affective disorder and its milder form, "the winter blues." What is happening is a seasonal form of depression, one of many illnesses now referred to as mood disorders. A high percentage of the elderly suffer from this disorder and benefit from phototherapy. The use of this therapy on the unit and after discharge can mitigate many symptoms of depression through the fall and winter and diminish the need for pharmacologic intervention.

Energy/healing therapies are gaining favor along with the other types of natural healing. Most often utilized in geropsychiatry are therapeutic touch and Reiki, either of which can be combined with massage.

To be therapeutic, *structured activities* must support the remaining abilities of the patient and minimize failure. The program should support dignity and encourage pleasure.

Activities should not make people anxious but be purposeful and stimulating—an opportunity to play a role within the community to which they currently belong.

The best activities are those that:

Affirm dignity
Break tasks down into steps
Communicate purpose and meaning to the participant
Provide opportunities to give to others
Establish new roles and re-establish old ones
Fulfill basic needs
Use remaining skills
Provide opportunities for success
Promote identity and self-esteem
Involve cultural and religious customs
Respect the individual
Are voluntary
Are fun.

When using any of the therapies, it is important to document the patient's emotional and physical response.

The HUC keeps a calendar of events for the unit, which usually includes a schedule of therapies. If outside people are involved, the HUC will make appointments and coordinate the reservation of space and equipment for the event.

Equipment

The equipment and supplies found on the geriatric unit are also available on the geropsychiatric unit. Commodes, incontinence supplies, walkers, handrails, geriatric chairs, grab bars, and canes are among the items needed (Fig. 6–3). Typically there are fewer of them, and they are more discreetly displayed to create a less institutional and more user-friendly environment. Medications and supplies for IVs and dressing are safely locked close to the nurses' desk.

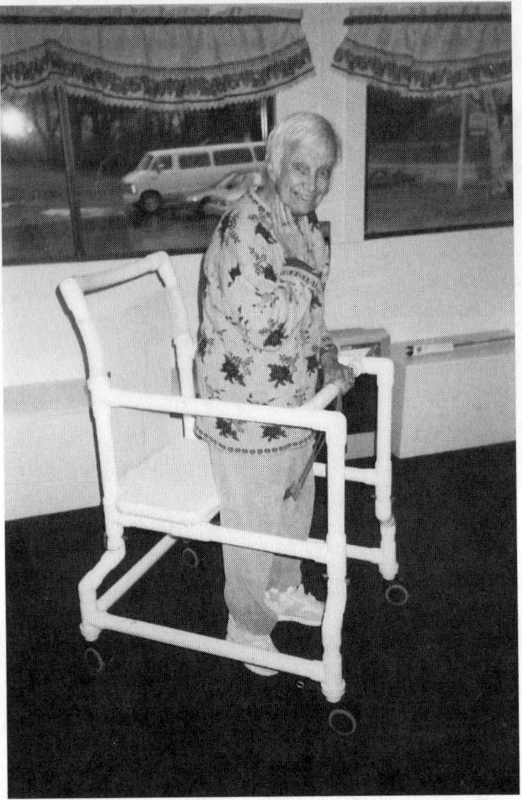

Figure 6–3
Restraint-free ambulator. (Courtesy of The Inn at Deerfield, Deerfield, NH.)

In some institutions, the HUCs are responsible for taking inventory and ordering supplies. They maintain the equipment log for the department and coordinate the scheduling of repairs when necessary.

Communication

With the Geropsychiatric Patient

The HUC is usually positioned in an area where he or she can be seen and approached by the patients. The patients, for the most part, have no concept of who is who and what job is assigned to whom. They are typically friendly and will try to carry on a conversation with the HUC. Communication is a problem in ADRD. Affected elders may not be able to make themselves understood and may not be able to understand what others are trying to tell them. When they do not remember a word, they will substitute one that sounds similar. If they cannot come up with a word, particularly to describe something, they will invent a new one.

In the early stages of the disease, communication can be made easier by the use of signs, labels, and written or printed messages. As the disease progresses, communication will be more difficult, and eventually the patient may be unable to speak at all. Nonverbal communication, such as light touch and laughter, is extremely effective. Although the patient with dementia is unable to communicate, this does not diminish the need for affection and touch.

General hints for effective communication with the patient are:

1. Always identify yourself and call the person by name. Don't quiz the patient or ask "Remember me?"
2. Attract their attention by approaching slowly from the front.
3. Maintain a comfortable, nonthreatening distance.
4. Listen well.
5. Limit how much you say on any one topic.
6. Maintain eye contact, looking calm and interested but not intense.
7. Watch and wait for a response; repeat the same words if necessary.
8. Respond to the feeling behind what is said or the behavior exhibited.
9. If the person does not respond to verbal direction, point, smile, touch, demonstrate, or initiate the motion.
10. Reduce background noise or confusion when trying to communicate.
11. If you don't understand, ask the person to point or demonstrate.
12. Speak slowly and distinctly at a low pitch.
13. Be aware of patients with hearing deficits.
14. Use POSITIVE terms.
15. Use familiar terms and short sentences.
16. Use cues.
17. Do *not* argue, confront, correct, moralize, or offer long explanations.
18. Limit choices. The best questions are those answerable by "yes" or "no."

About the Geropsychiatric Patient

The HUC will schedule the tests for the geropsychiatric patient. The tests are usually done in the general hospital area of the institution. It is important to pass on information to the other departments about current behaviors or things that will decrease the patient's frustration level. These may be as minor as telling the x-ray department that the color red will bring about a violent reaction from patient A, or that patient B cannot stand being in small spaces, or that patient C will become aggressive if a young person calls her by her first name.

The HUC will often be approached by family members for assistance and should bear in mind that they are often in denial or carrying misplaced guilt. This might make them difficult to communicate with. The HUC's training and experience in communicating under duress will be an asset in this situation.

Quality Assurance

In the integrated facility, someone from the geropsychiatric team will be on the quality assurance committee to provide whatever data are needed. In the freestanding and segregated units, data collection is necessary as well. Typically, data are collected to demonstrate effects and side effects of medication combinations and of the outcomes of various therapies. Incident reports of combative behavior as well as fall and accident logs are kept and reviewed by the appropriate committee. Based on the committee reports, plans are made to improve the care and conditions.

Closing Thoughts

The geropsychiatric unit by its physical layout alone will present a different type of challenge to the HUC. It is one of the patient care areas where a great deal of communication will go on between patients and HUCs. A HUC with patience and understanding and one who can redirect himself or herself after interruptions will do well in this unit.

It must be understood that this unit does not make people well in the standard medical tradition of "cure." It is frustrating and difficult to accept that an endearing patient will never get well. On the other hand, the appreciation you will receive for the kind attention you pay to this clientele is very rewarding. Working on the geropsychiatric unit affords an opportunity to be where there is constant change and new information to deal with. It is a unique challenge.

Review Questions

1. List three other names by which geropsychiatric units might be known.
2. Name three diseases seen in patients admitted to a geropsychiatric unit.
3. Explain what is meant by polypharmacy, and state its impact on the gerospsychiatric patient.
4. Describe six types of therapy that may be used to treat the geropsychiatric patient.
5. Discuss the role of the health unit coordinator in communicating with the geropsychiatric patient.

Bibliography

American Health Care Association and Alzheimer's Association: Care of Alzheimer's Patients: A Manual for Nursing Home Staff, 1985.

Brown IJ: Coping with the Winter Blues, 1992.

Guyther LP, Rabins P: Practical approaches for treating behavioral symptoms of people with mild to moderate Alzheimer's disease. Primary Psychiatry, 1996.

Levy M, Baumel BM: Alzheimer's disease. Primary Psychiatry, 1992.

Levy M, Baumel B, Rabins P, Gwyther LP: Part II, Images of aging.

Mace NL, Rabins PV: The 36 Hour Day. Baltimore, Johns Hopkins University Press.

Primary Psychiatry, 1996.

The Alzheimer Association Patient and Family Services: Family Guide. Chicago, 1992.

7

The Hematology/ Oncology Unit*

M. Mairata Frankwick

Objectives

At the completion of this chapter, the reader should be able to:

1. Explain how physicians use diagnostic procedures in the care of cancer patients.
2. List five types of diagnostic imaging studies performed to assist in evaluating cancer patients.
3. Identify the most definitive means of diagnosing all cancers.
4. Explain the primary purpose of chemotherapy.
5. List the three primary treatments for cancer.
6. Explain why many cancer patients require placement in protective isolation.

Vocabulary

Adjuvant therapy: Treatment that is added to a primary therapy to increase its effectiveness. This usually refers to chemotherapy or radiotherapy administered after surgery to increase the likelihood of cure.

Alopecia: Hair loss

Androgen: A male sex hormone that is sometimes used to treat recurrence of breast cancer

Anemia: A low red blood cell count, which can cause symptoms of fatigue, dizziness, or shortness of breath

Antibody: A blood protein developed by the body that fights against an antigen. Each **antibody** works against a particular antigen.

Antigen: A foreign substance introduced into or formed by the body that stimulates the formation of antibodies

Antimetabolites: A classification of anticancer drugs that prevent cell division by interfering with the DNA production process

Continued

* The editors would like to express special thanks to Bev Reed of Kirkland, Washington, for her early contribution as a consultant to the hematology/oncology chapter.

Vocabulary *Continued*

Asymptomatic: Without symptoms or obvious signs of disease. In its early stages, when the chances of cure are highest, cancer often develops without producing symptoms. Screening tests attempt to discover cancer at the **asymptomatic** stage.

Atypical: Abnormal or not usual. Cancer results from **atypical** cell division.

Autologous: Something that has its origin within an individual. It is a term used to describe blood transfusions and bone marrow transplants whereby the tissue is collected from an individual and stored to be transfused to the same individual at a later date.

Biopsy: The excision (by surgery or other procedure) of a small piece of tissue for microscopic examination of the cells. Biopsy is the definitive process for diagnosing cancer.

Bone marrow: The soft, fatty tissue that fills bone cavities. The body's blood cells are produced in the **bone marrow**; therefore, it is microscopically examined to diagnose and monitor treatment of cancers that affect the blood cells, such as leukemia, lymphoma, and multiple myeloma.

Bone marrow or stem cell transplant: The procedure of transplanting, by infusion, donor or autologous bone marrow as a treatment for certain types of acute leukemia and recurrent breast cancer

Brachytherapy: A cancer treatment that uses radioactive material implanted at the tumor site

Cancer: A general term for more than 100 diseases, all of which are characterized by uncontrolled growth and spread of abnormal cells to other parts of the body by way of the lymph system or bloodstream

Carcinoma: A form of cancer that develops in the surface layer of the tissue covering or lining organs of the body. This cancer often metastasizes.

Chemotherapy: The systemic treatment of cancer by oral or injected administration of drugs

Clinical trial: A carefully designed and executed investigation to evaluate the effects of a means to prevent, detect, diagnose, or treat a disease in humans. It identifies the benefits and the risks. All new drugs used in the United States are required to complete this process prior to being approved for use as therapeutic agents.

Cytology: The microscopic examination of the formation, structure, and function of cells; used to diagnose cancer

Continued

Vocabulary *Continued*

Endoscopy: The visual examination of the inside of body organs or cavities through a natural body opening or small incision by the use of a tubelike, lighted, optical system that also has the capabilities of obtaining tissue for **biopsy**

Estrogen: A female hormone sometimes given to inhibit tumor growth in breast cancer

Hepafilter: High-efficiency particulate air filter

Hyperalimentation: The total nourishment of the body with intravenous infusion of a solution of amino acids, glucose, vitamins, and minerals sufficient to sustain life. Also called total parenteral nutrition.

Incidence: The extent to which a disease occurs in the population; the estimated number of new cases diagnosed each year

Informed consent: Sufficient, understandable information regarding the benefits and risks of proposed treatment provided to the patient to make decisions regarding treatment and care

Interferon: A natural protein produced by normal cells that has been found to have antiviral and anticancer properties

Lesion: A change in body tissue; often used as a synonym for tumor

Leukemia: A cancer of the blood-forming tissues characterized by the overproduction of abnormal, immature, white blood cells. Leukemias are classified according to the dominant cell type and the severity (acute or chronic) of the disease.

Leukocyte: White blood cell. There are a number of types of **leukocytes**, but their common function is to combat infection throughout the body. A decrease in the number of leukocytes indicates a high risk for infection. An increase in the number of leukocytes may indicate the presence of an infection or malignancy.

Lymph: A clear fluid containing leukocytes and antibodies that circulates throughout the body via the lymphatic system

Lymphoma: A form of cancer that affects the lymph system. It has two varieties: Hodgkin's and non-Hodgkin's.

Magnetic resonance imaging: A noninvasive diagnostic technique using magnetic fields and radio frequency to produce images of internal areas of the body. It is useful in diagnosing diseases such as cancer.

Mammography: A screening and diagnostic technique using low-dose x-rays to visualize tumors in the breast too small to be felt on clinical examination

Continued

Vocabulary *Continued*

Metastasis: The spread of cancer cells via the lymph system or bloodstream from an original (primary) site to distant areas of the body. The newly formed (secondary) cancer sites are called metastases.

Melanoma: An aggressive type of skin cancer that is quick to metastasize if not treated early

Mortality rate: The number of deaths in a given population. For example, the **mortality rate** of lung cancer is higher in populations of smokers than nonsmokers.

Neoplasm: Any new abnormal growth. **Neoplasms** may be benign or malignant, but the term is generally used to describe cancer.

Nuclear scan: A diagnostic technique using radioactive materials, injected or ingested into the body, to produce an image of abnormalities or disease processes. The lungs are commonly scanned to detect pulmonary emboli; the brain, bones, and liver are commonly scanned to detect cancer.

Neutropenia: Low white blood cell count, which creates high risk for infection

Oncologist: A physician who is trained to specialize in the treatment of cancer. Some physicians specialize in a certain area of oncology, such as GYN oncology or neurologic oncology.

Oncology: The science dealing with the physical, chemical, and biologic properties of the causes and disease process of cancer

Paracentesis: A procedure using a large-bore needle to aspirate body fluid, usually from the abdominal cavity

Pathology: The study of the nature and causes of disease. It often refers to the microscopic examination of tissue used in diagnosis.

Platelets: A blood component that is essential to the clotting process. **Platelet** transfusions are given to cancer patients to prevent or control bleeding when chemotherapy or the disease process has caused the patient to have a low platelet count.

Primary site: The site in the body where a cancer originated

Radioactive implant: See *Brachytherapy*

Radiotherapy: The treatment of cancer with high-energy radiation. It includes brachytherapy and teletherapy.

Recurrence: Reappearance of a cancer at its original site after a period of remission.

Remission: The complete or partial disappearance of the signs and symptoms of a disease after treatment, also the period of time that a disease is under control.

Continued

Vocabulary *Continued*

Sarcoma: A type of cancer that forms in the supportive tissues (bone, cartilage, fat, muscle) of the body

Secondary: A term to describe a process or symptom that develops as a result of another (primary) process.

Screening: The search for disease processes, such as cancer, in individuals with no known symptoms

Side effects: The significant **secondary** effects of a specific treatment. **Alopecia** is a common side effect of some chemotherapy.

Staging: An evaluation of the extent of a cancer; necessary in determining treatment

Thoracentesis: A procedure using a large-bore needle to aspirate fluid from the chest cavity

Thrombocytopenia: A low platelet count, which creates a high risk for bleeding

Tissue: A collection of similar cells. The four basic types of body **tissue** are epithelial, connective, muscle, and nerve.

Tumor: An abnormal swelling or mass of tissue that can be either benign or malignant

Ultrasound: An examination that uses high-frequency sound waves to produce images of organs and abnormalities inside the body, also called echography

Venous access device: A catheter implanted into a vein and sutured in place to provide long-term venous access for drawing blood samples and administering IV fluids, chemotherapy, or blood products

Common Abbreviations

ABG	Arterial blood gas (lab)
Acid p'tase	Acid phosphatase (lab)
Adv. Dir.	advance directives
AIDS	Acquired immunodeficiency syndrome
Alb	Albumin (lab)
Alk p'tase	Alkaline phosphatase (lab)
ALL	Acute lymphocytic **leukemia**
AML	Acute myelocytic leukemia
ANLL	Acute nonlymphocytic leukemia
APML	Acute promyelocytic leukemia
Ax	Axillary
Baso	Basophile (lab)
B.E.	Base excess (lab)
Bili	Bilirubin (lab)
BMT	Bone marrow transplant
BSE	Breast self-examination
BSO	Bilateral salpingo-oophorectomy
Bx	Biopsy
C	Cervical
CA	Cancer, carcinoma
CAT	Computerized axial tomography (x-ray)
CK	Creatine kinase (lab)
CL	Central line
CLL	Chronic lymphocytic leukemia
CML	Chronic myelocytic leukemia
CPR	Cardiopulmonary resuscitation
CT	Computerized tomography/ chest tube
CVP	Central venous pressure
DIC	Disseminated intravascular coagulopathy
D.O.	Doctor's order
DPOA	Durable power of attorney (for health care)
DRG	Diagnostic related grouping
DVT	Deep vein thrombosis
Dx	Diagnosis
EGD	Esophagogastroduodenoscopy
ERCP	Endoscopic retrograde cholangiopancreatography
ESR	Erythrocyte sedimentation rate (lab)
Flex Sig	Flexible sigmoidoscopy
HC	Home care
Heme	Hematology
HSV	Herpes simplex virus (lab)
Hyperal	**Hyperalimentation**
IgA (D,E,G)	Gamma (A) immunoglobin (lab)
IS	Incentive spirometry
ITP	Idiopathic thrombocytopenic purpura
LAF	Laminar air flow
LDH	Lactic acid dehydrogenase (lab)
LN	Lymph nodes
LS	Lumbosacral/liver-spleen/lung sounds
Lymphs	Lymphocytes (lab)
MCH	Mean corpuscular hemoglobin (lab)
MCHC	Mean corpuscular hemoglobin concentration (lab)
MCV	Mean corpuscular volume (lab)
Mono	Monocyte (lab)
MPI	Modified protective isolation
MSS	Metabolic support service
Neb	Nebulizer
NH	Nursing home
NSA	Normal serum albumin
NSAID	Nonsteroidal anti-inflammatory drug
O_2sat	Oxygen saturation

Abbreviations and symbols are also essential to effective and efficient communication. Their use increases both speed in writing and speed in reading. For example, "1000 cc D5W" can be written and read much faster than "one thousand cubic centimeters of five percent dextrose in water." Strict guidelines developed by the Joint Commission on Accreditation of Healthcare Organizations (JCAHO) and each institution's medical records committee apply regarding the use of symbols and abbreviations in the medical record. The health unit coordinator must be aware of the guidelines and proficient in the use of approved symbols and abbreviations to ensure effectiveness of all communication. This list contains abbreviations and symbols most commonly used on the Hematology/Oncology Unit.

Common Abbreviations *Continued*

Onc	Oncology
OT	Occupational therapy
Path	Pathology
PC	Packed cells
PCA	Patient-controlled analgesia
Plt	platelets
PPN	Peripheral parenteral nutrition
PPR	Platelet pack, random donors
PPS	Platelet pack, single donor
PRBC	Packed red blood cells
Pro time	Prothrombin time (lab)
PSA	Prostatic-specific **antigen**
PT	Prothrombin time/physical therapy
t**PTT**	Partial thromboplastin time (lab)
Px	**Prognosis**
Rad Tx	Radiation therapy
RBC	Red blood cells (lab)
RNA	Radionuclide angiogram
RT	Respiratory therapy
SBO	Small bowel obstruction
SGOT	Serum glutamic oxaloacetic transaminase (lab)
SGPT	Serum glutamic pyruvic transaminase (lab)
SPEP	Serum protein electrophoresis (lab)
Staph	Staphylococcal
Strep	Streptococcal
SVCS	Superior vena cava syndrome
TC	Throat culture
T&C	Type and crossmatch
TF	Tube feeding
TPN	Total parenteral nutrition
TSCD	TED sequential compression device
US	**Ultrasound**
VAD	**Venous access device**

Medical Terminology Related to Hematology/Oncology

Medical terminology is the language of the medical field and the basis of communication in health care. The ability to thoroughly understand and effectively utilize current terminology is a skill essential to efficient health unit coordinating. The health unit coordinator (HUC) is often called on to translate complex medical terms into understandable language when dealing with patients, their families, and the public.

In addition to basic medical terminology, each unit or department uses terms that are specific to the diagnoses and treatments of the patients cared for and the services provided. Technological advancements and changes in procedures frequently add to the medical terminology related to cancer patients; therefore this list of terms is meant to be broad but not necessarily complete. The terms found in this section are not found in the body of the chapter but are, nonetheless, important for anyone considering a hematology/**oncology** career.

Adenocarcinoma—A form of cancer involving cells lining the walls of various organs in the body

Axillary nodes—Lymph glands located in the armpit (axilla). Certain cancers metastasize to these nodes; therefore, they are usually removed during surgery to determine the need for adjuvant chemotherapy.

Basal cell carcinoma—A common form of skin cancer that grows slowly and seldom metastasizes. It is easily cured when detected and treated promptly.

Benign tumor—An atypical growth that is not cancer and does not metastasize

Biologic response modifiers—A class of compounds produced in the body (e.g., interferon) that stimulate the body's immune system to naturally fight disease

Bone marrow **aspiration** and biopsy—A procedure in which a needle is inserted into the sternum (breastbone) or iliac crest (hip bone) to remove a small amount of bone marrow for microscopic examination. Bone marrow aspiration is the procedure used to harvest **autologous** or donor marrow for use in bone marrow or stem cell transplants.

Brain scan (nuclear)—An imaging examination utilizing intravenously injected radioactive material to detect primary and metastatic cancers

Cancer screening—Periodic health examination to detect **cancer** at an early, curable stage in asymptomatic individuals

Carcinogen—Any substance or agent that produces or increases the risk of developing cancer

Carcinoma in situ—An early and highly curable stage of cancer wherein the disease is still confined to one layer of tissue

Chemoprevention—Attempt to prevent disease by the use of drugs, chemicals, vitamins, or minerals. This concept is under study and is not yet widely accepted.

Combination **chemotherapy**—The use of two or more chemicals to achieve more effective treatment results

Combined modality therapy—The use of two or more types of treatment (surgery, radiation therapy, chemotherapy, or immunotherapy), alternatively or together, to achieve maximum effect

Computerized tomography scan—Specialized x-ray studies (also called **CT** or **CAT** scans) that produce cross-sectional views of the body and are helpful in detecting cancer and metastases

Epidemiology—The study of disease incidence and distribution in populations and the relationship between environment (physical surroundings, occupational hazards, and personal habits) and disease

Erythroplasm—Smooth or grainy red lesion on the mucous membranes of the mouth that may indicate an early cancer

Etiology—The cause(s) of disease

Five-year survival—A term used for the statistical basis of successful treatment. A cancer patient is generally considered cured if the disease has not recurred within 5 years.

Frozen section—Tissue excised, frozen, and cut into thin slices to be microscopically examined

Growth factor—A hormone-like medication that stimulates the production of blood cells in the bone marrow; also called colony-stimulating factor

Hodgkin's disease—A cancer that affects the lymph system and may invade other tissues. It is successfully treated in the majority of patients.

Hospice—In-patient and outpatient psychosocial and supportive care of patients and their families during the terminal stages of illness

Immunotherapy—A treatment that stimulates the body's own immune system to combat diseases such as cancer

In situ—Localized and confined to one area; a very early and highly curable stage of cancer.

Leukoplakia—White plaques on the mucous membranes of the mouth or gums that may indicate early stage cancer

Lymph gland or node—An accumulation of lymphatic tissue found at various intervals throughout the lymph system. Lymph nodes act as filters, keeping particulate matter, especially bacteria, from entering the bloodstream. They may also stop cancer cells but can become a site for metastasis.

Malabsorption—Impaired intestinal absorption of nutrients, common in diseases such as cancer, affecting the mucous membranes of the digestive tract

Monoclonal antibodies—Antibodies designed to seek out chosen targets on cancer cells. They are under study for use to directly deliver chemotherapy or radiotherapy to a cancer, thus sparing the healthy tissue, and for use to diagnose cancers at a early, curable stage.

Mucous membranes—Tissues that line the passages and cavities in the body that communicate with air.

Nodule—A small solid mass

Oncogene—The type of gene that contributes to the malignant transformation of a healthy cell when inappropriately activated

Palliative treatment—Treatment that relieves symptoms of a disease but does not alter the course of the disease

Polyp—A nodular growth of tissue in the lining of a body cavity; it may be benign or malignant

Precancerous—Abnormal changes in the cellular tissue that have the potential of becoming cancerous

Prognosis—A prediction of the course and end of a disease, the future prospects for the patient, and the estimated chance of recovery
Prosthesis—An artificial replacement for a missing part of the body
Radiation **oncologist**—A physician who specializes in the use of x-ray energy to treat cancer
Radiation therapist—A technologist with special training in the operation of the equipment used to treat cancer patients with radiation
Squamous cell carcinoma—A form of skin cancer that can metastasize if not treated
Stomatitis—Oral mucosa inflammation and/or sores resulting from chemotherapy or head and neck radiation; also called mucositis.

Description of the Unit

History

The hematology/oncology unit is a relatively recent addition to the standard nursing units in a modern hospital. Although cancer has been an acknowledged medical problem for much of recorded history, most treatment was unsuccessful and confined to radical or mystical methods before the 18th century. During the 18th century scientists began observing an above-average **incidence** of cancer in certain populations (breast cancer in nuns, scrotal cancer in chimney sweeps, and oral cancer in snuff users) and began to refute some long-held theories. Cancer became an illness worthy of study so as to develop better methods of treatment. Although cancer facilities were built in France, England, and America during the 18th century, most care was delivered in the home with the sole purpose of providing comfort; it wasn't until the 19th century that advancements in treatment were made. By the end of that century the use of anesthesia, the adoption of antiseptic procedures, the discovery of x-ray and radium, and the concept of chemical therapy were established. These set the basis for modern diagnosis and treatment of cancer.

At the beginning of the 20th century only 10 percent of cancer patients survived 5 years after diagnosis. Surgery was the primary method of treatment, and nursing care consisted mainly of care and comfort for the surgical patient. Many hospitals refused terminal care for chronic illnesses such as cancer, so most cancer care was delivered in the home. This offered no opportunity to develop standards of care for cancer patients. By the 1930s, 20 percent of cancer patients survived 5 years after diagnosis. This decade brought advancement in education, both of the public and in the medical field. Public health departments focused on cancer as a public health issue and encouraged the public to recognize and report cancer symptoms early. The federal government established the National Cancer Institute in 1937.

By the 1940s, 25 percent of cancer patients survived 5 years after diagnosis. With the shortage of nurses during World War II, the hospital became the primary site for the delivery of health care. Surgery and radiation therapy were still the primary methods of treatment, but chemotherapy was established as a credible treatment for cancer with the first chemotherapy-induced **remission** of disease. Other advancements in technology increased the complexity of cancer treatment. Just as doctors needed specialized education to treat cancer patients, so too did nurses.

The 1950s brought further progress with cobalt radiation therapy and national testing programs for the development of chemotherapy. Physicians were treating cancer patients with multiple therapies instead of single methods. Cancer nursing education expanded, and a team approach to cancer treatment was developed. By the 1960s over 30 percent of cancer patients survived 5 years after diagnosis. The new specialty of medical **oncology** was established, and these along with other specialty units (coronary care, medical and surgical intensive care units, burn units) were being created in hospitals. In the following 20 years great sums were provided to fund research and development of better ways to diagnose and treat cancer. By the 1980s half of all cancer patients survived 5 years after diagnosis, and hematology/oncology units were a well-established entity in almost all hospitals.

The end of the 20th century finds cancer diagnosis and treatment advanced to include high-tech diagnostic tests offered by radiology, **magnetic resonance imaging**, ultrasound, nuclear medicine, and laboratory, and high-tech, complex treatments including combinations of chemotherapies, immunotherapy, **brachytherapy**, teletherapy, and surgeries. Cancers are being diagnosed earlier and treated more aggressively, which is leading to more successful treatment and longer periods of survival.

Services Provided

As so many things have contributed to the progress of cancer diagnosis and treatment, so too have many things affected the services and operations of hospital hematology/oncology units. At their inception, these units mainly provided postsurgical care and some rudimentary chemotherapies for the newly treated patient, and palliative care for those patients no longer able to be treated; they looked and operated much like any other medical-surgical unit. Today hematology/oncology units may be quite varied in both their look and their operations as they provide the inpatient services of a constantly changing medical specialty. They not only must serve the physical needs of cancer patients but also provide emotional, social, and spiritual support for them and their families.

Today's hematology/oncology unit can offer any number and combination of services depending upon its size, the size of the hospital, and the population that it serves (general community or comprehensive cancer). These services may include some diagnostic and pretherapy work-ups; specialized (GYN, neuro, colorectal) or general pre- and postsurgical care; chemotherapy and immunotherapy; teletherapy and brachytherapy; evaluation of treatment; management of complications from the disease process or the treatment; outpatient or ambulatory care; and palliative care and terminal care. No matter how broad or narrow the scope or how brief or lengthy the duration of service, every hematology/oncology unit provides its patients and their families with focused emotional, social, and spiritual support. Cancer generally is a chronic illness with acute stages; throughout its duration a patient may experience many hospitalizations and will receive services in many different health care settings. The hematology/oncology unit strives to maintain a continuity in all aspects of the patient's care.

Role of the HUC on the Hematology/Oncology Unit

Because much of today's health care is delivered in outpatient settings, the acuity of patients in almost all hospital units is high and most inpatient treatment is complex. Therefore, HUCs working in hospitals must be knowledgeable about all aspects of the services provided and highly skilled to perform their jobs accurately, efficiently, and effectively. The HUC working on a hematology/oncology unit is no different. The remainder of this chapter will give the reader an overview of the services provided on the hematology/oncology unit and of the HUC's role and responsibility regarding those services.

Diagnostic Procedures

Diagnostic procedures are used with great frequency on the hematology/oncology unit. They are used to assist the physician in initially diagnosing, **staging**, and determining the treatment of cancer. They are used throughout treatment to monitor the patient's response. They are used to identify complications of the disease process, **recurrence** of disease, and side effects of treatment. Every body system can be affected, and almost every diagnostic procedure can be utilized. It is important to note that no single diagnostic procedure is conclusive in itself.

Categories and Purposes of Diagnostic Procedures

The following are the categories and purposes of the diagnostic procedures used on the hematology/oncology unit, with a list of frequently used tests in each category.

Laboratory

Clinical laboratory studies may be performed on blood, urine, sputum, feces, and other body fluids or tissues, which are obtained by simple collection or through invasive procedures. They provide information regarding the functioning of specific organs and the alteration of the body's metabolic process. As such, they are an integral part of diagnosing cancer and monitoring treatment. Abnormal test results can have various causes (no test is specific or sensitive to only one type of disease). Therefore, the significances listed pertain only to hematology and oncology.

Biochemistry Tests	Significance
Acid phosphatase **(acid p'tase)**	Acute leukemia, multiple myeloma, metastatic (bone) breast and prostate cancer.
*Alkaline phosphatase **(alk p'tase)**	Liver and bone cancer, leukemia and **lymphoma, tumors** causing extrahepatic biliary obstruction.
*Amylase	Lung and ovarian cancer.
*Calcium (Ca)	Leukemia, lymphoma, and multiple myeloma, lung (squamous), liver, esophagus, parathyroid, bladder, kidney, pancreas, and metastatic bone cancer.
Cholesterol	Prostate, liver, pancreas, and bone cancer.
Ferritin	Acute myeloblastic and lymphoblastic leukemia, Hodgkin's lymphoma, breast cancer.
*Glucose (BS)	Pheochromocytoma, glucagonoma, pancreas, islet cell, adrenal gland and stomach cancer, fibrosarcoma.
Haptoglobin	Lymphoma, metastatic cancer.
Immunoglobulins (IgA, IgD, IgE, IgG, IgM)	Myeloma, advanced neoplasms.
*Lactic dehydrogenase **(LDH)**	Liver and metastatic cancers, acute leukemia, lymphoma.
Lysozyme	Acute monocytic and myelomonocytic leukemia, chronic myeloid leukemia.
Parathyroid hormone (PTH)	Kidney, pancreas, ovary, and lung (squamous) cancer.
Progesterone	Adrenocortical and leuteinizing tumors.
*Serum alanine aminotransferase (**SGPT**, ALT)	Metastatic liver cancer.
*Serum aspartate aminotransferase (**SGOT**, AST)	Metastatic liver cancer.
Serum gamma glutamyl transferase (SGGT)	Pancreas and metastatic liver cancer.
*Uric acid	Leukemia, multiple myeloma, Hodgkin's lymphoma, lung, and disseminated cancer.

Tumor Markers	Significance
Alpha-fetoprotein (AFP)	Germ cell testicular cancer, pancreas, colon, lung, stomach, and biliary system cancer.
beta human chorionic gonadotropin (βHCG)	Choriocarcinoma, germ cell testicular cancer, stomach, pancreas, liver, lung, and colon cancer.
CA-125	Ovarian cancer.

Tumor Markers	Significance
CA-15-3	Metastatic and recurrent breast cancer.
CA-19-9	Pancreas, stomach, and colorectal cancer.
Calcitonin	Thyroid, lung (small cell), breast cancer.
Carcinoembryonic antigen (CEA)	Colon, rectal, stomach, pancreas, prostate, lung, and breast cancer.
Prostatic acid phosphatase (PAP)	Metastatic prostate cancer.
Prostatic-specific antigen (**PSA**)	Prostate cancer.

Hematology	Significance
*Hematocrit (Hct)	Nonspecific **anemia**.
*Hemoglobin (HgB)	Nonspecific anemia.
*Leukocyte count (WBC)	Leukemia, lymphomas, tumors involving peripheral blood marrow.
*Leukocyte differential (diff.) Basophils, eosinophils, lymphocytes, monocytes, neutrophils (banded and segmented)	All leukemias, lymphomas, including myelomas, **sarcoma**, and metastatic cancer.
*Platelet count (**Plt** ct)	All leukemias, lymphomas, multiple myeloma, carcinoma.

The laboratory tests listed above with an asterisk (*), along with the following tests, are affected by chemotherapy and thus necessary in monitoring treatment.

Bilirubin, total, direct, indirect (**bili**)
Blood urea nitrogen (BUN)
Creatinine (creat)
Creatinine clearance (creat cl)
Magnesium (Mg)
Partial thromboplastin time (**PTT**, APTT)
Potassium (K^+)
Prothrombin time (**PT**)
Reticulocytes (retic ct)
Sodium (Na^+)

Diagnostic Imaging

Diagnostic Imaging includes radiography, xerography, tomography, computerized axial tomography (CT, CAT), ultrasound (**US**) or echography (echo), magnetic resonance imaging (MR, MRI), and nuclear medicine imaging. Most of these procedures are noninvasive, but many call for the use of contrast agents requiring preparations that may include cathartic medications, enemas, and meal restrictions. These procedures provide information regarding the presence or absence of tumor, the character of tissue, the extent or spread of disease, and the staging of disease. They can also be used to localize a tumor for biopsy. Technology continues to dramatically advance this aspect of health care, creating many diagnostic options that formerly were unavailable or available only with surgical procedures. Each type of procedure is preferred for certain types and location of disease, and different procedures are selected according to this preference and the specific circumstances that each case presents.

Conventional radiology continues to be utilized in initial work-ups, with the use of external radiation for chest, abdomen, and bone. Contrast studies such as upper gastrointestinal (UGI) and barium enema (BE, Ba En) for the digestive tract, intravenous pyelogram (IVP) for the urinary tract, myelogram for the spinal canal, and angiography for the brain and lymph system are useful initial exams. Contrast studies remain the best diagnostic imaging examination for stomach and colon cancers.

Xerography is the method and **mammography** the examination of choice for early detection of breast cancer.

Tomography is utilized to identify small **lesions** in the kidneys, chest, and mediastinum.

Computerized axial tomography combines external radiation with computers to produce images. It is utilized most frequently in the following circumstances:

Head and neck cancers	Tumor identification, staging, follow-up.
Esophageal cancers	Extent of penetration (tumor measurement), and staging.
Lung cancers	Parenchyma and mediastinal nodes: identify nodes for biopsy; eliminates need for surgery.
Liver cancers	Some physicians prefer the MRI.
Kidney cancer	Staging and follow-up.

Magnetic resonance imaging uses strong magnetic fields to visualize areas that are normally obscured by bone. It is the examination of choice for brain and central nervous system (CNS) cancers and is used for staging and in follow-up of musculoskeletal cancers.

Ultrasound employs high-frequency sound waves to produce images; it is used most frequently to visualize abdominal, peritoneal, and pelvic tumors. It is often the method of choice in localizing tumors for fine-needle aspiration biopsies.

Nuclear medicine scans utilize an internal source of radiation, administered either orally or intravenously, to identify disease processes in both bone and soft tissue. They are used to identify bone metastases and thyroid, brain, and liver cancers. The molecular coincidence detection (MCD) scan can detect metabolically active tumors and metastases throughout the body.

Other Diagnostic Procedures

Endoscopy is an invasive procedure that allows internal visualization of body cavities and organs. Patients may require conscious sedation or general anesthesia. During these procedures, tumors can be located, biopsied, and sometimes excised. Areas of the body include esophagus, stomach, and duodenum (UGI endoscopy); biliary tract and pancreas (endoscopic retrograde cholangiopancreatography, **ERCP**); larynx, upper airway, and bronchial tree (bronchoscopy); anal canal, rectum, and sigmoid (sigmoidoscopy); large intestine (colonoscopy); cervix and vagina (colposcopy); peritoneal cavity (laparoscopy); and mediastinum (mediastinoscopy).

Biopsy is the most definitive means of diagnosing all cancers and of staging and grading many of them. Since cancers in the same organ but of different types require different treatments, it is necessary to not only locate the tumor but also identify it. Once a tumor had been located, histologic (tissue) or cytologic (cellular) specimens are obtained through a variety of methods, placed in the proper collection medium (preservative), and transported to the laboratory, where they are processed for microscopic examination by a pathologist. The validity of the results depends initially upon the quality of the specimen and the accuracy of the collection process. The **pathology** report will identify the type of tissue, the presence or absence of malignancy, the grade of the malignancy (how the tumor cells compare with normal cells of that type) and stage, if possible. These results are essential in diagnosing, determining treatment, assessing response to treatment, and establishing cure or recurrence of disease. The following are methods of obtaining specimens for biopsy.

Cytologic

Tissue scrapings	Usually of external (skin) or internal (cervical) linings. Pap smears are the common method of obtaining cervical scrapings for **cytology**.
Secretions	Sputum is one of the most common secretions and may be obtained by spontaneous or induced collection. Secretions may also be obtained during endoscopic procedures.
Washings	Cells obtained when applying a wash solution to the surface area of a body cavity. Usually obtained in endoscopic procedures, such as bronchoscopy.

Aspirations	Body fluids obtained during procedures such as **thoracentesis** (pleural fluid), **paracentesis** (abdominal fluid), and lumbar puncture (cerebrospinal fluid). Fine needle aspirations from a tumor site may be obtained under direction by ultrasound.

Histologic

Aspirations	The most common aspiration process that produces tissue is a sternal puncture, which obtains bone marrow.
Needle biopsy	Core tissue from a tumor site is obtained either during surgery or percutaneously during a sterile procedure using a topical or local anesthetic.
Excisional biopsy	The entire mass with only a small amount of surrounding tissue is removed. These are minor surgical procedures performed on the skin (lip, nose, ear, mole lesion site) on the breast, or on internal surfaces during endoscopy. Excision biopsies of the skin may also be the only necessary therapy.
Incisional biopsy	A portion of a large tumor, with some adjacent normal tissue, is removed using a small incision during a surgical procedure.

In addition to all these tests to diagnose, determine, and monitor treatment, many other diagnostic tests are performed on **heme/onc** patients to assess their ability to tolerate aggressive treatments (cardiac studies such as EKG, echocardiogram, radionuclide angiography, sestamibi, and pulmonary function studies). Tests are also done to identify side effects of treatment and complications of disease process, such as bacterial, viral, and fungal laboratory studies of blood and body fluids, chest and sinus x-rays to identify infections, and peripheral vascular studies (Dopplers) and **nuclear scans** (VQ lung scan) to identify blood clots.

The HUC Role and Responsibility Regarding Diagnostic Procedures

Heme/onc HUCs must be familiar with a broad range of diagnostic procedures and the methods of scheduling, sequencing, specimen collection, and patient preparation. They must know all the contraindications for the various exams so as to facilitate fast and effective testing and prompt reporting of results. Inaccuracy in arranging diagnostic procedures can create delays or errors in treatment and have grave consequences for the patient. New diagnostic methods are continually being developed to aid in the treatment of cancer, and heme/onc HUCs must keep their knowledge current.

Medications Specific to Hematology/ Oncology Units

Cancer has become primarily a medically treated disease; although there are other methods of treatment, most are used in combination with chemotherapy and other medicines. Cancer is often a disease of adults and older adults who frequently have additional health problems (e.g., diabetes, pulmonary disease, cardiovascular disease) that require medication. Cancer is a disease that secondarily affects many body systems, which then require medication. And cancer treatment has many **side effects** that require medication to prevent or palliate. For these reasons it would be impossible to discuss the services of the hematology/oncology unit without mentioning medications. And, for the same reasons, it would be impossible to discuss all the medications frequently used there.

Categories and Purposes of Medications

In an attempt to give the reader an idea of the multitude of medications specific to the hematology/oncology unit, the following are the categories and purposes of the frequently used medications with a list of some medications in each category.

Chemotherapy

The primary purpose of chemotherapy is to cure or arrest the progression of disease. It is given alone or in combination with other medications or treatments.

Alkylating Agents
- Busulfan
- Cyclophosphamide
- Chlorambucil
- Mechlorethamine

Antimetabolites
- Cytosine arabinoside
- 5-Fluorouracil
- Methotrexate
- 6-Thioguanine

Antibiotics
- Bleomycin
- Daunorubicin HCl
- Doxorubicin HCl
- Mitomycin

Plant Alkaloids
- Vinblastine
- Vincristine

Nitrosoureas
- Carmustine
- Semustine
- Streptozocin

Hormones
- **Androgens**
- Corticosteroids
- **Estrogens**
- Progestins
- Antiadrenals
- Antiandrogens
- Antiestrogens

Biotherapy
- Hematopoietic growth factors
- **Interferons**
- Interleukins

Miscellaneous
- Asparaginase
- Cisplatin
- Hydroxyurea
- Procarbazine

Antimicrobials

Antimicrobials are given to fight infections that result either from the disease process or secondarily from the side effects of cancer treatment. These medications are listed by the type of infection that they are used to treat.

Bacteria
- Aminoglycosides
- Cephalosporins
- Penicillins
- Clindamycin
- Erythromycin
- Vancomycin

Fungus
- Amphotericin B
- 5-Fluorocytosine

Protozoa
- Trimethoprim-sulfamethoxazole
- Pentamidine isethionate

Virus
- Acyclovir
- Alpha-interferon
- Vidarabine

Analgesics

Analgesics are used for pain management in cancer patients. Pain is a commom symptom of cancer (especially advanced cancer) and a frequent side effect of cancer treatments.

Narcotics
- Codeine

Hydromorphome
Levorphalol
Meperidine
Methadone
Morphine
Oxycodone
Oxymorphone

Non-narcotics

Acetaminophen
Nonsteroidal anti-inflammatory drugs (NSAIDs)
Salicylate

Antiemetics

Antiemetics are used to control nausea and vomiting, which are common side effects of cancer treatment.

Chlorpromazine HCl
Dexamethasone
Diphenhydramine
Dronabinol
Lorazepam
Metoclopramide
Ondansetron
Prochlorperazine
Promethazine
Synthetic cannabinoids
Trimethobenzamide HCl

Miscellaneous

Cancer patients may develop hypo- or hypercoagulation problems for which coagulants, such as phytonadione (AquaMEPHYTON, vitamin K), and anticoagulants, such as heparin and warfarin (Coumadin), are used. They also experience nutritional problems such as loss of appetite and anorexia for which corticosteroids and progestational agents are used to increase appetite and total parenteral nutrition (**TPN**) or hyperalimentation given to provide complete nourishment.

The HUC Role and Responsibility Regarding Medications

The heme/onc HUC must be familiar with a broader range of medications and their common dosages and routes than HUCs who work in most other specialty units. Since many chemotherapies are given in combinations and with adjuvant medications and in cycles with set schedules, heme/onc HUCs must be aware of these combinations and the cycles and schedules. Additional biologic and chemical therapies are being developed daily, and many heme/onc units are involved in the clinical investigations to determine their efficacy. They may also be involved in the **clinical trials** of newly proposed combination therapies. The heme/onc HUC must be knowledgeable about the protocols involved with these investigations.

Patients receiving chemotherapy must be closely monitored. Since many of the monitoring studies will be the same for each patient, as well as the other treatments surrounding the chemotherapy, physicians often prepare preprinted orders for each type of therapy (Fig. 7–1).

Treatments and Procedures Specific to the Cancer Patient

The goal of cancer treatment is cure, with cure defined as patient survival for 5 years following diagnosis. Some cancers have a higher cure rate than others, but, generally, 50 percent of all cancer cases diagnosed today can be cured. When cure is not possible, the goal of treatment may be to prolong life or to improve the quality of remaining life. Response to treatment is assessed as follows: complete remission, wherein all signs and symptoms disappear for a minimum of 4 weeks, and normal function returns; partial remission, wherein tumor size is reduced by at least one half; improvement, wherein tumor size is reduced by one quarter to one half, and some improvement in function is realized; no response, wherein there is no change in tumor size or functional status; and progression, wherein there is new tumor growth, new metastases, or reappearance of an old lesion. Even when cure or complete remission is obtained, some cancers can recur after an extended period of time. Clinical trials to determine the effectiveness of types and combi-

PREPRINTED PHYSICIAN'S ORDERS
HIGH DOSE CISPLATIN WITH AMIPOSTINE (PH-803)
Page 1 of 3

Date	Time	ORDERS	Physician	Nurse
		ANY ORDERS CROSSED OFF ARE NOT TO BE IMPLEMENTED.		
		Diagnosis:		
		Cycle: Karnofsky PS (0-100) ____________		
		Height (cm): ____________ Weight (kg): ____________		
		BSA ____________ m^2 BSA used: ____________ m^2		
		Treatment initiation plan/Protocol #		
		Platelet = ____________ Absolute neutrophil (ANC) = ____________		
		Baseline calculated creatinine clearance = ____________		
		1. Dr. Six Status: ____________		
		2. Allergies: ____________		
		3. Consults: ____________		
		4. Daily weight.		
		5. Regular diet.		
		6. DO NOT WRITE/ORDER ANY P.O. OR I.V. MEDS WITHOUT NOTIFYING DR. ____________.		
		7. PATIENTS SHOULD NOT BE PRETREATED WITH ANTIHYPERTENSIVES OR DIRUETICS FOR AT LEAST 24 HOURS BEFORE OR AFTER AMIFOSTINE/CISPLATIN without prior approval from the above physician.		
		8. The following medications are not to be administered for four days prior to and until 24 hours after the cisplatin/amifostine course of treatment: Nonsteroidal Anti-Inflammatory Agents: Nephrotoxic Agents: aminoglycosides, lithium, Bactrim trimethoprim/ sulfamethoxazole, loop diuretics, etc. I.V. Contrast for Radiographic Studies.		
		9. Vital signs q. 4^0 after chemo on day 1; then q. 8^0		
		10. Check bed for availability Trendelenburg position.		
		11. Take three supine systolic blood pressures during the 2 hours prior to drug administration. Use the average and determine grouping of systolic blood pressure prior to amifostine on table below.		

Guidelines for Interrupting Amifostine Infusion:

Baseline systolic BP (mmHg):	<100	100-119	120-139	140-179	>180
Decrease in systolic BP requiring interruption of amifostine infusion	20	25	30	40	50

Rev: 6/16/97 S
White - Hospital Chart *Yellow - Pharmacy* *Pink - History Section of Chart*

PREPRINTED PHYSICIAN'S OR
HIGH DOSE CISPLATIN WITH A

Date	Time	
		12. Determine thresh relevant decrease shown in the table
		13. Measure the blood druing amifostine finished.
		14. Insert foley cathet
		15. I & O q. 4 hours.
		16. Check blood gluc physician if blood
		17. Establish 2 IV site
		18. Have 2 IV pumps
		19. Labs - STAT befo creatinine and Mg
		20. Na, K, BUN, Crea
		21. Have available 3
		22. NS 1000 cc/hour
		23. Continue NS thro
		24. Discontinue NS in cisplatin infusion.
		25. No other drug or I with amifostine. A
		26. Mannitol 12.5 gm cc/hour and/or I > If no response wit
		27. Granisetron 1 mg
		28. Dexamethasone 2 Dexamethason 10
		29. Lorazepam 1 mg 12 hours after Cis
		30. Diphenhydramine
		31. Administer amifos solution as acontinuous infusion over 15 minutes. Flush the line with 20 cc NS. Total infusion time of amifostine plus the 20 cc NS flush should take 15 minutes. The patient must remain supine during the amifostine infusion.

Rev: 6/16/97 S
White - Hospital Chart *Yellow - Pharmacy* *Pink - History Section of Chart*

PREPRINTED PHYSICIAN'S
HIGH DOSE CISPLATIN WIT

Date	Time	
		32. Amifostine sh threshold valu cerebral or ca
		33. If hypotension normal saline BP returns to b
		34. If the patient's within 5 minute asymptomatic perfusion, ther times as nece should be mor infusion.
		35. Cisplatin (120 saline solution infusion and a
		36. Mannitol 25 gr
		37. Vinblastine (3. immediately fo
		38. Other chemoth ______ mg ______ mg ______ mg
		39. Resume IV hy after vinblastin until discharge
		40. Magnesium su gm IV, if Mg++
		41. Peri-Colace 1
		42. Compazine 10 PRN after che

Rev: 6/16/97 S
White - Hospital Chart *Yellow - Pharmacy* *Pink - History Section of Chart*

Figure 7–1
An example of preprinted physician's orders. (Courtesy of St. Joseph's Hospital, Marshfield, WI.)

nations of treatments are run throughout the United States at various hospitals and cancer centers under the auspices of many organizations (e.g., the Eastern Cooperative Oncology Group, the Southwest Oncology Group, the Cancer and Leukemia Group, M.D. Anderson, Pharmaceutical Oncology or Hematology, and the National Cancer Institute). When institutions cooperate in these trials, strict rules of protocol must be followed to ensure the accuracy of results.

Many factors contribute to the decision regarding treatment, some of which are age and general health of the patient, type of cancer, stage and grade of cancer or how early diagnosed, variety of treatments available, side effects of treatment, and wishes of the patient. Primary treatment may be a single type or a combination of different methods. Secondary treatment is often included as a planned aspect of treatment or as a response to the side effects or complications of primary treatment. The following is a list, including a brief description, of the primary treatments, some secondary treatments, and some related procedures.

Primary Treatments

Surgery is a localized treatment and the oldest known treatment for cancer; it remains an important component of cancer treatment. It may be used as the definitive treatment or in combination with chemotherapy or radiation therapy. It may be an open procedure or done with the use of a laparoscope or endoscope. The type of surgical procedure depends upon the site and the cellular classification of the tumor. Local excision is used when the lesion is small and the entire tumor can be removed along with a sufficient margin of surrounding healthy tissue. This includes tumors of the skin, lip, and ear. Major resections are used when the tumor (whether primary or metastatic) can be reached and removed in its entirety along with sufficient surrounding healthy tissue and associated lymph nodes. These resections can alter the patient's appearance and affect body functions (e.g., colostomy for colon cancer, amputation for bone cancer, mastectomy for breast cancer, laryngectomy for throat cancer). Surgery may be combined with adjuvant therapies to enhance the cure rate. These therapies include chemotherapy for control of metastases (e.g., in breast and ovarian cancer) and radiation therapy for local tumor control (e.g., in brain cancers). They may be administered before, during, or after surgery.

When cure is not feasible, palliative surgery becomes part of cancer treatment. This can include a number of surgeries to relieve obstruction throughout the body (e.g., airway, gastrointestinal, and urinary obstructions), surgeries to relieve compression by tumor on vital body structures (e.g., brain and spinal column tumors causing paralysis), and surgeries to control pain, such as nerve blocks and cordotomies.

Surgery is also used to treat complications of cancer and its treatments, to implant devices used to administer chemotherapy, and after cancer treatment as a method of rehabilitation to restore body function or appearance (e.g., surgically implanted prosthetics after limb amputation and breast reconstruction after mastectomy).

Medical treatment for cancer includes chemotherapy and biotherapy (see under *Medications Specific to Hematology/Oncology Units*). Although their mechanisms are different, they are both systemic treatments that cure cancer in its cellular stage. Biotherapy has only recently come into its own, with development and trial in the last two decades and more prevalent use in the current decade.

Chemotherapy can include a single drug or combinations of two or three drugs. It may be the definitive treatment or **adjuvant therapy** with surgery or radiation. Many kinds of cancers can be cured by chemotherapy alone or with multimodal treatment. These include acute leukemias, Hodgkin's and non-Hodgkin's lymphomas, myosarcoma, Ewing's sarcoma, choriocarcinoma, neuroblastoma, ovarian cancer, small cell lung cancer, testicular cancer, breast cancer, colorectal cancer, and osteogenic and soft tissue sarcomas. Many other cancers respond to but are not cured by chemotherapy. Some cancers do not respond well to chemotherapy. These include liver cancer, **melanoma**, non–small cell lung cancer, pancreatic cancer, renal cancer, and thyroid cancer.

Because chemotherapy destroys a certain percentage of cancer cells with each administration, it must be administered at intervals over an extended time (months) to be effective. It can be administered by a variety of methods, with the chosen method being the most effective. These methods include *intravenous,* to achieve rapid therapeutic blood levels and because many chemotherapies are not absorbed in the GI tract; *intrathecal,* to cross the blood-brain barrier; *intracavitary,* within the bladder, peritoneum, pleura, or pericardium, to treat malignant effusions and well-localized tumors; and *intra-arterial,* with a large amount of drug given through the artery that supplies the area of a localized primary or metastatic tumor.

A variety of equipment is used to administer chemotherapy (see under *Equipment and Supplies used in the Hematology/Oncology Unit*) along with a number of catheters, lines, and tubes. Chemotherapy is a caustic agent, some drugs being classified as irritants (producing pain and inflammation at the administration site and along the course of the vein) and some as vesicants (causing cellular damage or tissue destruction if they come into contact with subcutaneous tissue). Care must be taken in the handling, administering, and disposing of these drugs. Nurses who work with chemotherapy are specially trained.

Because chemotherapy is a caustic and systemic treatment, it has many side effects that must also be treated. It is important to note that not every drug has the same side effects and not every patient responds in the same manner. Some of these side effects are bone marrow suppression resulting in leukopenia, which makes the patient susceptible to serious infections; and **thrombocytopenia**, which makes the patient susceptible to hemorrhaging.

Gastrointestinal irritation results in nausea and vomiting (in only 30 percent of patients receiving chemotherapy), stomatitis, alteration in taste, anorexia, and diarrhea, which all affect nutritional balance and may place the patient at an increased risk for infection. Alopecia may result in an emotional reaction to the change in appearance, and germinal tissue effects may cause problems with sexual function and reproduction. Because chemotherapy works systemically, it can have an effect on various body organs resulting in cardiotoxicity, hepatotoxicity, neurotoxicity, pulmonary toxicity, and nephrotoxicity. Close monitoring of patients receiving chemotherapy is essential in the prevention and early treatment of side effects.

Radiotherapy (also called radiation therapy) has been used as a localized treatment for cancer since the early 1900s. Although effective early on, it was very rudimentary and often caused as many problems as it cured. Advancements in technology throughout the century allowed for improvements in treatment and reduction in damage to healthy tissue and other side effects. By the 1970s, radiation therapy had become an established discipline within oncology, and the last decade of the century finds 60 percent of all cancer patients being treated with **radiotherapy** at some time during their illness. Cancers curable by radiation include skin, early-stage Hodgkin's, early-stage breast following lumpectomy, seminoma, stage II uterine, vocal cord–laryngeal, thyroid, prostate, bladder, and anal canal. Cancers treated by adjuvant radiation include bladder, later stage breast, head and neck, brain, lung, esophagus, rectum, and soft tissue sarcoma. Radiotherapy can prevent brain metastases from lung cancer, and it is used to palliate pain, bleeding, and pressure caused by treatment or disease. Radiotherapy is the use of high-energy ionizing rays or particles to cure disease, control its growth, prevent metastases, or improve the quality of life. It can be administered externally or internally and is used as both primary treatment and adjuvant treatment with surgery or chemotherapy. The method and duration of treatment depend upon many considerations: type, location, and extent of disease; intent of treatment; the patient's general state of health; and the patient's wishes, among others.

External radiation (*teletherapy*) is the most common method of radiotherapy and is delivered by a radioactive source from a machine placed some distance from the patient. It is usually given in small doses once or twice a day, 5 days a week, for 6 to 8 weeks. The duration may be shorter if the treatment is for palliation instead of cure. Although in-patient treatments may be necessary initially (especially if used adjuvantly with surgery or chemotherapy), most external radiation is administered as an outpatient service, with patients being hospitalized only to treat complications or side effects. Some protocols call for radiation and chemotherapy to be administered concurrently. One-time, high-dose external radiation may be administered intraoperatively during a surgical procedure, with or without a follow-up series of lower dose treatments.

Internal radiation (*brachytherapy*) employs encapsulated (implanted) or unencapsulated (oral or intravenous) radioactive isotopes to deliver a higher total dose of radiation over a shorter time. With encapsulated implants, a container of radioactive material is placed in a body cavity (e.g., uterus, cervix); alternatively, needles, tubes, or seeds of radioactive material are placed directly into the tissues (e.g., brain, breast, prostate, head and neck). Placement is most often done in surgery or under the direction of ultrasound or CT. The container is kept in place for a number of days, during which time the patient is hospitalized in radioactive isolation. Strict procedures are followed regarding visitors (no children under the age of 18 and no pregnant women) and length of exposure to visitors and staff; the patient may not leave the room. When the implant is removed, the restrictions no longer apply and the patient is discharged.

When unencapsulated radioisotopes are administered by injection or orally (e.g., iodine-131 treatment for thyroid cancer), the radioactivity travels throughout the patient's system to the tumor site. As a result, for a time the patient's body secretions are radioactive. A standard protocol is followed to protect against contamination (see Fig. 7–12), and the patient remains hospitalized in strict radiation isolation for 3 to 7 days. Each day the level of radiation diminishes; when a safe level is reached, the patient is discharged. Most institutions employ a radiation safety officer to monitor care and procedures associated with radiation exposure.

The side effects of radiotherapy may include skin breakdown, bone marrow suppression, infection, and fatigue; nausea, vomiting, stomatitis, and anorexia resulting in malnutrition; esophagitis, cough, pneumonitis, and fibrosis; gastritis, diarrhea, and cystitis; and cerebral edema, alopecia, and tooth decay. Side effects are specific to the area of the body being treated, the type of treatment, and the reaction of the individual patient; they may occur early in treatment or may be delayed reactions. Treatment or prevention of side effects and complications requires supportive therapy and may necessitate longer hospitalization or rehospitalization.

Bone marrow or stem cell transplant is one of the newest forms of cancer therapy. The first transplants were performed in the 1950s, with no survival success but with enough effect on disease that further study was warranted. Clinical trials resumed in the 1970s, with the success rates increasing each decade as improved aspects of treatment reduced the frequency and intensity of graft-versus-host disease, enhanced engraftment, and made more types of transplants available. In 1987, a national donor registry was created, enabling more patients to locate donors with matched marrow.

Bone marrow transplant (**BMT**) is a lengthy, complex, highly intensive, expensive therapy that carries higher risks of those complications mentioned in connection with standard chemotherapy and radiotherapy. It is the treatment of choice in only a small number of cancers. It is used to treat leukemias (**AML**, **ALL**, **CML**), multiple myeloma, lymphomas, and Hodgkin's and non-Hodgkin's lymphoma and may be considered in breast and germ cell cancers and neuroblastoma. The treatment carries with it a very high risk of long-term side effects and lethal complications but offers the only chance of cure for many patients.

There are three types of marrow transplants: *syngeneic* (marrow donated from an identical twin), *allogeneic* (closely matched marrow donated from a related or unrelated person), and *autologous* (marrow from the patient's own system harvested during a remission phase). Although the regimens vary somewhat among the different types of transplants, they all have these same six stages:

1. *Preparation,* which includes medical evaluation, orientation, **informed consent**, education for patient and family, marrow harvest for autologous transplants, and central venous access establishment. Some of this stage may be done on an outpatient basis.
2. *Conditioning,* which includes the administration of extremely high dose chemotherapy and/or total body irradiation; it prepares the patient's body for successful grafting by eliminating all malignant cells and ablating the patient's immune system. During this time the patient is monitored closely to control immediate side effects and seri-

ous, life-threatening complications. Side effects of this stage of treatment remain a long-term possibility.

3. *Transplant,* which includes an intravenous infusion of the bone marrow or stem cells. Strict protocol is followed, and the patient is monitored for any signs of reaction (Fig. 7–2).

4. *Waiting for engraftment,* which includes continued close monitoring, supportive treatment, and management of complications while awaiting signs of engraftment.

5. *Engraftment and early recovery,* which includes evidence of engraftment and immune system and hematopoietic function recovery. Again, close monitoring, supportive treatment, and management of complications are a vital aspect of this stage. Graft-versus-host disease is a possibility from this stage on.

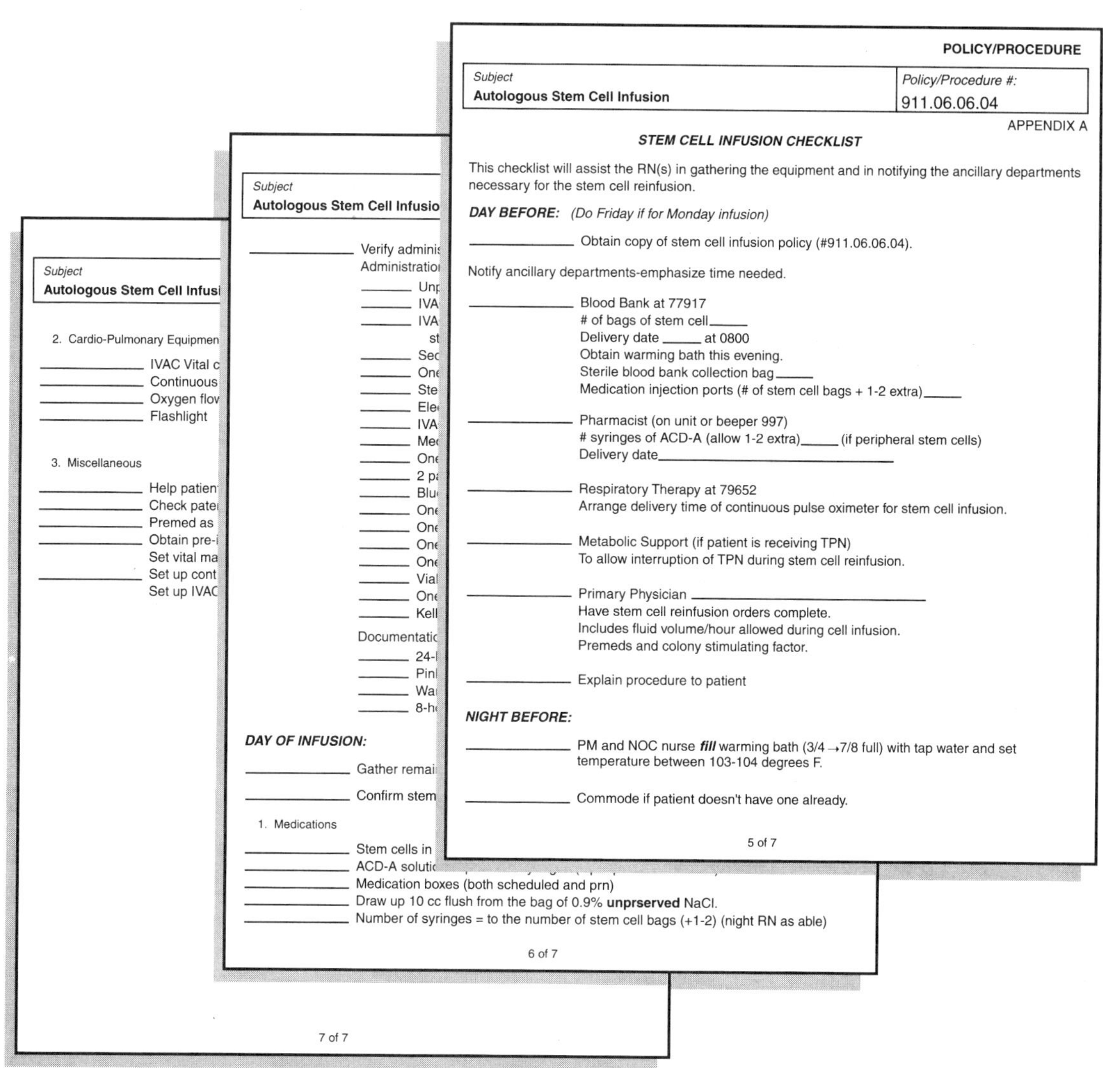

POLICY/PROCEDURE

Subject Autologous Stem Cell Infusion	*Policy/Procedure #:* 911.06.06.04

APPENDIX A

STEM CELL INFUSION CHECKLIST

This checklist will assist the RN(s) in gathering the equipment and in notifying the ancillary departments necessary for the stem cell reinfusion.

DAY BEFORE: *(Do Friday if for Monday infusion)*

________ Obtain copy of stem cell infusion policy (#911.06.06.04).

Notify ancillary departments-emphasize time needed.

________ Blood Bank at 77917
\# of bags of stem cell____
Delivery date ____ at 0800
Obtain warming bath this evening.
Sterile blood bank collection bag____
Medication injection ports (# of stem cell bags + 1-2 extra)____

________ Pharmacist (on unit or beeper 997)
\# syringes of ACD-A (allow 1-2 extra)____ (if peripheral stem cells)
Delivery date________

________ Respiratory Therapy at 79652
Arrange delivery time of continuous pulse oximeter for stem cell infusion.

________ Metabolic Support (if patient is receiving TPN)
To allow interruption of TPN during stem cell reinfusion.

________ Primary Physician ________
Have stem cell reinfusion orders complete.
Includes fluid volume/hour allowed during cell infusion.
Premeds and colony stimulating factor.

________ Explain procedure to patient

NIGHT BEFORE:

________ PM and NOC nurse ***fill*** warming bath (3/4 → 7/8 full) with tap water and set temperature between 103-104 degrees F.

________ Commode if patient doesn't have one already.

5 of 7

Subject
Autologous Stem Cell Infusio

________ Verify adminis
Administratio

DAY OF INFUSION:

________ Gather remai

________ Confirm stem

1. Medications

________ Stem cells in
________ ACD-A solutio
________ Medication boxes (both scheduled and prn)
________ Draw up 10 cc flush from the bag of 0.9% **unprserved** NaCl.
________ Number of syringes = to the number of stem cell bags (+1-2) (night RN as able)

6 of 7

Subject
Autologous Stem Cell Infusi

2. Cardio-Pulmonary Equipmen

________ IVAC Vital c
________ Continuous
________ Oxygen flov
________ Flashlight

3. Miscellaneous

________ Help patien
________ Check pate
________ Premed as
________ Obtain pre-i
Set vital ma
________ Set up cont
Set up IVAC

7 of 7

Figure 7–2
Stem cell infusion checklist. (Courtesy of St. Joseph's Hospital, Marshfield, WI.)

6. *Long-term recovery,* which includes discharge and outpatient monitoring for possible late complications. Subsequent complications may require rehospitalization.

Long-term therapies such as BMT require the most frequent use of supportive treatments.

Secondary Treatments

Blood Products

Blood product support is one of the most common types of secondary treatment in cancer care, because bleeding, coagulation problems, and anemia occur as an aspect of the disease process and as a side effect of the many treatments.

Packed red blood cells (**PRBCs**) are treatment for anemia (low hemoglobin) and active bleeding. They may need to be filtered or washed to remove leukocytes (leukopoor PRBCs) in transfusions for patients who have had previous transfusion reactions. They may also require irradiation to inactivate lymphocytes for severely immunosuppressed patients. Transfusion reaction (chills, fever, severe itching) is common in hematology/oncology patients; therefore, they often receive medications prior to transfusions to help prevent reaction. Cytomegalovirus (CMV) negative blood products may be necessary for patients who are severely immunosuppressed and have not been exposed to CMV. These patients risk death if they develop CMV pneumonitis.

Platelet concentrates are treatment for thrombocytopenia (low platelet count) and active bleeding and are given prior to some procedures that have a blood loss potential. Random donor (RD) platelets are collected from six to ten donors and pooled into one bag for transfusion. They are used for patients who have had either no previous transfusions or no previous transfusion reactions. Once the platelets have been pooled, they must be infused within 4 hours. Single donor (SD) platelets are collected from one donor. They are used for patients who have not had a therapeutic response from RD platelets or who are at risk for developing an allergy to transfusions. Human leukocyte antigen (HLA) platelets are collected from one donor who matches the patient with more than the standard ABO antigens. They are used for patients who no longer experience a therapeutic response to RD or SD platelets. This is a common problem in hematologic cancer patients who have received multiple transfusions. Fresh frozen plasma (FFP) is used for patients with abnormal clotting factors and patients who have received multiple transfusions. Albumin, cryoprecipitate, and clotting factors are additional blood components given to hematology/oncology patients.

Pain Management

Pain management is a highly complex aspect of cancer care. Not every patient with cancer experiences pain, but a high percentage of patients with advanced cancer do. Both the disease and its treatments can be the source of pain. Because this pain has so many dimensions and is a subjective experience, it requires a multidisciplinary approach.

Several factors determine whether pain occurs: location of the tumor or **metastasis** (bone and neural cancers produce the most severe pain), stage of disease (advanced cancer results in more severe pain than early stages) emotional and psychological state, history of past pain, and the cultural and religious background of the patient. Cancer pain can be acute and chronic, and when severe, can be intractable with normal methods. However, advancements in technology and studies focused on cancer pain management have made it possible to control over 95 percent of pain in in-patient settings. The following are some of those methods.

Analgesic administration of opiates, given alone or in combination with other drugs, is the most successful method of treating chronic, severe cancer pain. There are a number of methods of administration, but continuous infusion seems to provide the most constant level of relief. The administration may be subcutaneous, intravenous (continuous or patient-controlled **PCA**), or spinal (epidural or intrathecal) (Fig. 7–3). It often requires the surgical placement of an access line

PREPRINTED PHYSICIAN'S ORDERS
CHRONIC PAIN CONTROL/LONG TERM EPIDURAL CATHETER — Page 1 of 2

Date	Time	ORDERS	MD	RN
		1. **Consult the Pain Nurse** via Phamis under nurse consult screen.		
		2. **Consult Discharge Planner** "Pain Service Patient."		
		3. **Notify the Pain MD-on-call:** ¥ before starting patient on anticoagulant therapy. ¥ before starting patient on medications which may potentiate the narcotic e.g. diazepam, lorazepam. ¥ if patient's pain does not respond to medication or if there is an acute escalation in patient's discomfort. ¥ if fluid is leaking from the epidural infusion site. ¥ immediately if patient experiences numbness or tingling in lower extremities or trunk. ¥ immediately if respiratory rate <8 per minutes or systolic BP <90mmHg.		
		4. **Existing narcotic orders** (check one): ( ) A. Discontinue all previous narcotics. ( ) B. Continue previous narcotic with the following changes: ______ ( ) C. Taper previous narcotics in the following manner: ______		
		4. **PUMP MUST BE PROGRAMMED IN MICROGRAMS FOR EPIDURAL USE.** (Conversion Reminder 1 mg - 1000 mcg.) USE ONLY PRESERVATIVE-FREE AND ANTIOXID-FREE PRODUCTS. ***Cross out Medication below NOT prescribed.***		

Drug	Concentration/ml	Program As:	Cont. Rate	Demand Dose	Lockout Time	Max # Doses per Hr.
Morphine Sulfate	100 mcg/ml	mcg	mcg/hr	mcg	min	
Fentanyl	10 mcg/ml	mcg	mcg/hr	mcg	min	
Hydromorphone	40 mcg/ml	mcg	mcg/hr	mcg	min	
+ Bupivicaine	1 mg/ml					
Other:						

Date	Time	ORDERS	MD	RN
		5. **For breakthrough pain,** administer: ¥ Clinician Bolus ______ x 1 per event. ¥ Other Medication: ______		
		6. **For nausea/vomiting,** administer *(Cross out medication NOT prescribed):* ¥ Metoclopramide (Reglan) 10mg IV Q 6 hours prn OR ¥ Ondansetron (zofran) 4 mg IV Q 6 hours pern OR ¥ Droperidol 0.625mg IV Q 6 hours.		

Rev: 10/2/96 S

PREPRINTED PHYSICIAN'S ORDERS
CHRONIC PAIN CONTROL/LONG TE

Date	Time	
		7. **For mild pruritis** administ ¥ Diphenhydramine HCl 2
		8. **For respiratory depressi** ¥ Keep Naloxone 0.4 mg v ¥ Naloxone HCl 0.1 mg IV
		NURSING CARE (process a
		1. Check BP and respirations increase in rate and conce
		2. Change pump tubing Q 72
		3. Assess pain, level of consc
		4. Do not irrigate catheter.
		5. Every 4 hours document: F Demand doses Given: Atte Attempts data.

Rev: 10/2/96 S

Figure 7–3
Pain management preprinted physician's orders. (Courtesy of St. Joseph's Hospital, Marshfield, WI.)

and the use of alarmed infusion pumps. Close monitoring is necessary to ensure pain control yet avoid life-threatening side effects and complications.

Nerve blocks are used when all other methods of pain management have been attempted and the patient's pain remains intractable. There are two types: anesthetic (nondestructive and temporary) and neurolytic (destructive and permanent). These are invasive procedures that involve the injection of agents into or near the affected nerve.

Neurosurgical procedures are also used only when all other methods of pain management have been unsuccessful. Some procedures are: perip eral neurotomy, rhizotomy, cordotomy, myelotomy, and tractotomy. The procedures destroy the pain pathway by severing the appropriate nerve and are permanent. They may result in motor and sensory loss.

Nutrition

Proper nutrition is essential in the success of all cancer treatment. The disease process and many of the treatments have an adverse effect upon the patient's appetite and ability to consume and/or metabolize foods. Even when no problems exist, patients are educated in the principles of proper nutrition for cancer patients, including the use of oral nutritional supplements. Dietitians interview patients regarding their preferences and continue to monitor their caloric intake. When problems arise and patients are not able to maintain an adequate oral intake, various metabolic measures can be employed.

Total parenteral nutrition (TPN) is the continuous intravenous infusion of a concentrated solution containing glucose, proteins, vitamins, minerals, electrolytes, trace elements, and sometimes insulin. An intermittent infusion of lipids is also given. It can be administered through a peripheral IV but most often requires a central venous catheter, usually placed in the superior vena cava. Pumps are used to regulate the infusion rate. Orders are written for routine lab studies to assist in adjusting the content of the TPN, catheter care, and vital sign monitoring to guard against infection as well as precise instructions should sepsis be suspected (Fig. 7–4). TPN is used when the patient's GI tract is not functioning normally.

Enteral nutrition is used when the patient's GI tract is patent and functioning well but the patient is unable to consume an adequate amount of nutrition. Liquid formulas may be used as an oral supplement to an inadequate solid intake, as an oral replacement for the solid diet, or as a tube feeding. Tube feedings can be administered through a nasogastric tube placed by a nurse or GI technician or through esophagostomy, gastrostomy, or jejunostomy tubes usually placed by a surgeon. Pumps are sometimes used to regulate the infusion rate. Standard orders are written to monitor the patient's progress, electrolyte balance, and blood glucose.

Additional supportive treatments are often provided for hematology/oncology patients as a preventive measure or as specific needs arise, by the standard services of respiratory care, physical therapy, and occupational therapy.

Procedures

Cancer patients require a number of procedures to facilitate their diagnosis, treatment, and management on a hematology/oncology unit. The following discussion describes and gives the purpose of many of the common procedures.

Venous access device **(VAD)** placement is the insertion of a catheter to provide an access for administering chemotherapy, pain medication, antibiotics, antiemetics, TPN, and blood products and for withdrawing blood specimens. There are a variety of catheters; the type used depends upon the intended use and the length of time needed (Table 7–1). The catheters are inserted through the subclavian vein and terminated in the superior vena cava; they can have one, two, or three lumens that extend externally (Fig. 7–5). Some (Hickman, Groshong, Broviac, Quinton) are tunneled through the chest during a surgical procedure and are sutured securely into place (Fig. 7–6); they are intended for long-term use. Some (central lines) are not tunneled but are inserted directly into the subclavian vein by a physician (Fig. 7–7) and held in place with a single stitch, a dressing, and tape; they are intended for short-term use. Some are inserted through the basilic or cephalic veins by a trained RN (Fig. 7–8) and are held in place with a dressing and tape; they are intended for longer term use than a central line but less than a tunneled catheter. Some catheters (Port-a-Cath, OmegaPort, A-Port) are surgically implanted entirely under the skin and may terminate in various sites (e.g., hepatic artery, peritoneum, superior vena cava); they are intended for long-term use and are often used when outpatient treatment is planned (Fig. 7–9).

Thoracotomy is the placement of tubes into

PREPRINTED PHYSICIAN'S ORDERS
CENTRAL PARENTERAL NUTRITION

Date	Time	
		12. **LABORATORY ORDERS** a. In A.M. after TPN star Glucose, Liver Panel, Triglycerides, Uric Aci Reason ______ b. Days 2-4: Na, K, Cl, E Reason ______ c. Every Monday: Na, K Liver Panel, Triglyceri Mg, Prealbumin, Proti Reason ______ d. Every Thursday: Na, I Reason ______
		13. Daily weights.
		14. Strict I and O.
		15. Temp. q. 4 hours.
		16. Chemstrip q. 8 hours and than _____ or les than __
		17. NO PIGGYBACKING OF BLOOD DRAWING, OR (EXCEPTION PER PHYSI
		18. For suspected TPN cathe a. Obtain one blood cult **ASEPTIC CONDITIO** Obtain periperal blooc If catheter is removed tip cultured.
		19. If scheduled for MRI, call TPN and lipids.

Rev: 12/23/96 S

PREPRINTED PHYSICIAN'S ORDERS
CENTRAL PARENTERAL NUTRITION
Circle the numbers of the desired orders, and fill appropriate blanks. Page 1 of 2

Date	Time	ORDERS	Physician	Nurse
		1a. Consult Metabolic Support Service Dietitian and Pharmacist for assessment, recommendation and monitoring. 1b. Consult Metabolic Support Service Physician.		
		2. Central venous catheter to be placed by ______________ .		
		3. Central line cart from SPD.		
		4. Chest x-ray for catheter placement (tip of catheter must be in mid Superior Vena Cava).		
		5. Standard Heparin flush for capped lumens.		
		6. FORMULATION: ( ) STANDARD — ( ) CUSTOM Dextrose 12% — Dextrose _____ % Amino Acids 3.5% — Amino Acids _____ % Na+ 40 mEq/L — Na+ _____ mEq/L K+ 44 mEq/L — K+ _____ mEq/L C1- 55 mEq/L — C1- _____ mEq/L PO4- 15 m mole/L — PO4- _____ m mole/L Ca++ 8 mEq/L — Ca++ _____ mEq/L Mg++ 8 mEq/L — Mg++ _____ mEq/L Acetate 50 mEq/L — Acetate _____ mEq/L Gluconate 8 mEq/L — Gluconate _____ mEq/L Heparin 100 units/liter — Heparin _____ 12 component Vitamins/bag — Vitamins _____ 4 component Trace Elements/bag — Trace Elements _____ Insulin _____ Other:		
		7. Starting rate of infusion _____ ml/hr. per infusion pump.		
		8. Phytonadione 10mg IM every Monday. First dose:		
		9. Fat emulsion **(circle)** 10% 20% via Y-connector into TPN line below filter at rate of _____ ml/hr.		
		10. Peripheral IV of __________ to run at __________ ml/hr.		
		11. If TPN catheter is accidentally removed start IV of D10 at same rate of TPN.		

Rev: 12/23/96 S

Figure 7–4
Metabolic support preprinted physician's orders. (Courtesy of St. Joseph's Hospital, Marshfield, WI.)

the chest to treat pneumothorax. The tubes are inserted by a physician or physician's assistant under sterile conditions at the patient's bedside and are attached to suction.

Lumbar puncture (spinal tap) is the needle aspiration of cerebrospinal fluid from the patient's spinal column for the purpose of obtaining a specimen for diagnosis and/or monitoring treatment. It is performed by a physician under sterile conditions at the patient's bedside. *Sternal puncture (bone marrow biopsy)* is the needle aspiration of bone marrow from the patient's sternum for the purpose of obtaining a specimen for diagnosis and/or monitoring treatment. It is performed by a physician under sterile conditions at the patient's bedside.

Thoracentesis and paracentesis are needle aspirations of pleural and abdominal fluid, respec-

Table 7–1 VENOUS ACCESS DEVICES

Type	Uses
Short Term	
Peripheral catheter	Good for multiday therapy. Allows mobility without fear of infiltration.
Nontunneled central venous catheter	Good for emergency use. Can be inserted at the bedside by a physician. Can augment existing device.
Peripherally inserted central venous catheter (PICC)	Used for continuous infusion over longer periods of time. Can be inserted by nurses who are specially trained. External site care and routine flushing are required.
Long Term	
Tunneled central venous catheter	Used for long-term continuous or intermittent treatment. Good for TPN and vesicant infusion therapy. Requires site care and flushing.
Implantable port	Used for long-term intermittent therapy. Good choice for patients who are unable to perform site care, as none is needed when not in use. Must be inserted and removed by surgical procedure.
Peripheral port	Used when frequent, intermittent access is required. Preferred for patients with active lifestyles. No site care required between uses.

tively, from the patient's chest or abdomen for the purpose of obtaining a specimen or a treatment to remove excess fluid (ascites) from the patient's body. These procedures are performed by the physician under sterile conditions at the patient's bedside.

The HUC Role and Responsibility Regarding Treatment and Procedures

It would be unusual for any one hematology/oncology unit to offer every type of treatment listed here. They may offer a single type of service (e.g., medical, or surgical, or bone marrow transplant), a combination of two services (medical/surgical), or a specialty service (e.g., GYN oncology). No matter what the services of a specific unit, heme/onc HUCs must be knowledgeable about the policies and procedures that govern those services and familiar with the treatments and procedures offered elsewhere so as to facilitate effective patient care. They must be knowledgeable about possible side effects and complications so as to recognize critical situations, and they must keep their knowledge current as treatments and procedures are updated.

Equipment and Supplies Used in the Hematology/Oncology Unit

Special Rooms

Hematology/oncology units are equipped with specialized rooms to meet the needs of the various types of services offered. They may have a combination of the following:

Neutropenia rooms, which provide protective or reverse isolation for patients who are immunocompromised. These are private rooms with complete bathroom facilities that have ante areas, where staff and visitors can wash their

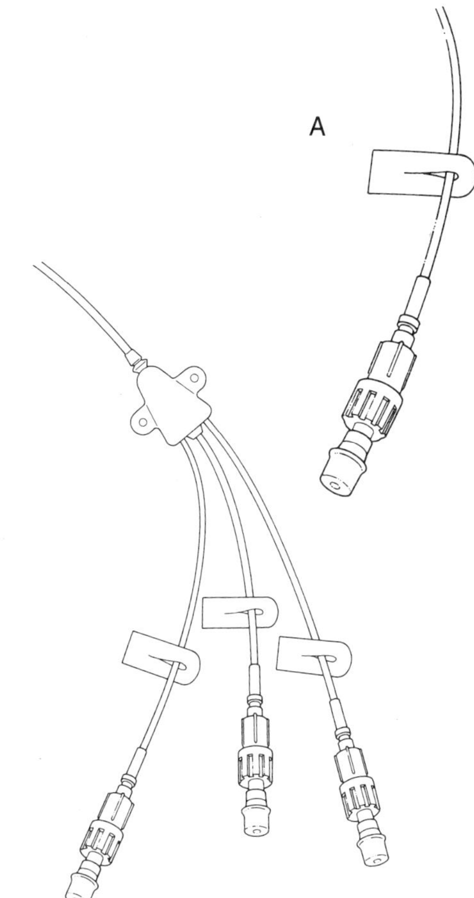

Figure 7–5
Single (*A*) and multiple-lumen (*B*) catheters. (From Bagnall-Reeb H, Ryder M, Anglim MA: Venous Access Device Occlusions [Independent Study Module]. Abbott Park IL, Abbott Laboratories, 1992.)

hands and obtain a mask, if necessary. They are equipped with positive-pressure ventilation to ensure that contaminates remain outside the room. They often include a calendar used to make entries regarding the patient's progress as demonstrated by lab values. Because patients may be confined to these rooms for an extended period, they are often larger to accommodate the longer stays of a family member or close friend, and they have additional furniture, exercise equipment, or entertainment equipment such as a VCR or CD/tape player.

Hepafilter rooms, which have the same features as the neutropenia rooms, with the addition of a ventilation system that filters bacteria from the air before it enters the room. These rooms are used for bone marrow transplant patients or patients receiving very high dose chemotherapy.

Radiation isolation rooms, which provide supplies for brachytherapy treatment and protection from the radiation source to the staff, other patients, and visitors. These rooms are private, with complete bathroom facilities, and generally are located at the end of halls or not adjacent to other rooms. The floors are marked designating the safe distance for visitors. In some cases all areas of the room that the patient might come in contact with are covered with protective plastic. There are lead shields for staff to work behind and disposal containers marked with radiation precautions. The rooms may be used for nonradiation patients when cleared by the radiation safety officer.

General isolation rooms, which provide protection from a patient's infectious process to the staff, other patients, and visitors. These rooms also have anterooms, where staff and visitors can wash their hands and obtain the supplies (gloves, gowns, masks) needed to enter the room. They are equipped with a negative-pressure ventilation system to ensure that room contaminates are not expelled into the hall or surrounding areas. These rooms are used for patients diagnosed with infectious processes such as active tuberculosis or methicillin-resistant *Staphylococcus aureus* (MRSA) infection and may be used by other patients when not needed for isolation.

Outpatient treatment rooms, which may be included to offer an area for patients to receive care when their outpatient facility is closed. These rooms are stocked with supplies for giving chemotherapy, blood products, and IV antibiotics. They may have recliners instead of beds.

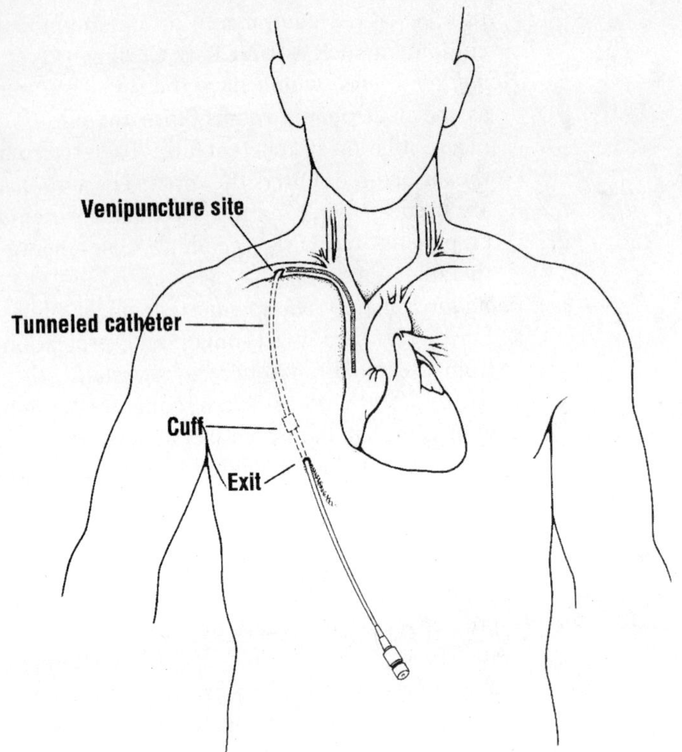

Figure 7–6
Tunneled central venous catheter. (From Bagnall-Reeb H, Ryder M, Anglim MA: Venous Access Device Occlusions [Independent Study Module]. Abbott Park, IL, Abbott Laboratories, 1992.)

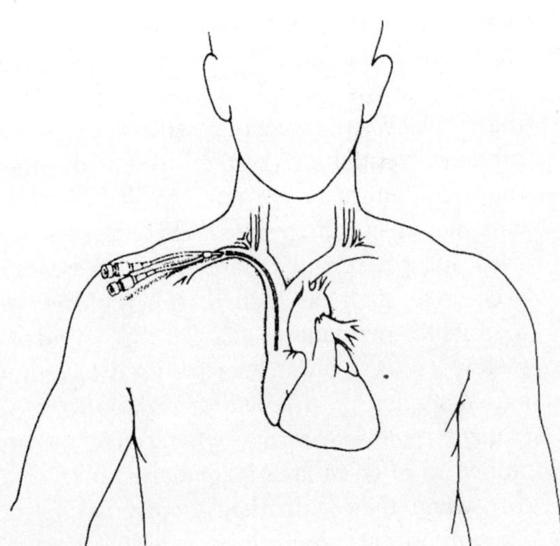

Figure 7–7
Subclavian or jugular insertion of nontunneled venous catheter. (From Bagnall-Reeb H, Ryder M, Anglim MA: Venous Access Device Occlusions [Independent Study Module]. Abbott Park, IL, Abbott Laboratories, 1992.)

Wellness/entertainment rooms, which are decorated to provide an atmosphere alternative for hospitalized patients. These rooms may have areas for reading or listening to music, meditation, or inspirational tapes; they may have exercise equipment such as treadmills or stationary bicycles; they may have informational brochures regarding wellness or support groups; they may have a selection of videotapes of movies or comedy routines; and they may have a selection of wigs or turbans for temporary use (Fig. 7–10).

Lounges, which offer a gathering area for larger groups and an alternative waiting area for patients' relatives and visitors. They are usually equipped with a number of sofas and chairs, some tables, magazines, a television set, and informational brochures. They may have a supply of toys, puzzles, or an aquarium to entertain small children. Some are equipped with coffeepots and refrigerators. These rooms are often

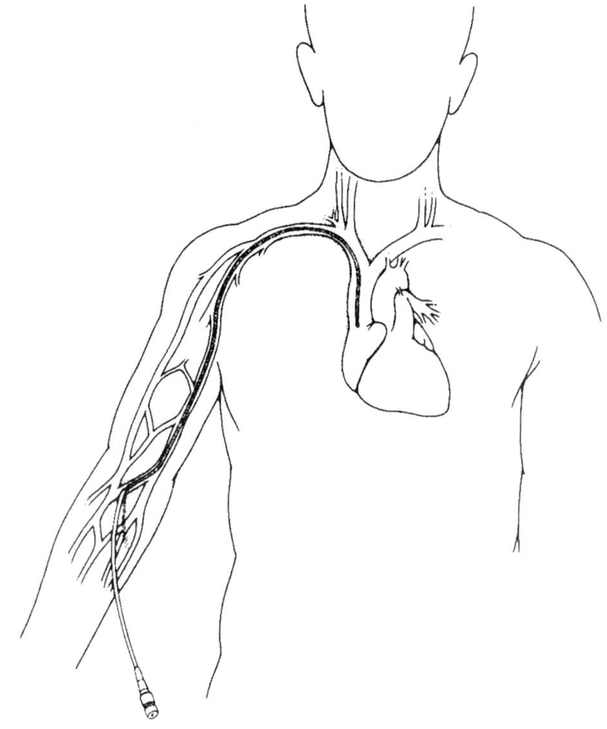

Figure 7–8
PICC (peripherally inserted central catheter). (From Bagnall-Reeb H, Ryder M, Anglim MA: Venous Access Device Occlusions [Independent Study Module]. Abbott Park, IL, Abbott Laboratories, 1992.)

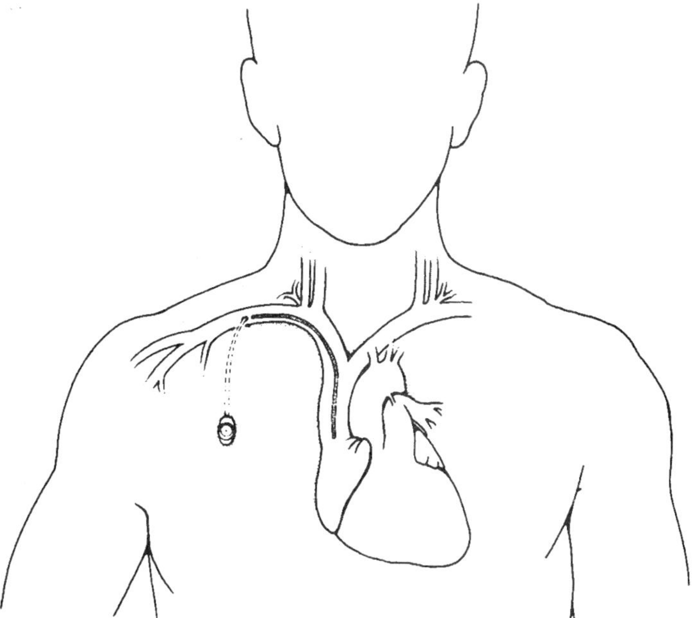

Figure 7–9
Catheter with implanted port. (From Bagnall-Reeb H, Ryder M, Anglim MA: Venous Access Device Occlusions [Independent Study Module]. Abbott Park, IL, Abbott Laboratories, 1992.)

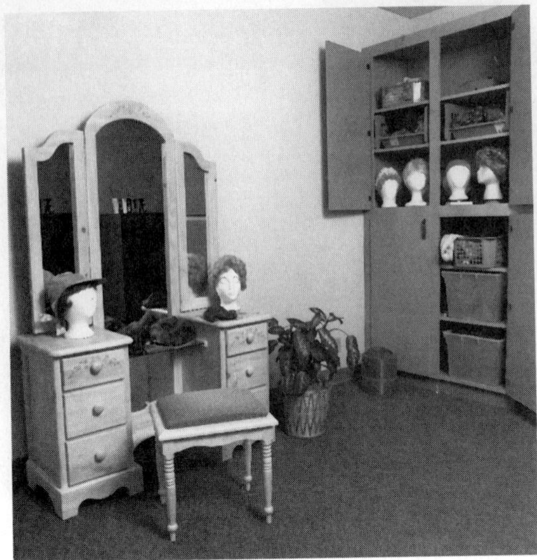

Figure 7–10
Wig area of wellness room.

decorated by the staff or volunteers for holidays or patients' birthdays and anniversaries.

Equipment and Supplies

Cancer patients may require monitoring of various types; therefore, heme/onc units may be equipped with cardiac monitors at the nurses' station to provide telemetry readouts of the patients' cardiac status. They may also have television monitors for observation of patients who are disoriented and at risk of injury.

Supplies that are specific to the heme/onc unit include biohazard equipment for the handling and disposal of chemotherapy materials and procedure trays or carts with supplies for central line placements, bone marrow biopsies, lumbar punctures, paracentesis and throacentesis, and thoracotomies.

Educational information provides assistance to the patients, relatives, and staff. Numerous brochures are published by organizations such as the National Cancer Institute, the American Cancer Society, the Leukemia Society of America, and the National Institutes of Health to provide information on all aspects of cancer prevention, diagnosis, and treatment; some are general, and some are specific to each type of cancer. Also, each hospital publishes informational brochures regarding instructions specific to its methods of procedure. These are all written in language devoid of technical medical jargon and are helpful to patients and family. In addition to public educational information, heme/onc units have educational information that allow their staff to remain current in general topics of cancer and specific policies and procedures that affect the operation of the unit.

The HUC Role and Responsibility Regarding Equipment and Supplies

As with every unit, the heme/onc HUCs are in charge of the management of all supplies and equipment. They must see that equipment is in safe working order and that supplies are well stocked. They must be aware of the supplies and equipment that are not kept in stock but that may be needed. Being familiar with all the supplies and equipment makes the heme/onc HUC an invaluable resource to patients, family, and staff.

Communication With and About Patients in the Hematology/Oncology Unit

In 1988, the American Cancer Society published the Cancer Survivors' Bill of Rights. Among other things, it states that cancer survivors have the right to the assurance of lifelong medical care through the efforts of their health care providers. This continuity of care requires clear and concise communication on the part of all the patient's health care providers.

Cancer is a chronic disease that requires long-term care delivered in a wide variety of settings (e.g., physician's offices, diagnostic clinics, community hospitals, major cancer centers, rehabilitation facilities, home care, nursing homes, and hospice). Patients move back and forth between these settings as different needs arise; they can be admitted and readmitted to the hospital at various stages of their care. The hematology/oncology unit provides only a portion of the complex, multidisciplinary care that cancer patients require throughout the course of their disease. Ongoing, effective communication by the heme/onc unit with all these settings as well as with the patient, the family, and numerous hospital departments is required to ensure that continuity of care is maintained.

Spiritual Services

Medical science has established the strong effect of the spiritual, emotional, and psychosocial state of patients on their physical well-being, their response to treatment, and their ability to recover. Cancer patients often turn to their religion or other spiritual guidance for strength or support during their illness. Some may struggle with feelings of anger and hopelessness. Many heme/onc units have staff clergy available who provide spiritual guidance or assist patients to cope. These chaplains are trained in illness counseling and can provide support to the families and staff as well as the patients. They can suggest that patients or their families attend support groups such as "I Can Cope," "Coping With Cancer Challenges," and "Cancer Survivors' Day," which are sponsored by the American Cancer Society. It is important that the patient's spiritual needs be recognized and addressed during the hospitalization period.

Psychological Services

Patients dealing with the diagnosis and treatment of a potentially terminal disease can experience fear, anxiety, depression, and hopelessness. These responses, although normal, hinder the patient's ability to benefit from treatment and recover from illness. Most heme/onc units provide routine psychological services to assist their patients. Psychiatrists are available to make assessments and prescribe necessary medication. Psychologists or psychiatric social workers are available to provide counseling and teach methods of coping to patients; group support sessions may be held. Family dynamics are also considered. The patient may be scheduled for follow-up care on discharge and continue to be seen with each readmission to the hospital.

Therapeutic Recreational Services

Patients who experience stress, anxiety, or depression related to their hospitalization or diagnosis and who do not respond well to spiritual or psychological services may benefit from therapeutic recreation. This service combines theories and modalities from physical therapy, occupational therapy, and psychology to develop activities that improve the patient's sense of well-being. It is especially beneficial to patients who experience long hospital stays.

These three services offer different methods and approaches to assist cancer patients in adjusting to their diagnosis, tolerating their treatment, and adapting to the changes in their family and social relationships. Good communication among the departments is essential in providing this interdisciplinary care.

Social Services and Discharge Planning

Patients who are diagnosed with a chronic, potentially terminal disease are faced with a number of changes in their lives that require making difficult decisions throughout the course of their illness. The social services and discharge planning departments are available to assist in many of these cases.

Institutions are required by law to provide their patients with information regarding living wills and medical powers of attorney. These are advance directives stating the patient's wishes regarding the extent of medical care should he or she need artificial means to be kept alive, and the designation of someone who will make decisions regarding future medical care when the patient is no longer able to do so. Social service personnel can assist patients and families in filling out these forms and providing the notarized signatures.

Cancer treatments are expensive. Insurance companies categorize some treatments as experimental and deny payment. Many patients become unemployed and lose their medical insurance. For a variety of reasons, patients can have serious financial problems with which the social services department can assist.

Patients are discharged from the hospital very early in their treatment and require continued care that may be delivered in a variety of settings. Discharge planners work to evaluate the patients' medical needs, equipment needs, and family situation to determine the discharge disposition that provides the best continuity of care. These can include transfer to a hospital closer to the patient's home and family; transfer to a skilled nursing facility, nursing home, or rehabilitation facility; transfer to an in-patient hospice facility; arrangement of ambulatory care appointments; and arrangement of home care that can include nursing care (complex treatments, lab tests, medications), home health aides (hygiene, simple treatments, ambulating), respiratory care (oxygen, breathing treatments), and equipment (walker, wheelchair, hospital bed). The discharge planner works closely with social services to facilitate discharge plans. Extensive written communication is necessary to ensure that high-quality care is maintained during these transfers.

Patients and Families

The most important communication in providing effective continuity of care is with the patient and the patient's family. It is essential that each staff member take the time to explain procedures in clear and concise language that can be easily understood. Because the stress of any illness hinders the patient's ability to concentrate, it is important that information and instructions be given more than once and also provided in writing.

It is important that patients and their families be provided with as much information about the diagnosis and treatment as they desire. Brochures published by the National Institutes of Health, the American Cancer Society, and the American Leukemia Society are available on every type of cancer and every aspect of treatment.

It is also important that staff take the time to listen to patients and their families. The knowledge that someone listens, someone hears, someone understands, and someone cares has an immeasurable effect on the patient's well-being.

HUC Role and Responsibility Regarding Communications

The spiritual, emotional, and psychosocial aspects of the patient's treatment are crucial to its overall success. These aspects of cancer care are necessary at every stage of treatment. Because of the interdisciplinary approach to cancer treatment and its duration, it is essential that good communication practices be used by all staff.

HUCs carry the greatest responsibility for maintaining good communication on the hematology/oncology unit. They must be knowledgeable about all the services available to their patients and the communication required to procure those services. They must be able to communicate with all the physicians, unit staff, personnel in other departments, visitors, family, and patients. In verbal communication, this requires making continuous adjustments for intellectual level, educational level, emotional state, culture, age, and gender; it also requires the use of proper grammar. In written communication, this requires clear and concise composition, correct spelling, proper grammar, and legible penmanship.

HUCs often answer the patient call-light systems; they must be aware of the patients' conditions and their ability to hear and speak in order to understand each patient's request and assess its urgency. Family members often bring their concerns or complaints to the HUC. It is important that undivided attention be given, empathy expressed, and action taken. The HUC's ability to communicate in a clear, concise, and effective manner helps ensure quality and continuity of care for the cancer patient.

Quality and Risk Management

As with any other unit in the hospital, quality and risk management issues are a concern on the hematology/oncology unit. The issues addressed in this discussion are specific to the types of patients treated in this specialized area. Knowledge of institutional policies in dealing with these issues is imperative.

Oncology Nursing Certification

As was discussed earlier (see *History*), advances in the diagnosis and treatment of cancer patients have brought about significant changes in the care given. This has required a much higher level of knowledge and skill on the part of the nurses who care for cancer patients. This need led to the establishment of the Oncology Nursing Society in 1975 and the development of *Standards of Oncology Nursing Practice*, which were most recently updated in 1996. The Oncology Nursing Certification Corporation was founded for the purpose of enhancing professional practice and patient care through oncology nursing certification, which validates competence and raises nursing standards of care.

Safe Handling of Cytotoxic Drugs

It is important for personnel on the hematology/oncology unit to take safety precautions when handling chemotherapeutic agents. Protections such as gloves, gowns, and masks are often necessary during preparation, administration, and disposal. Special areas are designated for the handling and preparation of many of the drugs. Health care workers must follow specific guidelines when handling bodily fluids of patients who have received cytotoxic agents. It is also necessary to give special attention to linens that may have been contaminated with any type of bodily fluids from patients receiving chemotherapeutic drugs in order to limit the exposure of the individuals handling them.

Spill Kits

Spill kits must be available in areas where cytotoxic drugs are prepared, dispensed, administered, transported, and disposed of. The contents of the spill kit and the directions for use are determined by OSHA regulations. The kit contains all the necessary supplies for the safe handling and cleanup of any accidental spills.

Blood and Blood Products

Because cancer and many of the treatments that cancer patients receive have adverse effects on the blood-producing mechanisms of the body, the administration of blood and blood products is a frequent, important, and integral part of cancer therapy.

Although administration of blood and blood products is a common therapy in many areas of medicine, it remains a risky procedure. Every effort is made on the part of organizations that collect blood and produce blood products to ensure safety. However, despite all precautions, an element of risk always exists.

HBV and HIV

Hepatitis B virus (HBV) and human immunodeficiency virus (HIV) are pathogens that have been known to be transmitted through blood products. Tests have been developed to identify these organisms, and careful **screening** of potential blood donors to determine their possible exposure have been instrumental in eliminating most of these contamination problems.

Administration

Great care must be exercised in the administration of blood components to prevent crossmatch errors. All hospitals must have procedures in place to safeguard the patient. These may include such practices as allowing only 1 unit of blood per patient to be released from the blood bank at a time, and not allowing blood for more than one patient on the nursing unit to be dispensed at the same time. Identification of the patient and comparison of the patient's ID information with the information on the blood bag should be confirmed by two people. Documentation of the transfusion is required.

Transfusion Reactions

A transfusion reaction is defined as any adverse or unfavorable effect on the patient from the transfusion of blood components. There are many symptoms of transfusion reaction that nurses are trained to recognize. These can include flushing of the face, fever, chills, wheezing, shortness of breath, hematuria, or renal failure. Prompt attention to these symptoms and appropriate intervention are vital, as some transfusion reactions can be fatal.

Infection Control

The need to protect against infections is twofold on a hematology/oncology unit. Since many patients receiving chemotherapy and/or radiation therapy are in an immunocompromised state, it is important to protect them from infectious agents that may be present in the environment. Patients with infections are placed in the appropriate isolation and cared for according to the institution's infection control policies.

Protective Isolation

Patients who are immunocompromised lack the ability to ward off any type of infection. Therefore, measures must be taken to reduce the risk of introducing infectious microorganisms into their environment. These measures include placing patients in a positive-pressure airflow room to reduce the risk of airborne pathogens entering when the door is opened; restricting visitors who have had recent infections (e.g., colds or flu); requiring meticulous hand washing on the part of anyone who will come in contact with the patients; requiring the use of masks, gloves, and gowns, when necessary, by health care workers and visitors; requiring the patients to wear masks if they must leave their room; and maintaining dietary restriction of fresh fruits and fresh vegetables. Fresh flowers and plants are also prohibited in the patients' rooms (Fig. 7–11). Statistics have shown that diligent hand washing is the single most effective mechanism in the prevention of infection.

Standard Precautions

The first line of protection for health care workers against bloodborne pathogens is inoculation. All personnel who are at risk of exposure to these agents should be vaccinated for HBV. Standard Precautions, formerly known as Universal Precautions, are a set of guidelines established by the Centers for Disease Control that are in place in all hospitals. These guidelines require that all blood and body fluids from any patient be considered potentially infectious and handled in a manner that would protect against contamination. Protective clothing, such as gloves, should be used by all personnel when handling these substances. In addition, proper disposal of waste and sharp objects, such as needles, is imperative. All accidental punctures should be reported immediately. As in protective isolation, good hand washing is the best defense against the spread of infections. These practices protect patients and health care workers alike. Hospitals provide proper equipment and training for the safety of their workers. It is often mandatory for employees to attend these sessions on a regular basis.

Radiation Safety

Radioactive materials are frequently used in the diagnosis and treatment of cancer patients. For diagnosis, the materials are taken orally or injected. For treatment, the materials are placed internally.

Radioactive materials may contaminate any-

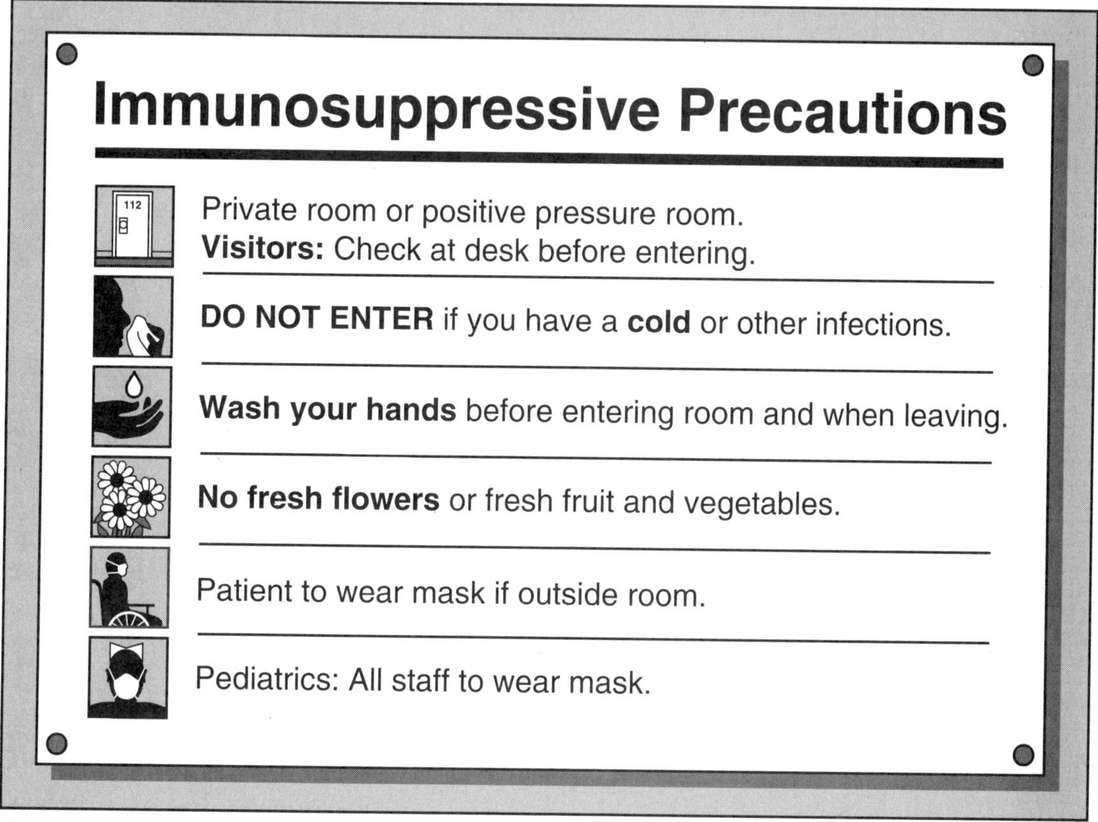
Immunosuppressive Precautions
112
Private room or positive pressure room.
Visitors: Check at desk before entering.
DO NOT ENTER if you have a cold or other infections.
Wash your hands before entering room and when leaving.
No fresh flowers or fresh fruit and vegetables.
Patient to wear mask if outside room.
Pediatrics: All staff to wear mask.

Figure 7–11
Immunosuppressive precautions placard. (Courtesy of St. Joseph's Hospital, Marshfield, WI.)

thing with which they come in contact. They can be inhaled, ingested, or absorbed through the skin. These circumstances produce a hazard, since the materials emit radiation and can cause great harm. Proper storage of these materials is vital.

Certain safety procedures should be in place for any health care worker who works with radioactive materials. These precautions include wearing protective clothing when handling the materials and hand washing with soap and water after working in an area where radioactive materials are present. Badges are worn by workers to monitor their level of radiation exposure.

When radioactive materials are used for diagnosis or treatment, the patients and their bodily fluids may become radioactive. Therefore, special guidelines must be followed when caring for these patients. In diagnostic procedures, the radioactivity decreases rapidly; thus the risk is low. When used for treatment, the materials are longer lasting and more hazardous. This increases the risk to the staff caring for the patient. Care is taken to minimize exposure. Precautions include entering the patient's room only to perform necessary duties and having the patient provide self-care as much as possible. Anything that has come in contact with the patient must be clearly labeled as radioactive; this includes specimens, linens, and waste. The patient's room must also be identified as containing radioactive materials (Fig. 7–12). The radiation safety officer must be notified immediately if a patient receiving **brachytherapy** dies.

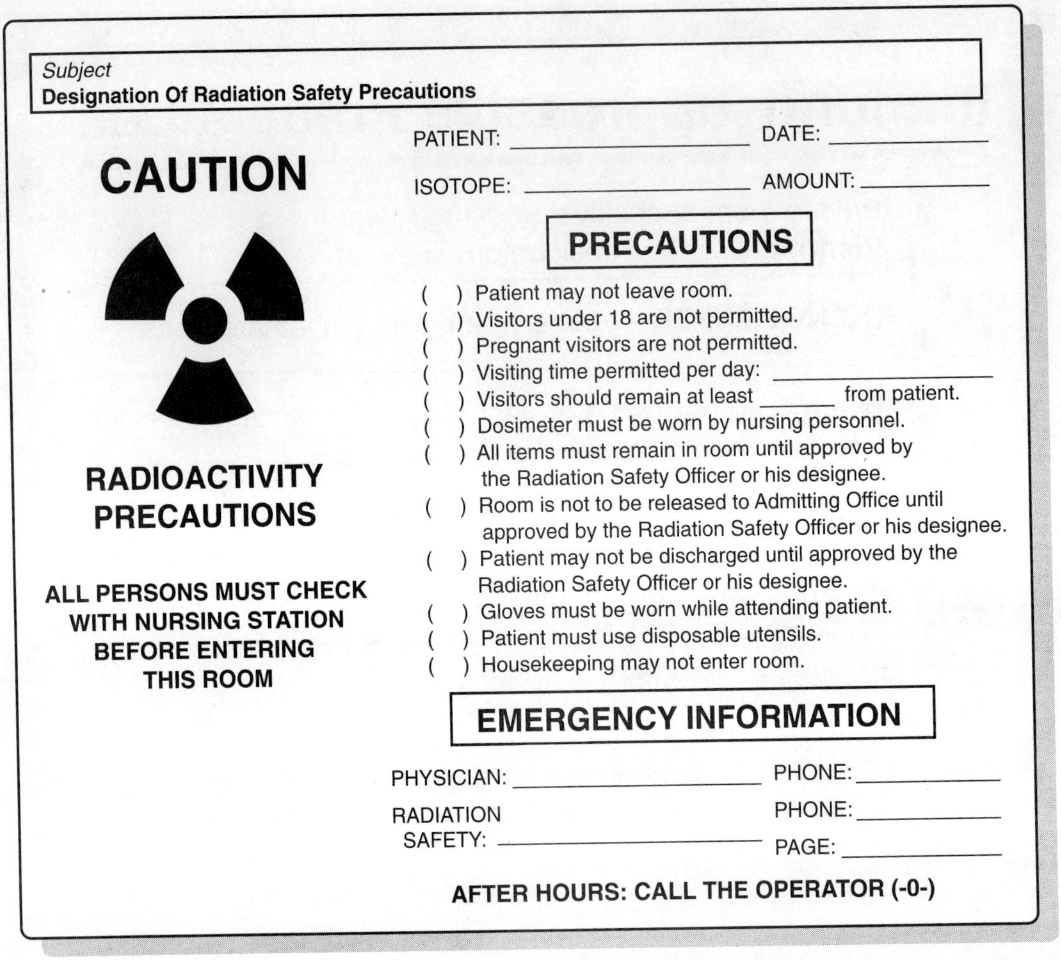

Subject
Designation Of Radiation Safety Precautions

CAUTION

PATIENT: ____________ DATE: ____________

ISOTOPE: ____________ AMOUNT: ____________

PRECAUTIONS

( ) Patient may not leave room.
( ) Visitors under 18 are not permitted.
( ) Pregnant visitors are not permitted.
( ) Visiting time permitted per day: ____________
( ) Visitors should remain at least ______ from patient.
( ) Dosimeter must be worn by nursing personnel.
( ) All items must remain in room until approved by the Radiation Safety Officer or his designee.
( ) Room is not to be released to Admitting Office until approved by the Radiation Safety Officer or his designee.
( ) Patient may not be discharged until approved by the Radiation Safety Officer or his designee.
( ) Gloves must be worn while attending patient.
( ) Patient must use disposable utensils.
( ) Housekeeping may not enter room.

RADIOACTIVITY PRECAUTIONS

ALL PERSONS MUST CHECK WITH NURSING STATION BEFORE ENTERING THIS ROOM

EMERGENCY INFORMATION

PHYSICIAN: ____________ PHONE: ____________

RADIATION SAFETY: ____________ PHONE: ____________ PAGE: ____________

AFTER HOURS: CALL THE OPERATOR (-0-)

Figure 7–12
Radioactivity precautions placard. (Courtesy of St. Joseph's Hospital, Marshfield, WI.)

The HUC Role and Responsibility Regarding Quality and Risk Management

HUCs play an important role in quality assurance and risk management. They are knowledgeable about all the policies and procedures that pertain to quality and safety on the hematology/oncology unit. It is their responsibility to enforce those policies as they pertain to the staff, the patients, and the visitors. In addition, many heme/onc HUCs play a role in establishing the policies that govern quality improvement (QI) in their hospitals and on their units by being members of QI committees. Because their position requires thorough knowledge of the operation systems, they are important members of these committees. They may also assist the heme/onc nurse manager in collecting data to assess unit procedures. Lastly, heme/onc HUCs ensure quality by performing their duties with a high level of accuracy, efficiency, and integrity.

Closing Thoughts

Working as a HUC on a hematology/oncology unit is demanding, challenging, interesting, and rewarding. The position requires a person with flexibility and stamina who can adjust to the frequently changing circumstances that exist on a unit that provides intensive, complex care to acute patients and constant supportive care to chronic patients.

Hematology and oncology are dynamic fields of medicine in which treatment advances, technology, legislature, and cost-containment efforts have an ongoing effect on the types of health care and the methods of providing it to cancer patients. The heme/onc HUC is given the ever-present opportunity to learn and develop new skills.

Although there is continuing change on the heme/onc unit, what remain constant are the patient and the patient's family. Family members are an extension of the patient and an important component of care and treatment (Fig. 7–13). The heme/onc HUC is a member of a health care team that delivers care to patients diagnosed with a potentially terminal illness. Fifty percent of patients diagnosed with cancer today can be cured, but the other 50 percent will not survive. Providing care and support to these patients and their families throughout the course of the illness is frequently emotionally demanding. Heme/onc HUCs must be able to face these demands. Even though working on the heme/onc unit can be emotionally demanding, it can also be emotionally rewarding.

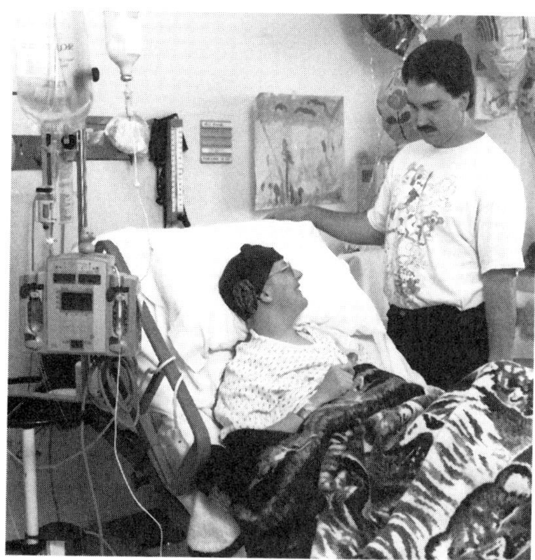

Figure 7–13
Patient and spouse.

The trend in in-patient care at the end of this century is toward short-term hospitalizations. Patients in most hospital units move through the system so quickly that there is little opportunity for them to get to know their health care providers. Because patients are discharged early and must continue their treatment and recovery in outpatient settings, in-patient staff are often not aware of the patient's progress or the treatment outcome. Frequently there is no opportunity for the staff to establish the type of relationship with the patients or their families that helps provide the sense of a job well done.

The nature of cancer and its treatment affords the staff on hematology/oncology units the opportunity to get to know the patients and their families and follow their progress through the course of the illness. This is especially true of long-term leukemia treatments and the bone marrow transplants. Even with the short, 2- to 3-day admissions for chemotherapy, the patients return every 4 weeks for a number of months to complete their treatment, and time is allowed to establish a relationship with both the patients and the patients' families. Hematology/oncology staff feel privileged to share the experience. Special relationships are also often formed between the HUCs and the patients' families. Many cancer survivors or the families of patients who do not survive continue a dialogue with the unit staff long after treatment has ended. Being a part of the heme/onc health care team is a rewarding experience.

Review Questions

1. Explain how physicians use diagnostic procedures in the care of cancer patients.
2. List five types of diagnostic imaging studies performed to assist in evaluating cancer patients.
3. Identify the most definitive means of diagnosing all cancers.
4. Explain the primary purpose of chemotherapy.
5. List the 3 primary treatments for cancer.
6. Explain why many cancer patients require placement in protective isolation.

Bibliography

Blood Borne Pathogens, Virginia Beach, VA, Coastal Video Communications, 1993.

Brant JM: Statement on the Scope and Standards of Oncology Nursing Practice. Washington, DC, American Nurses Publishing, 1996.

Clark JC, McGee RF: Core Curriculum for Oncology Nursing, 2nd ed. Philadelphia, WB Saunders, 1992.

Dow KH, Hilderly LJ: Nursing Care in Radiation Oncology. Philadelphia, WB Saunders, 1996.

Groenwald SL, Frogge MH, Goodman M, Yarbo CH: Cancer Nursing, Principles and Practice, 4th edition. Boston, Jones & Bartlett, 1992.

Making Your Credential Work for You: Pittsburgh, Oncology Nursing Certification Corp, 1997.

McCorkle R, Grant M, Frank-Stromborg M, Baird SB: Cancer Nursing, 2nd ed. Philadelphia, WB Saunders, 1996.

Medical Waste Handling, Virginia Beach, VA, Coastal Video Communications, 1993.

Otto SE: Oncology Nursing, 2nd ed. St. Louis, CV Mosby, 1993.

Radiation Safety. Virginia Beach, VA, Coastal Video Communications, 1993.

Tenenbaum L: Cancer Chemotherapy and Biotherapy. Philadelphia, WB Saunders, 1994.

Welch J, Silveria JM: Safe Handling of Cytotoxic Drugs, 2nd ed. Pittsburgh, Oncology Nursing Press, 1997.

8

Mental Health Unit

Gayle Levi-McLouden

Common Abbreviations

CT	Computed tomography
DSM-IV	*Diagnostic and Statistical Manual of Mental Disorders*, 4th edition
DST or DEX test	Dexamethasone suppression test
ECT	Electroconvulsive therapy
EST	Electroshock therapy
EEG	Electroencephalogram
GAD	Generalized anxiety disorder
MAOI	Monoamine oxidase inhibitor
MRI	Magnetic resonance imaging
OCD	Obsessive-compulsive disorder
PET	Positron emission tomography
PTSD	Post-traumatic stress disorder
SAD	Seasonal affective disorder
SSRI	Selective serotonin reuptake inhibitor
TCA	Tricyclic antidepressant

Objectives

Upon completion of this chapter, the reader should be able to:

1. Explain the difference between depressive disorders and ordinary sadness.
2. Name four depressive disorders listed in the DSM-IV other than depression.
3. List five anxiety disorders as identified in the DSM-IV.
4. List five studies that may be ordered to aid in the diagnosis of mental disorders.
5. Explain what is meant by bipolar disorder.
6. Describe what electroconvulsive therapy is and how the procedure is carried out.

Vocabulary

Agoraphobia: Fear of being alone or in open spaces

Anxiety: A feeling of uneasiness, apprehension, or dread resulting from a real or perceived threat whose actual source is unknown

Bipolar: Pertaining to an affective disorder in which both manic and depressive episodes occur

Cognitive: Pertaining to the mental process of comprehension, judgment, memory, and reasoning, as contrasted to emotional processes

Compulsion: An irresistible impulse to perform some act contrary to one's better judgment

Delusions: False beliefs that are rigidly held even in the face of strong evidence to the contrary

Depression: Emotional dejection greater and more prolonged than that warranted by any objective reason

Electroconvulsive therapy: The induction of a brief convulsion by passing an electric current through the brain for the treatment of affective disorder

Electroshock: The same as electroconvulsive therapy

Continued

Vocabulary *Continued*

Hallucinations: Sensory (sight, sound, touch, taste, or smell) impressions that have no basis in external stimulation

Mania: An unstable elevated mood in which delusions and poor judgment are present

Monoamine oxidase B (MAO-B): An enzyme that breaks down certain neurotransmitters

Norepinephrine (noradrenaline): A neurotransmitter that plays a role in mood and pain, and possibly in learning and memory

Neurotransmitter: A specialized chemical messenger, produced and secreted by nerve cells

Obsession: Preoccupation with an idea that dominates the mind

Panic: Sudden, overwhelming anxiety that causes loss of rational thought

Phobia: A persistent, abnormal fear or dread

Seasonal affective disorder: A syndrome characterized by fatigue, weight gain, and irritability during winter months. It affects primarily women.

Schizophrenia: A severe disturbance of thought characterized by delusions, hallucinations, and retreat from reality

Serotonin: A compound occurring in the brain, intestines, and platelets that induces vasoconstriction.

History

Physicians in the Western world began specializing in the treatment of the mentally ill in the 19th century. They were known as alienists and worked in large asylums, practicing what was then called moral treatment, a humane approach aimed at quieting mental outbursts and restoring reason. In the second half of the century, psychiatrists abandoned this mode of treatment and with it, the recognition that mental illness is influenced by both psychological and social issues. Drugs and other forms of somatic treatment were common as psychiatrists concentrated almost entirely on biologic factors as the cause of mental illness.

In the early 20th century, the writings of Sigmund Freud caused a change in thinking, with movement away from biologic factors to an emphasis on the psychiatric practice of psychoanalysis as the preferred mode of treatment. The 1940s and 1950s brought about another change in emphasis, this time to the social and physical environment. Somatic forms of treatment such as **electroconvulsive therapy** (ECT; electric shock) and psychosurgery were being used by some psychiatrists who were studying biologic influences as the cause of mental illness.

In the mid-1950s, the introduction of the first effective drugs for treating psychotic symptoms led to a change in the treatment of the mentally ill. New and more humane policies and treatment regimens were introduced into mental hospitals.

Drugs also allowed more patients to be treated in community settings in the 1960s and 1970s, a trend that continues today. Advances in the development of new medications have continued to assist patients in the recovery from and stabilization of their illness, enabling them to live successfully in the community.

Description of the Unit

A mental health unit is an area where the medical study, diagnosis, treatment, and prevention of mental illness takes place. In the mental health unit, patients with a wide variety of mental illnesses and mental health issues are treated in an environment designed to make them feel comfortable and safe. In this setting, patients can be observed, assessed, and helped by professionals such as psychiatrists, psychologists, social workers, nurses, occupational therapists, recreational therapists, and spiritual counselors. The goal of this multidisciplinary team is to provide the sort of environment in which every person, regardless of background or life experience, can receive the maximum benefit from his or her stay.

Patients coming to the mental health unit are both diverse and similar. The greatest similarity is that at the time of admission they are all experiencing difficulties in coping with their everyday lives. All patients bring their individual life experiences, biases, and perceptions, which affect their selected coping style.

In-patient programs are designed to support and protect the fundamental human, civil, constitutional, and statutory rights of individual patients. Treatment staff also ensure and protect the personal privacy of all patients hospitalized on a mental health unit.

On a mental health unit, certain precautions are taken to ensure the safety of both patients and staff. The precautions can include locked units, intensive monitoring, time-out rooms, and restraints. Time-outs give the patient an opportunity to calm down, especially if the patient has exhibited out-of-control behavior. Time-outs can be either unlocked or locked (seclusion). When behavior reaches the point where staff or other patients could be harmed, it may be necessary to place the patient in restraints. Medications may be used to assist in calming the patient so that behavior can be managed safely out of restraints or seclusion. Intensive monitoring and locked units may be necessary to manage suicidal patients to prevent them from inflicting self-harm.

Central Nervous System Anatomy and Physiology Related to Mental Health

The central nervous system consists of the brain and spinal cord. For purposes of this chapter, we discuss the brain and its functions. The brain is divided into three major sections: the brainstem, the cerebellum, and the cerebrum (Fig. 8–1). They are interconnected by a network of nerve cells called neurons in order to work in a coordinated manner.

Brainstem

The brainstem regulates internal organs and controls vital functions such as blood pressure and heart rate. It also serves as the initial processor of sensory information that ultimately goes to the cerebral cortex. The brainstem also regulates the sleep–wake cycle.

Cerebellum

The cerebellum is located posterior to the brainstem. It regulates skeletal muscles and controls coordination.

Cerebrum

The cerebrum is located above and around the brainstem and is responsible for mental activities and a conscious sense of being. The cerebrum is responsible for emotional status, memory, language, and the ability to communicate. The cere-

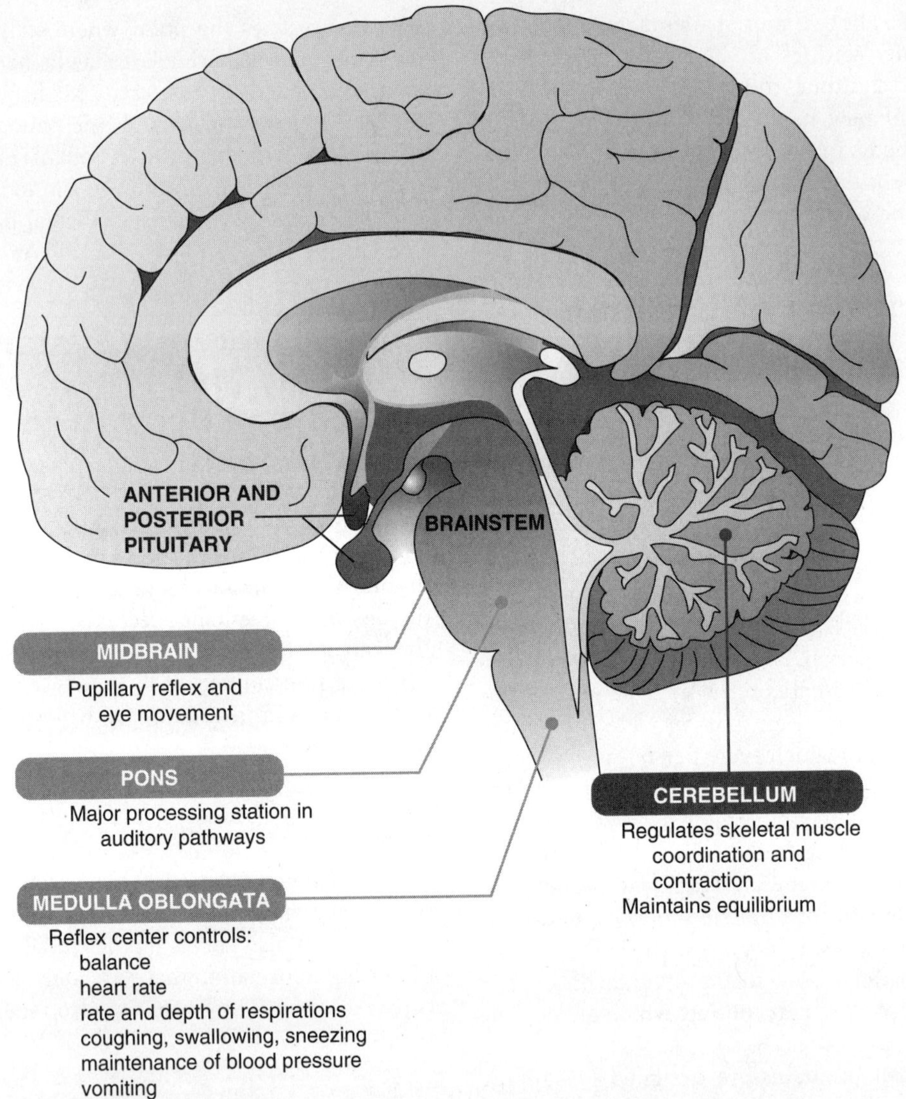

Figure 8–1
The functions of the brainstem and cerebellum. (From Varcarolis EM: Foundations of Psychiatric Mental Health Nursing, 3rd ed. Philadelphia, WB Saunders, 1998.)

brum is divided into lobes, and each lobe is responsible for different functions (Fig. 8–2).

Neurotransmitters

Neurotransmitters are chemicals that mediate the transmission of messages along nerves and across the synapses, which are the junctions between two nerve cells. They are produced and secreted by the nerve cells. Neurotransmitters play complex roles in the body, many of which are still the subject of research.

Acetylcholine is a neurotransmitter that appears to be involved in learning and memory. Dopamine is a neurotransmitter that is essential for motor functions. **Norepinephrine**, also known

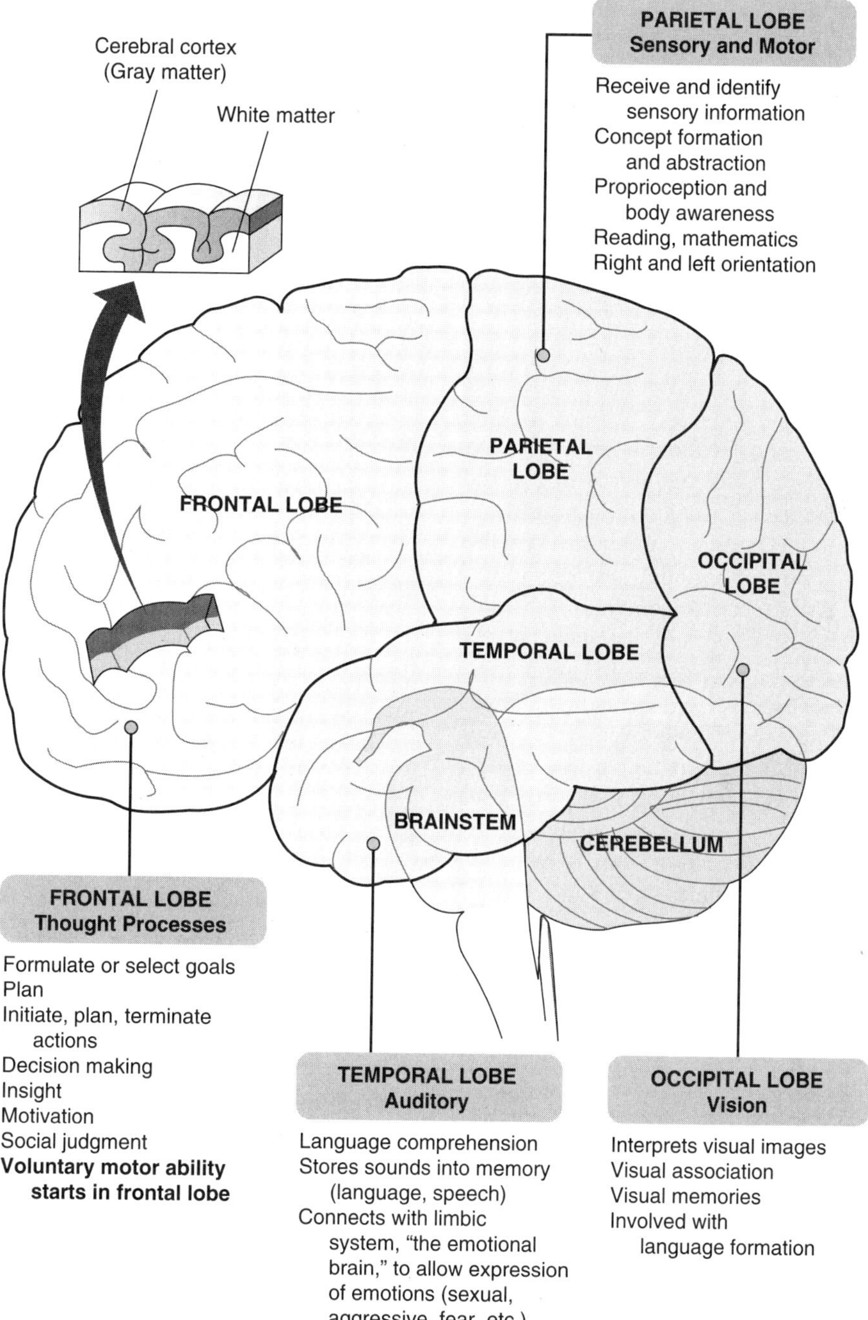

Figure 8–2

The functions of the cerebral lobes: frontal, parietal, temporal, and occipital. (From Varcarolis EM: Foundations of Psychiatric Mental Health Nursing, 3rd ed. Philadelphia, WB Saunders, 1998.)

as **noradrenaline**, plays a role in mood, pain, and possibly learning and memory. **Serotonin** is a neurotransmitter that plays a role in sleep, mood, pleasure, and pain. **Monoamine oxidase B (MAO-B)** is an enzyme that breaks down certain neurotransmitters (see Chap. 6).

Common Mental Disorders

Depressive Disorders

Depression

Depression is the most common problem seen by mental health professionals. According to the *Diagnostic and Statistical Manual of Mental Disorders,* 4th Edition **(DSM-IV)**, published by the American Psychiatric Association, in community studies, 10 to 25 percent of women and 5 to 12 percent of men seen by family physicians suffer from a major depressive disorder. In prepubertal ages, the incidence for boys and girls is the same. The highest incidence occurs between the ages of 25 and 44 years. For those patients who experience a major depressive episode, up to 15 percent die by suicide. In the United States, on any given day, 20 percent of patients hospitalized on nonpsychiatric units are suffering from depression that goes undetected and untreated.

It is important to separate depressive disorders from the normal phenomena of "blues" or sadness, which are not depression. Normal grief accompanying the death of a loved one is not depression either. People with the "blues" or normal grief may experience short-lived symptoms of depression, but usually they continue to function almost normally and soon recover without undergoing treatment. Prolonged grief that interrupts a person's ability to function may signal the need for professional intervention.

Bodily or "vegetative" functions may be affected in depression. Patients commonly experience appetite disturbance (either a decreased appetite with resulting weight loss or, less frequently, increased appetite with weight gain); sleep disturbance (usually difficulty falling asleep, frequent awakening, or early morning awakening with the inability to fall asleep again, but sometimes increased sleep); fatigue; decreased energy; lessening of interest in or enjoyment of usual activities, including sex; and gastrointestinal symptoms such as dry mouth, nausea, constipation, or, less commonly, diarrhea. Pains sometime mysteriously appear and may migrate from one site to another and disappear when the depression lifts. Behavioral changes associated with changes in mood, thinking, and bodily function may vary from those that are minor (e.g., social withdrawal) and largely unrecognized to profound problems with obvious tearfulness, sad expressions, stooped posture, and slowed-down or agitated movements (e.g., pacing, restlessness, wringing of hands). Some people are able to work normally but feel horribly depressed, whereas others are unable to perform daily activities like dressing.

Depressed thinking often takes the form of negative thoughts about one's self, the present, and the future. Depressed people frequently complain of poor concentration and memory and difficulty making decisions. **Anxiety**, a sense that something unspecified, but dreadful, may happen, is often present in depressed people. Exaggerated fears about specific situations may also occur. As depression becomes more severe, patients often think they are helpless and worthless and their situation is hopeless. They often think of suicide. In the most severe depressions, **delusions** may appear, sometimes involving excessive guilt for past behavior, serious physical illness that is not present, or impoverishment, when that is not the case. Occasionally **hallucinations** may occur. These are usually experienced as hallucinations that are heard (usually voices, but sometimes music, clicks, or other noises) or seen (images of people or flashes of light), and occasionally as hallucinatory experiences of taste, touch, or smell. These most severe depressions are classified as depressions with psychotic features or psychotic depressions. The hallucinations, delusions, and poor judgment indicate that the person may have "lost contact with reality." People experiencing command hallucinations (voices) are at risk to act impulsively on the commands.

Religious preoccupations and worries about the meaning of life may contribute to or aggravate depression. Religion may also be a source of support and comfort, and provide meaning for life that might not otherwise be present during a depression. Many environmental stressors, such as financial problems, new jobs, legal problems, retirement, or other changes, can contribute to the development of depression. Medical illnesses can also cause or contribute to depression. Genetic predisposition; developmental factors, such as early loss of a parent; psychological factors, such as intense grief reactions; and stress, such as coping with physical illness, can combine to produce a final common pathway to depression.

Bipolar Disorder

Bipolar disorders are those mood disorders that are characterized by one or more manic episodes and usually one or more depressive episodes. Between episodes, patients may have long periods of normal moods, or they may cycle between manic and depressed states.

Other depressive disorders defined in the DSM-IV include cyclothymic disorder, dysthymic disorder, and mood disorder. Each disorder has specific criteria for making the diagnosis. The process of diagnosis can be complicated because of the number of factors that must be considered and the possibility of a differential diagnosis.

Anxiety Disorders

It is important to recognize that anxiety is a normal response to circumstances that are threatening. It is only when that response is excessive or persistent or when it no longer functions as a warning sign that it is considered pathologic. People who suffer from anxiety disorders find it difficult to function in personal, occupational, or social situations. People with these disorders experience symptoms that are often disabling.

Anxiety disorders as identified in the DSM-IV include **panic**, phobias, obsessive-compulsive disorder (OCD), post-traumatic stress disorder (PTSD), and generalized anxiety disorder (GAD).

Panic Disorder

Anxiety in its most disabling state is called panic disorder. Patients with panic disorder experience recurrent panic attacks. Some patients have an accompanying **agoraphobia.** They become fearful of being alone at home, traveling in a car or plane, or any circumstance where they would find it difficult to escape. These unreasonable fears create a situation that becomes crippling. As an example, consider the mother who is not able to take her child to the dentist because the office is on the 24th floor and she is afraid to get into the elevator.

Phobias

People who suffer from a **phobia** experience an irrational fear of a specific object, activity, or situation. This leads to them avoiding, or trying to avoid the circumstance that arouses the fear. Common phobias include fear of things such as dogs, cats, bridges, water, storms, heights, and closed spaces.

Obsessive-Compulsive Disorder

Obsessions are thoughts or impulses that the person recognizes as senseless but is unable to put out of his or her mind. They cause the person to suffer severe anxiety.

Compulsions are repetitive, ritualistic behaviors that the person feels driven to perform in an effort to reduce anxiety. The anxiety is relieved temporarily but, because the relief is only temporary, the act must be repeated over and over in an attempt to gain further relief.

Most frequently, obsessions and compulsions occur together, although they can be experienced independently. Many people who do not suffer from mental disorders experience some behavior that could be considered mildly obsessive-compulsive. For example, consider the person who has doubts about locking the door or turning off the lights at bedtime and has to check to see that those things actually have been done.

These can be considered "normal" behaviors. When obsessive-compulsive behaviors cause severe distress and interfere with normal life, they would be considered pathologic. When OCD is severe, it occupies so much of the person's thought process that cognitive performance may be affected.

Post-traumatic Stress Disorder

Post-traumatic stress disorder occurs after a person has witnessed or been part of a traumatic event that is outside the usual, such as a plane crash, tornado, or crime. The person experiences recurrent and intrusive recollections of the event. The symptoms of PTSD may not appear until several months or years after the event. People who suffer from this disorder often have difficulty in personal, social, and occupational situations. They may become abusive to a spouse or child, and chemical abuse is also seen.

Generalized Anxiety Disorder

People with **GAD** experience excessive worrying about many things that lasts for 6 months or more. They may be restless, irritable, or tense and suffer from sleep disturbance. They often have trouble concentrating and complain of fatigue. Their worry is out of proportion to the actual situation about which they are anxious. They have difficulty making decisions because of their poor concentration ability and because they are afraid of making a mistake.

Schizophrenic Disorders

Schizophrenia is a disease that interferes with a person's ability to communicate, perform simple, everyday tasks, or even take care of basic needs. It is a psychotic disorder. That means that the patient, as previously described in psychotic depression, has "lost contact with reality." Symptoms include hallucinations and delusions. Symptoms usually begin to appear in early childhood or adolescence. Patients with chronic schizophrenia occupy a high percentage of hospital beds designated for mental health because of their impaired ability to function.

It was originally believed that the causes of schizophrenia were psychological, but more recent theories suggest that the causes may be found in neurobiologic abnormalities. People with these abnormalities tend to be vulnerable to life events that are stressful.

Patients with schizophrenia often become depressed and are at risk for suicide. Hospitalized patients often drink excessive amounts of water, creating a fluid imbalance that can lead to serious problems such as seizures, cerebral edema, and even death. A health unit coordinator (HUC) should be alert to the patient who is constantly seeking something to drink and report it to the nursing personnel. The schizophrenic patient may also engage in violent or aggressive behavior.

Cognitive Disorders

The cognitive disorders were formerly called organic mental disorders. They include delirium and dementia.

Delirium is a disturbance of consciousness that develops over a short period of time. It is always secondary to another condition such as a medical condition or substance abuse. When the underlying cause is removed, the problem resolves.

Dementia is addressed in detail in Chapter 6, and is not discussed here.

Diagnostic Studies

As a basis for determining a diagnosis, the psychiatrist usually conducts a thorough mental status examination. The psychiatrist (or other physician) collects a thorough medical history and performs a complete physical examination, including a complete neurologic examination. A variety of diagnostic studies can be conducted to confirm the diagnosis.

Diagnostic Imaging

Computerized Tomography Scan

A computerized tomography (CT) scan of the head reveals any abnormal structures present and indicates the nature of the abnormality. It is a particularly useful evaluation tool in the investigation of dementia syndromes.

Magnetic Resonance Imaging

Magnetic resonance imaging (MRI) scanning can be used in place of a CT scan. Indications are that brain imaging will become an increasingly important aspect of psychiatric assessment in the future.

Positron Emission Tomography

Positron emission tomography (PET) is a state-of-the-art imaging technique that provides a means of examining actual brain function. It is useful in studying psychiatric disorders such as OCD, depression, and schizophrenia. However, because it is so new, it is not available in all hospitals at this time.

Laboratory Studies

Several laboratory tests can be used to identify depression. These tests attempt to identify "markers" of abnormalities in biologic function that suggest a likelihood of depression. Blood, urine, and sometimes spinal fluid or skin are used in these tests. These tests include the TRH (thyrotropin-releasing hormone) stimulation test and thyroid function studies.

Dexamethasone Suppression Test

The dexamethasone suppression test (DST) has been found to be an effective diagnostic tool in the identification of depression. However, in approximately half of the people with major depression, the DST is normal, and these people usually respond as well to standard antidepressant medications as do those who have abnormal DST results.

In addition to the diagnostic laboratory studies, drug monitoring studies are conducted to determine the adequacy of blood levels of the therapeutic agents being given.

Other Diagnostic Studies

Electroencephalogram

Measurement of brain waves by electroencephalogram (EEG) is being used as a diagnostic tool in psychiatric illnesses. It is very helpful in assessing toxic and infectious causes of confusion.

Lumbar Puncture

Lumbar puncture may be performed if there is a suspicion of hemorrhage, infection, or cancer involving the central nervous system.

Medications

Medications for Depressive Disorders

All of our feelings and thoughts, both pleasant and distressing, are the result of many electrochemical reactions that occur throughout our brains and bodies. Most depressions can be treated with chemicals called antidepressant medications. We do not fully understand the mechanisms of action of these drugs, but it seems fair to conclude that antidepressant medications work by correcting chemical imbalances.

Selective Serotonin Reuptake Inhibitors

Selective serotonin reuptake inhibitors (SSRIs) are an important advance in the treatment of depressive disorders. These drugs enhance the neurotransmitter's effects by preventing the reabsorption of serotonin in circulation. They are the first-choice treatment for many depressed people because these drugs have a lower incidence of side effects and act more quickly than the tricyclic antidepressants (TCAs). They have also been shown to be effective in treating other disorders such as anxiety disorder, OCD, and panic disorder. Because of the lower incidence of side effects, patients are more willing to remain on the therapy. The more commonly used SSRIs are shown in Table 8–1.

Tricyclic Antidepressants

The oldest medications, TCAs, are used to help relieve the symptoms of depression. Patients must take these drugs for 10 to 14 days before any effect may be seen or appreciated. Side effects can include dry mouth, blurred vision, tachycardia, constipation, urinary retention, and esophageal reflux. They are not usually serious and are often short in duration, but urinary retention and severe constipation warrant immediate attention. An important point for the HUC to know about these drugs is that the entire dose should be scheduled at night, for two reasons. TCAs have a sedative effect, and thus they aid in sleep. Second, the minor side effects occur during sleep, thus causing less discomfort for the patient. Table 8–2 lists the more common TCAs.

Monoamine Oxidase Inhibitors

Monoamine oxidase inhibitor (MAOI) antidepressants are usually taken in divided doses throughout the day. Patients are monitored carefully because of side effects such as extreme elevations in blood pressure. Diet also has to be carefully watched when taking these medications because substances such as wine, cheese, and liver can cause severe hypertensive reactions in patients taking MAOIs, with the possible development of intracranial hemorrhage. Table 8–3 lists the MAOIs currently in use in the United States.

Table 8–1 SELECTIVE SEROTONIN REUPTAKE INHIBITORS

Generic Name	Brand Name
Fluoxetine	Prozac
Mirtazapine	Remeron
Paroxetine	Paxil
Sertraline	Zoloft
Venlafaxine	Effexor

Table 8–2 TRICYCLIC ANTIDEPRESSANTS

Generic Name	Brand Name
Amitriptyline	Elavil, Endep
Desipramine	Norpramin, Pertofrane
Doxepin	Adapin, Sinequan
Imipramine	Tofranil
Nortriptyline	Aventyl, Pamelor
Protriptyline	Vivactil
Trimipramine	Surmontil

Medications for Bipolar Disorder

Lithium has been the drug of choice in controlling bipolar disorder. This drug tends to stabilize mood at a normal level, eliminating the high level of euphoria and the crushing level of the depressive state. Lithium also is used for people who have only **mania**.

It is important for the HUC to be aware that

Table 8–3 MONOAMINE OXIDASE INHIBITORS

Generic Name	Brand Name
Isocarboxazid	Marplan
Phenelzine	Nardil
Tranylcypromine	Parnate

a number of diagnostic studies are needed before lithium therapy is begun. These include thyroid studies and a baseline electrocardiogram. Serum levels of lithium are monitored to ensure adequate therapeutic action. Special diet teaching is required because lithium competes with sodium (salt). Dietary and fluid adjustments are necessary during summer months when people perspire more. This can affect their fluid intake and consequently their lithium level.

More recently, anticonvulsants are being used to achieve stabilization in patients with bipolar disorder. They may be given alone or in conjunction with lithium. A list of antimanic drugs can be found in Table 8–4.

Medications for Anxiety Disorders

Medications can be helpful in reducing the somatic and psychological symptoms of anxiety disorders. When the anxiety is reduced, patients are better able to participate in the therapies that are directed at the underlying problems.

The drugs used to treat anxiety disorders include antianxiety drugs and antidepressants. Many of these drugs have the potential for addiction. The HUC should be aware of this and be alert to recognize drug-seeking behaviors on the part of ambulatory patients who may approach the desk. The most commonly used drugs are those mentioned in the preceding tables, as well as those found in Table 8–5.

Antipsychotic Medications

Antipsychotic drugs are used for cases of acute schizophrenia or when psychotic symptoms are present. They are effective 3 to 6 weeks after the medications have been started. Many of these drugs have major side effects, and a decision on which drug to use is often made on the basis of its side effects. Some of the commonly used antipsychotic drugs can be found in Table 8–6.

Table 8–4 ANTIMANIC DRUGS

Generic Name	Brand Name
Lithium	Lithane, Eskalith, Lithonate
Carbamazepine	Tegretol
Valproic acid	Depakane

Table 8–5 ANTIANXIETY DRUGS

Generic Name	Brand Name
Alprazolam	Xanax
Clonazepam	Klonopin
Diazepam	Valium
Lorazepam	Ativan
Oxazepam	Serax
Hydroxyzine hydrochloride	Atarax
Hydroxyzine pamoate	Vistaril
Busipirone hydrochloride	BuSpar
Propranolol	Inderal

Table 8–6 ANTIPSYCHOTIC DRUGS

Generic Name	Brand Name
Chlorpromazine	Thorazine
Thioridazine	Mellaril
Risperidone	Risperdal
Trifluoperazine	Stelazine
Fluphenazine	Prolixin
Olanzapine	Zyprexa
Clozapine	Clozaril
Quetiapine	Seroquel
Haloperidol	Haldol

Treatments

Psychotherapy

Psychotherapy is referred to as the talk therapy. The patient and doctor talk about past experiences the patient has had or current experiences the patient is having. They talk about important relationships and future goals, as well as the feelings, thoughts, and behaviors that these experiences or relationships produce. Psychotherapies are helpful in improving thinking patterns, relationships, or behaviors that may lead to depression, or intensify depressive symptoms.

Dynamic Psychotherapy

Dynamic therapies seek to understand unresolved and unconscious conflicts that may lead to depression. Depression is often described as anger turned inward, and it is thought that helping the person uncover, understand, and deal more appropriately with angry feelings may lead to recovery from depression. Patients are helped to understand themselves, develop insights, and explore new ways of dealing with their feelings and with other people.

Cognitive Therapy

Cognitive therapists help patients by focusing on their negative thoughts about themselves, the world, and their future. Negative thoughts about oneself often lead to lower self-esteem. Negative thoughts about the world can lead to excessive caution and guardedness. Negative thoughts about the future can lead to pessimism and hopelessness. The goal of cognitive therapy is to change the way the patient thinks, and in doing so, relieve the depressive symptoms.

Behavior Therapy

Behavior therapy is based on the assumption that changes in negative behavior can occur without insight into the underlying cause. It is directed at specific problem behaviors. Positive reinforcement is used to increase the frequency of desired behaviors and negative consequences are used to decrease the frequency of undesirable behaviors.

Light Therapy

Some people get depressed in the winter because of the limited availability of sunlight. This syndrome, which is characterized by fatigue, weight gain, and irritability, is known as **seasonal affective disorder** (SAD). Daily treatments of 2 to 3 hours' exposure to bright lights have been shown to be effective in managing the symptoms of this disorder.

Electroconvulsive Therapy

One of the most effective ways of treating depression and certain other psychiatric conditions is ECT, more commonly known as **electroshock** (EST). This treatment is for patients for whom antidepressant drugs have been ineffective, whose depression has become life threatening, or who might otherwise require prolonged hospitalization.

Patients receiving ECT must sign an informed consent. Each state specifies the local conditions for voluntary informed consent and how circumstances for committed patients or those with guardians are managed.

The procedure is performed while the patient is under general anesthesia, so the patient does not experience any discomfort or pain. The procedure is carried out in an area specifically designated for that purpose, away from the rest of the unit (Fig. 8–3). In many hospitals, ECT is administered in the postanesthesia care unit. The psychiatrist administers ECT using a multiple-monitored electronic instrument. One electrode is placed on each of the patient's temples. A small, carefully controlled electronic current is passed between the two electrodes. This causes a short, generalized convulsion. Because of intravenous medication to relax the muscles, only a slight twitching of the muscles is usually seen. The seizure usually lasts anywhere between 45 and 60 seconds. The therapeutic action is related to the

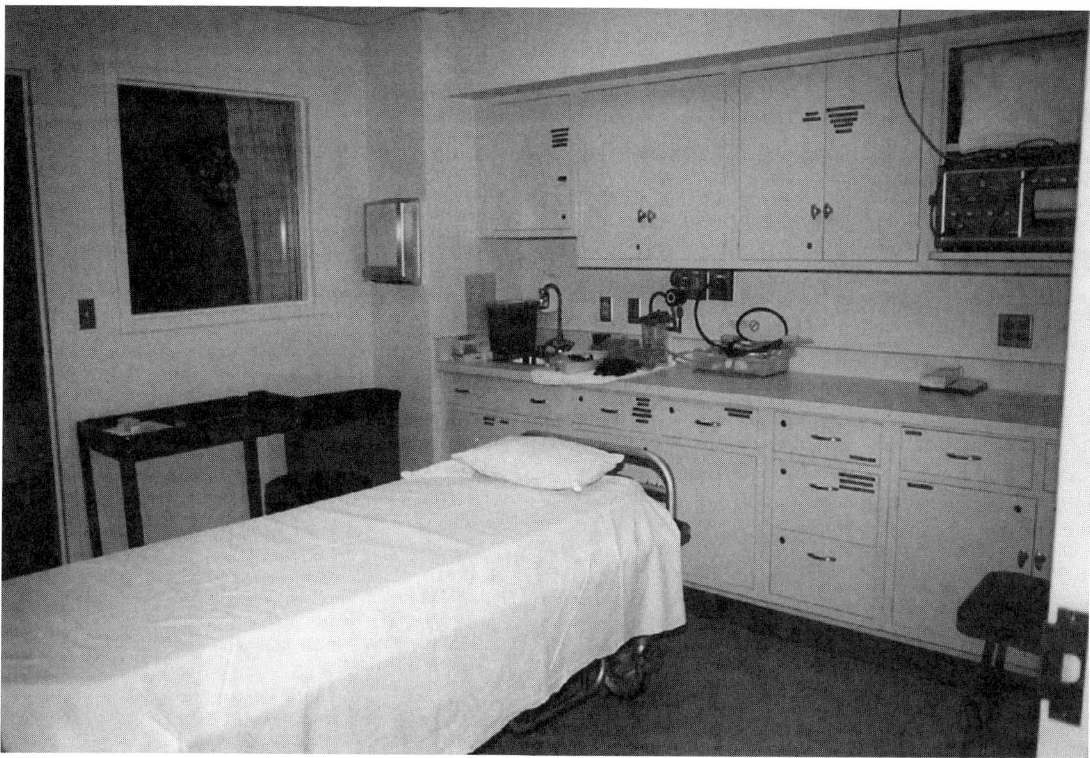

Figure 8–3
An ECT treatment room.

seizure activity itself, and not to the inducing agent, which is the electric current. Because the heart also operates using electrical conduction, a continuous electrocardiogram is recorded throughout the treatment and recovery phase.

Minutes after treatment, the patient slowly awakens in the recovery room (Fig. 8–4) and may experience transitory confusion similar to that seen in patients emerging from any type of brief anesthesia. Vital signs, such as blood pressure and pulse, are checked at regular intervals and the patient remains under continuous observation by the trained nursing personnel. When the patient is stabilized, he or she is returned to the hospital room. Because ECT is done under general anesthesia and the patient has been in a fasting state, breakfast is then served. The patient is then permitted to be up and around. Sometimes headaches, mild muscle soreness, or nausea occur, but usually these symptoms respond to simple treatment.

The number of treatments in any given case varies with the condition being treated, the individual response to the treatment, and the medical judgment of the psychiatrist giving the treatments. A typical course of therapy may consist of four to six treatments. The treatments are usually given two to three times a week. A certain amount of haziness, memory loss, and confusion may develop. This memory impairment is temporary and clears up usually within 1 to 3 weeks after the last treatment.

The length of time needed to recover varies from person to person, but is usually a few days

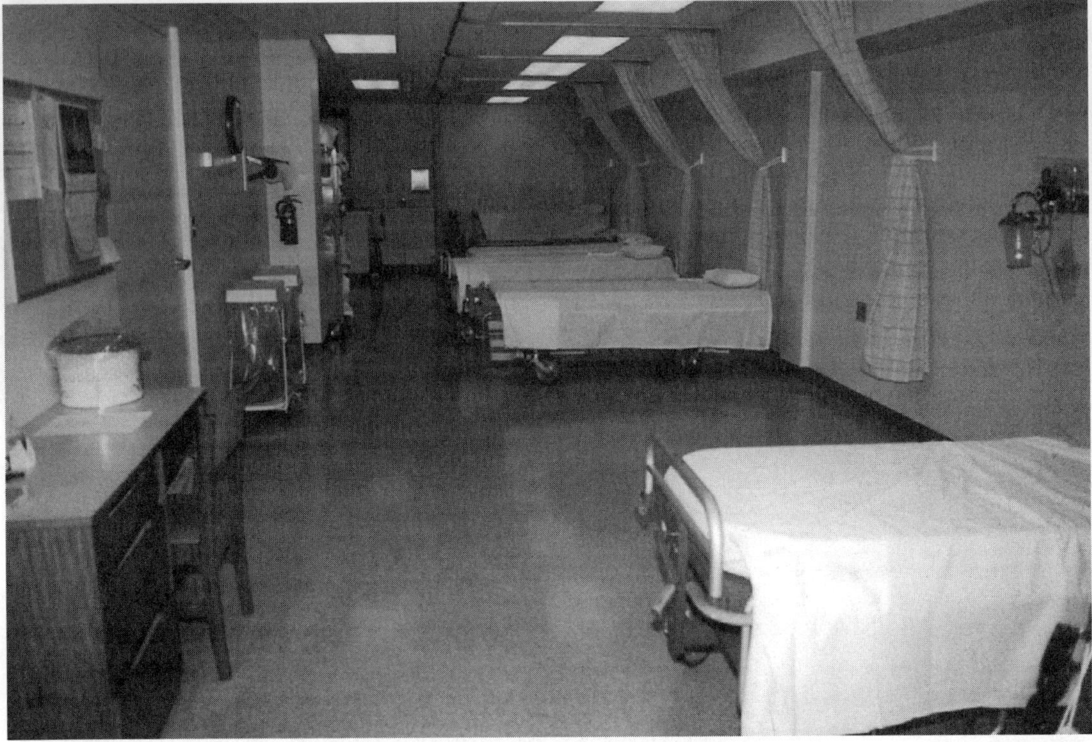

Figure 8–4
An ECT recovery room.

to 1 week. ECT is not considered a permanent cure, and maintenance treatment with medications decreases the relapse rate. Maintenance with ECT (once a month) may also be helpful in decreasing relapse rates for those patients who have poor success with antidepressant medications.

Communications

For the HUC, communication with the mental health patient is often on a much more personal level than in many of the other hospital units. Because many patients are ambulatory, they may frequently approach the desk for conversation. And, of course the HUC is the most readily available person. Being a good listener is very important because what the patient says, or perhaps leaves unsaid, may be a sign that a concern needs to be addressed. It is important for the HUC to be able to determine when the information needs to be turned over to the nursing staff.

The telephone presents another series of challenges. Confidentiality is taken to another level on the mental health unit. The HUC must be certain of the identity of callers and release no information inappropriately. In conveying information to appropriate people or departments involved with the patient's care, the HUC must be certain to convey only the necessary information.

Visitors seek the HUC for information regarding patients. It is important to recognize what information can be given to visitors. Any questions in regard to the patient's condition should be referred to the nursing staff. It is important to be aware that family members have concerns, and a willing ear may be very important to them as well.

Risk Management

Because mental health units are constructed with the idea of a treatment environment, everyone who works in the environment must be diligent in promoting patient safety. The need for patient safety focuses around specific areas of ensuring that patients can remain safe in the environment. For the HUC, there are specific implications for the role. The HUC is often the first person who patients and family meet. Many mental health units hold personal possessions on admission in order to go through them to ensure that there are no potential weapons or objects that patients might use to harm themselves. All staff members have an accountability to monitor patients in interactions with each other and the environment. As an example, this can mean that staff must count silverware on trays before and after meals to ensure that patients have not concealed contraband for self-harm activity. The nature of the psychiatric patient may include the potential for violence directed at others. Being aware of the potential for violence and knowing how to assist nursing personnel in the management of violent situations requires continuous training and practice to ensure a prompt response that promotes the safety of all people in the environment, patients and staff alike.

Closing Thoughts

A HUC who works in a mental health setting faces a multitude of treatment modalities that differ from those encountered in other nursing units. Duties are also different, requiring more clerical-legal activities than are found on other units. For example, many mental health patients are admitted against their will, through the courts; therefore, HUCs must become familiar with the proceedings for these types of admissions.

A mental health unit may be an environment where patients admit themselves on a voluntary basis or where patients may be detained against their will (per legal statutes when the patient is considered a danger to themselves or others). Each state has legislation or statutes that speak to how commitment is managed.

In many situations, the HUC working on a mental health unit may be involved in hands-on patient care as back-up to the nursing staff. This may include feeding, bathing, assisting with patient exams, or even making beds.

Many times, people are influenced in choosing a career path for personal reasons. When someone has had first-hand experience with mental illness in a spouse or other family member, he or she may find that working with this type of patient can be a way of dealing with the pain that these circumstances cause. It can become the way to a healthier and more peaceful way of life.

Review Questions

1. Explain the difference between depressive disorders and ordinary sadness.
2. Name four depressive disorders listed in the DSM-IV other than depression.
3. List five anxiety disorders as identified in the DSM-IV.
4. List five studies that may be ordered to aid in the diagnosis of mental disorders.
5. Explain what is meant by bipolar disorder.
6. Describe what ECT is and how the procedure is carried out.

Bibliography

American Psychiatric Association: Diagnostic and Statistical Manual of Mental Disorders, 4th ed. Washington, DC, American Psychiatric Association, 1994.

Fairview University Medical Center, Adult Mental Health Services, Adult Crises—30. Patient Information 61–8586, 1995.

Fairview University Medical Center: What You Should Know About Electroconvulsive Therapy. 61–7506, 1989.
Goldman HH: Review of General Psychiatry, 4th ed. Norwalk, CT, Appleton and Lange, 1995.
Greist JJ, Jefferson JW: Depression and its Treatment: Help for the Nation's #1 Mental Health Problem. Washington, DC, American Psychiatric Press, Inc., 1984.
Kraslecke DM, Tarkinou ML: Erasing the stigma of electroconvulsive therapy. Post Anesthes Nurs. 1992;7:84.
Tan MW, McDonough WJ: Risk management in psychiatry. Psychiatr Clin North Am. 1990;13:135.
Varcarolis EM: Foundations of Psychiatric Mental Health Nursing, 3rd ed. Philadelphia, WB Saunders, 1998.

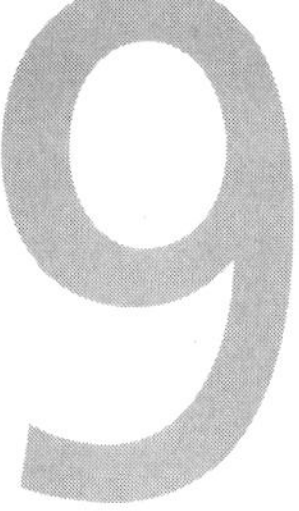

Neurology/Rehabilitation

Linda Winslow

Objectives

Upon completion of this chapter, the reader should be able to:

1. Identify the reasons why a patient would be hospitalized on a neurology unit.
2. List five imaging procedures used in diagnosing neurologic problems.
3. List five neurophysiology tests that might be conducted on a neurologic patient.
4. Name the scale used to assess the neurologic patient's level of consciousness.

Vocabulary

Cerebral angiography: Procedure to view the intracranial and extracranial blood vessel

Denervation: Deprivation of nerve supply

Digital subtraction angiography: Computer-assisted procedure to visualize extracranial or intracranial blood vessels

Doppler imaging: Ultrasound procedure used to trace blood flow

Glasgow Coma Scale: A standard measure used to evaluate a patient's level of consciousness

Neuron: Unit of nervous tissue that conducts impulses

Paralysis: Loss of voluntary muscle control

Paresis: Muscle weakness

Synapse: Site of contact between two neurons

Common Abbreviations

ADL	Activities of daily living
ALS	Amyotrophic lateral sclerosis
Amp	Amputation
BAER	Brainstem auditory evoked response
BMP	Bowel management program
CAOD	Carotid artery occlusive disease
CARF	Commission on Accreditation of Rehabilitation Facilities
CR	Communication rehabilitation
CVA	Cerebrovascular accident
DJD	Degenerative joint disease
DSA	Digital subtraction angiography
DTR	Deep tendon reflexes
EEG	Electroencephalogram
EMG	Electromyogram
ICP	Intracranial pressure
I	Independent
LOC	Level of consciousness/ laxative of choice
LOS	Length of stay
LP	Lumbar puncture
MRI	Magnetic resonance imaging
NWB	Non–weight bearing
Neuro	Neurology
NV	Neurovascular
OD	Right eye
OS	Left eye
OT	Occupational therapy
OU	Both eyes
Para	Paraplegic
PERRLA	Pupils equal, round, reactive to light and accommodation
PT	Physical therapy
PWB	Partial weight bearing
Quad	Quadriplegic
Rehab	Rehabilitation
ROM	Range of motion
RT	Recreational therapy
SCM	Sensation, circulation, movement
SEP	Somatosensory evoked potentials
Sx	Suction
SW	Social worker
TENS	Transcutaneous electrical nerve stimulation
TPN	Total parenteral nutrition
Tx	Traction
VA	Visual acuity
VEP	Visual evoked potentials
VF	Visual fields

Overview

Nursing units are the heart of the hospital. On these units, patients are provided with services unique to the unit. Most nursing units are designed to provide care for 18 to 50 patients. The neurology/rehabilitation unit is a combination of two unique services. In some hospital settings, these services are separate units, in others they are combined. This chapter provides you with the following information regarding these units:

1. Description of patient population served
2. Description of basic anatomy/physiology
3. Definitions of common abbreviations
4. Frequent medications
5. Diagnostic tests
6. Patient care delivery
7. Equipment and supplies
8. Documentation
9. Impact on health unit coordinating

Description of the Patient Population

The third edition of *Health Unit Coordinating* defines the neurology unit as an area devoted to the care of patients who are hospitalized for treatment of diseases of the nervous system. In general, the

The abbreviations listed for this chapter are those that a HUC working in this area would be expected to know. Only those in boldface type are used in the text and appear in boldface when they are used for the first time.

patient population served on this unit has suffered some type of alteration, either physiologic or psychosocial, because of changes in the nervous system function. These patients usually have experienced some type of change in one or more of the following: intellectual process, emotional response, sensory perceptions, fine and gross motor activity, communication systems, and the special senses (i.e., taste, smell, hearing, vision, touch). The goal of nursing care is to return the patients to lives that are as productive and independent as possible by assisting with their care. Each nursing team member should have a through understanding of the processes and resources available to assist the patients to meet this goal.

The rehabilitation nursing unit, also according to the third edition of *Health Unit Coordinating*, is defined as a unit that cares for patients who are hospitalized for physical handicaps; usually these patients need long-term treatment and care. The goal of the rehabilitation nursing unit is to facilitate the movement of patients toward independence. This goal is best accomplished by a multidisciplinary health care team that includes the patient and family members. These patients often have some type of physical handicap and are transferred from other nursing units. One of the units that transfers patients to the rehab unit is the neurology unit. To help the patients meet their goal of independence, the health care team members must have an understanding of anatomy and physiology, psychological responses to disability, and personal and community resources.

Anatomy and Physiology of the Nervous System

The nervous system is a complex bodily network that is usually divided into two parts (Fig. 9–1):

1. The central nervous system (CNS), which includes the brain and the spinal cord
2. The peripheral nervous system (PNS), which includes 12 pairs of cranial nerves, 31 pairs of spinal nerves, and associated ganglia.

The nervous system controls and integrates the activities of the different parts of the body, providing for normal voluntary and involuntary function of the body. Our view of the world, ourselves, and interactions with the world are greatly influenced by the correct functioning of the nervous system.

The basic structure of the nervous system is composed of nerve tissue. This tissue is made up of individual cells. The **neuron** is the unit of nervous tissue that conducts impulses. The basic function of the nervous system is to conduct impulses, and therefore the other cells in the nervous system provide support for the neurons, regulate the nerve cell environment, and feed the neurons. There are two types of neurons. Afferent neurons, also called sensory neurons or receptor neurons, receive incoming stimuli. They transmit impulses to the brain and spinal cord. Motor neurons transmit impulses away from the brain and spinal cord to other parts of the body that are capable of responding, such as muscle. These are also known as efferent neurons. The site of contact between two neurons is called a **synapse**.

Central Nervous System

Brain

The brain is located in the cranial cavity and is covered by the bony structure called the skull. The brain is the center for coordinating all body activity. It is divided into three main parts.

Cerebrum

The cerebrum is the largest part of the brain. It is divided into a right hemisphere and a left hemisphere. The following centers are contained in the cerebrum:

a. Sensory
b. Hearing
c. Sight
d. Motor
e. Memory
f. Intellect

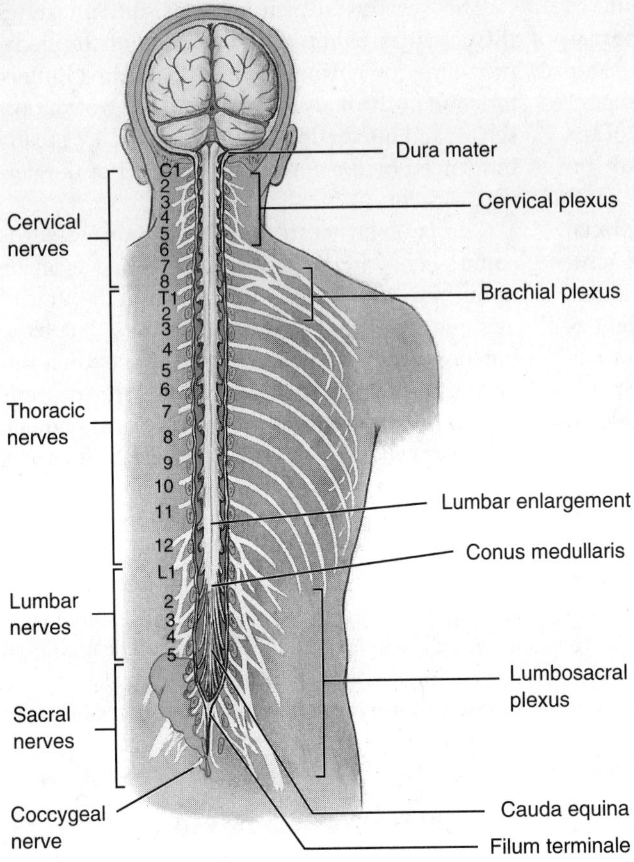

Figure 9–1
The nervous system. (From Applegate EJ: The Anatomy and Physiology Learning System: Textbook. Philadelphia, WB Saunders, 1995.)

g. Judgment
h. Emotion

Spaces in the cerebrum called ventricles produce cerebrospinal fluid (CSF). CSF surrounds the brain and the spinal cord. Its function is to cushion any shock that may occur in these areas.

Cerebellum

The cerebellum, also called the "hind brain," functions to assist in the coordination of voluntary muscles. It also maintains balance. It can be said that this area provides the fine tuning for motor activities.

Brainstem

The brainstem consists of three major divisions, the midbrain, pons, and medulla oblongata. In addition, cranial nerves 10 through 12 originate in the brainstem. This area is the final pathway between the cerebral structures and the spinal cord. It is an important area that has connecting links controlling three vital functions: heartbeat, blood pressure, and respiration.

Meninges

The brain is covered with three thin layers of membrane called meninges. They are located between the brain and the skull. The outer layer is called the *dura mater* or "hard mother" because it is shiny and tough. Its function is to form channels that drain blood from the brain.

The second layer is called the *arachnoid*. This is the pathway for reabsorption of CSF into the venous system. The *pia mater* or "tender mother" is the third layer of the meninges. It adheres closely to the brain. CSF flows between the arachnoid and the pia mater. This space is called the subarachnoid space.

Skull

The skull is composed of several bones fused together to form an immobile unit. The skull is divided into the brain skull and the facial skull. The function of the skull is to protect the vital organs inside. If an accident occurs and the brain is damaged, the skull's rigidity can prevent tissue expansion, thus causing problems.

Spinal Cord/Column

The spinal cord is the pathway for nerve tissue as it exits the brain. It is encased and protected by the bony structure of the spinal (vertebral) column. The spinal cord is the pathway for sensory impulses *up* to the brain, and motor impulses *down* from the brain. The spinal column is made up of 33 vertebrae joined together. These bones are separated by cartilage pads called *discs*. Any trauma to this area could result in injury that could lead to **paralysis**, the loss of voluntary muscle control.

Peripheral Nervous System

The PNS is any part of the nervous system outside the CNS. Peripheral nerves are usually interpreted to include the cranial nerves, the spinal nerves, and the autonomic nervous system. If a peripheral nerve is severed, the result is a loss of sensation and muscular activity to the area of the body served by the nerve. Note, however, that many nerves serve and overlap in a given area, so that the severing of one nerve may not be noticed. If many nerves are severed, the result is **paresis** or muscle weakness. There is some chance of regeneration of nerves, which can be facilitated by a surgical procedure. Success depends on the skill of the surgeon, the severity of the injury, and the postoperative care.

Autonomic Nervous System

The autonomic nervous system is also termed the "involuntary nervous system." Its major function is regulation of body organs and the internal environment of the body. There are two major subdivisions of the autonomic nervous system.

Sympathetic

The sympathetic system is the "fight-or-flight" regulator. This system provides the stimulation to activate those systems necessary in times of stress, emergency, or trauma. It inhibits those activities that are not needed at that time.

Parasympathetic

The parasympathetic system is the vegetative system. It is involved in those activities associated with the conservation and restoration of energy stores.

Both systems have great influence on the following organs and functions: eyes, heart, blood vessels, and lungs; bladder, gastrointestinal, and bowel control; and sexual functioning. The systems tend to balance each other.

Medications

Many patients with neurologic problems receive medications to help manage these problems. It is important to give patients and care providers information about the medications they will be taking. This information should include the medication name, dose and schedule of administration, common side effects, drug interactions, what to do if a dose is missed, what the drug is being given for, and when to call the physician. Some common medications and what they are given for include:

Drug	Reason for use
Coumadin	Blood thinner
Heparin	Blood thinner
Lovenox	Blood thinner
Surfak	Stool softener
Colace	Stool softener
Dulcolax tablets/ suppositories	Laxative
Urecholine	Urinary tract infection
Bactrim	Urinary tract infection
MS (Morphine sulfate)	Pain
Demerol	Pain
Dalmane	Sleep
Chloral hydrate	Sleep
Kefzol	Antibiotic
Tetracycline	Antibiotic
Elase	Pressure ulcers
DuoDerm/Op Sites	Pressure ulcers
Solu-Cortef	Reduce inflammation
Prednisone	Reduce inflammation

These are some of the medications you would most likely see ordered for patients on the **neuro/rehab** unit, but the list is far from complete. Each year, many new medications are made available for patient use. It is important for the health unit coordinator (HUC) to stay current with regard to new medications that are being used on the unit. The unit library, which usually includes references such as the *Physician's Desk Reference* and the *Hospital Formulary*, as well as the hospital pharmacists, are good resources for the HUC whenever there are questions regarding medication orders.

Diagnostic Tests

Most neurologic diagnostic tests provide general information on the presence of a problem in the area in question, but do not indicate the specific nature of the problem. For example, an echoencephalogram can confirm the presence of a lesion but cannot identify the nature of the lesion.

Imaging Procedures

Computed Tomography

Computed tomography (CT), or computed axial tomography, is a noninvasive diagnostic procedure that has had a significant impact on methods of diagnosis, especially in neurology and neurosurgery. This procedure has been refined and improved and is sure to continue in that direction. No special preparation is required and no special care is necessary after the procedure is completed. The advantages of using a CT scan are:

1. Much information can be collected in a short amount of time.
2. It is painless.
3. It reduces the need for more invasive tests that can be dangerous.
4. The amount of radiation exposure is low.
5. The scan can be performed on all patients who can remain still, whether they are conscious or unconscious.
6. The procedure is very accurate.

Magnetic Resonance Imaging

Magnetic resonance imaging (MRI) is an exciting new technology. This procedure shows sharp, detailed cross sections of living tissue. It provides anatomic information and information about the chemistry and physiology of living tissue. MRI is noninvasive and does not use radiation, thus eliminating exposure to the hazards of radiation. The procedure is painless and has no known risks to the patient. The patient is placed in a strong magnetic field and subjected to computer-programmed bursts of pulsed radio waves. MRI is effective in identifying small malignancies and degenerative diseases in the central nervous system. The MRI can serve as a very effective tool for diagnostic purposes because it can provide information very early in the disease process, even before other changes are noted.

Myelography

Myelography is a procedure in which a subarachnoid puncture is performed. CSF is removed (10 ml) and a contrast medium is injected. X-rays of the area are then taken. This procedure is ordered when the physician suspects a spinal cord tumor, herniated intravertebral disc, or ruptured disc.

Angiography

Cerebral angiography is a procedure performed to view the intracranial and extracranial blood vessels. The patient is injected with dye at either the carotid or vertebral artery directly, or indirectly through the femoral, brachial, subclavian, or axillary artery. X-rays are taken at various times after the injection. This procedure is used to diagnose intracranial lesions. Aneurysms and arteriovenous malformations can also be diagnosed. This procedure can be performed under local or general anesthesia.

Digital subtraction angiography (**DSA**) is a computer-assisted procedure used to visualize the extracranial or intracranial vessels, as well as other vascular conditions in the body. In this procedure, images are taken before and after injection of a contrast medium. The first image is then subtracted from the second. This procedure is useful in the diagnosis of arteriosclerotic disease, vascular lesions, and tumors, and in the postoperative evaluation of endarterectomy, aneurysms, and clipping.

Other Diagnostic Procedures

Lumbar Puncture

Lumbar puncture (**LP**) is a procedure used for diagnostic and therapeutic purposes. The procedure consists of placing a hollow needle into the lumbar subarachnoid space of the spinal canal. Diagnostic purposes may include:

1. Measurement of cerebrospinal pressure
2. Examination of the CSF for blood
3. Collection of the CSF for lab studies
4. Injection of materials to visualize parts of the nervous system
5. Evaluation of CSF flow

The procedure for therapeutic purposes may include:

1. Introduction of spinal anesthesia
2. Intrathecal injection of medication

This procedure requires careful medical judgment.

Doppler Imaging

Doppler imaging is a noninvasive procedure in which an ultrasonic probe is placed over the skin and slowly moved. This procedure uses sound waves to trace the flow of blood. The data are amplified and a graphic recording is made, as well as a sound recording. This procedure is painless, safe, and approximately 95% accurate. It is used to diagnose problems with carotid blood flow, plaque deposits in the carotid arteries, and **CAOD** (carotid artery occlusive disease).

Neurophysiology Tests

Electromyography

Electromyography (**EMG**) is a test used to detect the type and presence of neuromuscular disorders. This test records the electrical activity of the muscles and peripheral nerves. It can detect minimal **denervation** of a muscle. The test consists of inserting needle electrodes into the muscle to be examined. This test can be painful when the needles are inserted. The electrical activity of the muscle is recorded when the muscle is at rest and during contraction. The accuracy of this test depends on the skill, training, and experience of the person performing the test. This test is helpful in identifying compression or trauma to nerves.

Electroencephalography

Electroencephalography (**EEG**) is a test used in identifying seizure disorders and differentiating functional from organic brain disorders. An EEG can also aid in the diagnosis of stroke, head injury, drug overdose, brain death, and metabolic disorders. This test is a recording of the brain waves (electrical activity of the brain). Electrodes are placed on the scalp and the activity of the brain is recorded at rest, after hyperventilation, during sleep, and with light stimulation. This test takes from 40 to 60 minutes and prints out over 100 sheets of recordings. It is painless for the patient.

Evoked Potentials

Brainstem evoked potentials are tests classified into three categories. The categories are based on the type of stimuli provided and the sensory system stimulated. The three sensory systems are visual, auditory, and somatosensory. Evoked potentials are minute voltages that occur to brief stimuli and are recorded from the electrodes placed on the scalp.

Visual Evoked Potentials

Visual evoked potentials (**VEP**) are used in evaluating the optic nerves. This test can only be done on patients able to follow directions and cooperate.

Brainstem Auditory Evoked Response

Brainstem auditory evoked response (**BAER**) can be helpful in diagnosing posterior fossa tumors, stroke, and conductive hearing loss. This test can be done on conscious and unconscious patients.

Somatosensory Evoked Potentials

Somatosensory evoked potentials (**SEP**) is an unpleasant test using electrical stimuli to diagnose spinal cord function.

Laboratory Tests

Lab tests commonly ordered on patients with head/spinal cord injures include the following:

Study	Purpose
ABGs (arterial blood gases)	Assess arterial oxygen
WBC (white blood cell count)	Monitor development of sepsis
PT (prothrombin time)	Coagulation
Serum electrolytes	Assess fluid imbalance
BUN (blood urea nitrogen)	Assess renal function
UA (urinalysis)	Monitor for urinary infection/kidney disease
Glucose	Hypoglycemia/ hyperglycemia
Hemoglobin/ hematocrit	Blood loss due to hemorrhage

Neurologic Assessment

The neurologic exam focuses on determining the presence, absence, or lowering of function of sensory, motor, or reflex systems. This exam is performed by a physician initially. However, other health care team members may continue to perform and document findings periodically during the patient's hospitalization. The **Glasgow Coma Scale** (GCS; Table 9–1) is widely used in an attempt to standardize the professional's assessment of the patient's **LOC** (level of consciousness). The system's use is common throughout the United States and Europe because of its precision and use of clear terms. It then becomes easy to convey information from one health care provider to another. The scale was developed in 1974 at the University of Glasgow, Scotland. The scale is divided into three areas: eye opening, best motor response, and best verbal response. As a general rule, the lower the score on the scale and the longer the post-traumatic gap in the formation of memory, the more likely the patient is to suffer permanent cognitive and personality changes.

Patient Care Delivery

The patient is cared for by a patient care team. The team can be multidisciplinary or intradisciplinary, depending on the patient care delivery system in place at the health care facility. The team member-

Table 9–1 GLASGOW COMA SCALE

Assessment	Score
Eyes Open	
Never	1
To pain	2
To verbal stimuli	3
Spontaneously	4
Best Verbal Response	
No response	1
Incomprehensible sounds	2
Inappropriate words	3
Disoriented and converses	4
Oriented and converses	5
Best Motor Response	
No response	1
Extension (decerebrate rigidity)	2
Flexion abnormal (decorticate rigidity)	3
Flexion withdrawal	4
Localizes pain	5
Obeys	6
Total	3–15

ship is quite similar in both, but the function is different. In a multidisciplinary system, each discipline defines the goals for the patient, whereas in an intradisciplinary system, the team identifies the goals and all team members are involved in the process. This would mean that team members are involved in problem solving and goal setting outside of their disciplines. The model shown in Figure 9–2 is often used to illustrate the team concept.

Treatments

Treatments are provided by the patient care teams, and are specific to the patient needs. Treatments include beds, mattresses, pads, wound care products, medications, and surgical management.

Pressure Ulcer Care

Patients may require pressure ulcer treatments because often they have spent many days confined to bed. The health care marketplace offers a variety of devices to equalize pressure and distribute weight, including mechanical beds as well as mattresses filled with water, sand, or air. Mechanical beds are used to change pressure positions and reduce pressure on body areas that are at risk for breakdown. These devices, when used correctly, provide position changes safely. Included in this group are Stryker wedge frames, Circo electric beds, oscillating beds, and fluidized beds. Specialty mattresses are also used to reduce pressure on sensitive areas. These mattresses are filled with air, foam, and fluids.

Pads such as heel pads and elbow pads made of sheepskin can be used to reduce friction on sensitive areas. These pads do not reduce pressure.

Wound Care

Wound care products and medications are provided by several vendors. These products are used as prescribed by the physician. Surgical treatments are used when other options have failed or are not the best choice.

Oxygen

If oxygen therapy is ordered by the physician, respiratory care will deliver this service to the patient. Oxygen decreases the workload of the cardiopulmonary system, allowing the patient to breath easier, and reduces the effects of hypoxemia. Oxygen can be delivered through different

GENERAL HOSPITAL
Comprehensive Inpatient Rehabilitation Unit

FIM: Admission ____________ Present: ____________
Referred by: ____________
Date of Admission: ____________ Date of Plan: ____________
Contraindications: ____________
Diagnosis: ____________
Rehabilitation Problems: ____________

Estimated Length of Stay: ____________
Discharge Disposition: ____________

HOME HEALTH FOLLOW-UP/OUTPAITENT/TBI
☐ Nsg ☐ Aide ____ hours per day
☐ PT ☐ OT____ ☐ CR times per week

EQUIPMENT:
☐ Hospital Bed ☐ Cane ☐ W/C
☐ Walker ☐ Elevated toilet seat
☐ Tub bench commode ☐ Orthotics

I. TEAM REHABILITATION GOALS: | **PROJECTED TIME FRAME FOR ACHIEVEMENT**

GENERAL HOSPITAL
Comprehensive Inpatient Rehabilitation Unit

PATIENT/FAMILY IDENTIFIED REHABILITRATION GOALS | **PROJECTED TIME FRAME FOR ACHIEVEMENT**

Attest: Patient/family–this program plan has been discussed with me and my participation has been solicited and encouraged

____
Patient and/or Family Representative Date

____
Program Manager Date

Progress Conference Date: ____________

Comments:

Figure 9–2
Team plan for rehabilitation. (Modified from Marquette General Hospital: Comprehensive Inpatient Rehabilitation Unit, Marquette, MI.)

systems based on the patient's condition, oxygen concentration needed, and the patient's ability to comply with the therapy.

1. Low-oxygen systems include nasal cannulas or catheters, oxygen masks, and partial rebreathing masks.
2. T-pieces are used to deliver oxygen through a tracheostomy tube.
3. Transtracheal systems deliver oxygen directly into the trachea.

Bladder/Bowel Retraining

The retraining programs must be started when the patient is conscious, alert, and oriented, or success will not be achieved. Most hospitals have written protocols for these retraining or management programs. The following is an example of such a program:

If the patient is not able to gain bladder control, intermittent catheterization may be used. Patients can be taught this technique to use after discharge if needed.

Education

Patient education, including discharge instructions, can be challenging to present to patients with cerebral injuries. These patients may have special problems in learning because of cognitive deficits. These deficits might include memory loss, inability to think abstractly, easy distractibility, short attention span, poor judgment, and inability to transfer learning from one situation to another. Teaching materials need to be customized to each patient or family's learning style/needs. Often, older patients need written materials in large print or verbal instructions on audiotapes. Videotapes are excellent teaching tools.

Equipment and Supplies

As patients strive to return to their home environments, they are often faced with challenges that require the services of the orthotist, a professional who designs braces according to each patient's needs. Assistive devices often enable patients to return home at an earlier date and continue therapy on an outpatient basis. Other assistive devices that are commonly used on a neuro/rehab unit include the following:

Canes: These are available in many styles, with features for specific needs and lifestyles. Examples include straight cane, quad cane, broad-based cane, and tripod cane. Canes are held on the unaffected side.

Walkers: These devices vary according to structure and purpose. Reciprocal walkers are used by people who lose their balance and tend to fall backward. Pickup walkers can be lightweight and adjustable.

Bracing: This is used by patients who may need an assistive device to provide stabilization at the foot, knee, or ankle to make ambulation possible.

Documentation

Patient documentation is an important part of the patient's care. The documentation is the communication form used between team members. It charts a patient's progress, with different forms being used by various health care facilities to suit their particular needs. Flow sheets are easy to follow and charting by all team members can easily be retrieved. Critical pathways (patient plans of care with projected outcomes) are being used throughout the country (Fig. 9–3).

Closing Thoughts

As our population's life expectancy continues to extend into the eighth and ninth decades of life, rehabilitation services will continue to grow and be used by more and more people each year. Health care costs will encourage people to explore options and to focus on wellness activities. The HUC's position on the health care team will continue to expand with the technology of computers and equipment.

Adm Date: Nurse:

REHAB BRAIN INJURY
NSG Clinical Path 14 Day(s)

NSG DX: Functional Impairments: A, B, C, D, F, G, H, other

DRG's:
Improved Cognition/Memory/Judgement Improved Communication
Continent of Bowel and Bladder Safe, Adequate Nutrition
Improved Mobility Improved Psych/Soc Adj. Inc. Behav.

Eval-Days 1-2	TX I-Days 3-7	TX II-Days 8-12	Discharge Day
GOALS Oriented to Unit, Therapies, Schedule, Staffings Behavior Modification Nutritional Needs Being Met	GOALS Aware of Home Program (Pt. and Family) Behavior Modification Nutritional Needs Being Met Greater Independence w/ADLs and Mobility Improved Cognitive/Communicative Function	GOALS Knows Home Program (Pt. and Family) Behavior Modification, Tolerate Mod. Stim. Environment Nutritional Needs Being Met Greater Independence w/ADLs and Mobility Improved Cognitive/Communicative Functions	GOALS Knows Home Program Behavior Modification, Tolerate Mod. Stim. Environment Nutritional Needs Being Met Greater Independence w/ADLs and Mobility
ASSESSMENTS Q8*: Skin, Neuro, Psych/Soc., Agitation, Pain QD: Cardiovascular, Pulmonary, GI, GU, Equipment Needs, Teaching Needs Assessment by Therapists Additional Consults & Assessments PRN Neuro Psych Assessment PRN FIMS	ASSESSMENTS Q8*: Skin, Neuro, Psych/Soc., Agitation, Pain QD: Cardiovascular, Pulmonary, GI, GU, Equipment Needs, Teaching Needs Assessment by Therapists Additional Consults & Assessments PRN Neuro Psych Assessment PRN Fims Q Staffing	ASSESSMENTS Q8*: Skin, Neuro, Psych/Soc., Agitation, Pain QD: Cardiovascular, Pulmonary, GI, GU, Equipment Needs, Teaching Needs Assessment by Therapists Additional Consults & Assessments PRN Vocational Assessment FIMS Q Staffing	ASSESSMENTS WNL: VS, Skin, Neuro, Cardiovascular, Pulmonary, GI, GU, Psych/Soc., Agitation, Pain Teaching Needs Met Equipment Needs Met Assessments by Therapists Additional Consults & Assessments PRN FIMS
TEACHING Rehab Milieu Tour of Unit Therapy Schedule Provided and Reviewed Identify Support Network/Community Resources for D/C Planning Family Ed. re: B.I.	TEACHING Review Plan of Care Disease Process; Diabetes as indicated; Medication Admin.; Nutrition; Bladder & Bowel Mgmt; Skin Care; Tube Feedings PRN; Peg Tube Care PRN; Behaviour & Agitation Mgmt; Home Programs; TXs; Equipment Mobility-Ambulation; Transfers, Bed, W/C, Community ADLs (Basic) Family Ed.; Community Leisure Resources	TEACHING Review-Plan of Care, Disease Process, Diabetes PRN, Medication Admin., Nutrition, Bladder & Bowel Mgmt., Skin Care, Psych/Soc. Mgmt to include Mood, Behavior, Agitation, Home Programs, TXs, Equipment Mobility-Ambulation, Transfers, Bed, W/C, Community ADLs (Basic and High Level) PRN Family Ed. Community Leisure Resources	TEACHING D/C Instructions PMIs S&S to Report to MD TXs Activity Diet F/U Labs Family Ed.
KEY INTERVENTIONS V/S Bid Weight Monitor Labs and XR Intradisciplinary TX Identify Plan of Care w/ Pt./Family to include D/C Plans and Low. Stim. Protocol Low Simulation Protocal Initiated Behavior Modification Program Referral to B.I. Support Group Equipment Implemented, as indicated	KEY INTERVENTIONS V/S Bid Monitor Labs and XR Intradisciplinary TX Review Plan of Care w/ Pt./Family Community Resource Referrals PRN Memory Journal /Planner PRN Low Stim. Envir. Behavior Mod. Program	KEY INTERVENTIONS V/S Bid Monitor Labs and XR Intradisciplinary TX Review Plan of Care w/ Pt./Family Community Resource Referrals PRN Memory Journal /Planner PRN Mod. Stim. Envir. Behavior Mod. Program Opportunity for Community Reintegration	KEY INTERVENTIONS V/S Bid Equipment Ordered, as indicated Rx on chart and to patient TX Doc on D/C Summary Diet on D/C Summary Activity on D/C Summary F/U Appointments on D/C Summary F/U Therapy Scheduled Community Resource Referrals Arranged Vocational Rehab Referrals

Figure 9–3
Rehabilitation critical pathway. (Modified from Marquette General Hospital: Comprehensive Inpatient Rehabilitation Unit, Marquette, MI.)

The care of the patient will start before admission and continue into the home care environment. HUCs have been responsible for the clerical aspects of patient care. That care will continue with the patient as the focus of care. Technology will continue to provide care to people, but people will need to make up the "team" to provide the technology. In-patient ***LOS*** *(length of stay) will continue to decrease, and the home care environment will open new opportunities for the HUC.*

Review Questions

1. Identify the reasons why a patient would be hospitalized on a neurology unit.

2. List five imaging procedures used in diagnosing neurologic problems.
3. List five neurophysiology tests that might be conducted on a neurologic patient.
4. Name the scale used to assess the neurologic patient's level of consciousness.

Bibliography

Adams RD, Victor M, Ropper AH: Principles of Neurology, 6th ed. Princeton, NJ, McGraw-Hill, 1977.

Dittmar S: Rehabilitation Nursing. St. Louis, CV Mosby, 1989.

Hole JW: Essentials of Human Anatomy and Physiology, 4th ed. Dubuque, IA, William C. Brown, 1992.

Hoeman S: Rehabilitation Nursing: Process and Application, 2nd ed. St. Louis, CV Mosby, 1996.

La-Fleur Brooks M: Health Unit Coordinating, 3rd ed. Philadelphia, WB Saunders, 1993.

Rowland LP: Merritt's Textbook of Neurology, 9th ed. Baltimore, Williams & Wilkins, 1995.

Snell RS: Clinical Anatomy for Medical Students, 5th ed. Boston, Little, Brown, 1995.

Snyder M: A Guide to Neurological and Neurosurgical Nursing. New York, John Wiley and Sons, 1983.

10 The Operating Room

Cynthia Nault

Common Abbreviations

AORN	Association of OR Nurses
CRNA	Certified Registered Nurse Anesthetist
EUA	Exam under anesthesia
IS	Computer information systems
JCAHO	Joint Commission on Accreditation of Health Care Organizations
ODS	One day surgery
OR	Operating room
OSHA	Occupational Safety & Health Administration
PACU	Postanesthesia care unit
SS	Surgical Services

Objectives

Upon completion of this chapter, the reader will be able to:

1. List potential disruptions to the surgical schedule.
2. Describe various job positions in an operating room suite that a health unit coordinator might aspire to.
3. Explain ways that communication in the operating room suite might be different from that in patient care units.
4. Explain the statistical activities that a health unit coordinator might be required to do in an operating room.

Vocabulary

Arthroscope: Piece of equipment used to look into a bone joint

Endoscope: Piece of equipment used to look into a body cavity

Laparoscope: Piece of equipment used to look into the abdomen

Laparoscopic cholecystectomy: Removal of the gallbladder through a laparoscope

Managed care: Services determined by an insurance company

History

Operations have been been performed on humans and animals from the beginning of time. Unfortunately, documentation about the early days is scarce. Hippocrates may have been the first documented surgeon. He had a particular talent with fractures and splints. He developed a procedure for treating skull fractures that involved removing a circular area of bone. He was known as a great teacher of physicians, and his writings were used in teaching for centuries.

In the Dark Ages (400–800 A.D.) there are stories of hospitals. Written documentation of this was provided by monks of the Church of Rome. Churches and cloisters were the perfect places for

The abbreviations listed for this chapter are those that a HUC working in this area would be expected to know. Only those in boldface type are used in the text and appear in boldface when they are used for the first time.

hospitals. Lists of medicinal herbs could be found there. Many of the monks were encouraged to study medicine.

William of Saliceto (1210–1280) was instrumental in setting up a school of surgery. He recommended the use of a knife instead of the cautery in surgery (now we are going back to the cautery [laser]). He sutured severed nerves together surgically and worked toward bringing the disciplines of surgery and medicine closer.

Modern operating rooms (**ORs**) have come a long way since Hippocrates, both in theory and in practice. Surgical procedures continue to change with research and development of new tools and medications.

The operating room (OR) or surgical services may be the most mysterious part of any hospital. Most hospital employees would not have a reason to go into the OR on a routine basis. When they do go inside, they find that the rules are different. The people who work here are gowned and masked, so it may be impossible to recognize who they are.

Most ORs include more than just operating rooms, and for that reason this chapter will refer to the department as surgical services (**SS**), including the recovery room or postanesthesia care unit (**PACU**) and one day surgery (**ODS**) as part of the SS department. The actual operating rooms will be referred to as ORs.

Description of the Surgical Services Department

Sterile Center Core

Sterile center core is routinely not visible to anyone visiting Surgery. This area is located in the middle of the department, and the operating rooms surround or are attached to the core in some manner. This is a completely sterile area, and anyone entering must wear scrubs, shoe covers, and hat and, in some cases, a mask. Sterile supplies, equipment, and instruments are housed in this area and go into the ORs from here. At the end of a procedure, the same supplies, equipment, and instruments go out another way so that they will not contaminate the sterile core. Most hospitals send the used instruments to a central processing area away from the SS department. The OR staff will rinse off used instruments and send them to be cleaned, packaged, and sterilized. This can be a very involved process and, depending on the type of sterilization equipment, 24 hours may elapse before instruments are returned to surgery. The core will have some form of sterilization equipment that allows the staff to quick-flash some approved pieces of equipment and instruments. There are many guidelines for the proper sterilization of items used in the OR, and the infection controls are extremely strict. The core area is usually staffed by someone who is familiar with surgical cases, supplies, equipment, and instrumentation. This person is responsible for assisting the staff in preparing for each surgical case, ensuring that the appropriate supplies are available. It is a fast-moving pace and extremely stressful.

Control/Assignment Desk

The hub or heart of the department is the control, or assignment, desk. This desk may be in an area that can be accessed without scrubs, or it may be located in the sterile area. The control desk is staffed by several people with different duties and responsibilities. There is a board listing all the surgical cases of the day with the following information: (1) start time, (2) patient name, (3) patient age, (4) patient location, (5) surgical procedure, (6) surgeon, (7) type of anesthesia, and (8) names of the staff assigned to the case. A method is devised to determine the time that the patient arrives in the department, when the surgeon arrives, which staff people have had breaks or lunch, and anything else that the people at the desk may need to know. This can be done with colored magnets that are moved around the board. The board is usually in a handwritten, erasable form because as the day progresses it will be necessary to make changes in the rooms and assignments to allow for the unexpected and emergency cases (Fig. 10–1).

The surgery schedule is never final and may change many times in a day. The staff in the OR must always be prepared for the unexpected: (1) patients developing complications; (2) the case extending hours longer than planned; (3) the surgeon's being delayed at another hospital and getting bumped to the end of the day; (4) the emergency department calling with a multiple trauma case; and (5) staff members getting sick. These are just some of the unplanned events that can change the day. "Add on" cases are the most common cause of such changes. These are patients who the surgeon does not know about in advance but who need surgery *today*. The surgeon or the surgeon's office will call the control desk to get the case added to the day's schedule along with information about when the surgeon is available and the acuity of the case. If the case is threatening to life or limb, it takes priority over the scheduled cases, and one of those will be bumped back. If the patient can wait, the case is placed on a list of first-come, first-served. A tentative time may be assigned to the case, or it may have to wait until the end of the day and the surgeon will be called later with a time. On some days there may be many add-on cases, and on other days very few. Because it is totally unpredictable, the OR must be prepared.

Staff members working from the control desk may include a charge nurse, a HUC, a scheduler, and a supply coordinator. The charge nurse may remain at the desk or may roam the ORs to give assistance but still be available to the desk for guidance. There may be a HUC at the desk to answer the phones, put in orders, and handle issues that arise. The HUC may also put in charges and schedule cases, but in a busy hospital that may require several people. Often, answering the phones can be a full-time activity (Fig. 10–2).

One Day Surgery and Preop

It is not unusual for hospitals to separate the ambulatory or outpatient cases from the in-patient cases. An estimated 60 percent of all surgeries are done on an outpatient basis, and the number is rising quickly as insurance and managed care companies allow less and less time for in-patient care. Some institutions have separate ORs and others share ORs but keep the patients in separate areas. The reasons for this are that ambulatory surgery is generally shorter and less complicated and the patients have different needs. The outpatient may have had a preoperative visit

ROOM 1						
	Anes: *Taylor/Williams		OR: Moore/Jackson*			
0730	DR. SMITH*	APPENDECTOMY	GEN	DOE, JANE*	39	221
0830	DR. LAWRENCE	T&A	GEN	JONES, TOMMY*	4	ODS
0930	DR. APPLETON	BUNIONECTOMY	SPINAL	MYERS, MARY	52	ODS
ROOM 2						
	Anes: Hulle/Foster		OR: Wilson/Green*/Porter			
0730	DR. ROTH* HOOPER*	CABG	GEN	DAVIS, ARNOLD*	64	ICU

Figure 10–1
Entries on OR schedule.

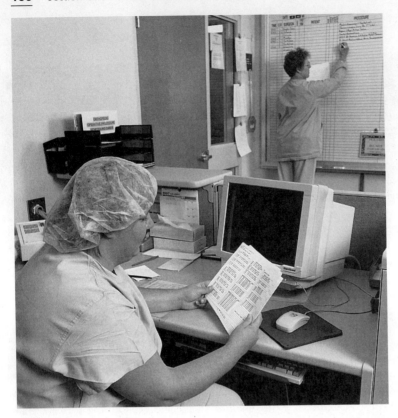

Figure 10–2
Control desk.

with anesthesia personnel prior to the surgery date. At this appointment a history of illness and previous surgeries is obtained. Necessary lab work, EKG, or x-rays are ordered so that the results can be reviewed prior to surgery. This visit also allows the patient to discuss different anesthesia agents and techniques with the staff. Patients are becoming more knowledgeable about their choices and need accurate information.

Outpatients arrive at the hospital 2 hours before the scheduled time of surgery. This allows time for registration and signing of hospital records. Occasionally the majority of the information is collected by telephone prior to the date of surgery, leaving only the signature to be obtained. The patient is prepared for surgery in the ambulatory or one day surgery preop area. If the patient did not have a prior visit with the anesthesia staff, that is done first so that any necessary testing can be ordered and completed before the scheduled start time.

The patient will undress and don a hospital gown, hat, and slippers if they are provided. He or she will be asked to sign the operative consent form once it is ascertained that patient and family understand the procedure scheduled. The surgeon will usually see the patient in this area prior to going into the OR. The nurse will start an IV line and give any necessary preop antibiotics or medications that are ordered. Anesthesia personnel may give the patient some IV medication for relaxation or to prevent nausea. Some patients may actually receive the anesthesia block for certain types of anesthesia; spinal blocks, regional blocks, and digital blocks all can be administered in the preop area, speeding up the surgical prep time in the OR. In many facilities families are allowed to stay with patients until they go into the OR.

The in-patient preop area may be staffed by the same personnel as the outpatient area, but usually there is a separate section for in-patients. In-patients usually have more serious conditions, and they may require a more detailed prep than outpatients. In-patients come to surgery with all the paperwork in order and usually already have an IV line. Preop medications have typically been given on the nursing unit. These patients may come to the area only 30 to 40 minutes prior to the scheduled start time. Both in-patient and outpatient preop areas have designated isolation and latex-free rooms.

Some hospitals have a special surgical observation area, where outpatients may go after PACU. They continue to rest and recover for several more hours (or overnight) before being discharged. For example, patients who have had their tonsils removed usually must eat and drink prior to discharge per order of the surgeon. Because this can take 3 to 5 hours, the patient is more comfortable resting in a regular bed with family to assist with care. More and more surgeons are utilizing this practice as in-patient stays are being discouraged after surgical procedures. This post-PACU observation area may be staffed with the same people who prepared the patient prior to surgery. In the A.M. they give preop care, and in the P.M. they give post-PACU care.

Postanesthesia Care Unit (PACU) or Recovery Room

PACU is the area that patients are taken to directly after surgery, the only exceptions being patients going directly to ICU or patients with local anesthesia for a minor procedure. All other patients are taken from the OR and monitored in PACU until they have met certain criteria. From PACU they may be discharged home, admitted to an observation or in-patient bed, or returned to the hospital room that they came from prior to surgery. Most PACU nurses have a special certification in postanesthesia care; they do not cross train with the OR nurses but may cross train with ICU nursing staff. The duties of HUCs who work in this area are much the same as those of an in-patient nursing unit.

Pathology Lab

There is usually a mini–pathology lab located in the SS area. This may be staffed with a pathologist, a lab tech, and a HUC either full-time or on call. The lab tech or HUC may stay in the mini-lab and call the pathologist when needed. Often the pathologist will go into the OR when called by the surgeon to receive a specimen that needs to be evaluated immediately, such as frozen sections. The pathologist will take the specimen to the mini-lab, do a preliminary exam, and call the results in to the surgeon. For example, when a skin lesion is removed and the tissue is found to be cancerous, the surgeon will want to remove tissue until there are clean margins all around the cancerous area. The pathologist will be able to determine whether enough tissue has been removed or whether further excision is necessary and relay this information to the surgeon. This is extremely valuable for both the surgeon and the patient. If unexpected findings from the pathologist necessitate removal of organs or body parts, the surgeon or assistant will break scrub to go out and talk with the patient's family. The family will be fully informed of the findings and be asked to sign additional surgical permits. This is done only in extreme situations, when both the family and the patient have been prepared to expect it. Preferably, circumstances would allow that the surgeon could wait until the patient and family could be informed together and further surgery could be planned on an urgent basis.

Unique Opportunities in the Surgical Services Department

Surgery Scheduling

Although surgery schedulers may also be HUCs, their primary duty is to schedule surgery. Usually the schedulers are located at the control desk or close by, where they have access to the daily board for reference. The desk should be convenient to surgeons wishing to schedule cases. The OR scheduler will use the charge nurse as a resource person when medical questions arise or nursing judgment is needed.

Many hospitals now schedule all their cases on the computer, but some still use the appointment book method. There are many advantages to using the computer, the primary one being that it saves time and is more efficient to use. The HUC who schedules surgery must have advanced medical terminology knowledge and understand the timing involved with scheduling cases. There is a very fine line to be drawn when assigning times to a case. Too much time causes holes in the day, when staff members are not busy. Too little time causes the next case to be delayed. Computer systems can usually give the average time needed for each procedure and can predict case time with accuracy. Dr. Jones may take 30 minutes to do an appendectomy, whereas Dr. Smith can do one in 10 minutes. When scheduling the case the scheduler will ask how much time is needed, knowing that all appendectomies take 10 minutes to set up and 10 minutes to tear down (information built into the computer). If the office wants a 10 A.M. scheduling and there is a 30-minute opening available, Dr. Smith could have that time, but Dr. Jones would be told that there was no opening and be offered alternative time slots of at least 50 minutes. This requires a great deal of tact and finesse. The scheduler must input accurate predictions of time while giving surgeons or their staff the service that they need to schedule their patients. This can be like walking a tightrope—one little deviation and you fall. The surgery schedule will never be perfect but should be a close prediction of the times.

The scheduler takes a lot of abuse when the schedule is not right or even when it is:

"Why did you schedule Dr. Jones at 10:00 when we have a 10:30 in that room? He will never be finished and I wanted out of here on time today!!"

"My office said you did not have any early openings, but I see one at 11:00. What is the deal here?"

"I want to start at 07:30 and I won't take no for an answer. You just give me Dr. X's time—I operate here more than he does!"

The position requires that situations be handled with a cool head and calm manner. The scheduler must be able to say "NO," even to a doctor, while using all the customer service skills to meet the needs of the staff, surgeons, and patients. This is not a position for everyone, and one that the HUC should consider very carefully before undertaking it (Fig. 10–3).

Inventory Management and Charge Control

Inventory management and charge control are two very critical areas in SS. This area may be staffed by one or more people. The staff may be nurses, surgical techs, or HUCs trained specifically for the position. It is important for anyone holding these positions to be knowledgeable in the process, supplies, and equipment of each surgical case. Disposable inventory may be maintained in the OR or ordered from central service, materiel management, warehouse, or the supplier who will deliver them each day. Someone must be in charge of seeing that the right items are in the department on the right day.

Some items are routine stock, while for others it is necessary to place a special order for a certain case or surgeon. The same is true for instruments and equipment. Inventory management is crucial to the success of the department. While it is important to see that the equipment, instruments, and supplies are available, it is just as necessary to control and contain costs to the department. Some hospitals have agreements with other area hospitals to lend special equipment to each other when available. This allows a piece of equipment that is seldom used to be loaned out, perhaps with a rental fee, to other facilities, saving them the expense of purchase.

Managed care has changed many of the practices formerly used in surgery. Before the introduction of managed care, if a surgeon wanted a special piece of equipment or special suture for all his or her cases, the OR would probably just

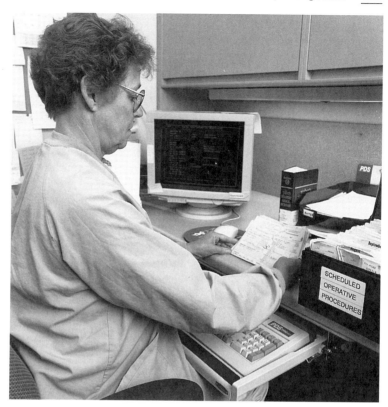

Figure 10–3
Surgery scheduling office.

order it (within reason) to make the surgeon happy. The cost was passed on to the patients (or insurers). This practice has been stopped, and hospitals are trying to standardize inventories by making contracts with suppliers for special pricing, e.g., using one product brand at a reduced cost. If the OR has a contract with suture supplier A and surgeon C likes the suture from supplier B, surgeon C will have to use suture A, since that is all that is available. Special requests may be honored only if they can be justified by the surgeon or if a group of surgeons all make the same request. Quality of supplies is the determining factor when making supplier decisions; cost is secondary. If supplier A and supplier B both have quality sutures that are comparable in types and sizes of needles and thread, but B is underpricing A, then B will probably get the contract. The supply coordinator must meet regularly with representatives from the different suppliers. The actual ordering may be handled from another area. The supply coordinator needs to be informed of pricing specials, supply orders that may be changed or back-ordered, and new items in production. Many suppliers will custom pack a group of common items into one tray for a reduced fee. These custom-packed trays require individual attention from the supply coordinator and manufacturer's representative.

The supply coordinator tracks department inventory on a daily basis. If supplies are ordered automatically via the computer, the inventory must be verified regularly to ensure that stock levels are set correctly. Even if supplies are ordered manually, routine inventories are made to maintain the proper quantities of stock items. Being out of critical stock items could cause serious harm to patients in addition to making the procedure more difficult for the surgeon and staff. The old Scouting adage applies: Be prepared.

In some computer systems all items associated with a surgical procedure are entered onto a surgeon preference card. When the computer recognizes the card, the procedure and all supplies are automatically placed on the patient billing record. This process is overseen by the charge control person in the OR. If automated preference cards are used, the charge controller will review each record to see that it has been edited properly. The card may call for four packages of suture while the surgeon needed six. The additional two packages need to be entered. If automated preference cards are not used, the individual charges for each supply item must be entered into the patient billing record. The charge controller must be familiar with surgical procedures and techniques in order to be able to review the accuracy of the items used or not used.

Clerical Support

There may be a variety of positions considered clerical support in SS. All of them may be filled by HUCs with different responsibilities for the various duties in the department, or there may be a combination of HUCs and administrative assistants. Some ORs may employ clerical support staff for typing and dictation, assisting the management with meeting minutes and letters, or staff scheduling duties. They may be HUCs or office-trained clerical support personnel. Surgery is a great area for Certified Health Unit Coordinators (CHUCs) because of the advanced level of medical terminology required.

Information System Coordinator

Hospitals that have advanced to a fully computerized operations system may have a special position for the management of all computer operations. The computer information system (**IS**) coordinator develops software for the department's use in scheduling surgery, recording the surgical case nursing notes, billing and inventory management, tracking trends, and reporting. The IS coordinator is also responsible for the upkeep of all computer hardware in the department.

Managed care providers, **OSHA**, **JCAHO**, and other regulatory agencies all demand a high level of accountability. This accountability is best managed with computer systems that can produce accurate data analysis. The data may be input by various people in the department. Schedulers input information prior to the surgical case; nurses or HUCs input information during or after the case. This information may contain the demographic details of the patient and doctor, the type of equipment used on the case, the outcome of the surgery, or any data that the department is interested in gathering. The information collected, which can be great or small, detailed or general, aggregate or microscopic, is valuable to health care and will be demanded more and more in the future.

Some common data outcome reports from the OR may be in the form of statistical analysis that will assist in making future staffing decisions. For example:

Case time	Calculated by patient IN room–OUT room
Surgeon time	Incision-Close time
Turnover time	#1 patient out of room–#2 patient in room

Based on these figures, SS management may decide that there is not enough staff to turn over the room fast enough, and extra staff may be hired. Surgeon times may be averaged to use as a guide for predictions of future cases. A surgeon with unusually long averages may be studied to find the reasons for the additional time.

Surgical equipment is monitored for safety to the staff and patients. Each piece of equipment has an identifying number, and this number is recorded in the patient case record notes. If a hazard is found in a piece of equipment, the computer can print out a list of all staff and patients who may have been exposed to the safety hazard in any given time frame. The same is true for drugs or implants that may be under a manufacturer's recall; a report can be printed in minutes as opposed to the noncomputer method of manually checking each chart.

The IS coordinator may have a HUC/CHUC background or computer experience or, ideally, a combination of both. The HUC background is helpful in understanding the nursing process. The computer background is needed to understand the computer logic process. Special training may be offered to the right person for this new area in health care. It is a challenging position with tremendous growth potential.

Surgical Services Management

Management in SS can be as varied as the many hospitals around the country. Larger hospitals may have several levels of management: director of surgery, nurse manager, business manager, head nurse, nursing coordinator, and clinicians. SS may operate with a higher level of management because this area generates a high level of revenue. Surgery is very competitive in pricing, and with the addition of sophisticated lasers, laparoscopes, and other high-tech equipment it is important to protect the revenue and at the same time keep current with the latest equipment.

Technology may be one reason that SS may employ clinical and nonclinical management. The clinical manager oversees the nursing staff and surgical procedures. The nonclinical business or inventory/supply manager may oversee the budget of the department; he or she makes decisions about which brand of equipment to purchase as well as when to purchase and when to lease equipment. Technology is changing faster than products can be manufactured. A busy surgery department is inundated with visits and calls about new products available today and in the future.

Frequently Used Medications

Medications used in the OR are usually not the same medications found on other nursing units, with the exception of antibiotics and pain control drugs. The majority of medications used in the OR are types of anesthesia and will be administered by the anesthesiologist or certified registered nurse anesthetist (**CRNA**) (Fig. 10–4).

Inhalation anesthetics are given through a mask and may be used alone or in combination with other forms of anesthesia. The most common types are as follows:

Nitrous oxide (N_2O)
Halothane (Fluothane)
Enflurane (Ethrane)
Isoflurane (Forane)
Desflurane (Suprane)
Sevoflurane (Ultane)

Intravenous anesthetics are the largest category, and most patients receive some type of IV anesthesia. The following are a few of the many that may be given in surgery:

Barbiturates (Brevital, Pentothal, Surital)
Benzodiazepines (Ativan, Valium, Versed)
Hypnotics (Amidate, Diprivan)

Some patients may receive a regional block rather than a general anesthetic. This means that the patient remains awake while parts of the body are made numb. A procedure such as a spinal block, Bier block, epidural block, or digital block can be used to achieve this state. The decision as to what kind of anesthesia will be used is made by a combination of surgeon, patient, and anesthesiologist depending on the type of surgery planned.

Diagnostic Procedures

Many patients coming into the OR have already had a number of diagnostic procedures either in the doctor's office or as an outpatient. By the time they arrive in the OR they have been diagnosed and are there for correction of the problem. Other patients have not been able to find the source of their problem and must rely on a surgical diagnostic procedure.

Scopes

Endoscopic procedures can be diagnostic or operative or, in some cases, both. Scopes are being

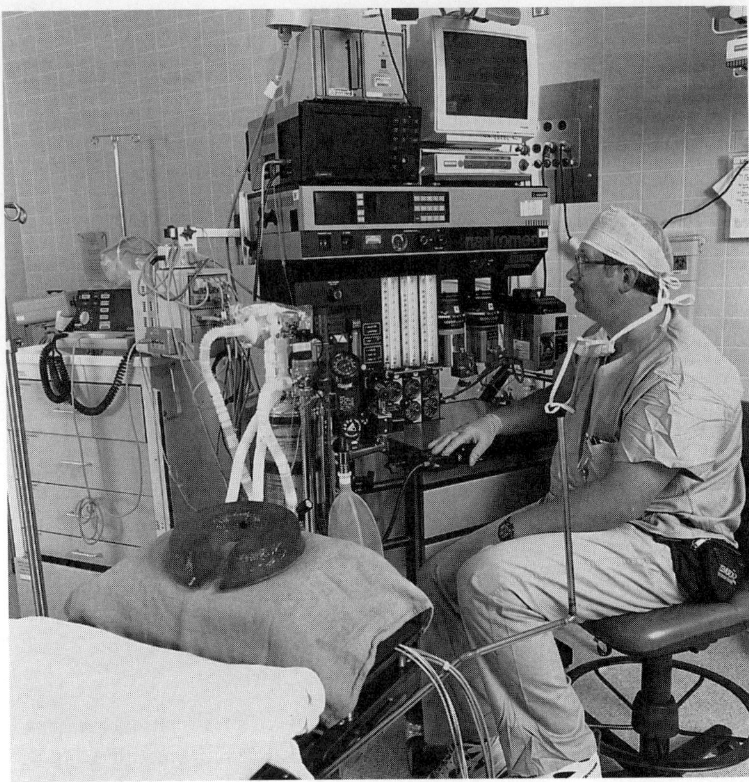

Figure 10–4
Anesthesia machine.

used in almost all surgical specialties from podiatry to cosmetic surgery. Scopes may be used to look into the body to see what the problem is, and, when necessary, the removal or repair is done through the scope. Ten years ago, if gallbladder disease necessitated removal of the organ, it was considered major surgery. The operation was lengthy; the incision was big; and recuperation was long and painful. Today, once the decision is made to remove the gallbladder, the process is very brief. The laparoscopic cholecystectomy takes less than 2 hours and requires only an overnight stay. In some cases the patient can go home 6 to 8 hours post surgery, and many return to work within a few days.

Another common scopic surgical procedure is arthroscopy, an orthopedic procedure that allows the surgeon to look at a joint through an arthroscope. Endoscopic sinus surgery may correct a breathing problem or chronic sinusitis. Endoscopic podiatry surgery corrects many foot deformities. Laparoscopes are used in gynecologic surgery for endometriosis and uterine fibroids, and cardiovascular surgeons use scopes to harvest leg vein grafts for heart surgery. Endoscopic plastic surgery is done for cosmetic repair and repair of tendons and nerves. Surgical procedures performed through a scope are increasing daily and will soon become the norm.

Exam Under Anesthesia (EUA)

Technically, all surgery is an **EUA**, since some form of exam is done either prior to or during the surgical procedure. The term EUA is used when that is the primary reason for the trip to the OR, such as for an orthopedic joint exam. For example, an injured shoulder may be difficult to diagnose if there is a high level of pain. Part of the diagnostic procedure may be range-of-motion testing on the shoulder and arm, which may be too painful if the patient is awake. Small children are difficult to examine when they are awake, because of their age, lack of understanding, pain, and fear. For these reasons, a surgeon may plan to remove tonsils but also does an EUA on the ears or other problem areas to see if surgical intervention is necessary at the same time.

Treatments and Procedures Specific to the OR

Most hospital facilities restrict surgical procedures to areas where strict sterile conditions can be maintained and monitored. The same is true for patients undergoing general anesthesia. Hospitals may have special sterile areas in labor/delivery (L&D), cardiovascular lab, GI lab, and radiology, where some invasive procedures or treatments are performed. These patients generally do not receive a general anesthetic (except possibly L&D) with an anesthesiologist present, but are given another conscious sedation medication. Most surgical procedures are restricted to the sterile OR.

Simple or minor lacerations are generally repaired in the emergency department (ED). If tendons or nerves are involved, however, the surgeon will want the sterility of the OR and may need a special microscope to repair the injury properly. The same is true for simple orthopedic fractures. Closed reductions are frequently taken care of in the ED, but if extensive manipulation or open repair is needed that patient will be brought into the OR.

Another procedure usually done only in the OR is the examination of organs and tissue by a pathologist using frozen sections to make an initial diagnosis of cancer. Many breast biopsy procedures could be done outside the OR, but the need to know if the tissue is cancerous requires the patient to have a surgical procedure. By the time the patient is awake the surgeon can deliver the results of the biopsy. At that time options can be discussed and plans made for further surgical intervention if necessary.

Equipment and Supplies Common to the OR

As technology grows, so does the mountain of equipment in the OR. Surrounded by the laparoscopes, video equipment (including screens and VCRs), cameras, portable x-ray machines, portable fluoroscans and microscopes, and more, it is hard to see the patient (Figs. 10–5 and 10–6).

Many hospitals would like to consolidate and modernize their operating suites, but what they really need is to be made larger, not smaller. Anyone who has been through remodeling or a move to new facilities knows that the planners and designers seldom create enough space for storage. It seems that planning storage space is non–revenue creating and therefore unnecessary. But the reality is that now there is twice as much equipment as there was 5 years ago.

This space-occupying equipment has made surgical procedures faster, cleaner, and safer but not cheaper. A laparoscopic cholecystectomy can be done in 60 to 90 minutes compared with 2 to 3 hours for an open gallbladder removal in the past. This represents a cost savings to the patient in time, but the cost of purchasing and maintaining expensive equipment is increasing.

Laser equipment is a prime example of growing technology. Lasers are obsolete the day that they arrive in the OR. Much like personal computers, new designs are released almost daily. The cost of a laser can be from $40,000 to over $200,000, and it changes daily. Because the range of what a laser can do is very wide, many facilities try to purchase the most general multipurpose laser possible. But owing to the many specialties now using lasers in routine surgical procedures it is almost impossible to purchase one model that meets everyone's needs. In the near future, every surgical procedure may involve the use of some kind of laser. This makes budget planning almost impossible. An attractive alternative for some hospitals is to lease lasers and other equipment from

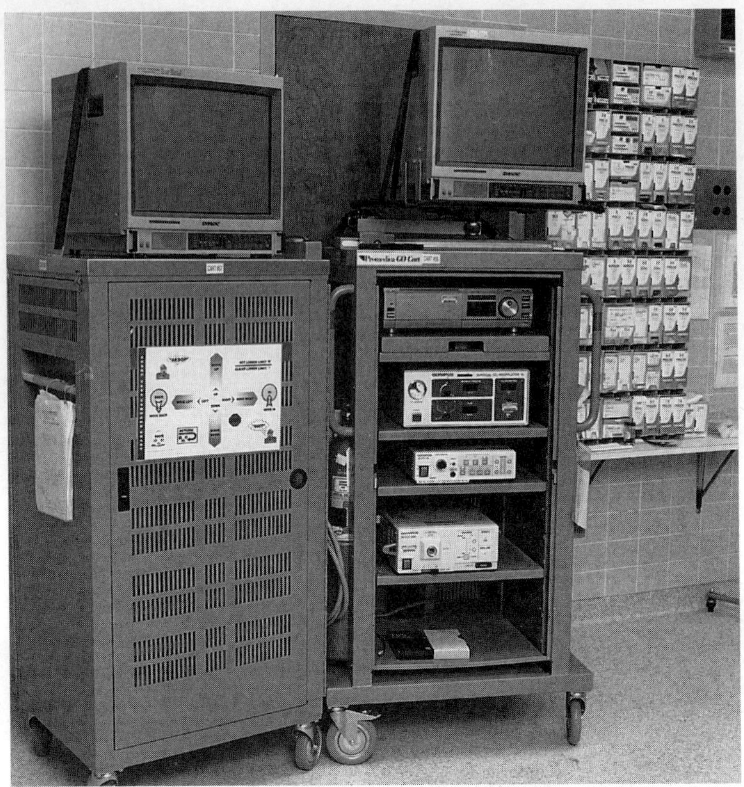

Figure 10–5
Video tower.

an outside company. It is not cost effective to purchase a piece of equipment for $50,000 when in 6 months it is obsolete. By leasing the equipment both money and space are saved. Leased equipment arrives the day of surgery and is picked up at the end of the day. Other expensive items leased for the OR are heart/lung machines and cell savers. The leasing companies find that it is to their advantage to provide trained personnel as part of the lease package.

Surgical instruments and trays may be located in the OR center core or may be stored in the central service or dispatch area of the hospital. Trays are generally a grouping of instruments that are used together. These trays and instruments may be reusable, disposable, or a combination of both. Many hospitals that began using some disposable items several years ago have switched back to reusable items to save money.

The majority of disposable items found in the OR consist of prep supplies for skin cleaning and shaving, sutures and staples, sponges used during surgery, paper drapes for isolating the surgical area, drains, tubings, catheters, dressings, and splints. This is a small sample of items needed for patient care in SS. These disposable items require a large amount of space and management. The critical point about disposable supplies is that they be charged to the patient and not lost in the shuffle. The person responsible for inputting patient charges must be familiar with what is commonly used in each surgical procedure in order to recognize what is missing.

Implants, which are used in a variety of surgical cases, are items frequently found in surgery. Human implants are usually bone, tissue, corneas, or organs. Organ transplants are major procedures with a wide range of possible complications. Arti-

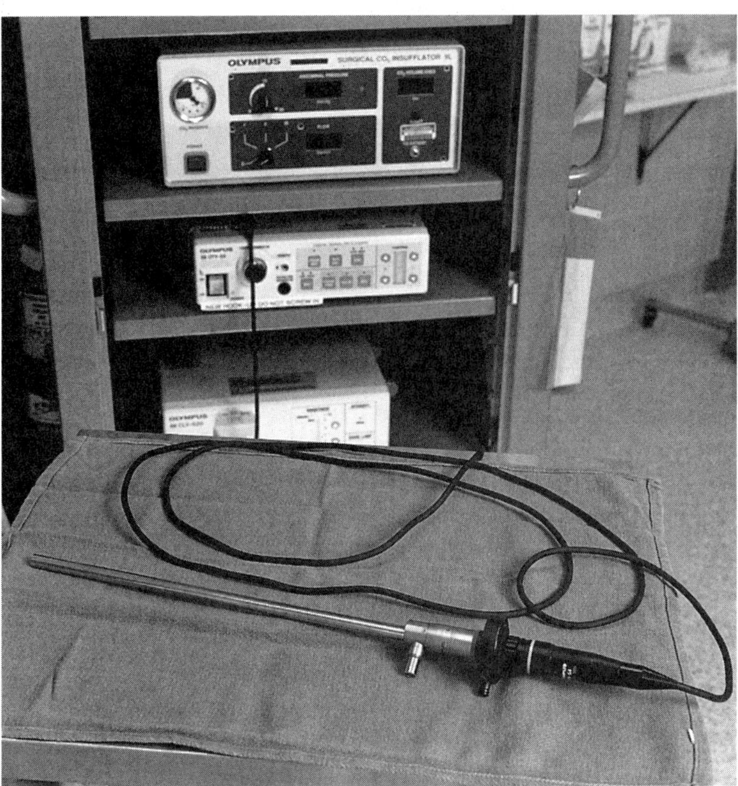

Figure 10–6
Scope with video camera.

ficial implants often require special ordering. Surgeons scheduling procedures that require an implant will leave instructions requesting the type, size, brand, or company desired. Many implants are artificial, made of steel or titanium. These are generally joint replacements and carry no risk of rejection. In some surgical procedures the patient may have a choice of artificial or nonartificial implants. Heart valves may be either artificial or animal (pig valves).

Some equipment found in the OR may not come to mind when the average person visualizes surgical equipment. One is some type of video paging system. The staff in and out of each OR need to know what is going on in the department. The desk wants to know the progress of the case: Is it running on time or will it be late? The staff in the room want to know if the next surgery has been delayed or canceled. Overhead paging and phone calls must be kept to a minimum so that the surgeon's concentration is not interrupted. A video pager is a series of TV monitors around the department and in the surgical suites. It operates from a computer and keyboard at the desk and pushbuttons in each room. Push a button and the CLOSE light comes on for your room; call a surgeon by pushing the SURG button; ready for pathologist, push the PATH light. When the button is pushed, all the TV monitors light up with the appropriate message, and a short "ding" is sounded to alert people to the changes. Messages that might be displayed are: 1—"SURG . . . Rm 1"; 2—"HK (housekeeping) . . . . . Rm 3"; 3—"CLOSE . . . Rm 11."

In message 1, the surgeon for Room 1 knows to go to the room; the patient is prepped and asleep. In message 2, the person at the desk knows that the next patient will be going into the room soon. In message 3, the PACU staff know to get ready for their next patient. The keyboard operator may type in free text messages for all to see, such as "Dr. Smith is delayed"; "Dr. Jones' case moved to Rm 10." Any SS that has this or a similar type of system knows how valuable it can be for communication within the department.

The last piece of equipment to discuss is the stereo and musical equipment found in the surgical suites. Many surgeons are more relaxed and efficient if they have their favorite music playing in the room. It helps keep them focused and working in a rhythm (not necessarily with the music). An OR may have built-in stereo equipment with a variety of CDs or tapes; some may use portable players; and in others the surgeons may have to bring their own equipment and choice of music. This equipment is treated with the same care as any other piece of surgical equipment. It is generally under lock and key when not in use.

Communication

Communication Within the Hospital

Communication in SS is a vital part of running the surgery schedule. Patients are scheduled for a set time, based on the amount of time that the surgeon ahead of theirs requested plus the amount of time that it takes to prepare the OR. These times are all based on estimates, and, therefore, the people working in surgery are either ahead of schedule or running behind. Either way, it takes lots of communicating to keep patients, staff, and surgeons on a schedule.

In-patients arrive in surgery 30 to 40 minutes prior to their scheduled start time. The person running the control desk calls the nursing unit to alert the staff that the transporter is on the way to pick up the patient. If the cases are running ahead of schedule, this call may come much earlier than the patient or unit nurse anticipated, and often there is some anxiety about getting the patient ready "early." If the day is running long and all the cases are behind schedule, it is essential to keep the unit nurse informed of the delay and the anticipated pickup times. Timing is crucial to the stress level of patients and families, especially the afternoon cases.

As the surgeon begins to close the skin and complete the surgical procedure the OR staff alerts the PACU staff to prepare for the patient. Patients going to ICU may arrive directly from the OR, and it is necessary for the ICU staff to be ready to receive the patient. This may be achieved by the HUC at the control desk as soon as the "close" signal comes from the OR. Patients who stop in PACU are usually there for 1 to 2 hours before going back to the nursing unit. The PACU nurse will call report to the nurse who will care for the patient on the unit to update him or her on the patient's present condition and the details of the surgical procedure. The process is much the same for outpatients in ambulatory surgery areas: to get the patient ready, go to the OR, get ready to receive the patient postop. The rule is to always communicate one step ahead of the patient.

The SS staff also utilize the services of others to assist with communication. The families waiting for news of the surgery are anxious for any information that gives them reassurance. Many hospitals have a pastoral care or chaplain staff to assist in the link of patient-staff-family information chain. A volunteer staffs the family waiting rooms and can identify the family of a patient. The surgeon or the OR nurse may call the waiting room and alert the volunteer to give the family a message:

Surgery is going well . . .
. . . taking longer than expected.
. . . having problems.
. . . will be out to talk with you soon.

The volunteer may alert pastoral care or the chaplain to visit when families are in distress or if the surgeon has information that will be upsetting. The pastoral care staff are specially trained in grief management and assume this stressful duty for the surgery staff so that they may concentrate on the patient. Only a very small percentage of patients die in surgery, but when it happens it is critical to have the staff communicate as much information as possible to the family about the patient's last minutes.

The HUC at the control desk may find it necessary to contact the admitting office during the course of the day to get bed assignments for patients in the OR. Occasionally patients are scheduled to be discharged after surgery, and they need to be admitted instead. The HUC will call to give the admission office the necessary information to admit the patient. This process also happens in reverse: Admission is planned, and patient is released upon discharge from PACU.

Communication with the Community

Generally within the hospital all communication regarding the patient is about present events, and some urgency surrrounds the exchange of information. Communications outside the hospital are for the future and can be handled in a more relaxed manner.

Scheduling surgery is ongoing, and calls come in all day from surgeons and their staff. The scheduling desk is like a hotel reservation desk—the customer needs a certain type of room for a particular day and time. The HUC who is scheduling surgery must have advanced communication skills. In addition to calls from surgeons' offices, there are calls from patients and families with a variety of questions: What time should they come to the hospital? When can they go home? Who can stay with them? How much will it cost, and what will the insurance pay? All these questions must be either answered or redirected to the appropriate person.

It may be necessary to call other hospitals in the area to locate and obtain equipment or supplies. Sometimes supplies do not arrive on schedule, or the inventory runs out before new supplies arrive. Technology has created a vast array of special equipment that may be used only once or twice a year. Some of this equipment is very delicate, and it breaks. Any one of these reasons may make it necessary to communicate with other area hospitals for the purpose of buying or borrowing what is needed to complete a surgical case. Hospitals may be competing for patients, but all are in the business of caring for people, no matter where they are located.

Most hospitals have some type of students, be they nursing, medical, pharmacy, radiologic, or HUC. Anytime there are students in direct contact with patients, patient care communication takes on a larger meaning. Students may not always understand the small details that experienced staff take for granted. In surgery this is often illustrated when new students arrive on the first day and are told to change into scrubs and come back to the desk. This may sound simple, but some of the students do not have the slightest idea what to do. They will return with the scrubs under their clothes, with scrubs on backward, wearing hats for shoe covers, and many other combinations. It is hard not to laugh, but it shows the trouble that poor communication can bring.

Documentation

Most patient care documentation is handled by the nursing staff on the surgical case record. The type of information found on this record is governed by hospital policy and procedures, OSHA, JCAHO, **AORN**, and other regulatory agencies. Case records may be computerized or handwritten, depending on the hospital. Regardless of how the information is entered into the case record it may be the HUC who pulls statistical analysis out of the record. This can be accomplished by entering certain information about the case into a computer and then having the computer pull out information or simply keeping a written tally of important events. Information that is helpful to have is the list of surgical procedures performed during a time period, the average case length, the average number of cases that one surgeon handled, or how many different surgeons operated in a time period. There is a magnitude of statistical data opportunities found in surgery. The key is to collect everything now that someone might want to know later. This is very difficult unless a computer is used for the collection and storage of data. Computer storage of data is more accurate and can be recompiled using new guidelines with much greater ease than hand calculated or stored data. Correct data can often mean the difference between increased budget allowance versus a decrease in budget because the documentation is not accurate or available.

Quality and Risk Management

Risk management and safety are crucial in SS for the surgical staff, medical staff, and students as well as patients. Technology has brought many advances into the OR, but at the same time the risk of injury is higher. More and more lasers are utilized, and many precautions must be followed to avoid injury. Laser injury can include lacerations, burns, eye damage, and fire. Many procedures are performed using electrical equipment, increasing the risks to the people in the room, if nothing other than getting tangled in all the cords on the floor.

Statistical tracking of all safety prevention and accidents may be handled by the HUC by filling out forms and reports. Logs are required for some special pieces of equipment for historical tracking. Lasers are inspected routinely to see if the beam is putting out too much light that might cause a burn or equipment failure. If a surgical patient is found to have a burn several days after surgery, the specific laser used in that case will be tested. The laser log is consulted to see which laser was used. This information may be the responsibility of the HUC in addition to many other statistics-gathering duties.

Closing Thoughts

Surgical Services has been the best and worst place that I have worked in health care. In the beginning it was the worst because I missed the contact with patients and families. Most of the contact in surgery is with staff and surgeons. Staff contact is in very short segments because they are on a schedule and are always running to the next case. This makes it hard to bond with people when you are new in the department. Even the surgeons are different in surgery from the way they are in the hospital setting. People from surgery tend to eat lunch in the department rather than in the cafeteria. There is an element of isolation that was very hard for me to deal with at first.

After I had worked in surgery for a while I realized that this department probably had more opportunities for the HUC/CHUC than any other in the hospital. I was very lucky, because the computer system was outdated, and soon after I began working I was asked to help choose a new system. Not only did I participate in researching but I was also taught to "build" the necessary dictionaries that operate the system and trained to maintain the system. It became clear that this would someday necessitate a full-time position. Shortly after the new system was implemented I submitted a written proposal to management creating the position I currently have in surgery, computer specialist.

I am totally responsible for all aspects of the software in surgery; the development of the basic system and screens; the creation of all the reports; all statistical analysis; developing presentation workshops; expanding our software use; all policy and procedures pertaining to computer use; policy and procedures pertaining to data analysis in the OR; and training the entire staff.

I have been to several computer software user conventions and meetings in other cities. People from other hospitals call and come to our hospital to talk about our system. I am recognized as the department resource and expert.

This is a very rewarding position, but I created it and made it mine. With the changes in health care moving quickly you must be alert to see your opportunity and go for it. If you have a good HUC background you can survive and grow with the changes. Join the professional organization, take the certification exam, and network with as many people as you can. Explore all the opportunities offered to you, take courses, go to seminars, attend meetings, join a committee, volunteer to help someone else. You never know where it may lead you . . . . maybe someday you will have your name in a book like this one.

Review Questions

1. Mention four ways in which a surgical schedule may be disrupted.
2. Name and describe two jobs/positions in the surgical suite that are available to HUCs.
3. Explain the communication that is involved when a surgical case is finishing in the OR.
4. List eight types of statistical activities that the health unit coordinator might become involved in.

Bibliography

Frenay A, Mahoney RM: Understanding Medical Terminology, 7th ed. St. Louis, Catholic Health Association, 1984.

Merck Index, 12th ed. Merck & Co, Rahway, NJ, 1996.

Stedman's Medical Dictionary, 24th ed. Baltimore, Williams & Wilkins, 1982.

Taber's Cyclopedic Medical Dictionary, 17th ed. Philadelphia, FA Davis, 1993.

The Orthopedic Unit

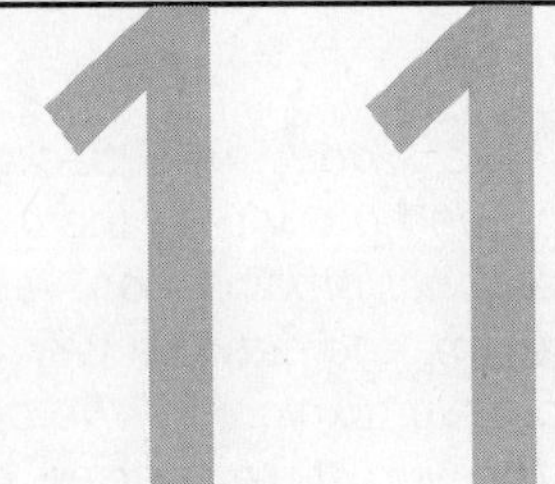

Lois Lawton

Objectives

At the completion of this chapter the reader should be able to:

1. List six diagnostic imaging procedures that would be conducted to identify orthopedic problems.
2. Explain what patient-controlled analgesia is.
3. Identify the surgical procedure performed to correct HNP.
4. Name the two types of traction and explain the difference between them.
5. Name three methods of immobilization other than traction.

Vocabulary

Amputation: Removal of part or all of a limb or other appendage of the body

Avascular necrosis: The death or decay of a bone due to the lack of blood supply

Cartilage: A specialized fibrous connective tissue

Dislocation: Displacement of a bone from a joint.

Doppler: A method of evaluating blood flow; used in assessing obstruction of the major blood vessels

Electromyography: Recording and study of the intrinsic electrical activity of the skeletal muscle

Fracture: The breaking of a part, especially a bone

Fusion: The merging or coherence of adjacent parts

Gallium scan: Nuclear imaging test using gallium as the dye

Halo: An apparatus used to apply traction to or immobilize the cervical spine

Internal fixation: Operative repair of fractures by placement of metallic implants on or in the fracture site

Ligament: A band of fibrous tissue connecting bones or cartilages, serving to strengthen and support joints

Myelogram: X-ray of the spinal cord using radiopaque dye

Continued

Vocabulary *Continued*

Open reduction: Surgical correction of a bone fracture or dislocation of a joint

Osteomyelitis: Bone infection

Periosteum: A specialized connective tissue covering all bones of the body and possessing bone-forming potential

Prosthesis: Artificial replacement for missing body part

Rotator cuff: A group of muscles and tendons that surround the shoulder joint

Sling: A suspension apparatus to provide support to an injured body part

Splint: A support used to immobilize an injured part of the body

Synovial fluid: Transparent viscid fluid found in joint cavities, bursae, and tendon sheaths

Tendon: A cord or band of strong white fibrous tissue that connects a muscle to a bone

Traction: The mechanical pull applied to a part of the body to maintain proper position and facilitate healing

Trapeze: A triangular bar attached to an overhead frame for the purpose of assisting the patient to move in bed

Common Abbreviations

ACL	Anterior cruciate ligament
ADL	Activities of daily living
AKA	Above-the-knee amputation
BKA	Below-the-knee amputation
CHD	Congenital hip dysplasia or dislocation
CPM	Continuous passive motion
CTS	Carpal tunnel syndrome
DJD	Degenerative joint disease
DVT	Deep venous thrombosis
EMG	Electromyography
EXT	External fixation device
FWB	Full weight bearing
Fx	Fracture
HNP	Herniated nucleus pulposus
L	Lumbar
MRI	Magnetic resonance imaging
NSAID	Nonsteroidal anti-inflammatory drug
NWB	Non–weight bearing
OA	Osteoarthritis
ORIF	Open reduction with internal fixation
O.T.	Occupational therapy
PCA	Patient-controlled analgesia
P.T.	Physical therapy
PWB	Partial weight bearing
ROM	Range of motion
SLR	Straight leg raises
TENS	Transcutaneous electric nerve stimulation
THR	Total hip replacement
TKR	Total knee replacement
TSR	Total shoulder replacement
TTWB	Toe-touch weight bearing

The abbreviations listed for this chapter are those a HUC working in this area would be expected to know. Only those in boldface type are used in the text and appear in boldface when they are used for the first time.

Related Terminology

Although the following terms do not appear in the text, they are terms that someone who works on an orthopedic unit would be expected to know.

Abduction—The pulling of a body part away from the midline

Adduction—The pulling of a body part toward the midline

Arthroscope—Fiberoptic endoscope used to examine the interior of a joint

Arthroplasty—Repair or replacement of a joint

Bryant's traction—An apparatus used for vertical skin traction to treat femur fractures in infants and young children

Closed reduction—Manipulative reduction of a fracture or dislocation without incision

Epidural steroid block—An injection of a corticosteroid agent into the epidural area

Ilizarov procedure—A process for internally lengthening bone fragments by slowly sliding the bone fragment until it is in the proper position

Meniscectomy—Surgical removal of meniscal cartilage (such as in the knee)

Orthotics—The field of knowledge relating to orthopedic appliances used to support, align, prevent, or correct deformities or to improve the function of movable parts of the body

Osteoporosis—A disease in which the bone becomes weak and brittle owing to loss of minerals

Osteotomy—The surgical cutting of a bone

Parallel bars—Two bars placed side by side to give assistance in walking

Tilt table—A table that can be tilted up or down; used in the rehabilitation of patients who have been confined to bed for a long time

Overview

The orthopedic department in the hospital is a specialized unit set up especially for the care and treatment of patients with deformities, diseases, and injuries of the bones, joints, and muscles. In hospitals that are designated as trauma centers the orthopedic unit will receive many of these patients directly from the ER, surgery, or ICU. The unit is supplied and equipped with special beds, **traction** equipment, walkers, crutches, casting materials, and other items needed for the care of these patients. The staff working in orthopedics have been trained to recognize symptoms and problems related to the musculoskeletal system in addition to general medical nursing skills. Patients may be admitted to this unit as a result of a traumatic event causing broken bones, or the admission may be a planned event such as joint replacement surgery. The majority of orthopedic patients undergo some type of surgical intervention at the beginning of their hospital stay. Orthopedic patients range in age from pediatric to geriatric.

Orthopedic units have undergone dramatic change in the past 20 years. In the 1970s it was not unusual for a patient to be kept in bed, under heavy sedation, for a week to 10 days after surgery. Patients remained hospitalized for weeks at a time, with bed rest as the only treatment ordered. Today, orthopedic patients get out of bed very soon after surgery, sometimes the same day. Heavy sedation is reserved for special circumstances. To justify hospitalization, all patients must be receiving some form of active therapy. Many may be admitted to an observation status, meaning that the physician plans to discharge the patient within the next 24 to 48 hours. In 1977, a patient having a laminectomy (back surgery) could expect to be hospitalized 2 weeks or longer. Today some laminectomy patients are admitted to an observation status, having surgery one day and going home the next.

Description of the Unit

Beds/Bathrooms

At first glance this unit may appear to be the same as other nursing units in the hospital; in fact, the arrangement of the patient rooms and nursing desk may be identical. A closer look may begin to show the differences. Most of the patient beds are equipped with an overhead frame. This is a metal bar that runs up the back of the headboard about 3 feet and extends the length of the bed and down the footboard. Attached to the upper bar with chain links (for adjustment) is a triangular piece of metal with a plastic handgrip called a **trapeze.** This frame is placed on orthopedic beds for several reasons. One is to assist the patient in moving in bed using the trapeze. Additional traction may be attached to the overhead frame if warranted by the extent of treatment. The overhead frame serves another valuable but less obvious purpose: By allowing the patient to assist with moving in the bed, it helps prevent skin breakdown and reduces the incidence of bedsores.

All bathrooms in the orthopedic unit are equipped with hand bars or rails to assist the patient in transferring from a wheelchair to the toilet. If the patient's bathroom has a shower there will be safety bars there also. In addition, there may be a shower chair so the patient may shower from a sitting position if unable to stand. The unit may have a tub room for the patient who needs a tub bath or whirlpool treatments. All these areas are equipped with safety equipment to aid the patient and staff so there is no slipping or falling.

Equipment

Orthopedic patients require a lot of bulky equipment. Traction frames, bed scales, wheelchairs, walkers, and bedside commodes are some of the everyday items that might be found in an orthopedic unit. Moving orthopedic patients about is not a simple task, and in many cases it takes extra equipment and people.

Staffing

Staffing may be increased, with a greater staff to patient ratio than some of the other nursing units. If the average staff to patient ratio is 1 to 5, the orthopedic unit may have a 1 to 4 ratio depending on the type of patients on the unit. If the unit is heavy with "full bed care" patients the 1 to 4 ratio may be in force, going to the 1 to 5 ratio on other days when the majority of the unit may be "assisted" patient care. The type of staff may also be different from the other nursing units. The orthopedic unit may be staffed with more nursing assistant positions. This position has many different names across the country: nurse assistant, orderly, nurse tech, orthopedic tech, orthopedic aid, and so on. These workers are a valuable addition to the unit and are necessary to accommodate the increased care and treatment that many orthopedic patients require.

Care of the orthopedic patient requires a team approach, and thus ancillary staff may be more evident on this specialty unit. Physical therapists, occupational therapists, social workers, and home health consultants are a few of the "extra" staff members who may be seen daily on the orthopedic unit. The HUC is an integral part of this team.

Anatomy and Physiology Related to Orthopedics

Musculoskeletal System

The musculoskeletal system consists of the bones and other soft tissues that assist the bones in performing their functions. These include muscles, **ligaments**, **tendons**, and **cartilage.** The musculoskeletal system provides support for the body; it acts as a protection for the internal organs; and it provides for movement. The musculoskeletal system also manufactures blood cells and acts as a storehouse for minerals, especially calcium.

Tissues of the Musculoskeletal System

The musculoskeletal system is made up of two types of tissue. These are connective tissue and muscle. Connective tissue includes tendons, ligaments, cartilage, and bone. The muscles are striated (striped) and are called voluntary muscles (as opposed to smooth muscle, which is not subject to voluntary control).

Muscle. Skeletal muscle makes up about half the body weight. It has the unique ability to contract, thus producing or preventing movement. There are over 600 voluntary muscles that enable the body to move (Fig. 11–1). Muscles are attached to bones by tendons.

Bone. The human skeleton consists of 206 bones (Fig. 11–2). Bones can be categorized as flat (pelvis), cuboidal (vertebrae), or long (humerus) based on their shape (Fig. 11–3). Bones contain bone marrow, where blood cells are manufactured, and are covered with a thin membrane called **periosteum**. Bones are connected to each other by ligaments. The ligaments function to stabilize joints, guide motion, and prevent excess motion.

Joints. Joints are classified as immovable, slightly movable, or freely movable. The freely movable joints are lubricated to prevent friction by a substance called **synovial fluid.** These joints include the hip, knee, ankle, shoulder, and elbow (Fig. 11–4). Cartilage covers the opposing ends of bones in the freely movable joints. Its purpose is to spread the loads applied to the ends of the bones over a larger area in order to decrease stress and minimize friction and wear within the joint.

Common Links

Orthopedic patients have one thing in common: They are incapacitated by a bone or muscle disease, illness, or injury. Because of this common link many orthopedic patients have many of the same symptoms and complaints as well as similar concerns.

Swelling. Swelling of the soft tissue surrounding an injury is the body's way of sending in reinforcements to protect the affected area. The increase of fluid often makes the patient very uncomfortable. Ice and elevation are commonly used to combat the swelling. In some cases treatment must be postponed until major swelling has diminished. In the case of a **fractured** ankle, if the swelling is severe a **splint** may be applied; in 48 hours, if the swelling has been reduced, a cast will replace the splint. The purpose of the cast is to immobilize the fracture and allow for healing in proper alignment, and this requires the cast to fit snugly. If the cast is applied over severe swelling, it will be too loose when the swelling is reduced. The same principle applies to severe injuries as well as the simple fractures. Major trauma and injury to any bony area also involves soft tissue damage and in some cases damage to muscles protecting the bones. Surgery to repair the damage may be postponed for 24 to 48 hours to allow these areas to recover. These cases are judged at the time of injury by the orthopedic surgeon, and a decision will be made to achieve the best outcome for the patient.

Loss of Freedom and Mobility. Loss of mobility and freedom are other results of orthopedic trauma. Whether the trauma is planned, as in scheduled surgery to replace a joint, or an unplanned traumatic injury, all patients will experience a life change. For most people this immobility and loss of personal freedom will be brief and will be tolerated well. For patients who find themselves immobile for an extended period, there may be a period of adjustment that will be difficult to handle.

Lifestyle Changes. The long-term orthopedic patient must learn to deal with a variety of lifestyle changes. Loss of independence and the accompanying loss of personal privacy may be difficult for some patients. Compounding these problems are the effects of pain medications that may cause constipation and diarrhea. These circumstances can create a situation of personal embarrassment for the individual.

Another lifestyle change may be personal modesty. In many situations (traction, for example) it is impractical for patients to be clothed in personal attire. Since the duration of treatment can be lengthy, this may result in patients' feeling a loss of dignity. This is a major lifestyle change. Fortunately, the orthopedic staff is aware of their discomfort and will assist in making them as comfortable (and covered) as possible.

Most adults are accustomed to feeding themselves, and having someone else feed them is embarrassing and requires some adjustment. Imag-

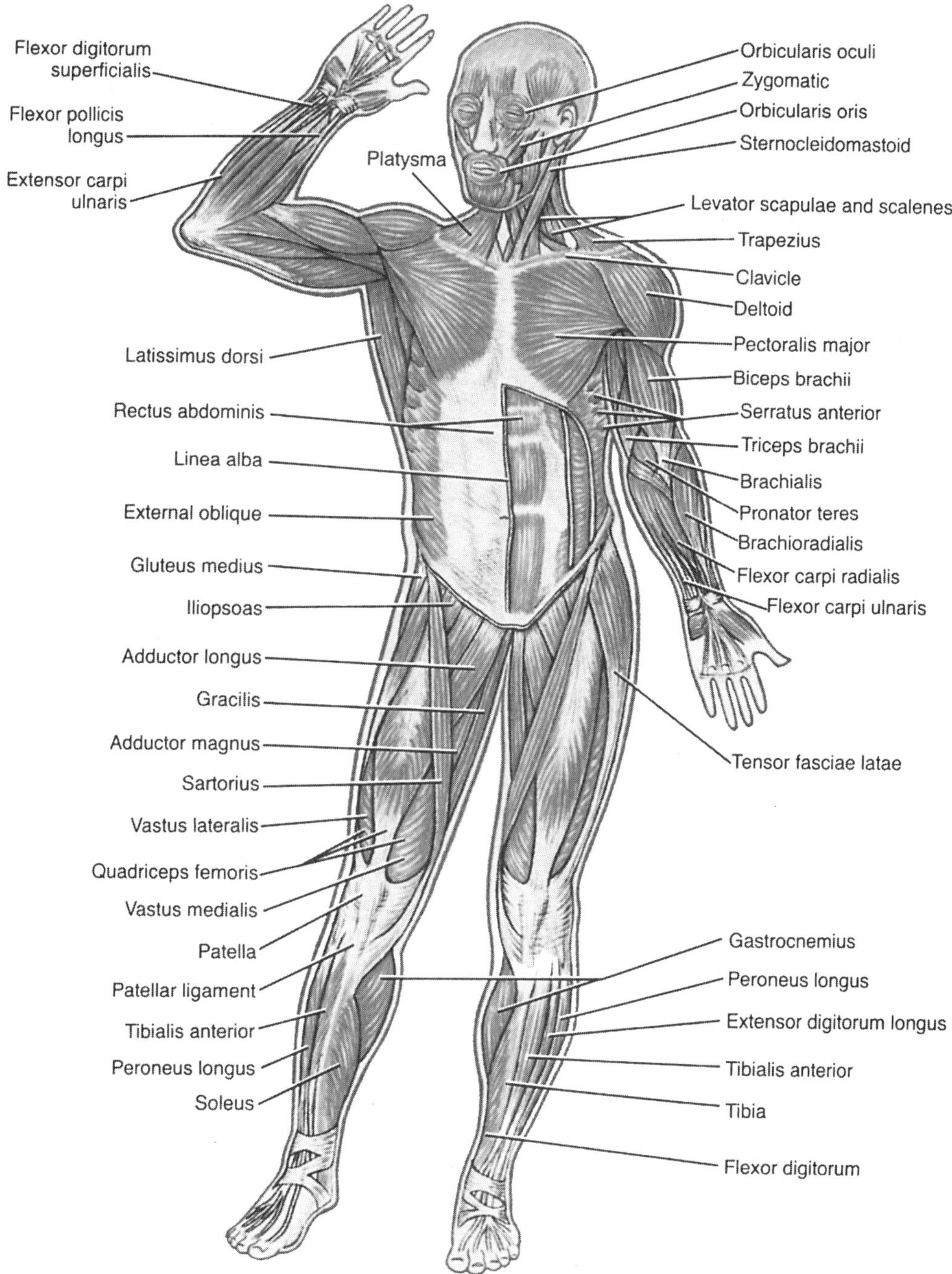

Figure 11–1
Skeletal muscles. (From O'Toole M [ed]: Miller-Keane Encyclopedia & Dictionary of Medicine, Nursing, & Allied Health, 6th ed. Philadelphia, WB Saunders, 1997.)

SKELETAL SYSTEM

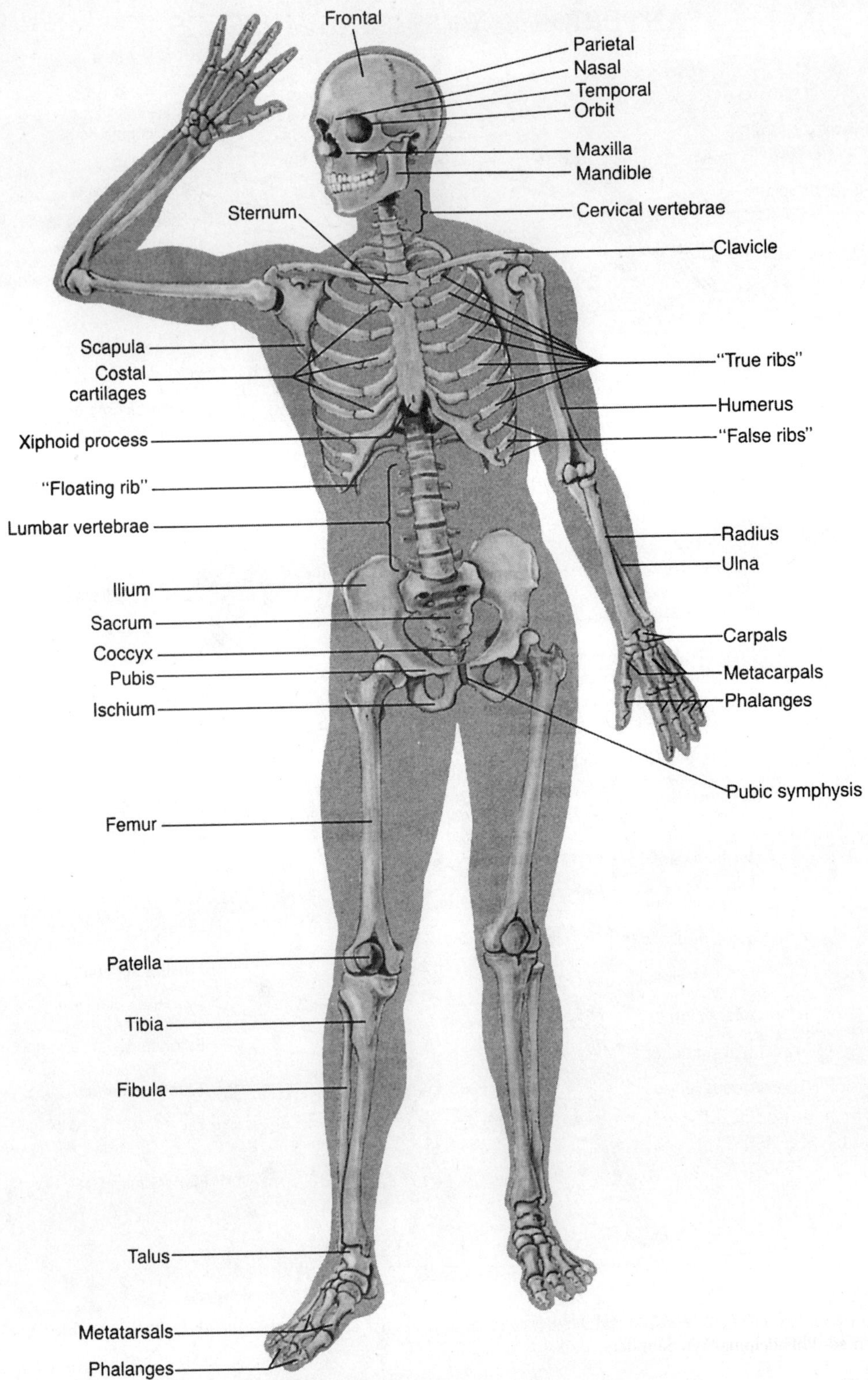

Figure 11–2 *See legend on opposite page*

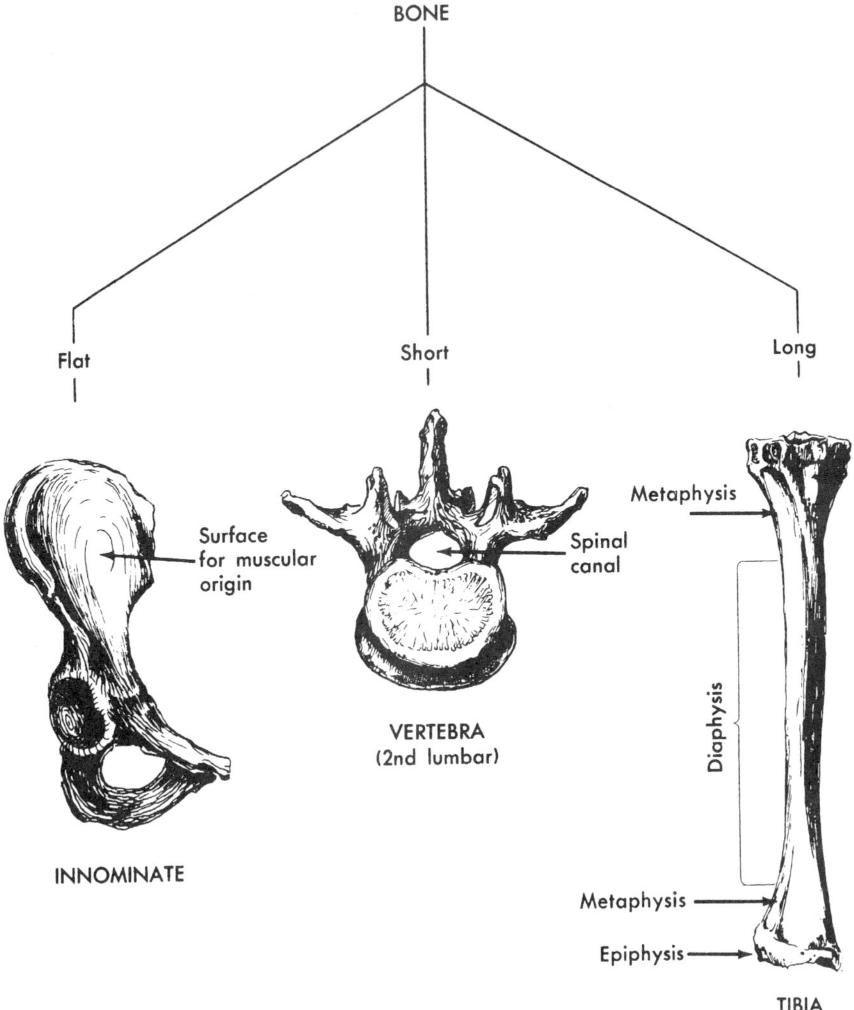

Figure 11–3
Bone types. (From Schneider ER: Handbook for the Orthopaedic Assistant, 2nd ed. St. Louis, CV Mosby, 1976.)

ine trying to butter a roll, cut up meat, or just get a spoon into hard ice cream with only one arm or while lying flat in bed. Now imagine having to deal with this problem several times each day for weeks or months. The frustration level for orthopedic patients can be very high for the smallest of tasks. It is sometimes easier for them to deal with the big frustrations than the small ones.

Rehabilitation. The average patient on the orthopedic unit will be treated for a period of time

Figure 11–2
The human skeleton. (From O'Toole M [ed]: Miller-Keane Encyclopedia & Dictionary of Medicine, Nursing, & Allied Health, 6th ed. Philadelphia, WB Saunders, 1997.)

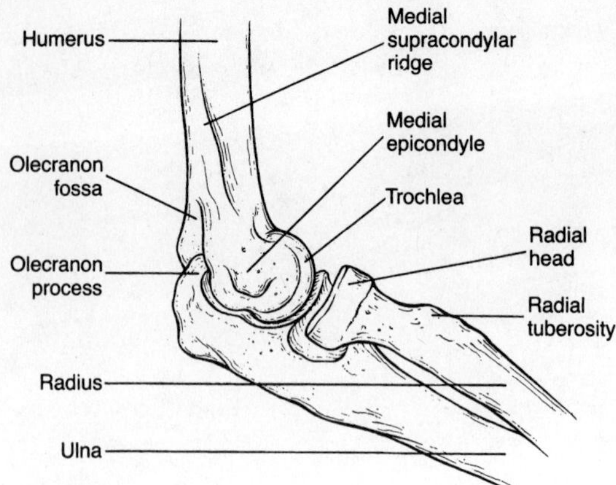

Figure 11–4
Elbow joint. (From Maher AB, Salmond SW, Pellino TA: Orthopaedic Nursing, 2nd ed. Philadelphia, WB Saunders, 1998.)

and then go home to complete the healing process. But for the major trauma patient an additional step may be required before discharge. This would be in a rehabilitation unit, either within the hospital or at a different facility. Patients who go on to rehab begin their therapy from the hospital bed. The majority of orthopedic patients receive some form of physical therapy: in the bed, in the room, in the hallways, and finally in the PT department. The extent of therapy is determined by the injury and the speed of recovery. Many patients continue therapy from home as outpatients. Patients who are to be transferred to a rehab unit may have a slightly different course of therapy in the hospital, since their progress may be slower and more intensive than that of other patients.

Medical Advances. Advances in medicine and changes in insurance reimbursement rules have changed the time frame for patients in the hospital, and this is no different for orthopedic patients. A few years ago it would not have been unusual to have many patients on the unit with a vague diagnosis of "back pain." Today insurance companies require many of the diagnostic tests to be obtained on an outpatient basis and reserve the in-patient status for people who need surgical intervention or treatments that are not available through home health services. Several years ago a hip fracture patient could expect to be in the hospital at least 2 weeks, if not longer; today that time is much shorter. Some patients are discharged to a short-term rehab unit within a week (or less) of surgery. Advances in therapy have made the recovery time shorter, and improvement in pain medications gives the patient the ability to participate in the therapy process, allowing faster healing and a shorter hospital stay.

Diagnostic Procedures

Diagnostic Imaging

X-Ray

An x-ray is the diagnostic study of choice to identify the presence of a fracture. Since bone is much denser than the surrounding tissue, it is very easy to see on the x-ray picture. However, x-rays are useful in other orthopedic conditions as well and many times may be used in conjunction with other studies to reach a diagnosis.

In addition to x-rays of affected bones some of the more common special procedures include:

Myelogram. The myelogram is a study of the spinal canal using a contrast material that is injected into the dural sac.

CT Scan. This is an x-ray that combines a high-powered computer with a rotating x-ray source to provide different views or slices of the area being studied.

Fluoroscopy. This test provides a continuous motion picture of a structure that can be viewed on a screen.

Nuclear Medicine Studies

Bone Scan. The most common diagnostic study done in nuclear medicine for orthopedic patients is a bone scan. It is indicated primarily to detect the presence of malignancies that metastasize to bone. These include breast, prostate, lung, lymph, thyroid, brain, and renal cancers. Bone scans can detect metastatic bone involvement much earlier than traditional x-rays. Bone scans can also be used when osteomyelitis, fracture, **avascular necrosis**, or rheumatoid arthritis is suspected.

Important points for the HUC to consider when transcribing orders for bone scans are the length of time necessary to complete the test and if hospital policy requires a consent form to be signed. Bone scans can be performed on an outpatient as well as in-patient basis.

Gallium Scan. A gallium scan is helpful in diagnosing tumors and abscesses. It is used primarily for imaging soft tissue rather than bone.

Magnetic Resonance Imaging. MRI is a noninvasive diagnostic study that uses a magnetic field and radio waves to produce an image. It is considered a more sensitive test than the CT scan. It is the preferred study when examining the spinal canal. It is particularly effective in diagnosing degenerated or herniated disks. It is also very useful in diagnosing tumors.

In scheduling patients for MRI the HUC must be aware of the limitations and contraindications for the study. Because the MRI tube is narrow the body size of the patient is an important factor. Patients with pacemakers are not good candidates for MRI. Patients on life support would also be excluded from this test.

Most hospitals will have a form for the patient to complete in order to determine eligibility. Length of time for the study is also a consideration for MRI. It is important that the patient be available for the duration of the study, which can last from 30 to 90 minutes. Therefore, no other tests or treatments should be scheduled during that time.

Laboratory Tests

Laboratory studies are the way a physician can measure what is happening with the patient, and for this reason a variety of lab tests will be performed on orthopedic patients. CBC, various blood chemistries, and urinalysis yield a great deal of information about the individual's overall health and are the beginning of any investigation into a problem.

Orthopedic patients must be watched for unusual soreness, swelling, and other signs of complications. These signs can mean a number of problems, including infections and other disease processes. The physician may order an ANA (antinuclear antibody), an ESR (erythrocyte sedimentation rate), or a RF (rheumatoid factor) to gain additional information.

When a blood clot is suspected, the doctor will order coagulation studies such as a prothrombin time (PT) and a partial thromboplastin time (PTT). If the patient is placed on anticoagulation therapy these studies will often be ordered on a daily basis to monitor the effects of the drugs. Many other laboratory studies may be ordered during the patient's hospital stay depending on the circumstances.

Other Diagnostic Studies

Electromyography (EMG). An EMG studies the electrical potential of muscles. It is used in orthopedic patients to help differentiate between musculoskeletal and neuromuscular problems. The procedure is performed by a physician.

Arthroscopy. This procedure is the examination of the interior of a joint using a small fiberoptic tube. The most common joint examined is the knee, but arthroscopy can be used on other joints as well. This procedure is generally carried out in the operating room and is done by the physician.

Doppler. The use of Doppler may be common on the orthopedic unit. If the patient has a suspected blood clot a Doppler will be used at the bedside to listen to blood flow. For further investigation an extensive Doppler study may be obtained in the diagnostic imaging department.

Medications Specific to Orthopedic Patients

Pain Control

Nonopioids

NSAIDs, Salicylates, and Acetaminophen

Nonsteroidal anti-inflammatory drugs (**NSAIDs**) have been added to the care and treatment of orthopedic diseases and injuries in the last 10 years. These medications offer several advantages, including the reduction of swelling. Anti-inflammatory medication helps the body keep soft tissue swelling to a minimum. Because soft tissue swelling is very painful, if the swelling is reduced, the pain will also be reduced. These medications do not contain steroids, which can cause many side effects in patients who do not require that additional treatment. A few of the more common NSAIDs are Feldene, Indocin, Motrin, Naprosyn, and Toradol. Some of these are available by injection as well as by mouth; some can be obtained over the counter, while others are available by prescription only. Studies have found that for many orthopedic patients this type of medication is as effective as medication containing narcotics.

Salicylates are chemically treated compounds, such as aspirin, once the most common nonprescription pain and fever reliever. Aspirin is used frequently in the treatment of rheumatoid arthritis (RA).

Acetaminophen (the most common brand is Tylenol) is used for the same symptoms as salicylates but contains no aspirin. Originally it was used only by people allergic to aspirin products or with gastric problems that are complicated by aspirin products. Today it is often used for patients with degenerative joint disease (**DJD**). Acetaminophen does not have anti-inflammatory properties and thus is not effective for reducing swelling. Any of these medications may be used to treat mild to moderate orthopedic pain, although those that also reduce swelling are used most often.

Opioids

Opioid analgesics are used for moderate to severe pain. The older term *narcotic* is being phased out because of its association with illegal drug use. This type of drug therapy has changed dramatically in the past few years. Thirty years ago many orthopedic patients would have received high doses of very strong narcotic medications for extended periods. Since that time the types and methods of narcotic drug therapy have changed many times. Currently the theory of opioid use is to give the stronger medications in the beginning and quickly taper to the nonopioid pain relievers.

One of the newer methods of opioid administration is IV patient-controlled analgesia (**PCA**). The doctor prescribes the amount of medication, and the patient can self-administer computerized, preset low-dose amounts whenever necessary. This system allows patients to manage their own pain and avoids the wait time associated with calling for the nurse to administer the medication.

Meperidine, morphine, hydromorphone, oxycodone, and codeine are the common types of opioid medications given to orthopedic patients.

Corticosteroids

Corticosteroids are hormones produced by the adrenal cortex, which is the outer portion of the adrenal gland. The hormones produced by this gland aid in controlling salt and water metabolism and regulating glucose metabolism. Corticosteroids may be given as adjuvant therapy to reduce inflammation. Common names for corticosteriods are hydrocortisone, prednisolone, and prednisone. Because of the potential for serious side effects, corticosteroid use is limited to specific situations.

Important points for the HUC to be aware of include dose scheduling and tapering. If possible, the medications should be given early in the day, when the body's natural steroid level is lowest. Corticosteroids are never stopped abruptly. Therefore, the doctor will frequently write an order that includes a series of decreasing daily doses to taper the amount of the drug that the patient is receiving before discontinuing it.

Antibiotics

One of the most serious complications that an orthopedic patient can face is an infection in or around the bone, known as **osteomyelitis.** Osteomyelitis is most frequently caused by *Staphylococcus* microorganisms. Infection may reach the bone through the bloodstream, from infection in adjacent soft tissue, or through a compound (open) fracture or other trauma. For the patient with a simple fracture of a small bone the risk of infection is low. If the fracture is compound, with an opening in the skin or in a large bone, the risk of infection goes up dramatically. The site and method of injury are taken into account when risk of infection is calculated. If osteomyelitis is not recognized and treated appropriately it may result in complications ranging from chronic pain to **amputation** and even death.

Almost all orthopedic patients going to surgery will receive IV antibiotics before, during, and after the operation. This includes surgery to repair traumatic injury and surgery for planned orthopedic correction.

Medications used to treat these serious infections include penicillin, nafcillin, ampicillin, amoxicillin, and the cephalosporins, such as cefazolin. However, many other antibiotics may also be ordered depending on the microorganism that is causing the infection.

Anticoagulants

Anticoagulants are substances that halt, prevent, or slow blood clotting. Blood clots that get into the bloodstream and travel to the lungs (pulmonary emboli) can cause severe complications and even death.

Orthopedic patients who experience trauma or undergo surgery are at risk for developing blood clots, especially deep venous thrombosis (**DVT**). Patients undergoing surgery for hip or knee reconstruction are at the highest risk. These patients may be given anticoagulants preoperatively to decrease the incidence of DVT. Heparin and Coumadin are the two most commonly used drugs to prevent and treat blood clots.

Treatments and Procedures Specific to the Orthopedic Unit

Surgery

The majority of patients in the orthopedic unit have had or will have some type of surgical intervention, because of either a traumatic injury or a planned repair. Traumatic injuries take all forms, from a simple bone fracture to multiple trauma with many injuries.

Traumatic injuries result from vehicular crashes, sports-related accidents, work or home accidents, and weather-related accidents. How the accident occurred may determine the severity of the injury. The seat-belted auto crash may produce less severe injury than the unbelted accident. The roller blader with arm and leg pads may have a simple fracture but without the protective padding may receive a complex fracture. Falling off a ladder at home may be more serious than falling the same distance at work when using a safety harness. Regardless of how severe the injury, if it requires surgical intervention and hospitalization, it is traumatic to the patient.

Orthopedic surgical repairs may include **internal fixation** of bones with the use of implants. Metal implants, which include pins, plates, rods, and screws may be removed after the bones have healed, requiring another surgical procedure. However, implants may also be plastic, ceramic, chemical, or biologic, such as allograft bone, and these may be permanent.

Placement of a joint **prosthesis** may be for a traumatic injury or may be due to degenerative changes in the natural joint. Older persons who fall and break a femur may need to have a hip prosthesis rather than having the hip repaired by pinning. This will be determined by the extent of damage, the age of the patient, and the presence of healthy bone. Degenerative changes to the joint and surrounding bone often lead to a total joint replacement, most commonly hips and knees. Many patients who suffer from severe arthritis may need to have both hips and/or knees replaced, whereas other patients may need only the right or left side replaced. People who suffer from rheumatoid arthritis may have many of their joints replaced, including the smaller joints in their fingers and toes, if the disease is causing crippling and immobility.

Sports injuries make up a large portion of orthopedic surgical cases. Shoulder or **rotator cuff** injuries are common in basketball, volleyball, swimming, weight lifting, and any other sport that requires an excess of upper body stretching or activity. Football, basketball, hockey, soccer, water/snow skiing, and other sports that use the lower body and involve a lot of twisting or pivoting will incur injuries to the hips, knees, and ankles. These injuries may not always involve bone but may affect the large muscles and tendons surrounding the bones. These muscles and tendons are what make it possible for our bodies to turn, twist, stretch, and pivot. If they become damaged or injured they will need to be repaired for normal activity and certainly for sports participation.

Patients in the hospital for back surgery are common in orthopedic units. Many of these patients will have a diagnosis of **HNP**, herniated nucleus pulposus. The lumbar spine is subject to tremendous forces and degenerative changes. The area most commonly affected by this force is in the lumbar spine, but injury can occur to the cervical spine as well. When the surrounding ligaments are also injured and weakened, the disk material begins to extrude through them (sometimes referred to as a bulging disk). These little pieces of disk can cause a great deal of pain and disability. After patients have exhausted the nonsurgical therapies or have an acute occurrence, surgical intervention may be necessary. The surgical procedure used for most HNP diagnoses is called a lumbar laminectomy, or cervical laminectomy if the problem is in the cervical spine. This is the removal of the disk material causing the problems. Patients with extensive disk involvement may require **fusion** of the vertebrae to provide the necessary stability.

Immobilization

Traction

Traction, a common form of treatment, uses pulling forces that are applied to areas such as neck, arms, feet, legs, and trunk in an attempt to relieve pain and promote healing. Traction may be applied to the skin or directly to the skeleton.

Skin Traction. Skin traction is applied directly to the patient's skin. It is often temporary, being used before surgery or to reduce muscle spasms. Patients may be in traction all the time or have an on/off schedule. Common types of skin traction include cervical traction, Buck's traction (Fig. 11–5), and Russell's traction. Ace bandages, belts, boots, and slings are commonly used in the application of skin traction. Massage is used to manually move the muscles and soft tissues of the body to improve circulation. This is often used in conjunction with whirlpool and ultrasonic therapy.

Skeletal Traction. In the case of unstable fractures, the placement of pins applied directly to the affected bone and extending externally may be necessary. Traction is then attached to the pins for a period of time. This allows stabilization of the bone for healing purposes. This type of traction is never removed without a doctor's order. Skeletal traction is commonly used for femur fractures (Fig. 11–6). If skeletal traction is used for cervical injuries it is applied to the head with tongs or **halo** (Fig. 11–7).

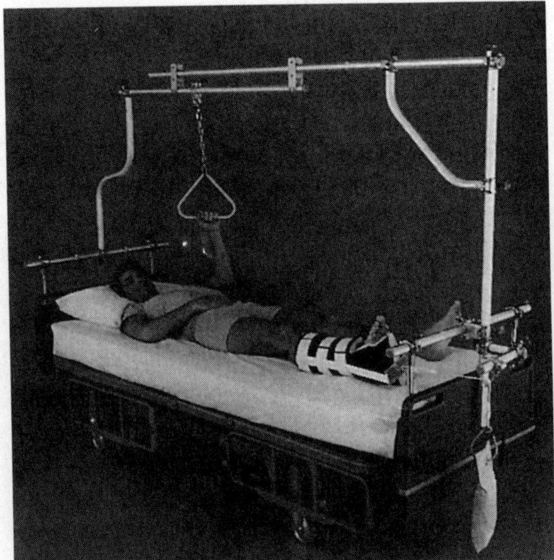

Figure 11–5
Buck's traction. (From Maher AB, Salmond SW, Pellino TA: Orthopaedic Nursing, 2nd ed. Philadelphia, WB Saunders, 1998.)

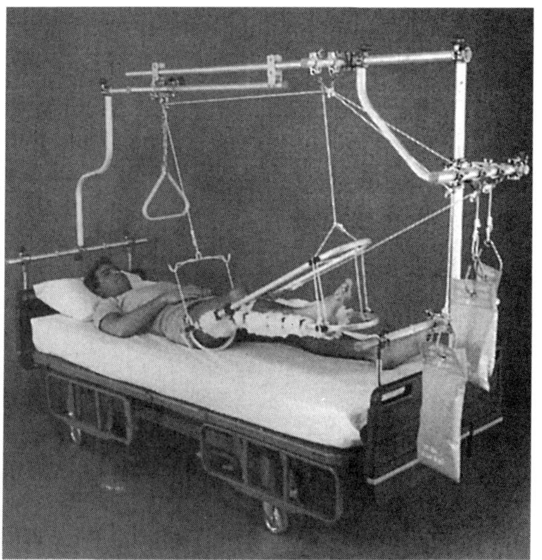

Figure 11–6
Skeletal traction. (From Maher AB, Salmond SW, Pellino TA: Orthopaedic Nursing, 2nd ed. Philadelphia, WB Saunders, 1998.)

Other Immobilizers

Casts and Splints. A cast or splint is a temporary measure for immobilizing a part of the body. Casts and splints are used to correct a deformity, maintain support, protect a realigned bone (as in a fracture), and promote healing. In some cases they can also facilitate early weight-bearing (Fig. 11–8). Casting materials include plaster of Paris and synthetic materials such as fiberglass.

External Fixators. External fixators are devices that immobilize a fracture using a system of wires or pins connected to a rigid external frame. They are used in situations of multiple trauma with a number of fractures. External fixators can be used for fingers (Fig. 11–9), limbs, and

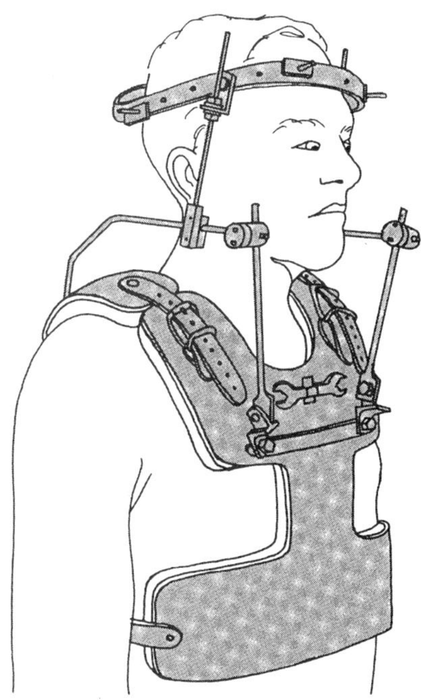

Figure 11–7
Halo traction vest. (From Maher AB, Salmond SW, Pellino TA: Orthopaedic Nursing, 2nd ed. Philadelphia, WB Saunders, 1998.)

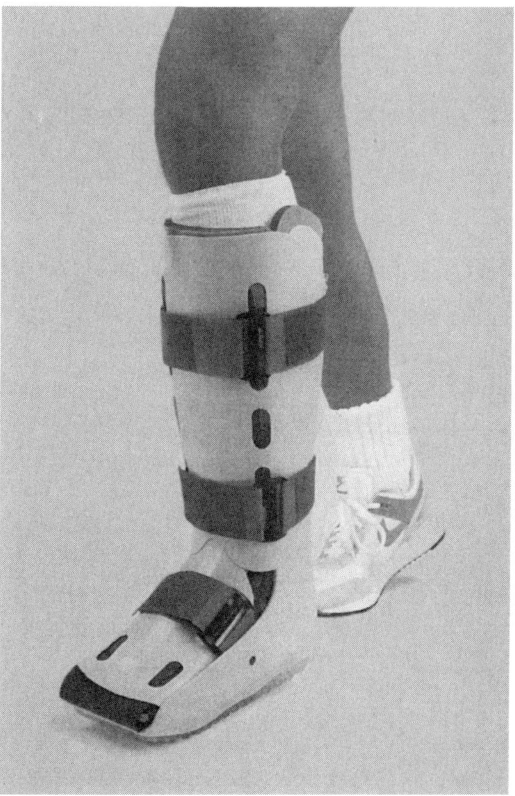

Figure 11–8
Pneumatic walker splint or castlike device. (Courtesy of Aircast.)

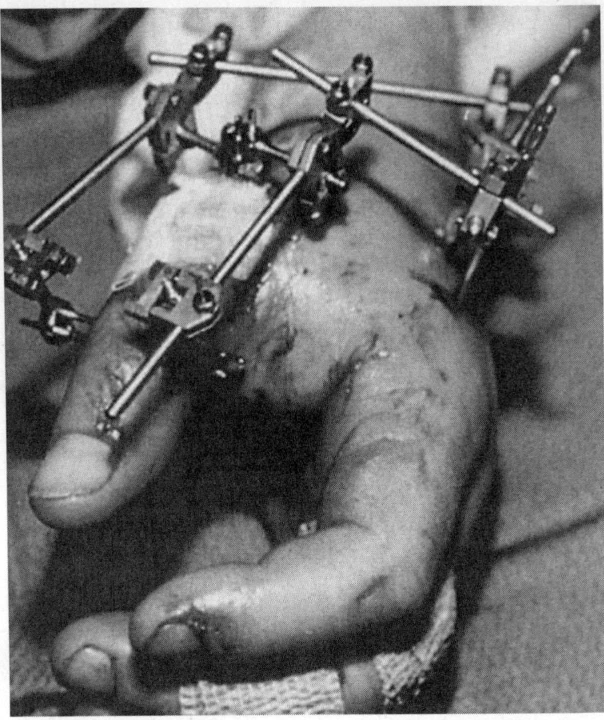

Figure 11–9
External fixator of the hand. (Courtesy of Howmedica, Inc., Pfizer Hospital Products Group.)

the pelvis. They are made of lightweight materials such as aluminum, titanium, graphite, and nylon.

Physical Therapy (PT)

Most patients will receive some form of physical therapy. For some it will begin immediately. Research has found that a broken body needs to get back into the normal routine of movement to heal. Once it was thought best to "let the body rest and recuperate. " We now know that that only makes it harder and causes the body to take longer to mend. Muscles, tendons, and ligaments become stiff and forgetful with inactivity. The different modalities of physical therapy include heat, cold, massage, light, electricity, ultrasound, and exercise.

Patients now prepare as much as possible for a scheduled surgery by learning simple exercises that they can do at home beforehand. Exercises that stretch and strengthen a knee, leg, or shoulder before surgery will make the healing process faster. Many patients will see a physical therapist as an outpatient and learn how to prepare for surgery. In addition to the exercises, the patient may learn the proper use of crutches, the safest way to go up and down stairs, and the best way to go from a sitting to a standing position. It is easier to learn how to do these things before the patient has a sore knee, leg, or shoulder.

Occupational Therapy (OT)

The physical therapist helps the patient learn to walk with a new knee replacement. The occupational therapist helps the patient learn to put on his or her socks during the healing process. Finding a way to accomplish day-to-day activities is very important to most patients. Learning to deal with what should be the simple task of putting on socks can be very frustrating to a person who cannot bend his or her knee. Patients want to care for themselves, and studies show that when they are allowed to participate in the activities of daily living they get well faster.

The occupational therapist may work with the patient several times a day. The therapist may arrive at the times of day when the patient needs the most help. If feeding is the lesson the therapist will try to be there when the trays are served.

The OT staff often have handy little "tools" that can help the patient with certain accomplishments. For example, a 3-foot-long shoehorn helps get feet into shoes if bending is a problem, and a long metal "grabber" can reach for high objects when stretching is difficult. Any time patients can be helped back into independent living they are much happier.

Equipment and Supplies Specific to Orthopedics

Assistive Devices

Ambulation

All orthopedic units have crutches, canes, and walkers. The more quickly patients can become mobile, the faster the healing process. Most patients will begin recovery with the device that offers the greatest assistance and gradually work their way to the device that offers the least assistance. For example, patients recovering from hip surgery may start out with a walker and work toward using a cane and then to walking alone, while a person recovering from a leg fracture may begin with crutches. The length of time that an assistive device is needed depends on the injury and the age and physical condition of the patient. Some patients may progress from walkers to canes in a matter of days, while others require additional time. Many older people may require the use of a walker or cane on a permanent basis.

Continuous Passive Motion

Continuous passive motion (CPM) machines are used for patients recovering from knee surgery, generally total replacement of the knee. The machine is used while the patient is in bed; it moves the leg slowly up and down, and back and forth (Fig. 11–10). It is designed to help the person gain mobility in a non–weight bearing manner. Patients may be on the machine many times during the day; the more it is used, the faster the healing process.

Communication With and About Orthopedic Patients

Professional

Communication is a major part of any HUC position and therefore one of the most important skills to master. The HUC has access to many forms of communication devices: telephones and computers as well as fax and copy machines. Proper communication via these devices is of utmost importance. The HUC is the first-line person on the nursing unit and carries a large responsibility for proper communication with the other health care professionals.

HUCs have many opportunities to communicate with physicians, both in person and on the telephone. When the physician is on the nursing unit the HUC may be asked when ordered tests are scheduled or to obtain the results of completed

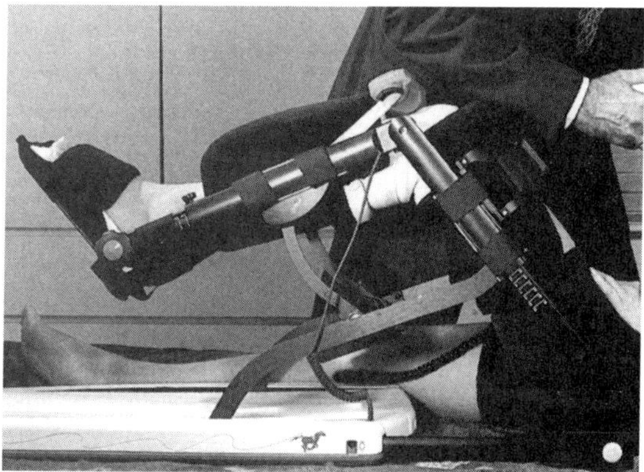

Figure 11–10
CPM machine. (Courtesy of Orthologic, Tempe, AZ.)

tests. The HUC may need additional information from the physician about written orders. It is important to maintain a friendly and helpful, but professional, manner with physicians. The HUC should know when to assist the physician with taking or receiving information and when to call for a nurse.

The HUC will communicate most with the staff working on the nursing unit. It is important to keep the staff informed of all new orders, changes in existing orders, patients' location off the unit, and new patients arriving from admitting, ER, or surgery. Keeping in close contact with coworkers will make the unit run more smoothly and efficiently.

Families, Visitors, and Patients

Family members and visitors often come to the HUC for information about the patient. The HUC should know exactly what information can be shared. The patient's location may be a frequent question. The HUC should be able to tell the family member or visitor when the patient left the unit and give an approximate return time. Information about the location of the patient depends on the situation: If the patient is having a scheduled test out of the department, the HUC could share that information, but if the patient was just rushed to surgery the HUC would want to call the nurse. The nurse might be able to answer questions that the HUC should not answer: the nature of the surgery, the condition of the patient, and so forth. The most important rule to remember is patient confidentiality.

Communication with the patient is another key aspect of the HUC role. If there is a call system at the desk it may be the responsibility of the HUC to answer patient calls. The HUC should answer these calls quickly and professionally. People in the hospital often feel isolated and frightened, in addition to having pain and discomfort. They may not behave in their normal manner; some patients may be angry and rude. They are taking out their frustrations on anyone who is around. The HUC should always maintain a pleasant speaking voice regardless of the patient's attitude. The HUC will get assistance for the patient in a timely manner and always assure the patient that the request is being taken care of as quickly as possible.

Order Entry

Transcription of physicians' orders is the process by which the HUC communicates information regarding the patient's care to the appropriate departments and personnel. Most hospitals use a computer system for the transmission of orders. It is crucial that these orders be 100 percent correct and complete. Giving the receiving department the right information can make a difference in the care of the patient. For example, if a patient needs to go to Radiology, the HUC needs to include accurate information about the method of transport (wheelchair, stretcher, bed), if oxygen is necessary, and if IV poles will be needed. If the person transporting the patient does not have the necessary equipment the test could be delayed and thus the treatment might also be delayed. Medicare and other insurances are allowing only a specific number of hospital days per diagnosis, meaning that delays are costly and not acceptable.

Quality/Risk Management

Infection Control

Since infection in the orthopedic patient can be debilitating and even life-threatening, steps must be taken to reduce the risk of infection in the environment. Many factors affect the patient's susceptibility to infection. Age, physical condition, nutritional status, and type of wound are all risk factors. It is important to include the patient in the effort to reduce the risk of infection. Education that stresses the importance of good hand washing is important for staff and patients alike. Proper reporting of all infections to the appropriate hospital department (Infection Control) is extremely important. This allows tracking of all infections and may help determine a pattern that can be identified and eliminated.

HUC Role

Policy and procedures are written and maintained for the purposes of quality and risk management. One of the goals of health care is to give good-quality care with minimal risk to patients and staff. The HUC should be well versed in the policies and procedures pertaining to the nursing unit. The HUC should know where the policy/procedure manual is located and how to use it. It should be in an area that is easily accessible to all staff members. Many times the HUC is the resource person when a question arises. The HUC may be the person on the unit who is responsible for typing new policies or changing existing policies and keeping the manual up to date.

Safety

Health care workers routinely put side rails on patient beds to prevent falls. The bathrooms are equipped with bars to help the patient maintain balance. There are double and triple checks when medications and blood are administered. Patient safety is part of health care.

Keeping the staff safe from injury is important as well. All hospitals have safety instruction and training in frequently performed tasks: the proper way to move and lift, the proper way to handle body fluids, and precautions on infection control and isolation. The restrooms may contain signs on the proper method of hand washing. There may be training on handling of hazardous material and how to determine if a substance is hazardous.

It is important to be prepared for emergencies at all times. Hospitals have codes that may be announced on the overhead page system for certain types of emergencies. Some of the common codes may be:

Code Red: fire
Code Blue: cardiac arrest
Code Gray: dangerous weather

The HUC should know what all the codes mean and the proper response to each. It is important to remain calm and collected during emergencies. If all personnel know what their task is and carry it out efficiently the emergency will be handled correctly.

Closing Thoughts

The health unit coordinator is a pivotal person in the unit, coordinating the patients and their activities, initiating the physicians' orders, communicating those orders to all the caregivers in the hospital setting. A vast amount of knowledge is required. Efficiency will be determined by the knowledge and the ability to function under pressure. The HUC should constantly seek new knowledge and strive for 100 percent accuracy.

Review Questions

1. List six diagnostic imaging procedures that would be conducted to identify orthopedic problems.
2. Explain what patient controlled analgesia is.
3. Identify the surgical procedure performed to correct HNP.
4. List the two types of traction and explain the difference between them.
5. Name three methods of immobilization other than traction.

Bibliography

Hoppenfeld S (ed): Orthopedic Dictionary. Philadelphia, JB Lippincott, 1994.

LaFleur-Brooks M: Health Unit Coordinating, 3rd ed. Philadelphia, WB Saunders, 1993.

Maher A, Salmond S, Pellino T: Orthopaedic Nursing, 2nd ed. Philadelphia, WB Saunders, 1998.

Mourad LA: Orthopedic Disorders. St. Louis, Mosby Yearbook, 1991.

O'Toole M (ed): Miller-Keane Encyclopedia & Dictionary of Medicine, Nursing, & Allied Health, 6th ed. Philadelphia, WB Saunders, 1997.

Thomas CL (ed): Taber's Cyclopedic Medical Dictionary, 14th ed. Philadelphia, FA Davis, 1981.

Internet

Wheeless CR: Wheeless' Textbook of Orthopedics, 1996.

Merck Manual, 1996–1997. Whitehouse Station, NJ.

12 The Pediatric Unit

Betty Lamb

Objectives

At the completion of this chapter the reader should be able to:

1. Explain how a pediatric unit differs from an adult unit.
2. Identify two staff members unique to pediatrics.
3. Explain the major difference in medication orders for children.
4. List ten of the indicators of child abuse.

Vocabulary

Child Life Specialist: A professional who is concerned with the psychosocial impact of illness and hospitalization

Child Life Aide: A staff member whose primary responsibility is to assist the Child Life Specialist in providing an environment and activities designed to meet the recreational, social, educational, and developmental needs of hospitalized children

Common Abbreviations

A.D.	Right ear
A.J.	Apple juice
ALL	Acute lymphocytic leukemia
BAER	Brainstem auditory evoked response
B.O.M.	Bilateral otitis media
Cal.	Calorie
C.F.	Cystic fibrosis
CHF	Congestive heart failure
CPS	Child protective service
FB	Foreign body
FTT	Failure to thrive
FUO	Fever of undetermined origin
fx	Fracture
G.C.S.	Glasgow Coma Score
GH	Growth hormone
GI	Gastrointestinal
gm	Gram
H.C.	Head circumference
HEENT	Head, ears, eyes, nose, throat
ISC	Isolette skin control
JRA	Juvenile rheumatoid arthritis
kg	Kilogram
lb	Pound
LBW	Low birth weight
LGA	Large for gestational age
lytes	Electrolytes
MMR	Measles, mumps, and rubella vaccine
MVA	Motor vehicle accident
NG	Nasogastric
NK	None known
N & V	Nausea and vomiting
PALS	Pediatric advanced life support
PKU	Phenylketonuria
RSV	Respiratory syncytial virus
R/O	Rule out
Sen.	Sensitivity
SGA	Small for gestational age
Sib	Sibling
SIDS	Sudden infant death syndrome
Synd	Syndrome
T.	Temperature
T & A	Tonsil and adenoids
T. bili	Total bilirubin
UAC	Umbilical arterial catheter
VZV	Varicella zoster virus

Medical Terminology Related to Pediatric Patients

The following medical terms are not found in the text, but they are terms that anyone working in a pediatric unit would be expected to know.

Acne—Inflammation of the skin with the formation of an eruption of papules or pustules

Adenoidectomy—Excision of the adenoids

Apnea—Absence of breathing

Anemia—A condition in which the blood is deficient in red blood cells or hemoglobin, or both

Appendectomy—Surgical removal of the vermiform appendix

Bradycardia—Slow heart beat; slow pulse

Bronchiolitis—Inflammation of the bronchioli

Circumcision—Surgical removal of all or part of the foreskin

Congenital—Present at or existing from the time of birth

Convulsion—Involuntary muscular contractions

Cystic fibrosis—An inherited disease, generally characterized by chronic respiratory infections and disorders of the pancreas and sweat glands

Dehydration—Occurs when output of water exceeds water intake

Diabetes mellitus—A disorder of carbohydrate metabolism characterized by hyperglycemia and glycosuria. The disorder is caused by inadequate production of insulin.

Encephalitis—Inflammation of the brain

The abbreviations listed for this chapter are those that a HUC working in this area would be expected to know.

Abbreviations related to medications for pediatric patients will be listed in that section of the chapter.

Epilepsy—A recurrent disorder of cerebral function characterized by sudden, brief attacks of altered consciousness, motor activity, or sensory phenomena

Febrile—Feverish

Fever—Elevation of temperature above normal

Fracture—A break or rupture in a bone; the breaking of a part, especially a bone

Gastroenteritis—Inflammation of the stomach and intestines

Hemophilia—A hereditary hemorrhagic disorder caused by deficiency of coagulation factor VIII

Hyperbilirubinemia—Excessive amount of bilirubin in the blood

Immunodeficiency—A deficiency in immune response

Pneumonia—Inflammation of the lung with consolidation

Description of the Unit

Physical Environment

Children are not little adults. The pediatric unit's environment is designed to be appropriate to pediatric patients, and the equipment and supplies are selected to meet their needs. Televisions (Fig. 12–1) and telephones are standard equipment. The decor of the unit is bright and cheerful. Rooms may be decorated with posters and personal items belonging to the patients. Carts stocked with toys for all ages are available. Video games are usually available for older patients. Television and games are used to provide education for patients and their families. There usually will be a playroom on the unit, which may be staffed by a **child life aide** who will offer organized play therapy for patients (Fig. 12–2).

Children from newborn up to age 18 years are cared for in the pediatric units and stand-alone pediatric hospitals. If the hospital has an adolescent unit, patients over the age of 12 years are admitted there. The pediatric unit must have many different types and sizes of beds and equipment for the patients and parents on the unit. There may be a limited number of private rooms to be used for older patients or for those with long-term illnesses. The private room enables the parents to spend the night with their child.

Patients are grouped by diagnosis, age, and sex. The small infant may be placed in a bassinet. There may be a sleeper chair in the room for a parent. If the mother is breast feeding, there will be a breast pump and an area for privacy. A small infant should not be placed in a room with a child over the age of 3 years. Patients from the age of 6 weeks to 3 years are placed in a crib with a plastic bubble over the top for protection. This will prevent the child from crawling over the top of the rail.

Children from 4 to 10 years of age are usually placed in a youth bed, which is shorter than an adult bed (Fig. 12–3). The 11- to 18-year-old is placed in an adult bed. This group should not be placed in a room with a younger child or infant.

Pediatric Staff

Although the staff in pediatrics is composed of RNs, LPNs, certified nursing assistants (CNAs), and HUCs, there are also other staff members who serve the particular needs of children and their families.

Child Life Specialist

The child life specialist (Fig. 12–4) is concerned with the psychosocial effect of illness and hospitalization. He or she works closely with families and health care providers to treat the whole child, making every effort to minimize the stressful and potentially negative impact of hospitalization and maximize opportunities for positive and supportive experiences. This professional works as an integral part of the health care team to provide opportunities for play, learning, preparation and support, medical play, self-expression, family involvement, socialization, and mastery of difficult experiences.

Child Life Aide

The child life aide is a professional who engages the children in age-appropriate activities, recog-

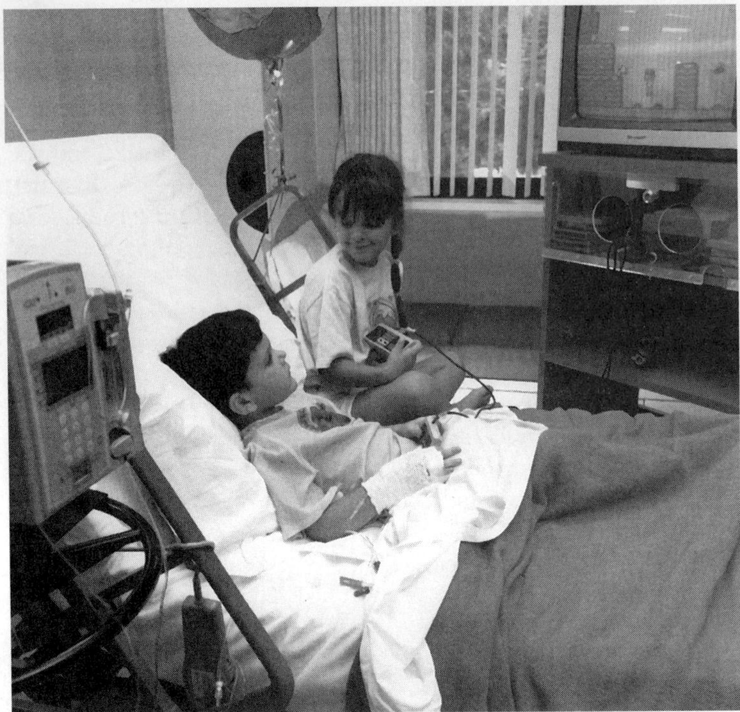

Figure 12–1
Pediatric patient playing TV games with his sister.

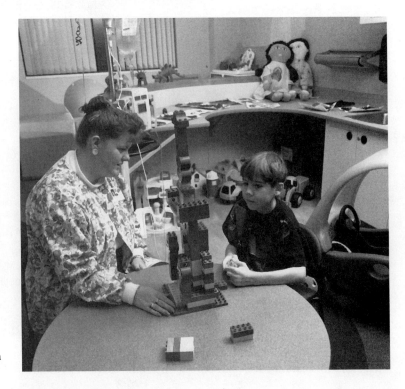

Figure 12–2
Child life aide in playroom with a young patient.

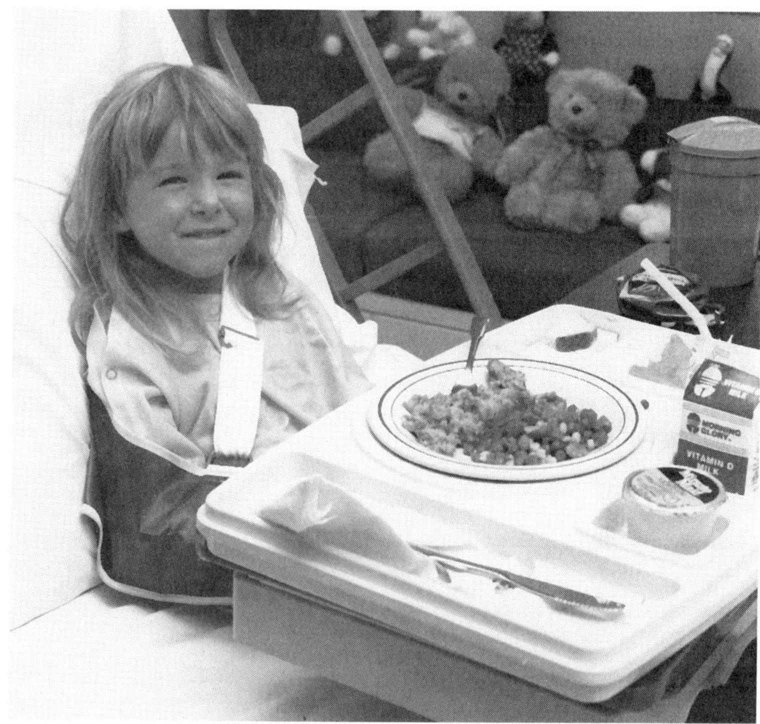

Figure 12–3
A preschool patient.

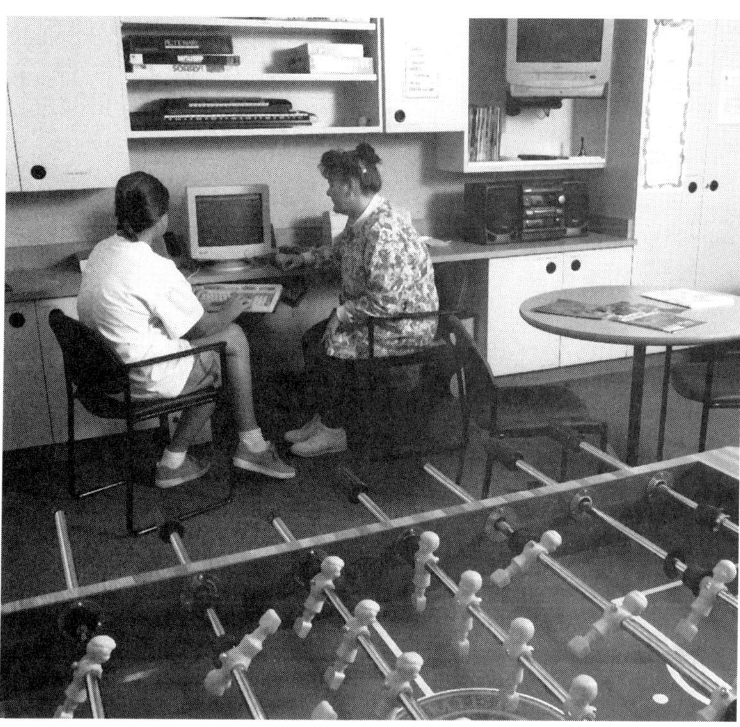

Figure 12–4
Child life specialist working with teenage family member.

nizing that play is an important part of a child's life, especially when in a strange and potentially threatening environment. The child life aide works under the direct supervision of the child life specialist.

Growth and Development

The staff of the pediatric unit is concerned not only with children's medical needs but also with their emotional and psychological well-being. They take the time to educate families and encourage them to get involved in the care delivery process. Erikson has described eight stages of development through which human beings pass in their lifetime (Table 12–1). Each stage allows the person to experience a central task or crisis, which must be resolved before moving on to the next level.

The nurse will interview the parents or guardian to determine the child's developmental level because the child's developmental growth may change the way that care is delivered. The nurse or play therapist will offer appropriate activities for the child's developmental age. The nursing staff should also include cultural and spiritual considerations in their care of the patient. An interpreter should be available if there is a language barrier.

Admission to the pediatric unit may be directly from the physician's office, or the child may have been treated in the emergency department and then admitted as an in-patient. The patient may come directly to the unit, bypassing the admission office. In this case, the parent will be asked to return to the admission office once the child is

Table 12–1 ERIKSON'S STAGES OF EGO DEVELOPMENT

Stage	Age	Bipolar Crisis	Successful Resolution	Unsuccessful Resolution
1	Infancy (birth to 1 year)	Trust versus mistrust	Hope and drive	Fear
2	Early childhood (1 to 3 years)	Autonomy versus shame and doubt	Will power and self-control	Self-doubt
3	Early childhood (4 to 5 years)	Initiative versus guilt	Purpose and direction	Unworthiness
4	Middle childhood (6 to 11 years)	Industry versus inferiority	Competency and method	Incompetency
5	Adolescence (12 to 20 years)	Ego identity versus role confusion	Fidelity and devotion	Uncertainty
6	Early adulthood (20 to 24 years)	Intimacy versus isolation	Love and affiliation	Promiscuity
7	Middle adulthood (25 to 65 years)	Generativity versus stagnation	Care and production	Selfishness
8	Late adulthood (65 on)	Integrity versus despair	Wisdom and acceptance	Meaninglessness and despair

Modified from Phares EJ: Introduction to Personality. Columbus, Charles E. Merrill, 1984.

in the room and has become acquainted with the sights and sounds as well as with the people caring for his or her needs. This allows the parent to feel comfortable leaving the child in order to complete the necessary paperwork. The admission counselor will obtain information such as age, date of birth, address, phone number, and type of insurance. The parent or legal guardian will sign the admission form.

The nurse will need to ask a parent or guardian specific questions about the patient. Detailed information required from the parents would include questions such as:

Do you know why your child is in the hospital?
Do you have a support system to help you care for the child?
What is the child's normal bedtime?
Does the child take a nap?
Does the child have a nickname?
Are the immunizations up to date?
Does your child have allergies to foods or medications?
Does your child take medications?

The nurse will complete a physical assessment of the patient, which includes the child's weight, height, temperature, pulse, respiration rate, and blood pressure. The nurse will document the patient's physical appearance, such as scars, rashes, or bruises. The nurse will ask the parents or patient what the child likes to do for fun and will ask about specific dietary likes and dislikes. The development information will be documented and entered into a care plan.

The HUC will be responsible for entering the information into the computer system. Hospital computer systems are used as a communication system from the nursing care unit to all departments in the hospital that provide services for patients.

Medication Information Specific to Pediatric Patients

Medications used on the pediatric unit are as varied as the patients. Most of the medications given to adults can also be administered to children. The big difference is the dosage. Because of the wide range of ages in pediatrics the dosages will have a wide range. Extreme care in administration is paramount. For the HUC that care is exercised in the transcription of the medication orders.

The Ordering Process

The physician or medical resident writes the order. The HUC transcribes the order to the Kardex and any other place that is required. The order must be communicated to the pharmacy. This should include a notation of any allergies and the weight of the patient. There are several ways to send the order to the pharmacy: It may be hand delivered or faxed; very often the order is entered into the computer system and transmitted immediately to the pharmacy. In some hospitals this is the responsibility of the unit pharmacist, whereas in others the HUC enters the order. In either case, accuracy is of the utmost importance.

The medication is delivered to the pediatric unit and placed in the medication room. In many hospitals there may be a satellite pharmacy on the pediatric unit that will dispense the medications. In addition to dispensing medications, the pharmacy provides the following services: IV additives, drug information, therapeutic monitoring, and pharmacokinetics consultation. Many hospitals use a unit dose system, in which drugs are dispensed in ready-to-administer form. The nursing personnel must chart when and how the medication was given.

The medication order should include the following information: name of the medication, route of administration, dose to be administrated, frequency, and length of time for administration. Orders for IV fluids should have the type of solution, additives (if any), and hourly infusion rate. IV pumps are used to regulate the rate of infusion. This avoids the possibility of a solution or medication infusing too rapidly while also ensuring that it does not infuse too slowly.

Abbreviations that are commonly used with medication orders include the following:

a.c.	Before meals
APAP	Tylenol

aq.	Aqueous
ASA	Aspirin, acetylsalicylic acid
Ca gluc.	Calcium gluconate
D.T.P.	Diphtheria, tetanus, pertussis
elix.	Elixir
gt.	Drop
gtt.	Drops
h.	Hour
HAL or Hyperal.	Hyperalimentation
IM	Intramuscular
Inj.	Inject
IV	Intravenous
IVPB	Intravenous piggyback
SC	Subcutaneous
syr	Syrup
TPN	Total parenteral nutrition

Treatments and Procedures Specific to Pediatric Patients

The pediatric patient may need to be immobilized during many treatments and procedures, and these should be explained to the patient and parents. The child life specialist may use puppets or dolls to illustrate the procedure. The child's room and the playroom should be considered safe areas, where nothing painful or threatening happens. All treatments and procedures should be carried out in the treatment room.

Procedures commonly performed on the pediatric patient include but are not limited to:

1. Blood gases, ABG/CBG, Arterial/Capillary
2. Bili lights for hyperbilirubinemia
3. Bulb syringe for suctioning and clearing out the nostrils
4. Urine pH by dipstick
5. Stool for guaiac
6. BAER
7. Spinal tap
8. Head circumference

Equipment and Supplies Specific to Pediatric Patients

Child-sized equipment and supplies must be the standard in the pediatric setting. Children suffer from a different spectrum of diseases and injuries than adults do. The unique physiologic responses to illness and injury demand specific equipment. In addition to ordering equipment, the HUC may need to order special supplies for patients who are sensitive to latex. Diets are ordered at the time of admission and updated as needed. A diet order may range from formula for a small baby to pizza for a 10-year-old. Patient allergies are listed at the time of admission.

Some of the common equipment and supplies that would be ordered for the pediatric patients include:

High chair/Playpens/VCR/Nintendo
Coloring books/Crayons/Toys
Baby bottles/Pacifiers
Arm splints/Arm boards
Diapers of various sizes from newborn to large
Feeding tubes/Urinary collection bags
Suction catheters/IV equipment
Formulas such as Similac, Enfamil, and ProSobee.
Formulas with iron are also available. Enfamil 20 means 20 cal per oz. Nipples come in an assortment of sizes.

Communication With and About Pediatric Patients

Children require special care and understanding from the nursing staff. When a sick child arrives in a strange environment, anxious and in pain, the child's reaction will depend on his or her age and previous care. A 10-month-old infant's perception of an examination is very different from that of an 8-year-old child. Prior experience with medical care will also affect the child's response. For example, a chronic asthmatic child who has been admitted to the hospital many times will have a different attitude toward being admitted than a child being admitted for the first time.

Infections

Patients admitted to the pediatric unit with infections will be isolated in a room. Departments providing services for the patient should be informed of his or her isolation. Disposable items should be used, if possible, to decrease the potential for contamination. All reusable supplies and equipment should be properly cleaned and/or disinfected before use with another patient. A HUC who is going to have hands-on contact with the patient may be required to wear a gown and gloves. It may be the responsibility of the HUC to instruct visitors about isolation procedures and the importance of gowning and hand washing. When the patient is discharged, the housekeeping department must provide terminal cleaning, making sure that all contaminated environmental surfaces and equipment are cleaned and wiped with a disinfectant.

Child Abuse

Child abuse can leave a scar that is carried throughout life. Many child abusers were abused as children. The cycle continues as long as the child abuse continues. As a health care worker a HUC may be involved in the process of reporting child abuse, which is required by state law.

Child abuse is legally defined as follows: physical injury that is inflicted by other than accidental means; willful cruelty or unjustifiable punishment of a child; cruel or inhuman corporal punishment or injury; neglect; and sexual abuse.

Indicators of Child Abuse

Neglect. Some indicators of neglect are the following: The child is lacking adequate medical and dental care. The child is always sleepy or hungry. The child may be dirty or inadequately dressed for the weather conditions. There may be evidence of poor supervision. Conditions in the home may be unsafe or unsanitary.

Physical Abuse. There are bruises, burns, abrasions, or lacerations caused by other than accidental means. The injury is unusual for a specific age group. There is evidence of handprints, bite marks, and pinches. There are unexplained or conflicting explanations or reasons given for the injury. The caretaker attempts to hide injuries. The child states that the injury was caused by abuse. The child is excessively passive, compliant, or fearful.

Sexual Abuse. The child is a victim of other forms of abuse. The child reports sexual activities to a trusted person. The child shows detailed and age-inappropriate understanding of sexual behavior. The child wears torn, stained, or bloody underclothing.

When a family is reported for child abuse, the family is usually referred to services such as counseling or parenting classes, except in serious abuse cases, in which the child may be removed from the home. If the abuse is neglect, the family may be referred to public assistance agencies. The goal is to keep the family intact unless the child is in danger.

Legalities

At the time of the child's admission the parents or guardian will be asked to sign the permission to admit the child to the hospital and authorize the staff to care for the patient. They will be informed of the patient's rights, the services that the hospital will provide, and how to access the patient relations services. Child passenger safety information for patients under the age of 4 years or less than 40 pounds should be given to the parents.

Surgery and procedures consents are signed at the time of admission if a patient is scheduled for surgery. Emergency surgery consents are signed on the unit. The physician must inform the parents of the surgery and expected outcome. The HUC may prepare the consent for the parents or guardian to sign. The complete procedure should be spelled out, with no abbreviations. Hospital policy will dictate if the HUC may witness the signing of the consent. The signed consent becomes a part of the medical record, with a copy given to the parents. If the patient is a ward of the court, a copy of the court order must be placed in the medical record.

Consents should be written in the language spoken by the parents. An interpreter may be used to explain the information to the parents. The interpreter must make a notation in the chart as to the information given to the parents.

Pediatric Death

The death of a child leaves an emptiness that parents cannot fill by other children or attachments; their grief is seemingly endless. Grieving is a part of healing. There is no relationship like that of parent and child. The bond between parent and child endures over time, distance, and strife. The relationship is threatened when a child's life ends. It is important to understand that the loss of a child to a parent is like no other loss. The parent is left with an empty space. The parent grieves for the wishes, the hopes, the dreams for all that child could be, and is. The parent grieves for the child as a separate person.

The process of grief has peaks and valleys, highs and lows, and periods of greater and lesser intensity. Some of the most important peaks and also some of the most painful times for families are the anniversary times: of the child's birth, and of the child's death. Families may want to continue to celebrate the birthday of the child by doing something special, such as planting a tree.

The family may have feelings of bewilderment, confusion, and self-blame. It is not uncommon for parents to question all that they believe in. Many families have a need to preserve the child's space in the home and hold onto clothing and possessions.

Anger is a very normal reaction. The parents may be angry with God, or they may be angry with the health care system for not saving their child. Health care professionals can respond to parents who are grieving; they need not personalize that anger.

Social workers and the hospital chaplain are trained to help the parents and staff cope with the loss of a child. The hospital may have a committee of people who are trained to work with the parents and offer workshops to help the staff deal with the death of a patient. The staff may want to, and should be encouraged to, attend the funeral. Parents should be encouraged to set aside time on each holiday to remember the child.

Closing Thoughts

The HUC is the cornerstone of the pediatric unit. You are responsible for ensuring that the unit functions smoothly. You will greet the patient and family when they arrive on the unit, and you may be the first person the patient and his or her family see. You will need excellent communication skills to work on a pediatric unit. You will need to communicate with the parents and the patient plus the staff of the hospital. You must establish the trust and respect of the people with whom you come in contact.

You will assemble the chart, ensuring that all the proper forms are in place. The processing of orders may be by means of paper requisitions or entered into the computer. It will be your responsibility to ensure that the proper tests, procedures, and equipment are ordered in a timely manner. The test results determine the care of the patient. You must keep your unit stocked with the necessary supplies for the nursing staff to perform the tasks of caring for the patient.

You must be able to work in an emergency situation; there is no room for error.

Children may be very ill when admitted to the hospital but usually recover more quickly than adult patients. Children are unique, as are their needs. The pediatric unit or hospital provides the care and expertise needed to care for children.

Review Questions

1. Explain how a pediatric unit differs from an adult unit.
2. Identify two staff members unique to pediatrics.
3. Explain the major difference in medication orders for children.
4. List 10 of the indicators of child abuse.

Bibliography

Behrman RE, Kliegman RM, Arvin AM (eds): Nelson's Textbook of Pediatrics, 15th ed. Philadelphia, WB Saunders, 1996.

Chabner D-E: The Language of Medicine, 5th ed. Philadelphia, WB Saunders, 1996.

Children's Health Network-CNE 7326: Communicating with the Hospitalized Child (video). Presenter: Elizabeth C. Poster, R.N., Ph.D., Assistant Clinical Professor, UCLA School of Nursing; Director, Nursing Research & Education, The Neuropsychiatric Institute, The University of California, Los Angeles.

Dorland's Medical Abbreviations. Philadelphia, WB Saunders, 1992.

Hospital Satellite Network: A Child Dies (video). Presenters: Penelope Buschman Gemma, R.N., M.S., C.S., Child Specialist in Child Psychiatric and Mental Health Nursing, Presbyterian Hospital, New York; Joan Hagan Arnold, R.N., M.A., Assistant Professor, Community Health Nursing, Adelphia University School of Nursing, Garden City, NY, 1987.

Leonard P: Building a Medical Vocabulary, 4th ed. Philadelphia, WB Saunders, 1997.

Overbeck B, Overbeck J: Helping Children Cope With Loss. Dallas, TLC Group, 1992.

Same Day Admission Unit

13

Louise A. Butterfield

Common Abbreviations

H&P History and physical examination

PACU Postanesthesia care unit

Preop Preoperative

Postop Postoperative

TENS Transcutaneous electrical nerve stimulation

Objectives

At the completion of this chapter the reader should be able to:

1. Explain the reason for the development of same day admission units in hospitals.
2. List five specific areas that may be found in a same day admission unit.
3. Name five types of pain that may be treated in the pain management area.
4. Describe the role of the Health Unit Coordinator in the same day admission unit in communicating with the community.

Vocabulary

Ablation therapy: Treatment that involves eradication of a problem area of tissue or an organ

Autologous: Related to self; belonging to the same organism

Calculi: Stones, usually composed of mineral salts, occurring within the body, chiefly in hollow organs or their passages

Lithotripsy: The crushing of calculi in the bladder

Preoperative: Time before going into the OR

Postoperative: Time after leaving the OR

Overview

Managed health care has created many opportunities for hospitals to rethink the old ways of doing things. The initial concept was to find a way to cut costs without jeopardizing the care and treatment that were considered best at that time. Along the way, hospitals realized that changing old practices not only saved money for the hospital, insurance providers, and patients but also often provided better service to the patient. Before managed care, the cost of health care was not a primary concern of most hospitals. Twenty-five years ago a person could travel from hospital to hospital and find that the majority of them operated the same way. This is no longer the case. In today's health care world hospitals are as diverse as the people they serve. Each hospital is struggling with new ways to meet the needs of the patient while holding down costs. The patients, or consumers, have had to adjust to the new ways. Managed health care has forced them to understand more about their health care treatments and to question each decision that affects that care.

The same day admission unit is a result of new ideas that serve the patient better while monitoring costs. In the old formula of health care, patients would have all the services provided to them on an in-patient basis. Today most services can be provided on an outpatient basis, reserving in-patient status for situations in which there is no alternative.

Description of Same Day Admission Unit

The same day admission unit is a centralized area for the nursing staff to prepare patients for surgery, testing, or ancillary procedures while affording a quiet environment for both patients and families. This unit can provide services for both outpatients and in-patients. It may be one unit or several specialized units. Some of the specialty units may be:

Same day surgery, including **lithotripsy**
GI lab
Pre-admission testing
Discharge/Holding
Pain management
Heart catheterization, including **ablation therapy**.

Same Day Surgery

Same day surgery implies that a patient will come into the unit in the morning and go home following surgery in the afternoon or early evening. The unit may be organized into patient care sections, special labs, anesthesia evaluation area, lounge, and central desk (Fig. 13–1.) The staff in this unit have additional training in their area of expertise.

Patients will arrive at least 2 hours prior to surgery. In most cases the registration information will have been obtained by telephone, so all the patient must do is sign the registration forms. The patient and family will be taken to the unit to prepare for surgery. This area may be one very large room with either glass partitions or curtains. Some hospitals offer individual rooms, where patients can get ready for surgery, where family members can wait during the surgery, and where patients, after leaving the recovery area, can return to prepare for dismissal. Whatever the physical setup, the patient and family are allowed to stay together as much as possible prior to surgery.

In the preoperative stage of treatment the patient dons hospital clothing and is evaluated by the preoperative (**preop**) nurse and anesthesia personnel. Depending on the findings of the evaluation, some testing may be required. Any preop testing will be done quickly so that surgery is not delayed. The surgeon will see the patient prior to going into the operating room; the patient and family have the opportunity to ask last-minute questions at this time.

Another function of the preop area is to provide postoperative (**postop**) teaching. Managed care has taught health care providers that the patient and family are better able to tolerate the surgical procedure and postoperative care if they have the proper information and education. Knowing what to expect during and after surgery and how to deal with the situations that arise will often shorten the healing process. Therefore, education is a big part of preoperative care. Education may be in the form of discussion with the patient and family, a video explaining the procedure, or hands-on training in using crutches or a walker. Family members may be instructed in changing dressings and taught how to recognize a postop infection.

After patients receiving general anesthesia move from the preoperative area into the operative area, little of their time is spent awake. Once the patient is on the operating table the anesthesia is administered. The staff caring for the patient during this time are specially trained in anesthesia and operating room procedures. When the surgical procedure is over, the patient will be quickly moved into the postanesthesia care unit (**PACU**, formerly known as the recovery room.) Patients remain in the PACU only as long as necessary to maintain a normal respiratory status. Pain medication may be administered in the PACU. When the desired level of alertness and respiratory func-

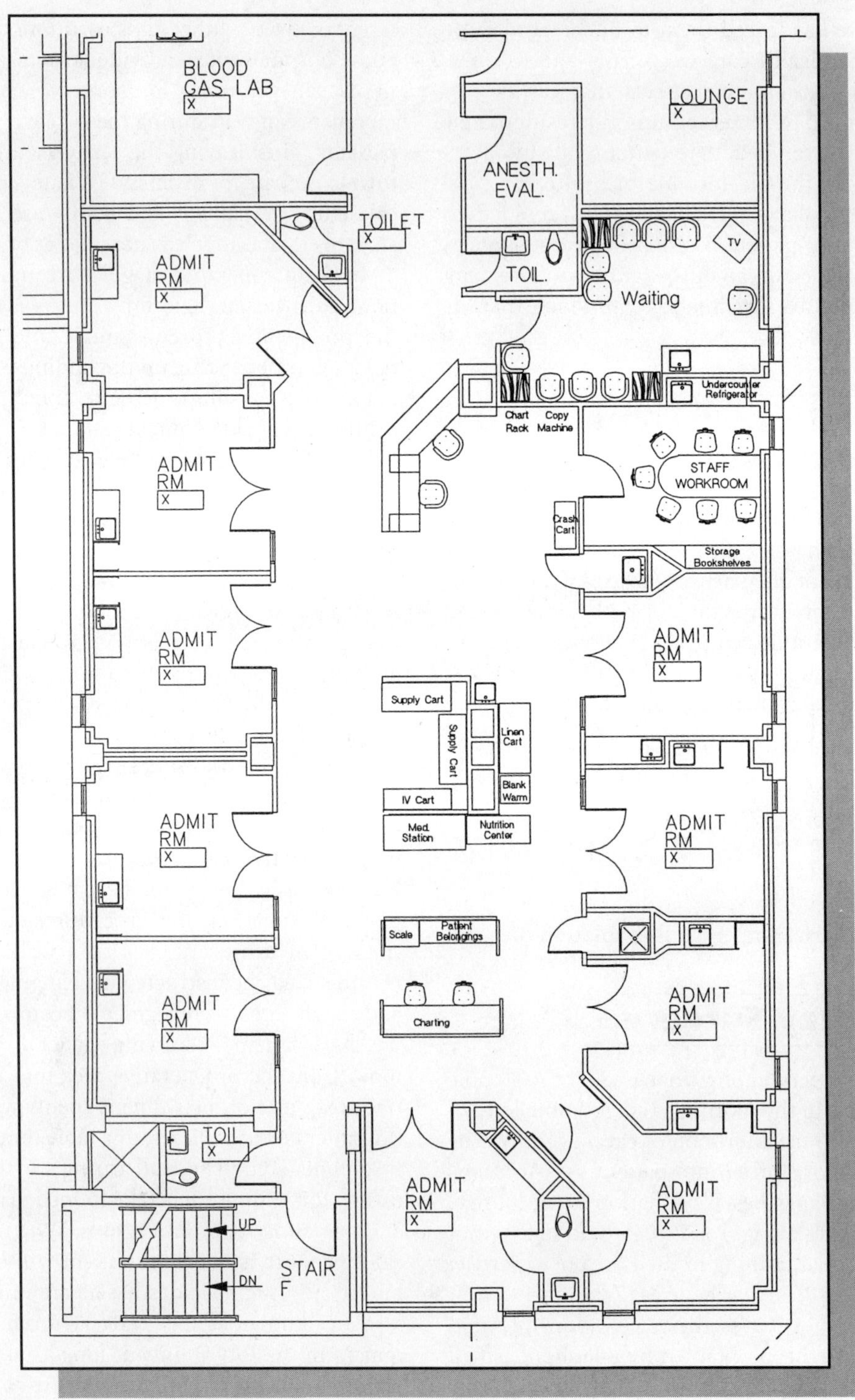

Figure 13–1
Layout of a typical same day admission unit.

tion has been reached, the patient is returned to the day unit to complete the recovery process.

The type of surgical procedure determines the length of time that the patient stays in the day unit before going home. A patient who had a breast biopsy may go home shortly after leaving the PACU, whereas a patient who had sinus surgery may stay several hours. Many factors are weighed in the amount of time required before dismissal. The doctor may write orders detailing the conditions. An example of some of these orders is:

"Pt may be dismissed when":

1. 6 oz of liquid can be swallowed without choking or vomiting.
2. Able to walk to bathroom without assistance.

Regardless of the orders, the staff in this area will keep close watch on the progress of each patient. In some cases the patient does not make the appropriate progress or develops an unexpected reaction. It is then necessary for that individual to spend the night as an observation patient. This may occur in the same day admission unit or in another area, depending upon the facility.

GI Lab

This unit operates in the same manner as the one day surgery area. Patients are prepared, have the procedure, and recover in the same unit. The GI lab serves both in-patients and outpatients. Patients seen in this area are generally adults, and all are undergoing routine or diagnostic gastrointestinal evaluation and treatments. Except for emergencies, this unit operates Monday to Friday during daytime hours.

Pre-admission Testing

This part of the unit provides professional staff and an area where patients can have all pre-admission testing done on an outpatient basis. The pre-admission testing unit may be combined with the same day surgery unit, or each may be separate. Insurance companies will no longer pay for a person to be admitted to the hospital 1 to 2 days early to have necessary testing done. Many of these individuals are surgical patients, but there will be other types of patients as well.

Patients who are having in-patient surgery often need preliminary studies prior to the operation. These may include blood and urine studies and x-rays, CT scan, MRI, or other radiologic imaging. The process may also include evaluation by a professional in rehab therapy, physical therapy, or speech therapy as well as consultation with a dietitian, social services worker, or spiritual guidance counselor.

It is not uncommon for patients to donate blood (**autologous** donation) that is saved for use if needed during or after surgery. This requires one visit for each donated unit of blood; the donations must be timed several days to a week apart. The patient may be instructed to take supplemental iron prior to each donation.

The following is an example of the services of the pre-admission testing unit: An individual is scheduled for total knee replacement surgery. This patient may have three appointments prior to the date of surgery.

First visit (3 weeks prior to surgery)

Evaluation by anesthesiologist
EKG, lab, x-ray, if necessary
Evaluation by rehab therapist
Autologous blood donation
Education on surgical procedure

Second visit (2 weeks prior to surgery)

Rehab therapy training
Evaluation by social services staff
Autologous blood donation
Education on postop hospital care
Tour of in-patient rehab nursing unit

Third visit (1 week prior to surgery)

Rehab therapy training
Visit with pastoral care counselor (if requested)
Visit with occupational therapist
Education about posthospital expectations

Finalize plans for posthospital care with social services staff

Patients going through this extensive training and education prior to surgery heal faster and with fewer complications than in years past when these services were not available. Education is the focus of the staff in this unit, and they have been trained to present this education in the best possible way.

The pre-admission unit may also see patients for reasons other than surgical. For example, patients may receive IV antibiotics or blood transfusions on an outpatient basis.

Discharge Planning and Holding Unit

Managed care dictates the number of hospital days that each diagnosis warrants. This is reviewed daily, and discharge planning begins the day of admission. This responsibility may be carried out in many different ways in various institutions. It may be attached to the pre-admission unit or be a separate area depending on the needs of the hospital and patients.

The discharge planner will start to outline the conditions for discharge on the first admission day; alternatively, the planning may begin at a pre-admission testing appointment. At that time, depending on the diagnosis, a time log is established. The discharge planner works closely with the physicians and nursing personnel and keeps the patient and family members informed of all plans and possibilities.

Once the discharge has been confirmed, arrangements are made for the type of transportation that is needed. Patients may have to wait for transportation or for the availability of appropriate caregivers. Many hospitals have a discharge/holding area set up, where patients are brought after they have been prepared for discharge by the nursing unit. The area is arranged for comfort and convenience, with comfortable places to wait, reclining and rocking chairs, reading materials, and light refreshments. It is a quiet area, so those patients who want to nap will not be disturbed. The discharge planner may go over last-minute instructions or teaching with the patient or family in this area.

By utilizing a discharge area the hospital is freeing the expensive nursing unit staff for direct patient care. It allows the housekeeping staff to clean the room and make it available for the next admission in a timely manner. If discharges are planned in advance, the hospital will know the time when most patients will depart the unit and will be able to staff accordingly. This is a cost savings to the institution.

Hospitals used to operate on a time in/time out basis, similar to a hotel. Patients were discharged in the morning, and new admissions came in the afternoon. Saving health care dollars has made it necessary to change that practice. Patients are discharged and admitted at all hours. It is not unusual for patients to be discharged late at night, if that is when their covered days expire. Hospital beds taken up with discharged patients are a drain on health care dollars.

Pain Management

Ten years ago people with chronic pain had two choices for pain management—take heavy narcotics or suffer with pain. Progress in this area of health care has been enormous. The way that health care providers look at and treat pain is completely different from years past.

Research studies have shown that people with chronic pain do not heal or improve as fast as people who are able to control pain. Studies also show that the use of strong medications may not be the answer. For example, historically the patient with a back injury would be put to bed with heavy medication. This approach might take weeks of therapy and drugs before the individual could resume some normal activities. In contrast, the pain management unit offers such treatment modalities as nerve blocks, transcutaneous electrical nerve stimulation (TENS) units, relaxation techniques, and imagery, so that today the same patient may be back to normal activities in a shorter time. The patient is spared the burden of dealing with narcotics that cause side effects and other complications.

The pain management unit treats both in-patients and outpatients. The patients may be treated for cancer pain, migraine headaches, degenerative arthritis, pain from injury, or postoperative pain. They may be seen either once or twice or on a long-term basis. This form of care has changed the lives of many people and has allowed them to return to normal activities.

Heart Catheterization Unit

Many advances have been made in the diagnosis and care of cardiac patients. One of the most dramatic advances is that patients can now access many treatments on an outpatient basis. The heart catheterization unit is an example of this progress, treating outpatients as well as in-patients.

All patients coming into this unit have been evaluated for some type of heart disease and are at the point in their care that the physician needs to look into the heart to see exactly what is happening. Heart catheterizations were once reserved for individuals who had already had a heart attack. With today's health care we want to prevent heart attacks. Investigation may begin when the individual first experiences any coronary irregularity. Patients may need EKGs, blood tests, radiologic testing, and possibly a monitored stress test before undergoing a heart catheterization. It is not necessary to experience a heart attack before investigation and preventive treatment can begin.

Individuals are smarter about their own health care—they know what may contribute to heart disease, and most people try and prevent it whenever possible. They know that diet and exercise, in addition to family history, play a major role. Because they are more knowledgeable about the causes of heart disease they are less fearful of cardiac testing and procedures.

The heart catheterization unit is staffed by people who have special training in diseases of the heart. Patients coming into this unit may develop a special bond with the staff and may have the same caregiver throughout the visit. Most of the procedures in this unit are performed on patients who are awake, giving the caregivers special opportunities to inform and educate.

Patients may move through the unit similarly to the same day surgery patient. There will be a preprocedure area, the procedure room, and a place to recover afterwards. In some facilities, patients scheduled for catheterization procedures are admitted and discharged through the same day admission unit.

After the procedure is complete, the in-patient returns to his or her room. For an outpatient a stay in the unit of several hours may be required before discharge. Family members are encouraged to be by the bedside both before and after the procedure.

Education is a priority of this unit, for both the patient and the family. While the patient is in the procedure room the family is given instructions and is educated on the type of treatment and postprocedure care. A staff member may speak with each family member individually; alternatively, the family may be asked to watch a video and read material that is made available to them. People with coronary artery disease must alter their lifestyle to improve their quality of living and extend their life expectancy. This may be a matter of simply changing the diet and enrolling in an exercise program. Family members are encouraged to make the same changes as the patient.

Patient Care Procedures

Nursing Staff

When the patient arrives in the unit the nursing staff works as a team to prepare him or her for surgery or procedure as quickly and efficiently as possible. The patient's ID band will be reviewed to be sure that the information is listed correctly. An allergy band will be attached to the wrist or ankle of an individual who has allergies. The patient will be told to undress and don hospital clothing. Dentures, hearing aids, contact lenses, and jewelry will be removed and given to a family member. Glasses are removed just prior to surgery.

The patient should have had a history taken and physical examination made prior to the surgery. A copy of the document should be in the chart ready to accompany the patient to surgery. If there is no **H&P**, the surgeon or anesthesiologist must be contacted to do one before the case can proceed. All preoperative test results are placed in the patient's chart. Tests done the same day as the procedure will be obtained STAT, to avoid delays to the patient, surgical staff, and physicians. The surgical permit must be signed and in the chart prior to surgery. The anesthesia staff will be called to perform a preoperative assessment if the patient is being administered anything other than a local anesthetic.

A nursing assessment of the patient's status is done initially to see that there are no new developments that could cause complications during procedure (Figs. 13–2 and 13–3). The assessment includes taking vital signs, discussing the medical history, and ascertaining the last time the patient had anything to eat or drink. Any question that arises concerning a patient's status is reported to the anesthesiologist and surgeon.

As soon as the patient has been cleared to proceed, the nursing staff assumes the role of case manager by initiating the patient care plan. The appropriate patient teaching will be reinforced with brochures, videos, and teaching cards. The education is documented in the patient record.

Preoperative orders are then completed and may include starting IVs, giving IV or IM medications, inserting a Foley catheter or nasogastric (NG) tube, and obtaining an EKG. Surgical skin preps are done in this area as ordered (Fig. 13–4).

Once the patient has been medicated, an ongoing physical assessment is carried out until he or she is transferred into the OR. Side rails on the bed remain up; the patient's respiratory status is monitored as is his or her comfort level.

When the patient is ready for transfer into the OR the nursing personnel will transfer the entire patient chart and give a verbal report to the OR nurse. Family members are allowed to remain with the patient whenever possible until the time to go into the OR. The OR staff will take responsibility for the patient, and the preoperative nurse will offer support and information to the family.

Health Unit Coordinator Responsibilities

The HUC may begin working on a patient chart days before the person is scheduled to arrive in the unit. Preregistration is carried out by the HUC or someone in the registration office. If preliminary testing is to be done, the results may begin to arrive long before the patient does. When information arrives, the HUC will see that the papers go to the proper area. The day before surgery, a patient chart is assembled, including any test results on hand. The chart also contains the forms that will be needed by the nursing or anesthesia staff. Labels may be put into the chart in anticipation of specimens going to the lab.

On the day of surgery the HUC will greet and welcome the patient and family on arrival. The registration process may be completed by obtaining the patient's signatures for insurance and payment arrangements. The HUC will direct the individual to his or her cubicle and notify the nursing staff of the patient's arrival in the department.

Once the patient has been assessed there may be orders to transcribe and enter into the computer. Testing will be ordered as STAT, so that results will be back in the department quickly. Test results done in the doctor's office may not be in the department, so the HUC will need to call the office to have them faxed.

The HUC is expected to know the patient's and family's whereabouts at all times to direct physicians and hospital personnel to the right area without delay. If a family is not in attendance, the HUC must anticipate one or many calls inquiring about the patient. When the patient returns to the unit from PACU, it is not unusual for the HUC to prepare the discharge instruction sheet based on the physician's orders.

Medications

Nursing Responsibilities

Registered nurses are responsible for the administration of all medications. Medications given for surgical patients fall into three categories: preop,

PREOPERATIVE ADMISSION/DISCHARGE UNIT

(INITIALS/SIGNATURES)

Page 1

NOTES	DISCHARGE
	Temp. Oral, Axillary, Rectal, Core
	IV Sites: No redness or irritation (Initial)
	If yes, explain
	DC'd at
	Patient has clothes and other valuables
	Home going Rx sent with patient (initial) or N/A
	Return appt. YES ☐ NO ☐
	Home Care Provider
	Driver
	Left via: Wheelchair ☐ Walked ☐ Carried ☐ Cart ☐
	Accompanied by: Secretary ☐ Nurse ☐ Volunteer ☐
	Patient Orderly ☐ Self ☐ Parents ☐
	Discharge score
	Discharge criteria met (initial)
	Date Time Initial

I UNDERSTAND THE HOMEGOING INSTRUCTIONS THAT HAVE BEEN EXPLAINED TO ME.

_______________ Instructions Given # _______
(Patient or Significant Other)

Homegoing instructions explained by _______________ Time _______

Instructions reviewed by _______ Time _______ Instructions Given # _______

Medication Card _______

Post-op Call (Follow-up phone call #) To be made (date)

Pain/Muscle Soreness
Nausea & Vomiting
Appetite
Drainage
Hematuria/Voiding
Fever
Spinal Puncture Site
Sore throat/Hoarseness
Cough
Color/Motion/Sensation
Encourage questions
Refer to M.D. Information obtained from Call made by

PREPROCEDURAL STANDARD RECORD

PREOPERATIVE ADMISSION/DISCHARGE UNIT

PREPROCEDURAL STANDARD RECORD Page 2

ADDRESSOGRAPH

#1 Needs complete review
#2 Needs Reinforcement/Repetition
#3 Demonstrates/Verbalizes understanding
#4 Not Applicable
#5 Unable to complete teaching

Phone Call

Date Arrival Time
Procedure
Phone # Home
Work
Age Physician
Instructions given to
Relationship

A NPO (Light Breakfast)
B Infant under 6 months awaken at and fed pop, apple juice or water (No milk or formula)
PREMATURE INFANT-NOTIFY ANESTHESIA
C Bath/Shower/Shampoo/Enema/Douche
D May Brush Teeth
Remove all makeup and nail polish
E Clothing/Accessories/Valuables/Money/Jewelry
F Current Health/Exposure to Chicken POx
G Pregnancy? (LMP_________)
Health Hx
H Current Meds
I Operative Site
J Number of visitors
K Length of stay
L Transportation-Driver
M Home Care
N 1. Do you live alone? Yes No
2. Are you currently caring for someone? Yes No
3. Does anyone (including your family) come to your home? Yes No
4. Are you or family concerned over how your care will be managed after you leave the hospital?
5. Do you have any financial concerns?
6. Social Services notified Date

FALL RISK STANDARD

Assess mobility: D/B:
0=Independent
1=assist of 1
2=assist of 2
3=total lift
4=bedrest

Mobility aid used: D/B:
aid

Assess gait: D/B:
0=straight
1=mild/mod path deviation or uses walking aid
2=marked path deviation

Assess balance D/B:
0=steady s support
1=steady c aid
2=unsteady/leans/sways/staggers

Comments/Phone

PREOP

ID Bracelet ☐ Consent ☐ H&P ☐ EKG ☐
Clinic Record ☐ Anesthesia ☐ Lab ☐ X-Ray ☐
NPO Since: Side Rails ↑ ☐ Allergy Band ☐
TEDS ☐ Thromboguards ☐ Call Light ☐ Brakes ☐
Preop Teaching:
Pain Level Scale ☐ Incentive Spirometer ☐
TCDB ☐ Types of Pain Management ☐
Preps/Shave/Foley/Other

Op Site
Preop Notes

Date Time Mode
ADS / SDS / DIRECT / INPT
IV Start/Maintenance

O_2 O_2 SAT
MEDICATIONS:

TOTAL: IV Meds IV Fluids
Glasses Hearing Aid
Dentures Other
To O.R. Time Mode
Family Personal Belongings
Initial/Signature:

Figure 13–2
Preprocedural standard record.

PREOPERATIVE ADMISSION/DISCHARGE UNIT

Page 1

Initial assessment:

Clergy to visit?:

Bill of rights to patient/family: (Initial) ____ BSI: (Initial) ____

Orient to room & routines: (Initial)

Temp(C)____ Oral Rectal Axillary Tympanic

B/P ____ Right left position ____

Pulse ____ Respiratory rate ____ /min

Height ____ Weight ____ lb. or kg. Actual/Stated

Recent weight changes: Diet:

Allergies– Identify and describe: (i.e. medications, food, other)

Allergy band on: ____ Yes Chart flagged: ____ Yes

Significant health history:

Medication–prescribed and over the counter: Taken:	Last dose:	Usual times

Disposition of meds: Home__ Pharmacy__ With pt.__ Not brought in__

Do you use alcohol beverages/drugs?____

When did you have your last drink?____

Have you or anyone in your family ever been concerned about your drinking or drug use?____

Date: ____ Time: ____

Admit from: ____ Via: ____

Name preference: ____

Can information be given to others? Yes ____ No ____

Who?

Community services used?

Discharge needs:

Do you feel safe in your home?

SUPPORT SYSTEMS

Name	Relationship	Phone #

BRADEN SCALE

SENSORY PERCEPTION	MOISTURE	ACTIVITY
1. No impairment	1. Rarely moist	1. Walks frequently
2. Slightly limited	2. Occasionally moist	2. Walks occasionally
3. Very limited	3. Very moist	3. Chair fast
4. Completely limited	4. Constantly moist	4. Bed fast
MOBILITY	**NUTRITION**	**FRICTION & SHEAR**
1. No limitation	1. Excellent	1. No apparent problem
2. Slightly limited	2. Adequate	2. Potential problem
3. Very limited	3. Probably inadequate	3. Problem
4. Completely limited	4. Very poor	TOTAL RISK SCORE

Belongings:	Glasses	Hearing aid	Contacts	Prosthesis	Dentures	Money	Jewelry (list)	Shoes	Coat	Slacks/skirt	Shirt	Dress
Family		R/L			U/L							
In room		R/L			U/L							
In safe												
Other/list												

Do you have an Advance Directive? Yes__ No__ Deferred__

If yes, where does the patient say this document is located?____

(If the patient says the document is in our medical record and the record is available, please confirm that the document is there. If the patient says the document is at some other location, invite the patient to have the document placed in their record at our institution.)

SIGNATURE R.N. DATE

SIGNATURE R.N. DATE

PATIENT DATA BASE/ASSESSMENT

PREOPERATIVE ADMISSION/DISCHARGE UNIT

Page 2

PHYSICAL ASSESSMENT

The following cues will be considered in a physical assessment. If the physical assessment is normal, indicate with a "√" in the box after the particular assessment area. A "blank box" denotes a finding that requires further elaboration on the lines to the right.

ASSESSMENT PARAMETERS

"Neurological assessment" – Awake and aware. Oriented to person, place and time. Behavior appropriate to situation. Verbalization clear and understandable. Swallows liquids and solids without difficulty. Moves all extremities to command with equal strength bilaterally. No sensory deficits. Denies numbness or tingling in all extremities. Pain free. ☐

"Cardiovascular assessment". Regular pulse. First and second heart tones brief and clear. Denies chest pain. Pedal and radial pulses present. Denies calf tenderness.; no calf redness present. No edema. ☐
Pacemaker set at ____

"Pulmonary assessment"–Respirations 10–24/min. at rest. Respirations easy, quiet and regular. Breath sounds present and clear throughout lung fields bilaterally. Absence of abnormal breath sounds. Sputum clear. Nailbeds and mucous membranes pink. No cough, nightsweats, weight loss or fever.Tobacco usage. ☐

"Gastrointestinal assessment"–Abdomen soft and flat or slightly rounded. Bowel sounds active in 4 quadrants (5–34/min). No pain with palpation. Tolerates prescribed diet without nausea and vomiting. Having BM's within own normal pattern and consistency.
Last BM ____ Prescribed diet ____
Ostomy ____ ☐

"Genitourinary assessment"–Able to empty bladder without difficulty or pain. Denies frequency. Urine clear and yellow to amber. No sexuality/ intimacy concerns. Ostomy ____
LMP ____ ☐

"Integumentary assessment"-Skin color within patient's norm. Skin warm, dry, and intact. Mucous membranes moist. Adequate wound healing. No evidence of inflammation, nodules, nail changes, ulcerations, or rashes.
COMPLETE DIAGRAM BELOW ☐

"Musculoskeletal assessment"-Absence of joint swelling and tenderness. Normal ROM of all joints. No muscle weakness. Steady gait. ☐
Assisstive device. ____

DIAGRAMMING CODE:
Abrasion-A
Bum-B
Confusion-C
Decubitus-D
Erythema-E
Laceration-L
Petechia-P
Rash-R
Scar-S

RN Signature

Date

RN Signature

Date

PATIENT DATA BASE/ASSESSMENT

Figure 13–3
Patient database/assessment.

MEDICATION AND DOCTORS ORDER FORM

UNIVERSITY HOSPITAL

PATIENT NAME

CLINIC NUMBER

Date and Time Ordered • Please Write Medication Orders Between the Dashed Lines

↓ Imprint Patient Name Here ↓

ADMITTING PREOPERATIVE ORDERS -- SURGERY DEPARTMENT

DATE: ____________ Admit Status: _____ IP _____OP

ADMISSION DIAGNOSIS: ______________________________.

1) Admit to Dr. ______________________________'s Service.
2) Notify on admission: ______________________________.
3) Allergies: ______________________________.
4) Code status: _____Y _____N
5) Vital signs: ______________________________.
6) Diet: ______________________________.
7) Activity level: ______________________________.
8) Parenteral fluids: ______________________________.
______________________________.
9) Medications: ______________________________.
______________________________.
______________________________.
______________________________.
10) Lab: Check tests to be performed:

_____ CBC	_____ K	_____ Creatinine	_____ Type & Cross
_____ Hct	_____ PTT	_____ Electrolytes	_____ units
_____ Hgb	_____ Glucose	_____ Urinalysis	

11) _____ ECG
12) _____ X-ray chest
_____ Other ______________________________
13) Other tests: ______________________________
____
____
14) Knee-high Thromboguards.
15) Anesthesia preop. check to be done today.
16) Treatments: ______________________________
____
____
17) Special teaching: ______________________________
____
18) Consent:. ______________________________

Revised: December, 1998

SIGNATURE: ______________________________

Under authorization from the P & T Committee another generically equivalent drug (identical in form and content) may be substituted for the drug ordered. ☐

Figure 13–4
Medication and doctor's order form.

interop, and postop. Preop meds will be given by both the preoperative staff and the anesthesia staff; interop meds are given by the anesthesia staff; and post-op meds are given by PACU and postop staffs.

The types of medications given in the preoperative admission same day surgical unit setting are:

Antibiotics

Ancef
Ceftizoxime
Ampicillin
Tobramycin

Drugs causing relaxation

Valium
Versed
Ativan

To prevent GI problems

Reglan
Zantac

For postoperative nausea and vomiting

Zofran

Parenteral pain medication

Demerol
Fentanyl
Morphine

Oral pain medication

Tylenol with codeine
Percocet
Vicodin
Darvocet

Health Unit Coordinator Responsibilities

The HUC is responsible for maintaining the supplies on the unit, including the pharmacy stock items. Stock items include IV fluid and tubing, generic medications, aspirin, Tylenol, milk of magnesia, saline, and ibuprofen. The supply list is monitored, and items are ordered as needed. The HUC is responsible for transmitting the medication orders from the physician order sheet to the pharmacy. This is done manually or by computer.

Communication

Within the Hospital

There is a need for open communication whether the unit is multifunctional or single service, such as a same day surgery unit. This is the only way that optimal patient care can be achieved. In the current health care climate, the need for streamlined process requires cooperation from each member of the team to carry out duties and responsibilities in a professional manner. Communication is the key to good patient care. The HUC is the hub of the communication wheel, receiving and relaying information among the appropriate areas. By remaining calm and unemotional, the HUC keeps the lines open, enabling information to flow from one area to another without problems. In this fast-paced environment, it is easy to become flustered when there is a breakdown in the line, but the professional HUC will know how to handle these situations and redirect the information to the right place without conflict or disagreement.

With the Community

HUCs may spend more time communicating with the community than do any other department personnel. The main reason for this is the telephone; the HUC is generally responsible for answering the telephone. The caller's first impression of the department or facility is made by the manner in which the phone is answered. The caller may be concerned about a family member or friend in surgery or may want information about an upcoming appointment. If the HUC answers the phone in a pleasant and professional manner, the caller will be put at ease. The HUC may have to refer the caller to another person, but the first impression will have been a positive one.

The HUC may have to maintain the educational library of books and brochures that is made available to the public. This library allows people to choose the information that they need. The department may also maintain a video library, and the HUC will be responsible for checking out videos to the consumer.

Hospitals that maintain a good relationship with the community are the same hospitals that will survive the current turmoil in the health care industry.

Documentation

There is an old saying, "If it is not documented, it did not happen." Any question asked of the patient—for example, a question about allergies—is worthless if the information is not documented or written down. The nursing staff is trained to document all nursing care information. This documentation, in some cases, may be the most important form of communication.

The HUC may be called upon to document information about calls that he or she places, including the time that the call was placed and to whom. The HUC notes the time that orders are transcribed or entered into the computer. Messages for the physicians, staff, or families must be recorded accurately and dispatched urgently. In some units the HUC maintains a log of the location of the families and the times in and out. Regardless of what the information is, the most important aspect is the documentation.

Closing Thoughts

This is a fast-paced and exciting unit that provides individualized care in a safe environment. This assists the patient to maintain his or her physical, emotional, and spiritual well-being. The unit is a combination of in-patient nursing units and an outpatient clinic. Every day is new and different, and being bored is never an issue. There is plenty of opportunity to use interpersonal skills with staff, visitors, and patients. This is a unit that is evolving quickly and constantly changing to be prepared for the future of health care. There are many opportunities for the professional health unit coordinator in these changing times.

Review Questions

1. Explain the reason for the development of same day admission units in hospitals.
2. List five specific areas that may be found in a same day admission unit.
3. Name five types of pain that may be treated in the pain management area.
4. Describe the role of the HUC in the same day admission unit in communicating with the community.

Bibliography

Skidmore R: Mosby's Nursing Drug Reference. St. Louis, CV Mosby, 1998.

Special Care Units

14

OVERVIEW

Sandy Ayres

Objectives

Upon completion of this chapter, the reader will be able to:

1. List and define abbreviations used in the special care units.
2. Explain the evolution of special care units.
3. Identify equipment that is common to most special care units.

Vocabulary

Oscilloscope: An instrument producing an instantaneous visual display of a waveform on a screen

Photodetector: A light-detecting device

Transducer: A device that transforms one form of energy to another

Volumetric: Capable of measuring volume.

Common Abbreviations

A/C	Assist/Control mode
AACN	American Association of Critical Care Nurses
ABG	Arterial blood gas
CI	Cardiac index
CMV	Control mode ventilation
CO	Cardiac output
CPAP	Continuous positive airway pressure
CVP	Central venous pressure
DBP	Diastolic blood pressure
EKG	Electrocardiogram
FIO_2	Fraction of inspired oxygen
H_2CO_3	Carbonic acid
HCO_3	Bicarbonate
ICU	Intensive care unit
IMV	Intermittent mandatory ventilation mode
LAP	Left atrial pressure
LVP	Left ventricular pressure
MAP	Mean arterial pressure
O_2	Oxygen
$PaCO_2$	Carbon dioxide pressure
PAD	Pulmonary artery diastolic pressure
PaO_2	Blood oxygen pressure
PAP	Pulmonary artery pressure
PAWP	Pulmonary artery wedge pressure
PCA	Patient-controlled analgesia
PEEP	Positive end-expiratory pressure
pH	Hydrogen ion concentration
RAP	Right atrial pressure
RVP	Right ventricular pressure
SaO_2 or O_2sat	Oxygen saturation
SBP	Systolic blood pressure
SIMV	Synchronized intermittent mandatory ventilation
SpO_2	Saturation of hemoglobin
VT	Tidal volume

Special care units are found in both small and large hospitals. Smaller hospitals tend to have one general intensive care unit (ICU) that houses patients with medical and surgical conditions. Larger hospitals may have a variety of specialized units, including separate medical surgical ICUs. The largest facilities and teaching hospitals have a wide variety of special care units that may include one or more of the following: cardiothoracic surgical ICU, coronary care unit, neonatal ICU, pediatric ICU, and surgical ICU.

This chapter describes special care units (Fig. 14–1). An introduction to special care is followed by a discussion of the evolution of special care units and the equipment common to these units. Then the chapter is broken down into six parts, each of which describes a different special care unit.

Introduction to Special Care

Special care involves grouping patients with similar life-threatening or potentially life-threatening conditions in a single area. According to the American Association of Critical Care Nurses (AACN), the "critical patient requires constant intensive, multidisciplinary assessment and intervention to restore stability, prevent complications, achieve/maintain optimal responses."[1] Because of the patients' needs, ICUs are staffed with nurses who have specialized skills.

Special care nurses have an increased awareness of the need for frequent assessments and of a patient's airway, breathing, and circulation. They also are knowledgeable about the advanced technology that is found in many special care units. The AACN has defined critical nursing as "that specialty within nursing which deals specifically with human responses to life-threatening problems."[17]

Special care units tend to offer similar services and functions, but the patients have different characteristics. In some units the patients are alert (coronary care units), whereas in others the patients may be totally dependent on nursing care (cardiothoracic surgical ICU). Most special care units are designed to give the nurses good visibility of their patients.

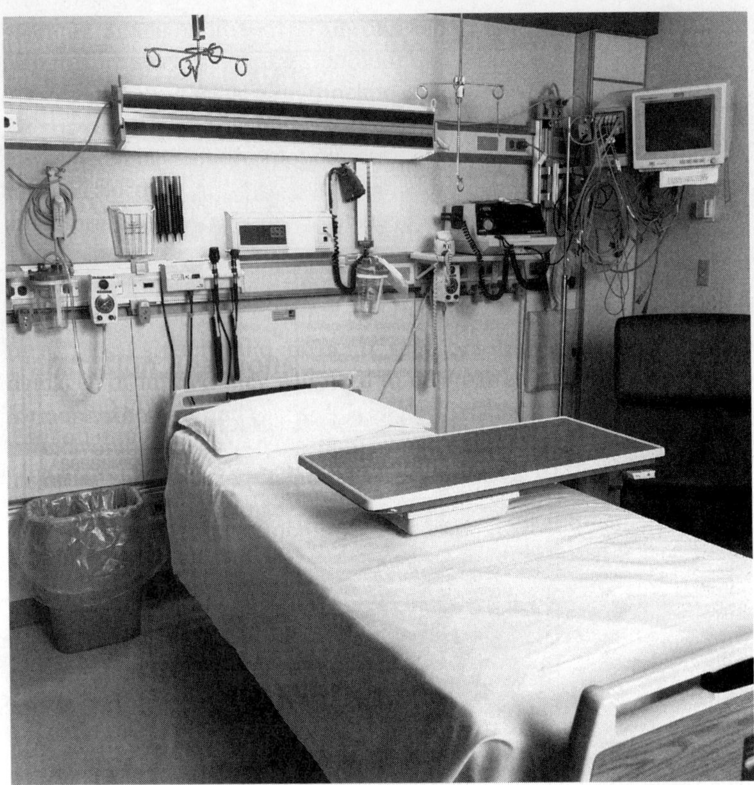

Figure 14–1
An intensive care unit.

Evolution of Special Care Units

The postanesthesia recovery room is recognized as the first special care unit. In the early 1940s the postanesthesia recovery room was created to treat World War II casualties. The unit allowed staff to watch patients closely for airway obstruction and postoperative hemorrhage. It was found that the mortality rate decreased with the use of the postanesthesia recovery room.

The burn unit was the second type of special care unit to be developed. In 1942 a burn unit was created to treat victims of the Cocoanut Grove fire in Boston. Massachusetts General Hospital found that this specialized care unit was valuable in the treatment of mass casualties. This unit was later disbanded, but since then hospitals specializing in the treatment of burn victims have been established.

A third type of special care unit was started for respiratory care. In the late 1940s and early 1950s the poliomyelitis epidemics created a need to have a special place to treat respiratory paralysis patients. Once again, the mortality rate decreased with the establishment of the respiratory care unit. The treatment of these cases advanced the development of respiratory methods, leading to the establishment of permanent ICUs.

In the 1950s other types of ICUs were created to closely watch patients. Brigham Hospital in Boston opened a cardiac surgical unit in 1951. In 1953 a North Carolina hospital set up a medical surgical intensive care unit (ICU). At this hospital, someone asked "[w]hy can't we put all of our critical patients in one room, have available everything we need for an emergency and give them the best care possible?"[4] In 1958, a Maryland hospital started an ICU for patients with respiratory insufficiencies. Baltimore City Hospital staffed this unit with physicians who specialized in life support techniques.

Advances in cardiac resuscitation equipment (pacemakers and defibrillators) resulted in the opening of coronary care units in 1962. The monitoring of heart rhythm and the treatment of life-threatening arrhythmias decreased the mortality rate in patients.

Even though premature infant nurseries were first established in 1896, it was during the 1960s when the neonatal ICUs grew in number.[2] This was a result of improved resuscitation methods and mechanical ventilation techniques. Further, pediatric ICUs have been created to provide specialized care to the critically ill child. It was determined that children of all ages have different needs from those of adults.

The number and type of special care units increased in the late 1960s and the 1970s. This increase has had an effect on the number of specialists in the various fields. Likewise, professional associations have been organized to help with clinical research and certification and to provide a network for the various specialty fields.

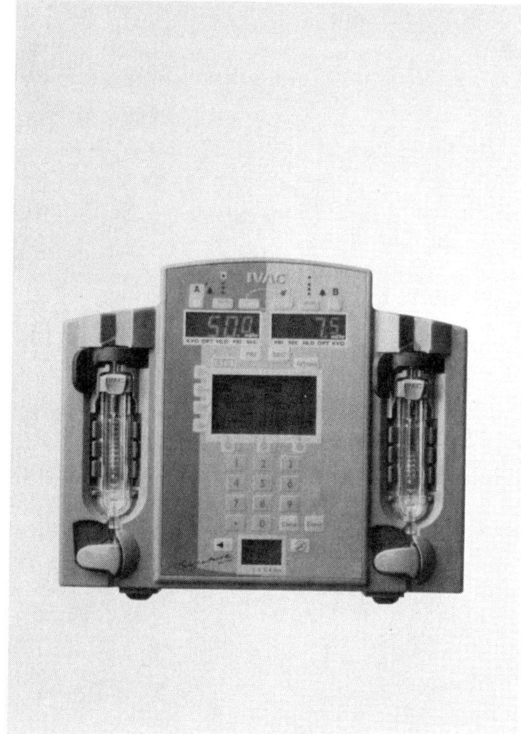

Figure 14–2
Volumetric infusion pump. (Courtesy of Gary Jellon.)

Equipment Common to Special Care Units

Infusion pumps, ventilators, monitoring equipment, and defibrillators are common equipment found in the different types of special care units.

Infusion Pumps

Various types of infusion pumps are used in ICU. First, patients may need fluids or intravenous medications. To ensure an accurate flow rate, volume-controlled infusion pumps are used (Fig. 14–2). The physician orders the amount of fluid to be given to a patient over a specific time (rate); the nurse sets the machine's rate according to the physician's orders; and a consistent flow of fluid is delivered to the patient. Further, some medications that are given intravenously need to be infused over a period of time (such as antibiotics, which are usually given over 1 hour). Using a **volumetric** pump to dispense this medication allows the nurse to provide other care at the same time.

Another type of pump is used to control dispensing of a pain medication by a patient. Patient-controlled analgesia, or **PCA**, pumps give the patient a mechanism to obtain pain relief without waiting for the nurse. The nurse presets the pump according to the physician's order; this allows the patient to press a control button as needed for pain relief. There is a time-delay mechanism that prevents overdosing.

Ventilators

Mechanical ventilators provide respiratory support care (Fig. 14–3). A ventilator takes over the breathing function for the patient. Patients with decreased lung capability or respiratory failure

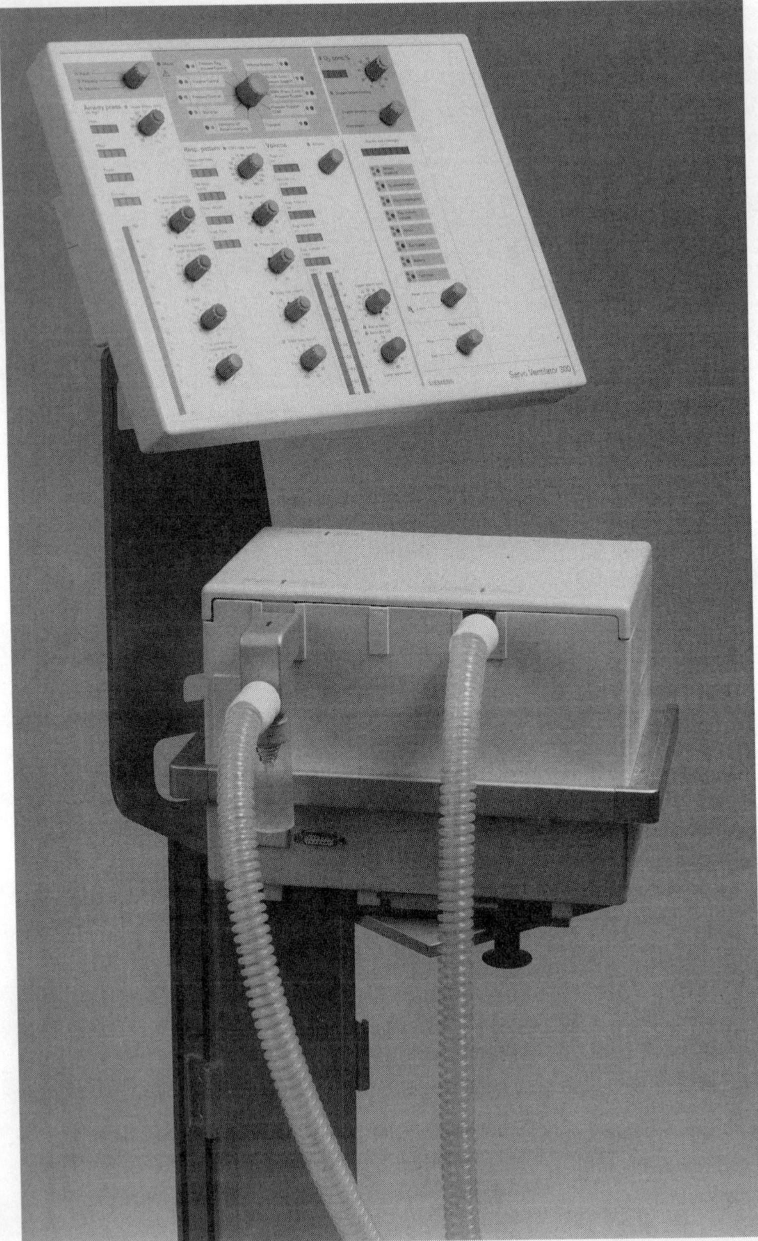

Figure 14–3
Ventilator. (Courtesy of Siemens Medical Systems, Electromedical Group.)

may have to be placed on a ventilator in order to move gas in and out of the lungs.

There are different types of mechanical ventilators—pressure-cycled, volume-cycled, and time-cycled. The choice of ventilator is determined by the patient's condition. A pressure-cycled ventilator can be used on patients who do not have a pre-existing pulmonary disease. This type of ventilator delivers a flow of gas at a preset pressure. Volume-cycled ventilators are the most common. The volume of gas that they deliver depends on the patient's lung volume. The time-cycled ventilator is used on the pediatric patient. It delivers a flow of gas over a specific amount of time.

The physician specifies the settings for the ventilator. The orders commonly include **FIO_2, VT,** and mode. FIO_2 is the fraction of inspired (inhaled) oxygen delivered to the patient. VT, or tidal volume, is the volume of air that is moved in and out of the lungs with each respiration (breath). There are various types of modes—**CMV, A/C, IMV,** and **SIMV.** CMV is control mode ventilation. The ventilator is set up to automatically deliver breaths for a patient, who is not allowed to breathe on his or her own. CMV is rarely used. With A/C (assist/control) mode, the patient initiates the inspiration and controls the frequency. Each breath, whether initiated by the patient or the ventilator, is the same volume. With IMV, or intermittent mandatory ventilation mode, the patient can spontaneously breathe between the mandatory breaths delivered by the ventilator. SIMV (synchronized intermittent mandatory ventilation) delivers mandatory breaths at the same time as a patient triggers the machine by inhaling (inspiratory negative trigger). SIMV is a set number and volume of breaths from the ventilator plus whatever breaths the patient initiates with his or her own volume. This mode helps wean the patient from the ventilator.

Other settings that are frequently ordered include **PEEP** and **CPAP.** PEEP refers to the positive end-expiratory pressure, and CPAP is continuous positive airway pressure. Both settings provide continued pressure in the airway and alveoli. The goal of both is to restore or maintain the functional lung capacity of a patient.

The settings on the ventilator are changed according to the patient's status. A test that is run to determine lung status is arterial blood gas **(ABG).** Blood is drawn from the patient's artery. The results show the blood oxygen pressure **(Pao_2)**, carbon dioxide pressure **($Paco_2$)**, carbonic acid **(H_2co_3)**, amount of bicarbonate in the blood **(Hco_3)**, hydrogen ion concentration **(pH)**, and oxygen saturation **(SaO_2)**.

Monitoring Equipment

Patients in special care units are connected to various types of hemodynamic monitoring equipment. Hemodynamics is the study of the forces involved in the circulation of blood. Monitoring a patient's condition can be done by either noninvasive or invasive procedures. In a noninvasive procedure, equipment is connected to different outside parts of the body, whereas an invasive procedure involves entering a part of the body through an incision. Noninvasive monitoring means a lower risk to patients.

Noninvasive monitoring equipment provides information to the nurse and physician about a patient's blood pressure, pulse, and heart. A noninvasive blood pressure monitor displays the systolic and diastolic blood pressure reading, heart rate measurements, and mean arterial pressure **(MAP)** readings. MAP indicates the pressure available for tissue perfusion. A cuff is placed on either the arm or the leg. It automatically pumps up at preset intervals to provide the readings (Fig. 14–4).

A pulse oximeter measures oxygen saturation, or O_2sat (Fig. 14–5). A sensor is placed on the patient's finger, toe, nose, or earlobe. The sensor has two sides—one side contains a red light source, the other an infrared light source. When this sensor is placed on the body, it transmits a constant red wavelength of light between these two sources. The hemoglobin in the patient's blood absorbs the light. The amount of light absorbed reflects the amount of oxygen in the blood. A photodetector registers the amount of light absorbed and sends it to a monitor that displays the percentage of saturation of hemoglobin **(SpO_2)** and pulse rate.

An electrocardiogram **(EKG)** monitoring system is a continuous display of heart conduction (Fig. 14–6). Electrodes are placed on the patient's chest to pick up the electrical impulses. Cables containing wires are connected to the electrodes to transmit the electrical impulse signal to a bedside monitor. The bedside monitor is also wired to a central monitor at the nurses' station.

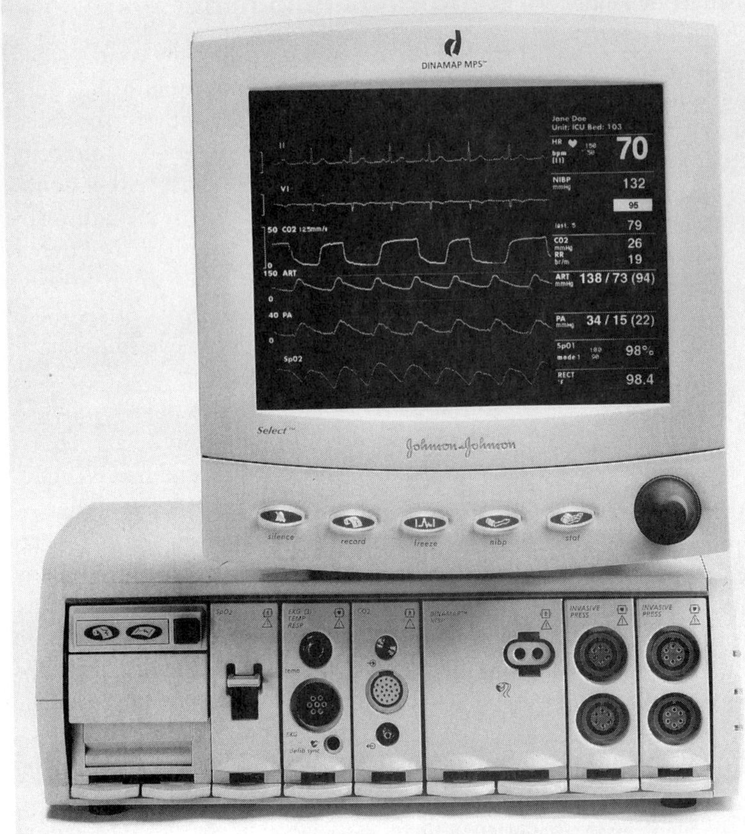

Figure 14–4
Noninvasive blood pressure monitor. (Courtesy of Johnson & Johnson Medical, Inc., Tampa, FL.)

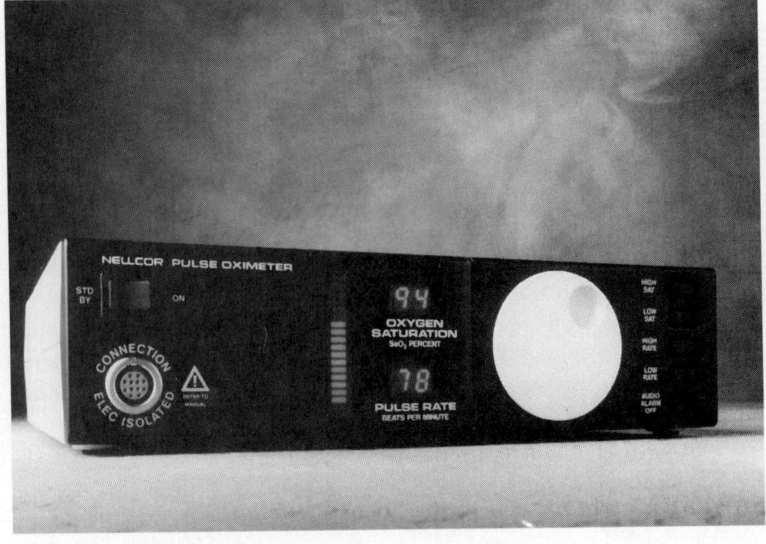

Figure 14–5
Pulse oximeter. (Reprinted by permission of Nellcor Puritan Bennett, Pleasanton, CA.)

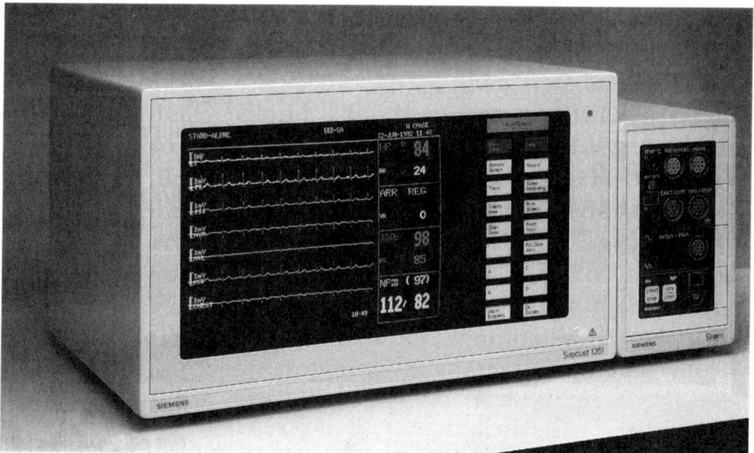

Figure 14–6
Bedside monitor system. (Courtesy of Siemens Medical Systems, Electromedical Group.)

Invasive monitoring is used to obtain information about a patient's cardiorespiratory status and the response to treatment. A physician inserts a catheter through a blood vessel. The catheter can include either a single- or a multiple-pressure transducer system. The transducer detects pressure changes and sends a signal to a monitor system. The system's recorder, or **oscilloscope**, displays the signals in digital and graphic form.

A single-pressure transducer system catheter is inserted into an artery in order to monitor blood pressure and to obtain arterial blood for testing. The monitor displays the patient's systolic blood pressure (**SBP**), diastolic blood pressure (**DBP**), and MAP. SBP measures the pressure when the heart is contracting. DBP measures when the heart is filling with blood (or expanding). MAP is the perfusion pressure, or the force, required for blood flow through the circulatory system. Using the catheter to obtain blood avoids the need to stick the patient with a needle. Many patients in special care units have their blood frequently tested.

More than one type of catheter uses a multiple-pressure transducer. Depending on the type of catheter used, the monitor may display pulmonary artery pressure (**PAP**), pulmonary artery diastolic pressure (**PAD**), pulmonary artery wedge pressure (**PAWP**), right or left atrium pressure (**RAP/LAP**), right or left ventricular pressure (**RVP/LVP**), central venous pressure (**CVP**), cardiac output (**CO**), and cardiac index (**CI**). The different pressure readings provide the physician with the tools to assess the patient's cardiovascular status, evaluate the response to treatment, and identify potential complications.

Defibrillator

The defibrillator is used to restore normal rhythm by sending an electrical current to the heart (Fig. 14–7). A patient's heart may need to be defibrillated if the heart stops or goes into a life-threatening arrhythmia (irregular heartbeat). The patient is connected to the defibrillator, and the nurse or physician electrically charges the machine. When the defibrillator reaches a specific voltage, the defibrillator paddles are placed on the patient's chest. The electrical current is then discharged from the machine through the patient. This procedure is repeated until the heart rate has been restored.

Closing Thoughts

Patients are placed in special care units in order to receive constant care provided by specially trained nursing staff in a highly technical

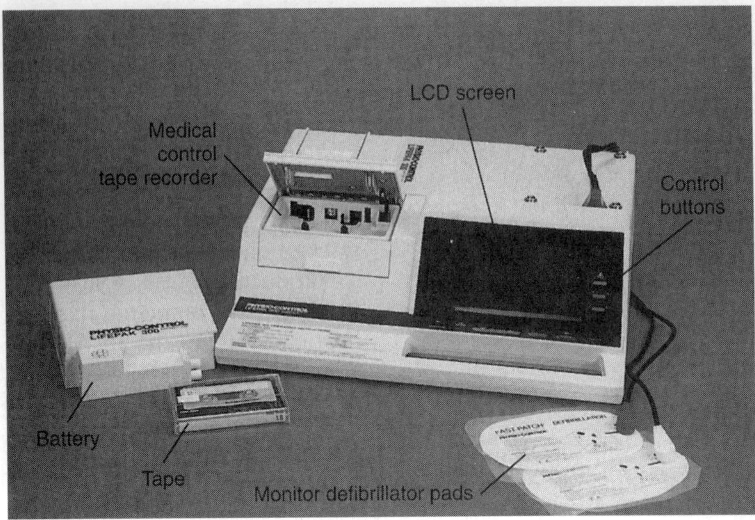

Figure 14–7
Components of an automated external defibrillator. LCD, liquid crystal display.

environment. Nurses are trained to monitor and analyze a patient's vital life functions. Technical equipment provides information to the nurses and physicians that is used to decide the course of treatment to achieve or maintain the optimal outcome.

The ratio of patient to nurse is lower in a special care unit than on a general unit. Patients in these units are generally dependent on nursing staff. A lower ratio allows the nurse to spend the required time to assess, treat, and care for the patient. Further, the families of patients in these units need extra attention from the staff.

The HUC is a vital part of the special care unit's staff. A HUC needs to be efficient, organized, and attentive. Efficiency is needed to transcribe the volume of orders written on the patient's chart. Also, the HUC is frequently interrupted by staff, physicians, and family. Organizational skills are needed to maintain the patient's chart. Volumes of paperwork are generated on patients in special care units. Finally, the HUC needs to be attentive to surrounding situations. If a patient's condition deteriorates, the HUC needs to respond to requests immediately.

Review Questions

1. Write the meaning of the following abbreviations: CMV, PAP, PCA, SIMV, and VT.
2. List in order of their development the following: Burn Unit, Post Anesthesia Unit, Neonatal ICU, Coronary Care Unit.
3. Differentiate between CMV, SIMV, A/C, and IMV.

Bibliography

1. Banner MJ, Lampotang S, Blanch PB, Kirby RR: Mechanical ventilation. *In* Civetta JM, Taylor RW, Kirby RR (eds): Critical Care, 2nd ed. Philadelphia, JB Lippincott, 1992, pp 1391–1417.
2. Barrett V: Caring for the respiratory patient. *In* Carey KW (ed): Nursing Photobook: Ensuring Intensive Care. Horsham, PA, Intermed Communications, 1981, pp 18–57.
3. Bryan-Brown CW: Pathway to the present: A personal view of critical care. *In* Civetta JM, Taylor RW, Kirby RR (eds): Critical Care, 2nd ed. Philadelphia, JB Lippincott, 1992, pp 5–11.
4. Cadmus RR: Intensive care reaches silver anniversary. Hospitals 1980; 54:98–102.
5. Clochesy JM: Historical development of technology and critical care nursing. *In* Clochesy JM (ed): Advanced Technology in Critical Care Nursing. Rockville, MD, Aspen, 1989, pp 1–10.

6. Committee on Hospital Care: Hospital Care of Children and Youth. Elk Grove Village, IL, American Academy of Pediatrics, 1986.
7. Goodnough-Hanneman SK: Ventilatory management. *In* Clochesy JM, Breu C, Cardin S, et al (eds): Critical Care Nursing, 2nd ed. Philadelphia, WB Saunders, 1996, pp 96–164.
8. Gozensky C, Mead S, Purcell JA: Caring for the cardiovascular patient. *In* Carey KW (ed): Nursing Photobook: Ensuring Intensive Care. Horsham, PA, Intermed Communications, 1981, pp 60–105.
9. Groh DH: Treatment or torture: Why critical care? *In* Fowler M, Levine-Ariff J (eds): Ethics at the Bedside: A Source Book for the Critical Care Nurse. Philadelphia, JB Lippincott, 1987, pp 1–21.
10. Hayne AN, Bailey ZW: Nursing Administration of Critical Care. Rockville, MD, Aspen, 1982.
11. Kaplow R, Wooldridge-King M: Infusion devices and techniques for administration. *In* Boggs RL, Wooldridge-King M (eds): AACN Procedure Manual for Critical Care, 3rd ed. Philadelphia, WB Saunders, 1993, pp 835–854.
12. Kern LS: Hemodynamic monitoring. *In* Boggs RL, Wooldridge-King M (eds): AACN Procedure Manual for Critical Care, 3rd ed. Philadelphia, WB Saunders, 1993, pp 281–367.
13. McKinley MG: Electrocardiographic monitoring. *In* Boggs RL, Wooldridge-King M (eds): AACN Procedure Manual for Critical Care, 3rd ed. Philadelphia, WB Saunders, 1993, pp 232–250.
14. Medina V: Advances in mechanical ventilation. *In* Clochesy JM (ed): Advanced Technology in Critical Care Nursing. Rockville, MD, Aspen, 1989, pp 29–49.
15. Miller LR: Hemodynamic monitoring. *In* Clochesy JM, Breu C, Cardin S, et al (eds): Critical Care Nursing, 2nd ed. Philadelphia, WB Saunders, 1996, pp 203–234.
16. O'Grady SG, Engstrom S, Fisher JA: Special pulmonary procedures. *In* Clochesy JM, Breu C, Cardin S, et al (eds): Critical Care Nursing, 2nd ed. Philadelphia, WB Saunders, 1996, pp 199–231.
17. Sanford SJ, Disch JM: AACN Standards for Nursing Care of the Critically Ill. East Norwalk, CT, Appleton & Lange, 1989.
18. US Department of Health, Education, and Welfare: Planning for General Medical and Surgical Intensive Care Units: A Technical Assistance Document for Planning Agencies. Washington, DC, Government Printing Office, 1979.
19. Walker CB: Precordial shock. *In* Boggs RL, Wooldridge-King M: AACN Procedure Manual for Critical Care, 3rd ed. Philadelphia, WB Saunders, 1993, pp 251–266.
20. Wright J, Doyle P, Yoshiham G: Mechanical ventilation: Current uses and advances. *In* Clochesy JM, Breu C, Cardin S, et al (eds): Critical Care Nursing, 2nd ed. Philadelphia, WB Saunders, 1996, pp 262–288.

Special Care Units

14

PART 1: CORONARY CARE

Kathryn Bymers

Objectives

Upon completion of this chapter, the reader will be able to:

1. Identify diagnostic studies carried out on CCU patients.
2. Describe treatments used on CCU patients.
3. List medications commonly used in a CCU.
4. Describe communications required in a CCU.

Vocabulary

Ablation: The process of eliminating or removing

Aneurysm: A weakening of a blood vessel wall or heart chamber wall resulting in a saclike protrusion

Angina pectoris: Chest pain that occurs when diseased blood vessels restrict blood flow to the heart

Angioplasty: A technique for treating blocked arteries by temporarily inserting a catheter with a balloon at the end into an artery and then inflating the balloon briefly to reduce the blockage in the artery

Antiarrhythmic drug: Medication to prevent or alleviate heart arrhythmias

Anticoagulant: Medication that keeps blood from clotting—often called a blood thinner

Aorta: The largest artery in the body, which exits from the left ventricle and carries oxygenated blood to all parts of the body

Arrhythmia: An abnormal heartbeat

Artery: Blood vessel that carries blood away from the heart

Atherectomy: Method of shaving or removing plaque from an artery with a specially designed catheter

Continued

Vocabulary *Continued*

Atherosclerosis: Fatty deposits in an artery producing narrowing and hardening

Atria: The upper holding chambers of the heart

Atrioventricular node (AV node): A group of cells found between the atria and ventricles that regulate the electrical current of the heart rhythm

Bradycardia: An abnormally slow heartbeat

Bundle of His: The band of cardiac nerve–like fibers that originates at the AV node and propagates the impulse originating in the SA node through the right and left bundle branches to the terminal Purkinje fibers

Capillaries: The smallest blood vessels

Cardiac arrest: Condition in which the heart stops beating and breathing ceases abruptly

Cardiac catheterization: Process in which a catheter is inserted into the heart to assess the condition of coronary arteries, valves, and heart muscle

Cardiac output (CO): The amount of blood that the heart pumps through the circulatory system in 1 minute

Cardiopulmonary resuscitation (CPR): An emergency measure that involves the use of artificial breathing and chest compressions to circulate oxygen and blood in a person whose breathing and heartbeat have ceased

Cardioversion: An electrical shock applied to the chest in an attempt to convert certain abnormal heart rhythms to a normal one

Conduction system: Special muscle fibers that conduct electrical impulses throughout the muscle of the heart

Defibrillation: An electrical shock applied to the chest to stop fibrillation and restore a normal heart rhythm

Depolarization: The process by which electrical impulses are spread throughout the cardiac conduction system and the heart muscle

Diastole: Period of the cardiac cycle when the heart relaxes to allow blood to flow into it

Edema: Swelling caused by fluid accumulation in body tissues

Effusion: The escape of fluid through the walls of a blood vessel into a tissue or body cavity

Endocardium: The smooth membrane that covers the inside surface of the heart

Enzyme: A complex chemical capable of speeding up specific biochemical processes in the body

Continued

Vocabulary *Continued*

Epicardium: The thin membrane that covers the outside surface of the heart

Fibrillation: The rapid and uncoordinated beating of the chambers of the heart

Informed consent: Signed permission from a patient for a medical procedure after he or she has been told about it and understands its risks and benefits

Intra-aortic balloon pump (IABP): A balloon attached to a catheter that is inserted through an artery into the aorta to produce alternating inflation and deflation, decreasing the work of the heart and increasing the flow of blood to the coronary arteries

Myocardial infarction (MI): A heart attack, an area of permanently damaged heart tissue

Pacemaker: A device that delivers an electrical stimulus to the heart to help regulate the heartbeat

Palpitation: An uncomfortable sensation within the chest caused by an irregular heartbeat

Pericardium: The membrane or sac that surrounds the heart

Pulse: The rhythmic expansion and contraction of an artery as blood is forced through it

Repolarization: A recharging of the myocardial cells so they may again respond to stimulation

Sinoatrial (SA) node: The natural pacemaker of the heart—a group of specialized muscle cells within the right atrium that emit electrical impulses that initiate the contractions of the heart

Stenosis: The narrowing or constriction of an opening

Stent: A device made of expandable metal mesh that is inserted into a narrowing artery and then expanded and left in place to keep the artery open

Swan-Ganz catheter: A monitoring catheter used to assess the cardiac output and pressures in the right heart chambers and pulmonary artery

Systole: Period of contraction in the cardiac cycle when the heart pumps

Tachycardia: An abnormally fast heartbeat

Trendelenburg: A position in which the patient's head is low and the body and legs are on an elevated and inclinedplane (used in treating shock)

Valve: A flap of tissue that prevents backflow of blood to keep it moving in the right direction through the heart

Vein: A blood vessel that returns blood to the heart

Ventricle: One of two large lower pumping chambers of the heart

Common Abbreviations

ACE	Angiotensin converting enzyme
AICD	Automatic implanted cardioverter defibrillator
AMI	Acute myocardial infarction
AV	Atrioventricular
CAD	Coronary artery disease
CCU	Coronary care unit
CF or **CFX**	Circumflex (artery)
CHF	Congestive heart failure
CO	Cardiac output
CPR	Cardiopulmonary resuscitation
CVP	Central venous pressure
DCA	Directional coronary atherectomy
DVT	Deep venous thrombosis
ELCA	Excimer laser coronary angioplasty
EP	Electrophysiology
IABP	Intra-aortic balloon pump
ICD	Implantable cardioverter defibrillator
LAD	Left anterior descending (artery)
LBB	Left bundle branch
LMCA	Left main coronary artery
MI	Myocardial infarction
MUGA	Multigated acquisition scan
NTG	Nitroglycerine
PAP	Pulmonary artery pressure
PET	Positron emission tomography
PTCA	Percutaneous transluminal coronary angioplasty
PCWP	Pulmonary capillary wedge pressure
RBB	Right bundle branch
RCA	Right coronary artery
SA	Sinoatrial (node)
SAECG	Signal averaged electrocardiogram
TEC	Transluminal extraction catheter
TEE	Transesophageal echocardiogram
TPA	Tissue plasminogen activator
TPN	Total parenteral nutrition

Description of the Unit

The coronary care unit (CCU) is a small unit that is well equipped and staffed with specially trained nurses and other health care professionals to care for the acutely ill patient with cardiac problems. There are usually 6 to 12 rooms depending on the size of the hospital. The patient is kept under close observation and constant monitoring that allows for continuous assessment of his or her condition. The patient's electrocardiogram is displayed on a monitor screen both at bedside in the patient's room and at the nurse's monitor desk. The nurses keep a constant watch so that any change in condition can be detected early and appropriate treatment initiated immediately.

The patient rooms are usually situated around the nursing desk area so that they can be seen from the desk. A typical patient room is ideally a private room. It has a bed with a special mattress that enables x-rays to be taken directly through the mattress using a C-arm. This way the patient does not have to be transported to radiology for x-rays for such things as confirmation of line placements and other procedures. The headboard should be removable to make it easier to do emergency intubations. It should be easily put in **Trendelenburg** and reverse Trendelenburg positions.

Each room is equipped with a monitor, which provides both a visible and an audible record of the patient's heartbeat and other vital signs, such as blood pressure. On the wall at the head of the bed are many electrical outlets, wall suction equipment, a stethoscope, and a sphygmomanometer for taking blood pressures. A patient call button is always accessible. Nurse call buttons and an emergency code alarm button to summon additional or emergency help are also found here. IV hangers are fixed to the ceiling. Stationary poles fitted with pumps to regulate IV fluids and drugs administration are in the room as well. A wall clock that starts timing when the code alarm button is activated is a necessity. Some rooms are equipped with a bedside defibrillator in case of emergencies.

Having a television or radio to counter the boredom of lying in bed is pleasant for the patient. When the patient's condition improves enough to get out of bed, a chair or rocker is placed by the bed so that he or she can continue to be monitored.

Other areas in a CCU include a medication room, where patients' medications, IV fluids, IV tubing and supplies, emergency drugs, and pain medications are stored; a central location, where all patient supplies such as dressings, catheters, and personal items are kept; and a laundry cart or room, where all the clean linens, gowns, and towels are stored. Most CCUs have a kitchenette for patient nourishments and an ice machine. There is a physician's dictating room, preferably close to a room or area where x-rays can be viewed on a computerized system or on an x-ray view box. Found close by are a family waiting room and a private consultation room, where families can meet with physicians.

One of the most important areas in the CCU is the health unit coordinator's desk. It is usually in the center of the unit and placed where visitors and hospital personnel enter. On the HUC desk, there is a computer, into which physician orders are entered, and a printer, where many reports and laboratory printouts are received. It is where most of the telephone calls are answered. It is the place to obtain information regarding the patient's location, for example, whether the patient has gone for a test or has transferred out of the unit. All the patient chart forms, test requisitions, and computer downtime forms are kept here. This is the appropriate place to have a fax machine and a copying machine. Reference books, a laboratory manual, HUC manual, dietary manual, and procedures for emergency codes and downtime are kept at the HUC desk.

Anatomy and Physiology of the Cardiovascular System

The human heart is a hollow, muscular organ roughly the size of a man's clenched fist. It is located in the middle of the chest between the lungs, with the lower part, the apex, to the left of center. The strongest and hardest working muscle in the body, the heart acts as a pump, constantly circulating blood to all parts of the body.

The **myocardium** is the muscular wall of the heart. It contracts to pump blood out of the heart and then relaxes as the heart refills with returning blood. It is the thickest of the three layers of the heart wall. It lies between the **endocardium**, the smooth membrane covering the inner surface of the heart, and the **epicardium**, the thin membrane covering the outer surface. The **pericardium** is the outer fibrous sac that surrounds the heart. Its smooth, well-lubricated lining provides protection against friction and allows the heart to move easily within it.

The interior of the heart consists of four chambers connected by valves. The upper chambers are divided into the left **atrium** and the right atrium. The thin-walled atria receive blood from the veins. The lower chambers, the left **ventricle** and the right ventricle, are thick-walled and pump the blood out through the arteries.

The two sides of the heart have distinct functions and together can be viewed as a dual pump. The right side of the heart receives oxygen-poor blood from the entire body and then pumps it to the lungs to be oxygenated and to lose carbon dioxide. The left side receives the oxygenated blood from the lungs, and then the blood is pumped to all the tissues in the body.

The muscular partition that divides the two sides is called the **septum.** Four heart **valves** allow the blood to move in only one direction. The mitral valve on the left side and the tricuspid valve on the right control the flow of blood from the atria to the ventricles. The aortic valve is between the left ventricle and the **aorta**, and the pulmonary valve is between the right ventricle and the pulmonary artery. These two valves control the flow of blood out of the ventricles.

There are three kinds of blood vessels: arteries, veins, and **capillaries**. An **artery** is a vessel that carries blood away from the heart to the body, and a **vein** is a vessel that carries blood from the body back to the heart. The capillaries are microscopically small blood vessels between arteries and veins that distribute oxygenated blood to all the body tissues.

The coronary arteries wrap around the surface of the heart and keep it supplied with oxygenated blood. The left main coronary artery (**LMCA**) splits into two branches, the circumflex (**CF, CFX**) and the left anterior descending (**LAD**), which supply blood to the front, left side, and back of the heart. The right coronary artery (**RCA**) supplies blood to the bottom right side and the back of the heart.

The two largest veins of the body are the superior vena cava, which carries the blood to the heart from the head and arms, and the inferior vena cava, which carries blood from the trunk and legs. The pulmonary vein carries oxygen-enriched blood from the lungs back to the heart.

The Cardiac Cycle

The cardiac cycle is the time from the beginning of one heartbeat to the beginning of the next one. In each heartbeat, first the atria and then the ventricles contract, followed by a pause.

The blood can be traced on its journey through the heart by following the blood returning from all parts of the body via the superior and inferior vena cavae into the right atrium. This blood passes through the tricuspid valve and empties into the right ventricle. Contraction pumps the oxygen-depleted blood through the pulmonary valve into the lungs, via the pulmonary arteries. Carbon dioxide is released and exchanged for oxygen. The oxygenated blood moves from the lungs via the pulmonary veins into the left atrium and is gently pumped through the mitral valve into the left ventricle. The powerful pumping action of the left ventricle sends it through the aortic valve into the aorta to be delivered to all the body tissues. This cycle is one heartbeat and is continuously repeated throughout a person's life. The typical heart beats approximately 72 beats per minute, and each beat lasts about 0.83 seconds.

Blood Pressure

Each heartbeat is composed of two phases—the contraction phase, or **systole**, and a relaxation phase, or **diastole.** Systole occurs when the blood is forced out of the heart. Diastole occurs when the heart relaxes between beats as it fills with blood. Blood pressure measures the force exerted by the blood against the arterial walls during these two phases. Systole indicates the maximum force exerted and diastole the weakest. Blood pressure is recorded as two figures separated by a diagonal line, with the systolic pressure followed by the diastolic pressure. For example, in a blood pressure reading of 120/80, the systolic pressure is 120 and the diastolic pressure is 80. Many factors influence the blood pressure, such as the resistance of the blood flow in the blood vessels, the pumping action of the heart, the thickness or quantity of blood, and the elasticity of the arteries. Elevated blood pressure is called hypertension, and low blood pressure is called hypotension.

The Conduction System of the Heart

The **conduction system** consists of nervous tissues that conduct electrical impulses throughout the heart. This conductive tissue consists of four masses of highly specialized cells—the **sinoatrial** (SA) node, the **atrioventricular** (AV) node, the **bundle of His**, and the Purkinje fibers.

The SA node is found in the upper portion of the right atrium and possesses its own intrinsic rhythm. It can initiate each heartbeat without being stimulated by any external nerves and sets the pace for the rate of the heart. It is commonly known as the natural "pacemaker" of the heart. The electrical impulse discharged by the SA node is transmitted to the AV node, which causes the atrium to contract. The AV node is located at the base of the right atrium. From the AV node, a bundle of special conduction fibers, called the bundle of His, relays the impulse to the Purkinje fibers. The bundle of His is extended by a right bundle branch (**RBB**) and a left bundle branch (**LBB**) about halfway down the two sides of the interventricular septum, where they continue as Purkinje fibers. These fibers then extend up the walls of the ventricles and transmit the impulse to both the right and the left ventricles, causing them to contract.

Blood is then forced out of the heart through the pulmonary artery and aorta. Impulse transmission through the conduction system generates weak electrical currents that can be detected on the surface of the body. These electrical impulses can be recorded on paper by means of an electrocardiogram (EKG). The impulses cause deflections of the needle of the EKG machine, and a record is made of the resulting waves. These waves are designated by the letters P, Q, R, S, and T; each is associated with a specific electrical event of the heart cycle. The P wave is the **depolarization** or contraction of the atria. The PR interval, the beginning of the P wave to the beginning of the QRS, is the time it takes from the beginning of the atrial contraction to the beginning of the ventricular contraction. The QRS complex is the depolarization of the ventricles. The T wave is the **repolarization**, or the recovery of the ventricles. As the blood is exerted through the arteries with each heartbeat, it can easily be felt as the pulse.

Cardiovascular Diseases

Many different types of cardiovascular diseases are responsible for patients being admitted to the CCU. Some are very serious, and others can be milder. Many different sorts of treatment are used depending on the type and severity of the disease. Treatment can range from drugs to surgery to simply altering some part of one's lifestyle, such as changing to a healthier diet, quitting smoking, or increasing exercise.

Coronary Artery Disease

Coronary artery disease (**CAD**) involves the progressive narrowing of the coronary arteries that supply nourishment to the heart muscle. The narrowing is due to fatty plaque deposits along the artery wall (**atherosclerosis**). As the coronary arteries become severely narrowed, the blockage limits the blood flow. This may cause chest pain, or angina, to develop. If the coronary arteries become completely blocked, a myocardial infarction (MI) or heart attack may occur.

Diagnosing CAD involves a physical examination by a physician, who will take a medical history, including symptom review, and order certain tests. The tests will include blood work, an EKG, and a chest x-ray. An exercise EKG, or stress test, is done to demonstrate the heart's response to exercise. An echocardiogram will check how the heart is functioning. Further tests that may be required are radioisotope scanning and an exercise thallium test to check the blood flow for blockage.

Treatment consists of medications to help relieve the chest pain. Some medications help open the coronary artery to improve the blood flow through the artery, such as beta-blocking drugs or calcium channel–blocking drugs. Aspirin may be helpful, too, since it tends to lessen the possibility of blood clot formation. Usually a combination of several medications is prescribed for people with severe angina.

Sometimes a percutaneous transluminal coronary angioplasty (**PTCA**) is done to try to open the artery to improve the blood flow. A **stent** can also be inserted in a coronary artery to keep it open. Those patients with severe angina not relieved by medications or those with blockages in several arteries may be candidates for coronary artery bypass surgery.

Angina or Chest Pain

Angina, or **angina pectoris**, is the medical term for chest pains behind the breastbone. It is a very common symptom of CAD. Usually it is due to a blockage in one or more coronary arteries; it may be precipitated by physical activity, stress, or cold temperatures. Most episodes last less than 15 minutes. Angina should never be ignored; a physician should be consulted for a complete physical examination. Often angina can be diagnosed from symptoms alone, but usually an EKG and a stress test are ordered.

The initial treatment for angina is rest. If this is not effective, nitroglycerin (**NTG**), taken under the tongue, should relieve the pain. Other treatments should include a change in lifestyle, such as stress reduction, exercise conditioning to increase endurance, smoking cessation, and weight reduction.

Myocardial Infarction

A **myocardial infarction (MI)**, or heart attack, occurs when there is a complete blockage of a coronary artery. This is due to either a clot in the artery or an accumulation of fatty plaque that shuts off the blood flow and prevents oxygen from reaching that section of the heart. Symptoms of an acute MI, such as crushing chest pain, especially if radiating down the arms, need immediate medical attention. Diagnosis of an MI is confirmed by an EKG and by having serial cardiac **enzymes** (LDH, CK, CK-MB, and TNI) drawn. An echocardiogram may also be done.

If the patient arrives at the hospital within 4 to 6 hours of the onset of chest pain, the emergency treatment is to administer a coronary thrombolytic drug such as streptokinase, urokinase, or tissue plasminogen activator (**TPA**). It is often possible to dissolve the clot using these drugs, which restore the blood flow and greatly decrease heart damage and mortality. **Anticoagulants**, initially IV heparin and later p.o. warfarin (Coumadin), are used. Other medications that are administered are morphine or meperidine, to eliminate pain and anxiety, and NTG, to relax the muscles in the blood vessels. Other treatment includes bed rest for the first day or two, supplemental oxygen, and a diet low in cholesterol and sodium. By following a cardiac rehabilitation program after an MI, the patient can learn how to make the lifestyle adjustments necessary to avoid recurrences.

Congestive Heart Failure

Congestive heart failure (**CHF**) is a condition in which the heart is not working adequately to pump enough blood. There is an accumulation of fluid in the lungs and other body tissues, especially the feet, ankles, and legs. CHF may be caused by prolonged hypertension, damage from an MI, CAD, diseases of the heart muscle or heart valves, or a congenital heart defect.

Diagnosis can often be made by a physician listening to the patient's complaints—typically, shortness of breath, swelling of the feet and ankles, and fatigue—and then listening to the chest with a stethoscope. A chest x-ray can reveal fluid in the lungs or an enlarged heart, indicating that the heart has tried to compensate for its inability to pump enough blood.

One of the first steps in treatment is to limit salt intake. Salt is a contributing factor to fluid retention. Medications most commonly used to treat CHF are diuretic drugs to help rid the body of excess sodium and water; vasodilator drugs to dilate blood vessels; and digitalis to strengthen the contractions of the heartbeat. The best way to avoid heart failure is salt restriction, weight control, and a routine exercise program.

Cardiac Arrhythmias

An **arrhythmia** is any abnormality in the rate or regularity of the heart's normal rhythm. Many arrhythmias are minor and do not require treatment, whereas others need to be controlled with medications or may require other procedures or possibly surgery. Arrhythmias can be divided into two main groups: the **tachycardias**, in which the heart rate is faster than normal—greater than 100 beats per minute; and the **bradycardias**, in which the heart rate is slower than normal—less than 60 beats per minute. The rhythm may be regular or irregular. Arrhythmias may be caused by an interruption of the normal pathway of the impulses, CAD, excessive caffeine or alcohol consumption, fatigue, stress, and certain medications.

Diagnostic tests for arrhythmias are an electrocardiogram (EKG or ECG) to show the heart rhythm. A signal-averaged EKG may be done to identify electrical signals that may predict arrhythmic events. Esophageal electrocardiography may be performed to better detect some arrhythmias. Another way to evaluate rhythm disturbances is the use of a Holter monitor, which continuously monitors the heart rate for a 24-hour period. Electrophysiology (**EP**) studies, performed in a **cardiac catheterization** laboratory, show how the heart reacts to a controlled electrical stimulus.

Treatments for different types of arrhythmias are drug therapy, **ablation** procedures, implantable devices, and surgery. Drug therapy is often the first method for treating an arrhythmia. There are many different **antiarrhythmic drugs** that are effective alone or in a combination of medications. Examples of medications used to correct irregular heart rhythms are quinidine, bretylium, lidocaine, and procainamide.

Persistent tachyarrhythmias can be corrected by **cardioversion,** which is a technique of applying an electrical shock to the chest. Another treatment option is radio-frequency ablation, using a catheter equipped with a device that permits mapping of the electrical pathways of the heart. The cardiologist can then use high-frequency radio waves to ablate, or eliminate, the pathways that are causing the arrhythmia. A **pacemaker** may be needed to regulate the heart rhythm in some cases of bradycardia from heart block. The implantable cardioverter-defibrillator (**ICD**) is an option for treating serious ventricular arrhythmias that could cause cardiac arrest (Table 14–1).

Table 14–1 CARDIAC RHYTHMS

Rhythm	Abbreviation
Atrial fibrillation	A. Fib.
Complete heart block	CHB
Heart block	HB
Normal sinus rhythm	NSR
Paroxysmal atrial tachycardia	PAT
Premature atrial contractions	PACs
Premature ventricular contractions	PVCs
Superventricular tachycardia	SVT
Ventricular tachycardia	VT or V. Tach.
Ventricular fibrillation	V. Fib.

Cardiomyopathy

Cardiomyopathy is a disease of the heart muscle. There are three main types of cardiomyopathy—dilated, hypertrophic, and restrictive. The most common form is dilated cardiomyophy, in which the heart muscle becomes weak and the chambers of the heart enlarge, stretch, and balloon out. Hypertrophic cardiomyopathy results from an abnormal thickening of the heart wall that obstructs the flow of blood to the heart. In restrictive cardiomyopathy, the least common type, the heart muscle grows inflexible, thus restricting proper stretching. This prevents proper filling of the heart with blood.

Diagnosis of cardiomyopathy is begun when a chest x-ray reveals an enlarged heart. Other tests include an EKG and an echocardiogram. The diagnosis can be confirmed by a biopsy of the heart muscle. Treatment of symptoms includes medications such as the diuretic drugs to help the heart failure and the antiarrhythmic drugs to correct any abnormal heart rhythm. In many cases the heart muscle continues to deteriorate, and the only remaining option is a heart transplant.

Endocarditis

Endocarditis is a bacterial infection of the lining of the heart chambers, valves, and main arteries. It occurs when a large number of bacteria enter the bloodstream, causing fever, chills, heart failure, and rapid destruction of a heart valve.

Diagnosis is made through blood samples, which are examined for bacteria or fungi and cultured so their sensitivity to antibiotics can be determined. An EKG and an echocardiogram, especially **TEE**, are also used for diagnosis. Treatment consists of high doses of IV antibiotic and/or antifungal drugs. If a heart valve has been extensively damaged, it may have to be replaced surgically with an artificial valve. Precautions must be taken by anyone who has a heart valve defect or an artificial valve whenever any procedure or surgery is done. Such procedures could cause bacteria to enter the bloodstream. Antibiotics must be prescribed prior to any surgical procedure as well as dental work, including cleaning.

Cardiogenic Shock

Cardiogenic shock occurs when the heart muscle becomes too weak to contract adequately to supply sufficient blood to the body and heart muscle. It can be a severe complication of acute myocardial infarction (**AMI**), occurring during the first few days, and of arrhythmias or other cardiac disease. Symptoms include cool, clammy, pale extremities; hypotension; and low **cardiac output** (**CO**). These symptoms may also be seen in pulmonary embolus, pneumothorax, valve thrombus, and dissecting aortic **aneurysm**.

Diagnosis is made by taking a history of the patient, especially of cardiac disease and blood pressure, as well as obtaining an EKG, CBC, electrolytes, arterial blood gases (ABGs), coagulation lab tests and blood cultures. Monitoring of the patient's vital signs, heart rhythm, urine output, and hemodynamics are important in order to treat the cardiogenic shock patient.

Initial treatment of the patient with cardiogenic shock consists of inserting arterial and PA lines and a urinary catheter. These will be used to closely monitor hemodynamics, blood pressure, and CO. Medications may include vasoconstrictors if the blood pressure is low, diuretics to assist in low urinary output, and inotropic agents to correct CO and arterial pressure readings. Patients who require such support for more than a day or two or are in severe shock are often put on an intra-aortic balloon pump (**IABP**). Patients experiencing cardiogenic shock from AMI may benefit from urgent coronary artery **angioplasty** or coronary bypass grafting surgery as soon as they are stable enough to withstand the procedure.

Sudden Cardiac Death Survivor

Sudden cardiac death occurs unexpectedly, shortly after the onset of symptoms or even without any symptoms, when the heart suddenly stops beating and breathing ceases. The victim collapses and becomes unconscious. However, if the cardiac arrest is witnessed by someone who knows **cardiopulmonary resuscitation** (**CPR**) and administers it immediately, that person can survive and brain damage may be avoided. If urgent help is not received and oxygenated blood flow restored to the brain within 4 to 6 minutes, brain death occurs.

The usual cause of sudden death is ventricular fibrillation, from which the heart rarely returns to a normal rhythm on its own. A defibrillator is needed to stop the fibrillation by delivering an electrical shock to the chest that helps re-establish a normal rhythm. In some cases a patient who is at risk for recurring dangerous rhythms may need to have an internal automatic cardioverter-defibrillator (**AICD**) implanted surgically.

Hypertension

Hypertension is the medical term used for elevated blood pressure. It is a leading risk factor for heart attacks and also the major cause of strokes. Most people do not have any symptoms at first and do not realize that they have hypertension. It usually takes years before it becomes apparent that the arteries to the heart have become damaged. Risk factors for developing hypertension are obesity and excessive use of salt. Heredity also appears to be a factor.

Diagnosis is made by keeping a written record of blood pressure readings. Blood pressure is measured with a sphygmomanometer and a stethoscope to hear the thumping sounds of blood flow through the artery. Consistent readings of greater than 140/85–90 mm Hg lead to a diagnosis of hypertension. Additional tests may be necessary to determine an underlying cause or to assess damage caused by hypertension.

Medication can be given to treat the underlying cause of hypertension and correct it. There are a large number of antihypertensive drugs that can be prescribed. These include diuretics, beta blockers, vasodilators, **ACE** inhibitors, and calcium channel–blocking drugs. If hypertension is left untreated, headaches, visual problems, shortness of breath, stroke, and kidney and heart failure are possible outcomes. High blood pressure can be controlled to a great extent by restricting salt, stopping smoking, limiting alcohol, increasing exercise, and controlling weight.

Medications Specific to the Coronary Care Unit

When patients are diagnosed with heart disease, they may be treated with a wide variety of cardiovascular drugs. At first a patient may have to try several different drugs to find one that is effective for the heart problem and has the fewest side effects. Often a combination of drugs is prescribed to increase the effectiveness of a treatment. Because each patient reacts differently to drugs, he or she needs to inform the physician of any symptoms and side effects so the appropriate drug and the correct dosage can be prescribed.

Each drug has three different names—a detailed, descriptive chemical name; a generic name, which is a shorter chemical name and officially approved; and a specific brand name, which is chosen and registered by the company that manufactures it. Table 14–2 shows some of the drugs used in a CCU.

Diagnostic and Special Procedures in the CCU

Laboratory Tests

Partial thrombolytic time (APTT) is done to evaluate clotting factors and to monitor heparin therapy; the prothrombin time (PT) is used to monitor oral anticoagulant therapy, such as Coumadin. Cardiac enzymes are ordered to evaluate causes of chest pain or whenever an AMI is suspected. Serial total creatine kinase (CK) and creatine kinase isoenzymes (CK-MB) are drawn every 8 hours the first 24 hours. Other indicators of cardiac muscle disorders are lactate dehydrogenase (LDH), myoglobin, troponin 1 (Tn1) and troponin T (TnT). Most blood tests do not require any preparation other than the need to have the patient fasting for a certain length of time. Tests such as total cholesterol and triglycerides, used to assess the risk of coronary artery disease, require a 12- to 14-hour fast before the blood is drawn (Tables 14–3 and 14–4).

Most of the other diagnostic tests and procedures are classified into either noninvasive or invasive categories. Noninvasive tests are those that do not involve entering the body by any means, for example, a needle puncture, entering an artery with a catheter, or performing a surgical incision. Invasive techniques are used when more advanced procedures are necessary that require a dye or contrast medium to show arteries or parts of the body that would not be seen on an x-ray.

Diagnostic Imaging Procedures

The chest x-ray is an important test in the evaluation and screening of heart disease. X-rays are a form of radiation, but there is minimal radiation exposure with a chest x-ray. The x-ray produces an image on film that outlines the heart, lungs, and other structures in the chest. The shape and size of the heart, the presence of abnormal deposits of calcium, and the accumulation of fluid in the lungs can all be visualized on the chest film. The bedside portable x-ray machine is very useful in the CCU, where the patient cannot always be moved to the radiology department. It can be used only when the bed has a special mattress. A portable x-ray machine is brought to the bedside, and the patient remains in bed while the x-ray is taken.

Moving images of the body at work can be taken with a fluoroscope. These images can be recorded on moving film or in a series of still pictures taken in rapid succession. The portable fluoroscope is very useful in the placement of Swan-Ganz catheters, temporary pacemakers, or central lines.

Cardiograms

An EKG is a very common test used to evaluate the electrical activity of the heart. Electrodes are attached to the chest, arms, and legs and connected to an EKG recording machine. The electri-

Table 14–2 MEDICATIONS USED IN THE CCU

General Name	Common Trade Name(s)	Functional Class(es)	Uses in CCU
abciximab	*ReoPro*	Platelet aggregation inhibitor	Prevent cardiac ischemia after PTCA
adenosine	*Adenocard, Adenoscan*	Antidysrhythmic	Paroxysmal superventricular tachycardia (PSVT)
alteplase	*TPA, Activase*	Antithrombiotic	Thrombi of MI and stroke
amiodarone	*Cordarone*	Antidysrhythmic	V. Tach., A. Fib., V. Fib., PSVT
anistreplase	*ASPAC, Eminase*	Thrombolytic enzyme	Acute MI
aspirin	*Ascroptin, Ecotrin, ZORprin*	Antiplatelet	Thromboembolic disease prophylaxis
atenolol	*Tenormin*	Beta blocker	Mild to moderate hypertension, angina
bretylium	*Bretylol, Bretylate*	Antidysrhythmic	V. Tach.
bumetanide	*Bumex*	Loop diuretic	CHF, hypertension
chlorothiazide	*Diuril, Diurigen*	Diuretic	Edema, hypertension
cholestyramine	*Questran, Cholybar*	Antilipemic	Primary hypercholesterolemia
clonidine	*Catapres*	Central alpha-adrenergic agonist	Mild to moderate hypertension
colestipol	*Colestid*	Antilipemic	Primary hypercholesterolemia, digitalis toxicity
digitoxin	*Crystodigin*	Cardiac glycoside, inotropic	CHF, A. Fib., PAT
digoxin	*Lanoxin*	Cardiac glycoside, inotropic	Atrial dysrhythmias, CHF
diltiazem	*Cardizem, Dilacor XR*	Calcium channel blocker	Angina, vasospasm, hypertension, atrial arrhythmias
dipyridamole	*Persantine*	Antiplatelet, coronary vasodilator	Coronary disease, angina, prevent TIAs
disopyramide	*Norpace*	Antidysrhythmic	PVCs, A. Fib., SVT, V. Tach.
dobutamine	*Dobutrex*	Direct acting adrenergic agonist	Cardiac decompensation, refractory heart failure
dopamine	*Intropin*	Vasopressor	Hypotension, shock

Table continued on following page

Table 14–2 MEDICATIONS USED IN THE CCU *(Continued)*

General Name	Common Trade Name(s)	Functional Class(es)	Uses in CCU
enoxaparin	*Lovenox*	Antithrombotic	Prevent pulmonary embolus, venous thrombosis
epinephrine	*Adrenalin*	Adrenergic	Cardiac arrest, anaphylaxis
esmolol	*Brevibloc*	Beta-adrenergic blocker	Hypertensive crisis, SVT
furosemide	*Lasix, Uritrol*	Loop diuretic	CHF, edema, hypertension
heparin	*Heparin, Liquaemin*	Anticoagulant	Pulmonary embolus, DIC, deep venous thrombosis
hydralazine	*Apresoline, Alazine*	Direct-acting peripheral vasodilator	Essential hypertension
hydrochlorothiazide	*Hydrodiuril, Esidrix, Thiuretic*	Thiazide diuretic	Edema, hypertension, chronic CHF
isoproterenol	*Isuprel*	Beta-adrenergic agonist	Heart block, shock
isosorbide dinitrate	*Isordil, Dilatrate-SR, Sorbitrate*	Nitrate antianginal	Angina pectoris
isosorbide mononitrate	*Imdur*	Nitrate antianginal	Angina pectoris
labetalol	*Trandate, Normodyne*	Beta blocker	Mild to moderate hypertension
lidocaine	*Xylocaine, LidoPen*	Antidysrhythmic, local anesthetic	Ventricular arrhythmias; local before procedures
lovastatin	*Mevacor*	Cholesterol-lowering agent	Mixed hyperlipidemia
mannitol	*Osmitrol*	Osmotic diuretic	Edema, acute renal failure, poisonings
methyldopa	*Aldomet, Amodopa*	Alpha-adrenergic inhibitor	Hypertension
metoprolol	*Lopressor, Toprol XL*	Beta blocker	Mild to moderate hypertension, angina
morphine sulfate	*Morphine Sulfate*	Narcotic analgesic	MI pain, pulmonary edema
nadolol	*Corgard*	Beta-adrenergic receptor blocker	Mild to moderate hypertension, angina
niacin	*Niacar*	Vitamin B_3	Adjunct in primary hyperlipidemia

Table 14–2 MEDICATIONS USED IN THE CCU *(Continued)*

General Name	Common Trade Name(s)	Functional Class(es)	Uses in CCU
nifedipine	*Adalat, Procardia*	Calcium channel blocker	Vasospastic angina, hypertension, atrial arrhythmias
nitroglycerin	*Nitrostat, Nitrol, Nitro-Bid*	Coronary vasodilator	Angina
procainamide	*Pronestyl, Promine, Procan SR*	Antidysrhythmic	PVCs, atrial arrhythmias
propranolol	*Inderal, Inderide*	Beta-adrenergic blocker	Arrhythmias, angina, hypertension
quinidine	*Quinaglute, Quinidex, Cardioquin*	Antidysrhythmic	Atrial arrhythmias
reserpine	*Serpasil*	Antiadrenergic	Hypertension
reteplase	*Retavase*	Thrombolytic enzyme	Acute MI
simvastatin	*Zocor*	Antihyperlipedimic	Adjunct in primary hyperlipidemia
sodium bicarbonate	*Sodium bicarbonate*	Alkalinizer	Metabolic acidosis in cardiac arrest
spironolactone	*Aldactone, Sincomen*	Potassium-sparing diuretic	Edema of CHF, hypertension
streptokinase	*Streptase, Kabikinase*	Thrombolytic enzyme	Dissolving clots, blockages in blood vessels
ticlopidine	*Ticlid*	Platelet aggregation inhibitor	Reduces risk of stroke
urokinase	*Abbokinase*	Thrombolytic enzyme	Dissolving clots, blockages in blood vessels
verapamil	*Calan, Isoptin, Verelan*	Calcium channel blocker	Angina, atrial arrhythmias, hypertension
warfarin	*Coumadin*	Anticoagulant	Pulmonary embolus, deep venous thrombosis

cal impulses are then recorded for each heartbeat on paper as wavy lines, known as the P, Q, R, S, and T waves. An EKG is useful in detecting cardiac arrhythmias and revealing conduction abnormalities, enlargement of the heart chambers, and evidence of an MI (Fig. 14–8).

An *exercise EKG* is performed when more information about what happens to the heart when it is stressed by exercise on a treadmill or stationary bike.This test is used to diagnose the cause of chest pain and to identify arrhythmias that develop during physical activity. The patient's

Table 14-3 LABORATORY TESTS AND VALUES*

Test	Full Name	Normal Values	Comments
BE	Base excess	0 (+/−) mEq/L	Arterial draw
BUN	Blood urea nitrogen	6–24 mg/dl	
Ca	Calcium (serum)	8.4–10.4 mg/dl	
Chol	Cholesterol (total)	100–200 mg/dl	
CK MB	Creatine kinase isoenzyme	0–5% of CK	
CK	Creatine kinase	30–170 U/L	
Cl	Chlorides (serum)	100–110 mEq/L	Part of electrolyte panel
CO_2	Carbon dioxide (serum)	23–30 mEq/L	Part of electrolyte panel
Creat	Creatine	0.8–1.4 mg/dl	
Bicarb	Bicarbonate	21–27 mEq/L	Arterial draw
Hct	Hematocrit	M 37–50 F35–47 mg/dl	
HDL	High-density lipids	30–80 mg/dl	Fasting required
Hgb	Hemoglobin	M13–18 F12–16 mg/dl	
K^+	Potassium (serum)	3.5–5.5 mg/dl	Part of electrolyte panel
LDH	Lactate dehydrogenase	81–170 U/L	
LDL	Low-density lipids	60–180 mg/dl	Fasting required
Na	Sodium (serum)	136–146 mEq/L	Part of electrolyte panel
O_2 Sat	Oxygen saturation	94–99%	
Pco_2	Carbon dioxide tension	35–45 mm Hg	Arterial draw
pH	Hydrogen ion concentration	7.3–7.49	Arterial draw
Plt	Platelet count	150,000–350,000/mm^3	
Pao_2	Partial pressure of oxygen	80–105	Arterial draw
PT	Prothrombin time	12–14 sec	Norm compared with standard
PTT	Partial thrombin time	27.3–38.9 sec	Norm compared with standard
RBC	Erythrocyte count	3.5 million–6.2 million/mm^3	Lower norms for females
Trig	Triglyceride level	35–160 mg/dl	Fasting required
WBC	Leukocyte count	4000–11,500/mm^3	

* Normal values may vary in different laboratories.

Table 14-4 CARDIOVASCULAR DRUG LEVELS

Medication	Therapeutic Range	Toxic Level	Comments
Amiodarone	1.0–2.0 μg/ml	>2.0 μg/ml	Drawn 8 hrs after dose
Digitoxin	15–25 ng/ml	>35 ng/ml	Drawn 12–24 hrs after dose
Digoxin	0.8–2.0 ng/ml	>2.4 ng/ml	Drawn >6 hrs after dose
Disopyramide	2–5 μg/ml	>7 μg/ml	
Lidocaine	1.5–5.0 μg/ml	>6 μg/ml	
Procainamide	4–10 μg/ml	>12 μg/ml	
Propranolol	50–100 ng/ml	variable	
Quinidine	2–5 μg/ml	>6 μg/ml	

blood pressure and pulse are closely watched. It is useful in determining guidelines for activity in patients with known heart disease and for patients after an MI (Fig. 14–9).

In *Holter monitoring*, several electrodes are placed on the patient's chest, and he or she wears a portable recording device for 24 or 48 hours. A continuous recording is made of the patient's normal daily activities. A similar device that can be used is known as the king of hearts. Instead of a continuous recording the patient pushes the record button only when symptoms of palpitation or irregular heartbeat occur. The king of hearts can be worn for several days or weeks. These ambulatory EKGs are useful for detecting arrhythmias and signaling the need for further therapy.

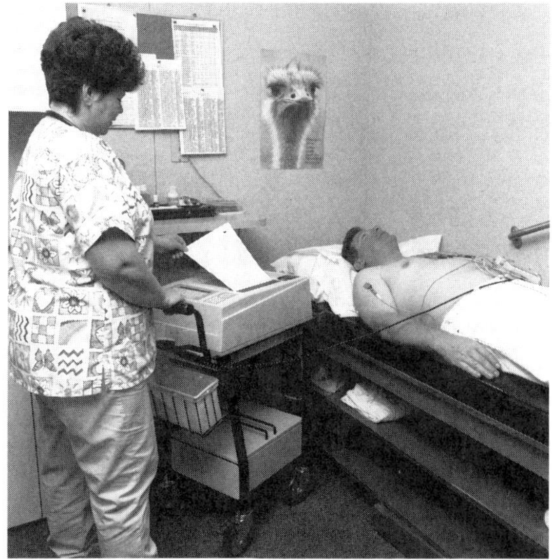

Figure 14–8
EKG machine.

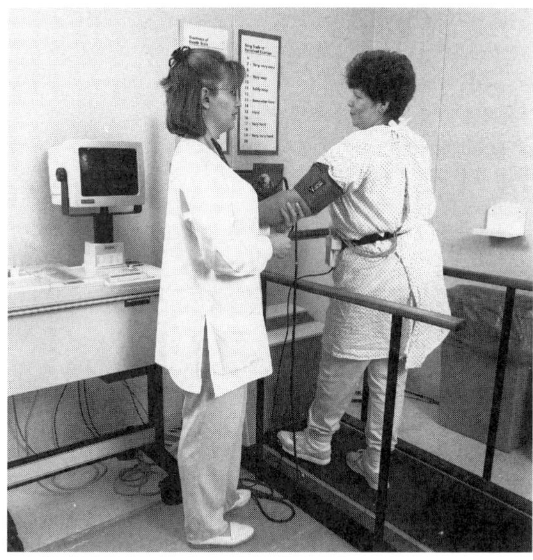

Figure 14–9
Stress lab.

A *signal-averaged electrocardiogram* (SAECG) picks up small electrical currents that are present long after normal heart muscle activity. These small currents are called late electrical potentials and are usually found in areas where there is injury to the heart muscle. A regular EKG is taken, and, with the aid of a computer, it is superimposed, creating a combination of signals known as an averaged EKG. The resulting record is analyzed to detect late potentials, which indicate an increased risk for arrhythmias after an MI.

An *echocardiogram* is a noninvasive procedure that makes it possible to look directly at the heart structure and valves. A transducer placed over the heart sends ultrasound waves through the body that are then reflected or echoed back from the heart structures. An echocardiograph machine determines how much time it takes for the sound waves to travel to and from the heart and then reconstructs an image of the heart to display on a video screen (Fig. 14–10).

There are several different ways to obtain an echocardiogram depending on the specific information needed. An M-mode echocardiogram measures heart structures using a single ultrasound beam and provides a narrow segmental view of the heart. It is helpful in measuring the size of a heart chamber or the thickness of the heart muscle. A two-dimensional (2-D) echocardiogram uses a planar ultrasound beam that shows an image in two dimensions. By changing the position of the transducer it is possible to see most parts of the heart and how they are functioning. This method is also used to evaluate valvular heart disease, cardiomyopathy, congenital defects, pericardial effusion, and intracardiac masses.

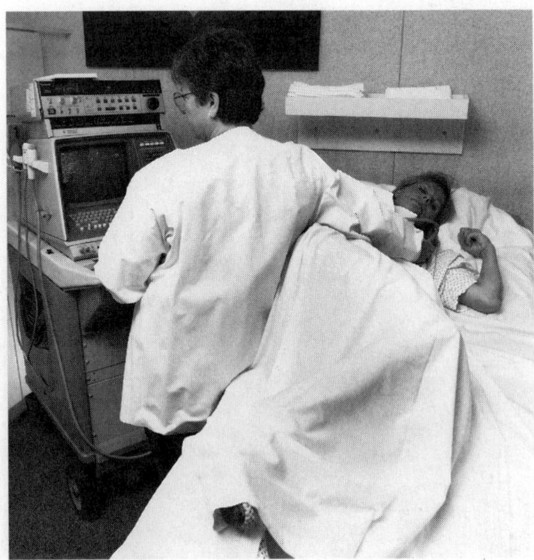

Figure 14–10
Echocardiogram lab.

The Doppler and color Doppler are two other types of echocardiograms. In a Doppler study, when the sound waves bounce off the blood cells as they move through the heart and vessels they change pitch in a certain way. This change in pitch can then be measured, and the direction and speed of blood flow can be calculated. Both the sound and the visual information can be displayed to show the flow of blood through the heart. Doppler echocardiography is especially useful in determining whether the heart valves are working properly. The color Doppler technique displays the direction of the blood through the heart, in color on a screen.

A *transesophageal echocardiogram* (TEE) is utilized to obtain better views of the back of the heart in patients who are obese or have thick chest walls. A TEE is performed by passing a endoscope containing a 2-D transducer through the patient's mouth and throat and into the esophagus. During the test a cardiologist may reposition the transducer at different sites in the esophagus. The sound waves are visualized on a screen and recorded and analyzed. This provides very clear views of the interior of the heart to locate blood clots, ascertain function of prosthetic valves, and assess aortic dissection. Transthoracic echocardiograms view the heart through the chest wall.

A *stress echocardiogram* is performed immediately after the patient exercises on a treadmill or stationary bicycle, while the heart rate is still high. It checks how well the heart works when it is stressed. This test is done to detect abnormalities in the heart wall motion in patients with CAD. If a patient is unable to exercise because of arthritis or some other condition, a similar effect can be achieved by using dobutamine or dipyridamole.

These medications mimic the effects of exercise by increasing the pumping action of the heart.

Scans

Nuclear scans show the heart's functioning as well as the blood flow through the heart. In nuclear scanning, a very small amount of radiation is introduced into the bloodstream to produce images of how the radioactive material is distributed in the body. The radiopharmaceutical is either swallowed or, more commonly, injected into a vein. A gamma camera is rotated around the patient, who is lying still, and the signals are used by a computer to generate an image of the heart and its circulation. Nuclear scans can show the size of the heart chambers, how effectively the heart is pumping, and if there is scarring from previous heart attacks. Additional information can be gathered when the scan is performed in combination with a exercise stress test.

A *multiple-gated acquisition scan* (**MUGA** scan) is a cardiac blood pool scan that is used primarily to check the size and function of the ventricles, including the presence of aneurysms. The doctor or technician administers an injection of red blood cells that are tagged with a small amount of technetium. A camera records the radioactivity as the technetium passes through the ventricle. Multiple images are made showing the heart in motion. Resting and after-exercise scans are taken. The stress MUGA scan can detect changes in the heart's pumping action.

Another type of nuclear scanning using technetium is called *infarct imaging* or *hot-spot myocardial imaging*. It is used to detect a recent heart attack and to determine the extent of damage to the heart. A scan is done 1 to 3 hours after the technetium is injected. Views are taken from several positions. The technetium accumulates in the damaged tissues of the heart; to help identify the size and location of a heart attack, the scan shows these areas of injury as hot spots.

Myocardial perfusion scanning is used to determine if any area of the heart is not receiving enough blood. This is called a thallium scan, cold-spot myocardial imaging, or sestamibi scintigraphy, depending on which radiopharmaceutical is used. The thallium or sestamibi accumulates in the normal healthy heart tissue, rather than in the damaged areas, and cold spots are produced on the screen. The cold spots indicate where the coronary arteries are blocked and where tissue has been damaged by a heart attack.

There are other sophisticated diagnostic imaging procedures used to visualize the heart, although the equipment is costly and not available in all facilities. *Computed tomography* (CT scan) is an x-ray technique but yields more information than a regular x-ray. A patient lies still on a table while part of the x-ray machine is rotated around the chest; this allows images to be obtained from different angles. A computer gathers all the information and constructs cross-sectional images of the heart. The physician can then view the internal structures of the heart either on a computer screen or on x-ray film.

Magnetic resonance imaging (MRI) uses magnetic fields and radio waves instead of x-rays to visualize the heart. This procedure shows details of the heart's anatomy and can be used to detect congenital defects and masses or tumors within and around the heart. Diseases of the pericardium, heart muscle disorders, and vascular disorders can be detected and evaluated. The patient must lie still on a narrow bed that slides into a large cylinder-like machine. Claustrophobic persons may experience anxiety in such a small space, so they may need a mild sedative to tolerate the test. Patients with pacemakers or internal metal objects cannot be scanned because of the magnetic environment. Patients who have artificial valves can be scanned safely.

Positron emission tomography (**PET** scan) is a technique similar to CT scanning. It uses a different substance tagged with a positron-emitting isotope to measure the blood pressure and blood flow through the heart chambers and the pulmonary artery. These data help diagnose intracardiac shunts, pericardial disease, and right-sided valve lesions.

A *cardiac catheterization* assesses the function of the mitral and aortic valves, patency of the coronary arteries, and integrity of the left ventricle. It can identify septal defects and other congenital heart disorders. The patient must be in a fasting state for at least 6 hours prior to the test, and an **informed consent** needs to be obtained. This involves an explanation of the procedure by the physician, including the benefits and risks. The risks include bleeding, damage to the artery or vein used, heart attack, and reactions to the contrast dye.

Preparation for the procedure involves starting an IV line in the arm to administer medications and fluids, preparing the site by shaving and scrubbing the area to be used, and attaching EKG electrodes to the chest for heart monitoring. The patient is generally given a mild sedative before going to the cath lab.

To begin the procedure, the cardiologist inserts a catheter into a blood vessel in the arm or groin and advances it into the heart. A radiographic dye is injected through the catheter. A television monitor shows an x-ray image of the catheter being advanced through the blood vessel. This helps the cardiologist position it so as to see where the contrast dye goes and which coronary arteries are occluded. A series of x-ray pictures are taken from different views and then evaluated (Fig. 14–11).

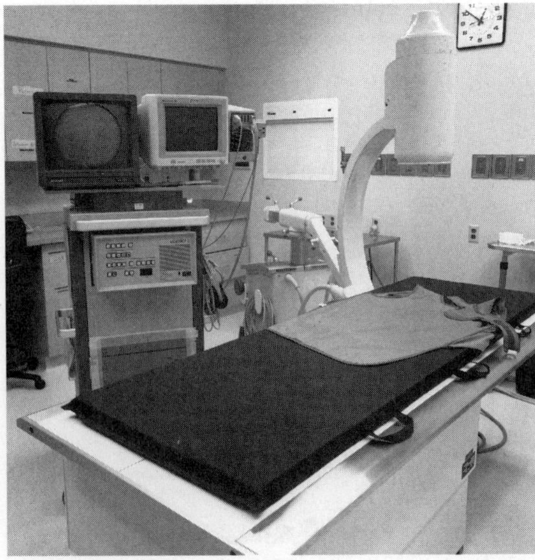

Figure 14–11
Cardiac catheterization lab.

Electrophysiology Studies

Electrophysiology (EP) studies are ordered when more detailed information is needed to evaluate unexplained syncopal episodes and other problems with the heart's rhythm. They are also used to assess the effectiveness and proper dosage of arrhythmia medications and are sometimes done prior to pacemaker insertion. People who have experienced sudden cardiac death and were resuscitated are good candidates for EP studies.

The procedure for EP studies is similar to a heart catheterization, and the preparation is the same. The test is performed by an electrophysiologist, who inserts one or several electrode catheters into the femoral vein in the groin. The catheters are advanced along the vein, into the heart, and along the conduction system.

The electrodes record the electrical impulses in various parts of the heart and measure how the heart conducts impulses from one area to another. During the test the electrophysiologist may stimulate the heart with different types of electrical impulses to mimic the arrhythmias that are causing problems. Various medications may be given to determine which ones best control the arrhythmia. When the study is over, the catheters are removed; pressure is applied to the skin to stop any bleeding; and a dressing is applied. Bed rest needs to be maintained for several hours.

Therapeutic Procedures

Ablation

One treatment option for arrhythmias is radiofrequency ablation, which is performed in the cath lab. The catheter that is used is equipped with a device at the tip that allows mapping of the electrical pathways of the heart. It is inserted into a vein in the groin and advanced into the heart. After seeing the whole map the cardiologist can determine where the problematic pathway is, and the catheter is placed close to that pathway. With the use of high-frequency radio waves the abnormal pathway that is causing the arrhythmia can be eliminated. This procedure is effective in managing selective arrhythmias. Radio-frequency ablation can also be used to slow the heart rate in rapid atrial fibrillation.

Coronary Angioplasty

Percutaneous transluminal coronary angioplasty (PTCA), or balloon angioplasty, is used in the treatment of **stenosis** in the coronary arteries. It is performed in the cath lab by a cardiologist—much like a cardiac catheterization and with the same preparation and risks.

This procedure uses a specially constructed catheter equipped with a small balloon on the tip. The cardiologist inserts a sheath, a short tube, into an artery in the groin. A catheter is inserted through the sheath under fluoroscopy. It is advanced, under direct visualization using contrast dye, into the coronary artery that has the blockage. A smaller catheter with the deflated balloon is inserted through the first catheter until it is at the blocked area. The balloon is inflated for 30 to 90 seconds and then deflated. This is repeated several times in order to stretch open the artery by compressing the plaque against the artery wall. After the balloon catheter is removed, additional pictures are taken to see how the blood flow through the artery has improved, and then the guide catheter is removed. The sheath usually is left in for 4 to 12 hours. To prevent bleeding, it is important to keep the patient on bed rest with the leg straight while the sheath is in and for several hours after the sheath is removed.

There are other procedures to open blocked arteries. One method is a *directional coronary atherectomy* (**DCA**), which shaves off and then removes plaque from a blocked artery. A catheter equipped with a nonflexible cylinder is inserted into the coronary artery. The cylinder has a window containing a cutter on one side and a balloon on the opposite side. By inflating the balloon, the cutter is pressed against the plaque; it shaves off the plaque, which is stored in a collection chamber and removed from the artery when the catheter is removed. The procedure is useful on large vessels with noncalcified lesions but cannot be used on small vessels or lesions on bends because of the nonflexible cylinder.

An *excimer laser coronary angioplasty* (**ELCA**) is performed by using a flexible laser-tipped catheter that vaporizes the plaque with a tiny laser beam. This leaves the artery with a smooth inner surface. ELCA is used on long lesions and occlusions that cannot be dilated or crossed with a balloon.

A *rotoblator* is an option for treatment of calcified lesions and total occlusions that can be crossed with a wire but cannot be crossed and dilated with a balloon. This instrument has a diamond-coated bur on a flexible shaft that rotates at high speed and grinds the hard plaque into microparticles. These particles can then pass through the coronary circulation.

A *transluminal extraction catheter* (**TEC**) is utilized in a similar way, but the catheter has a rotating hollow cutter with suction connected to it at the tip. The plaque or clot is cut into small particles and then suctioned out through the catheter. TEC is used on thrombus-containing lesions and degenerated vein grafts and when a large amount of plaque must be removed to open the blood vessels.

Other Catheterization Procedures

Sometimes, even after a successful PTCA, a blockage can recur in the same area. When this restenosis happens, or to minimize the chance of its happening, the cardiologist may recommend that a *coronary stent* be placed. A stent is a small, stainless steel, slotted tube placed on a balloon catheter. It is inserted into the artery immediately following a PTCA procedure and positioned at the site of the obstruction. As the balloon is inflated, the stent is expanded and pushed against the artery wall. Then the balloon is deflated and removed, but the stent remains permanently in the artery to keep it open. More than one stent can be placed in the same area if needed, as in a long lesion. The lining of the artery wall grows over the stent in a period of 4 to 5 weeks. Anticoagulants are required during the procedure and for at least a 6 to 8 weeks afterwards to prevent blood clots from forming on the stent.

A similar catheterization technique can be used to open heart valves. They may have become stenosed or narrowed, or the stiff valve leaflets may have become stuck to one another. *Valvuloplasty*, or reshaping of the valves, is a procedure done in a cath lab by a cardiologist. A balloon-tipped catheter is guided into the heart through a blood vessel and into the affected valve. The balloon is inflated to allow more blood to flow through and then is removed. If a balloon valvuloplasty is ineffective because of excessive calcium buildup or regurgitation of blood through the valve, a surgical repair or replacement is necessary.

Permanent Pacemaker

A permanent pacemaker is implanted in the upper chest in the operating room or cath lab, usually under local anesthetic. A pacing lead wire is inserted through a vein and into the heart. It is connected to a pulse generator surgically placed and inserted in a pocket under the skin. The generator contains the battery and electronic circulator, which produces electrical impulses as needed. The device is usually a demand pacemaker, so it fires only when the heart rate drops below a set rate. The pacemaker must be checked periodically to ensure that it is working properly. The battery life is usually 5 to 10 years. Indications for a permanent pacemaker are drug-resistant bradycardia, heart block from an MI, or complete heart block. A pacemaker will cause the heart rate to be restored to normal.

Temporary Pacemakers

A temporary pacemaker is used in an emergency situation for bradycardia or complete heart block. It is sometimes required after a patient has had an MI and is used for a short time. The procedure involves inserting an electrode catheter into the right ventricle under fluoroscopy. The battery-powered pulse generator is worn outside the body.

Defibrillation

In cases of cardiac arrest, CPR must be started immediately to restore the circulation of oxygen-carrying blood to the brain. CPR uses external chest compressions and artificial ventilations to try to circulate blood through the body to avoid brain damage, which can occur within 3 to 4 minutes if the brain does not receive oxygen.

In order to correct the life-threatening arrhythmia of ventricular fibrillation, which can occur following an MI, it is necessary to use a technique called defibrillation. Ventricular fibrillation produces an ineffective quivering action of the heart muscle. A brief electrical shock is administered to the patient's heart in an attempt to correct the rhythm. Two electrode paddles that have been charged by the defibrillator are positioned over the chest, to which conductive gel pads have been applied. The electrical current shocks the heart back into a more normal rhythm. The patient may need two or three shocks, which are usually administered using a higher amount of energy each time until the dangerous rhythm has resolved.

Cardioversion

Cardioversion is like defibrillation because it is used to deliver an electrical shock to the heart to correct an arrhythmia. The difference is that it uses a lower electrical current, and the shock can be synchronized to be delivered at a specific point in the cardiac cycle. To perform this procedure, two defibrillator paddles are charged and positioned over pregelled conductive pads placed on the chest. The current is delivered by pressing the discharge button on both paddles at the same time. Synchronized cardioversion is used to treat arrhythmias such as unstable atrial flutter, atrial tachycardia, atrial fibrillation and supraventricular tachycardia. It is usually done electively when drug therapy fails or when it is determined that the patient is clinically unstable from the arrhythmia.

Automatic Implantable Cardioverter Defibrillator (AICD)

Patients who have a history of ventricular tachycardia (VT or V. Tach.) and are sudden death survivors, may be a candidate for an automatic implantable cardioverter defibrillator (AICD). The placement of this device is performed in the operating room by a cardiovascular surgeon or cardiologist. It consists of a pulse generator implanted under the skin in the upper chest area or abdomen, cardiac leads placed in the heart, and tiny patch leads attached to the heart. The leads record the activity of the heart and when it detects life-threatening arrhythmias, the patch leads deliver an electrical shock to restore the heart to a normal rhythm.

Intra-aortic Balloon Pump

Intra-aortic balloon pump (IABP) therapy is used to assist the heart when it is working too hard because it is not receiving enough oxygen. The device can be placed at bedside under fluoroscopy, in the operating room, or in a cath lab. It consists of a balloon catheter that is inserted into a femoral artery, advanced into the aorta, and attached to an external pump machine.

The pump constantly inflates and deflates the balloon, alternating with the patient's heartbeat. When the balloon inflates, the heart receives help pumping freshly oxygenated blood through the coronary arteries into the heart muscle. When it deflates, the workload on the heart is lessened. Indications for this device are unstable angina, cardiogenic shock, and other complications from MI. IABP therapy is used to stabilize patients with severe left main coronary artery disease who will be requiring cardiac surgery.

Pericardiocentesis

Pericardiocentesis is a procedure used to remove blood or other fluid that has accumulated in the pericardial sac. The procedure, which can be done at the bedside, involves the use of an intracardiac needle to withdraw the fluid from the pericardium. The fluid that is extracted is analyzed by the lab to help diagnose the underlying disease. Most hospitals have a pericardiocentesis tray holding all the needles, specimen containers, and other sterile supplies that are needed.

The primary indication for a pericardiocentesis is cardiac tamponade. This is a life-threatening condition caused by fluid or blood accumulation in the pericardial sac, which compresses the heart. Following the procedure a portable chest x-ray is required immediately to rule out the presence of a pneumothorax. The patient is closely monitored for complications, such as arrhythmias or cardiac arrest.

Monitoring and Treatments in the CCU

There are many treatments and procedures specific to the CCU. Some are common to all patients admitted to the unit, and others are specific to the treatment of symptoms of different cardiovascular diseases. The initial orders for most admissions include keeping the patient at bed rest, taking frequent vital signs and daily weights, tracking intake and output, and providing a diet low in cholesterol and saturated fats with restricted salt. Cardiac enzymes and other laboratory tests are ordered to determine whether or not an MI has occurred.

Continuous cardiac monitoring of the rate and rhythm is done on all patients in the CCU. This is displayed in the patient's room and also at the central nurse's station, where a recording of the heart rhythm can be printed out. Visual and auditory alarms will sound if the patient has abnormal heartbeats or if the heart rate is higher or lower than the setting on the monitor alarm. Twelve-lead EKGs are performed frequently using an electrocardiograph machine or the patient's monitoring system if it has that function.

Respiratory monitoring is important in the treatment of the patient with chest pain. Oxygen is administered immediately. The oxygen is titrated according to the percent of oxygen saturation.

This parameter is derived from a continuous saturation monitor or a pulse oximeter placed intermittently on a finger or an ear.

In cases of respiratory or **cardiac arrest** it may be necessary for the patient to be intubated. An endotracheal tube is inserted through the mouth or nose, down the throat, and into the trachea and is then attached to a mechanical ventilator. The ventilator will provide assistance or control of respirations until the patient is capable of adequate rate and volume through spontaneous respiration.

Patients on a ventilator need frequent ABGs to help monitor their condition. ABGs can be drawn by a single arterial stick or by an arterial indwelling catheter (A-line). By utilizing an A-line, the nurse can draw a blood sample from the arterial line rather than having to do repeated arterial punctures.

Use of special catheters makes possible a variety of hemodynanic monitoring techniques. One example is the Swan-Ganz catheter. This has multiple lumens, which enable the monitoring of different hemodynamic parameters, such as *central venous pressure* (**CVP**), *pulmonary artery pressure* (**PAP**), *pulmonary capillary wedge pressure* (**PCWP**), and *cardiac output* (CO). With the aid of portable fluoroscopy, this special catheter can easily be placed at the bedside. A portable chest x-ray is taken after placement to ensure that the catheter is in the correct position in the heart.

Arterial pressure monitoring is an invasive technique by which an IV type catheter is placed in an artery (usually the radial artery). After the catheter is placed, areterial pressure readings are displayed on the screen of a monitor and can also be recorded on paper. Constant monitoring of arterial pressures is very important when intravenous vasoactive drugs, such as nitroprusside and dopamine, are needed to regulate the patient's blood pressure.

A *central venous line* is placed instead of a peripheral intravenous line, especially in the event of peripheral collapse or poor venous access. It is inserted through a major vein, such as the subclavian vein or internal jugular vein, at the bedside under sterile conditions. A follow-up portable chest x-ray is taken to check for proper placement.

Intravenous fluids in large volumes and irritating solutions, such as concentrated potassium chloride and total parenteral nutrition (**TPN**) solutions, can be given safely using a central line. It also allows monitoring of central venous pressure (CVP) and can be used to draw blood samples. CVP measurements are monitored with a manometer connected to the catheter and can also be monitored with a Swan-Ganz catheter. This parameter gives accurate information in assessing the pumping ability of the right side of the heart as well as blood volume returning to the right side of the heart from the systemic circulation.

Cardiac output is the amount of blood pumped through the circulatory system in 1 minute. Measuring the CO helps evaluate cardiac function. One method is thermodilution, which uses the balloon-tipped Swan-Ganz catheter. A solution, usually normal saline (N/S) or 5 percent dextrose in water (D5W) is injected through one port in the catheter. A computer then calculates the CO from the difference in temperature of the injected solution and that of the pulmonary artery.

Equipment and Supplies Used in the CCU

The most frequently used piece of equipment in the CCU is the cardiac monitor. Monitor supplies include the lead wires and cables, disposable pregelled electrodes, and EKG recording paper. There are numerous catheters and guide wires for intravenous use as well as the specialized catheters for arterial, central, and hemodynamic monitoring, such as the Swan-Ganz catheter.

Oxygen tubing, nasal cannula, and masks and emergency oxygen equipment, including a mechanical ventilator, must be readily available. An intubation tray, which is kept with other emergency equipment, contains endotracheal tubes, laryngoscope with straight and curved blades, hand-held resuscitation bag, and a local anesthetic spray, such as Xylocaine. Heparinized blood gas syringes are kept handy for use by respiratory therapists and nurses.

An emergency or crash cart and a defibrillator

must be on the unit near the patient rooms at all times. Pregelled conductive pads and defibrillation paddles are on the defibrillator cart. The crash cart contains all the emergency medications needed during a "Code" as well as supplies such as sterile towels, drapes, gloves, and gowns used to put in emergent intravenous lines, central lines, or Swan-Ganz catheters.

A portable fluoroscope is used when procedures such as pericardiocentesis, central line placement,and temporary pacemaker insertion are performed at bedside. Lead aprons must be available whenever any type of irradiation is being used. Most hospitals have central line carts, pacemaker insertion, and pericardiocentesis trays preassembled with all the necessary sterile supplies. Other supplies that are stocked in the CCU are for temporary pacemaker placement and include the pacer wire, generator, and electrode catheters.

Communication in the CCU

In a CCU there is constant communication with the patients, their families, and their nurses and physicians. The telephone is one of the main means of communicating at the HUC desk. Many of the calls received are from family members inquiring about the patient. Calls need to be directed to the patient's nurse or to the patient, if he or she is able to take calls. The telephone is also frequently used to page the doctors and residents with laboratory results or other information and messages.

The physician sometimes telephones an order for the patient. In some facilities the HUC receives and writes the order in the patient's chart. Facilities with policies that allow HUCs to take telephone orders usually have special requirements. These typically are that the HUC be experienced, trained in a formal program, and certified by NAHUC. In other facilities, the HUC must seek a nurse to take the order.

The next most utilized mode of communication is the computer. The HUC processes the physician's orders via the computer. This includes transcribing them to the nurse's treatment sheet and routing the orders to the appropriate departments. All patient charges generated in the CCU are entered into the computer by the HUC on a daily basis.

Since many tests and procedures need to be scheduled for specific times, the HUC communicates with many different departments in the hospital. For example, EKG, radiology, nuclear medicine, and echocardiography as well as the laboratory and the pharmacy are often contacted to order routine tests or to make a specific request. The HUC also communicates with the emergency room regarding admissions and transfers.

The HUC communicates with the family, who are often in the waiting room between visits. Telephone calls need to be connected to them or messages relayed to them. The family often leaves word with the HUC about where to locate them.

The spiritual services department is very important in helping deal with the emotional needs of the patient and family or just to visit. They also provide Holy Communion or other sacraments for the sick.

Social services and discharge planning nurses are sometimes contacted for advice on any financial worries or family concerns and if home help or nursing home placement needs to be arranged. Cardiac rehabilitation is generally ordered as soon as the patient is able and continues into the discharge phase (Fig. 14–12).

In a "Code" situation, a team will usually respond. The team typically consists of additonal critical care nurses, physicians, anesthesiologist or nurse anesthetist, respiratory therapist, pharmacist, EKG technician, phlebotomist, and chaplain. The HUC must coordinate activities surrounding their participation.

Quality Assurance

All patients admitted to coronary care, or anywhere in the hospital, have the right to expect quality care from everyone who is involved in their care. They have the right to receive all information from their physician and nurses in CCU

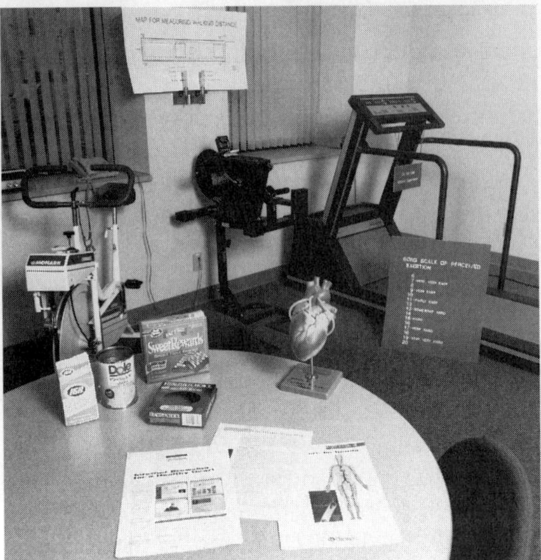

Figure 14–12
Cardiac rehabilitation.

regarding their diagnosis, what treatment options are available for them, and what kind of results they can expect.

They can expect the hospital staff to follow the rules and regulations and safety measures that have been set by the hospital, the state, and the Joint Commission on Accreditation of Hospitals (JCAH). The JCAH regularly audits hospitals to review the quality of care, evaluate the policies and procedures, and advise them if something needs to be improved in order to comply with their standards.

In order to maintain the quality of care in a CCU, committees are established to follow various aspects of care. Examples of what these committees follow are continuity of care, new product evaluation, development or revision of visiting policies, and research into developing more efficient and effective charting methods. The committees work to give the patient the best care possible and to help them and their families through this critical experience.

The CCU patients are sometimes monitored to determine whether the physician is ordering the procedures appropriate to the severity of their illness. This type of peer review is done to ensure that patients do not receive unnecessary, expensive, invasive procedures when simpler, noninvasive, and less expensive tests will result in the same diagnosis.

Closing Thoughts

In summary, a coronary care unit is a highly specialized, well-equipped unit that cares for the acutely ill cardiac patients and that is staffed by specially trained nurses. It is very important, particularly in a smaller critical care setting, that all the nurses, nursing assistants, and health unit coordinators work well together to make the unit run smoothly.

In a department of this level of activity, it is becoming more usual for the HUC to do such things as take orders over the phone and do independent transcription. It is recommended that these be done by certified HUCs with the additional training to do so.

Bibliography

Albert JS, Rippe JM, Booth TJ, Wilcox R (eds): Manual of Cardiovascular Diagnosis and Therapy, 4th ed. Boston, Little, Brown, 1994.

Alexander G: The battle against heart disease. *In* Zeleny R (ed): The 1984 World Book Year Book. Chicago, World Book, Inc, 1984.

Aster G, Roth V: The American Medical Association. New York, EP Dutton, 1980.

Bashore TM: Invasive Cardiology, Principle, and Techniques. Philadephia, BC Decker, 1990.

Billups NF (ed): American Drug Index, Facts and Comparisons, 41st ed. St. Louis, Kluwer, 1997.

Clayman CB: The American Medical Association Family Medical Guide, 3rd ed. New York, Random House, 1994.

Clayman C, Hough H: The American Medical Association Encyclopedia, Vols I and II. New York, Random House, 1989.

Cummings RO (ed): Textbook of Advanced Cardiac Life Support. Dallas, American Heart Association, Scientific Publishing, 1994.

DeAngelis R: Cardiovascular system. *In* Alspach JG: Core Curriculum for Critical Care Nursing, 4th ed. Philadelphia, WB Saunders, 1991.

DeBarkey M, Gotto A: The Living Heart. New York, David McKay, 1977.

English CA, English RJ, Giering LP: Introduction to Nuclear Cardiology, 3rd ed. Wilmington, DuPont Pharma, 1993.

Fowler NO: Diagnosis of Heart Disease. New York, Springer-Verlag, 1991.

Guyton AC: Textbook of Medical Physiology, 6th ed. Philadelphia, WB Saunders, 1981.

Gylys BA, Welding ME: Cardiovascular system. *In* Medical Terminology—A System Approach, 2nd ed. Philadelphia, FA Davis, 1983.

Hall JB, Schmidt GA, Wood LD: Principles of Critical Care, Vol I. New York, McGraw-Hill, 1992.

Shaw M, Cahill M: Handbook of Diagnostic Tests. Springhouse, PA, Springhouse Corp, 1995.

Braunwald, E (ed): Heart Disease—A Textbook of Cardiovascular Medicine, 5th ed, Vol 1. Philadelphia, WB Saunders, 1997.

Heger JW, Rath RF, Nieman JT, Satterfield T: Cardiology, 3rd ed. Baltimore, Williams & Wilkins, 1994.

Hillis LD, Lange RA, Winiford MD, et al: Meglet N, Wilcox R (eds): Manual of Clinical Problems in Cardiology, 5th ed. Boston, Little, Brown & Co, 1995.

Daly S, Ellis R, Falk D, et al: Nursing Procedures. Springhouse, PA, Springhouse Corp, 1992.

Kee JL: Laboratory and Diagnostic Tests with Nursing Implications, 3rd ed. East Norwalk, CT, Appleton & Lange, 1991.

Kerrod R: The Human Body, Vol 7. The World Book Encyclopedia of Science. Chicago, World Book, Inc, 1991.

Larson DE: Mayo Clinic Family Health Book, 1st ed. New York, William Morrow, 1993.

Margolis S, Moses H: The John Hopkins Medical Handbook. New York, Rebus, Inc, 1992.

Massie B, Amadon T: Heart. *In* Turney L: Current Medical Diagnosis & Treatment, 36th ed. East Norwalk, CT, Appleton & Lange, 1997.

McGoon MD: Mayo Clinic Heart Book, 1st ed. New York, William Morrow, 1993.

Moreau D: Nursing Drug Handbook. Springhouse, PA, Springhouse Corp, 1997.

Price SA, Wilson LM: Pathophysiology. *In* Ladig D (ed): Clinical Concepts of Disease Processes, 4th ed. St. Louis, Mosby Yearbook, 1992.

Riedman S: The working heart. *In* Zim HS: Heart. Racine, Western Publishing, 1974.

Rippe JM, Irvin RS, Fink MP: Procedures and Techniques in Intensive Care Medicine. Boston, Little Brown, 1995.

Shaw M, Cahill M: Handbook of Diagnostic Tests. Springhouse, PA, Springhouse Corp, 1995.

Shaw M, Cahill M: Everything You Need to Know About Medical Tests. Springhouse, PA, Springhouse Corp, 1996.

Shtasel P: Medical Tests and Diagnostic Procedure. New York, Harper & Row, 1997.

Skidmore RL: Mosby's Nursing Drug Reference, 1997. St. Louis, CV Mosby, 1997.

Sox HC: Common Diagnostic Tests, Use and Interpretation, 2nd ed. Philadelphia, American College of Physicians, 1990.

Thomas CL (ed): Tabers Cyclopedic Medical Dictionary, 17th ed. Philadelphia, FA Davis, 1993.

Tapley D, Morris T, Rowiand L: The Columbia University College of Physicians & Surgeons. New York, Crown Publishers, 1995.

Texas Heart Institute: Heart Owner's Handbook. New York, John Wiley, 1996.

The Human Heart—A Living Pump. Bethesda, National Institutes of Health, National Heart, Lung & Blood Institute, 1995.

Wright JE, Shelton BK: Desk References for Critical Care Nursing. Boston, Jones & Bartlett Publishers, 1993.

Zaret BL, Moser M, Cohen LS: Yale University School of Medicine Heart Book, 1st ed. New York, Hearst Books, 1992.

Special Care Units

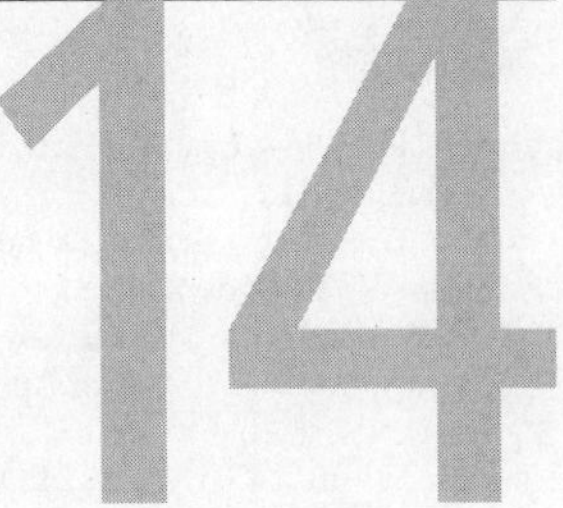

PART 2: NEONATAL INTENSIVE CARE

Patricia A. Hassan Ibrahim

Objectives

Upon completion of this chapter, the reader will be able to:

1. Describe the levels of neonatal care.
2. Discuss causes of and treatments for disorders of the neonate.
3. Explain procedures that are unique to the NICU.
4. Describe the role of the HUC in the NICU.

Vocabulary

Apgar score: A scoring system, developed by Dr. Virginia Apgar in 1952. The score is based on observation of the heart rate, respiratory effort, muscle tone, reflex irritability, and color. Each item is given a score of 0, 1, or 2. Evaluations of all five categories are made at 1 and 5 minutes after birth.

Apnea: The cessation of breathing

Cyanosis: A condition characterized by a bluish discoloration of the skin denoting lack of oxygen

Icterus: A yellowish discoloration of the skin and other organs due to an increase of bilirubin levels in the blood

Kangarooing: Also known as skin-to-skin contact. Offers the premature infant the chance to recover from the effects of interrupted intrauterine growth and development.

Oxycardiogram: Also known as a sleep study. A test ordered on patient-documented apnea or bradycardia. The neonatologist will interpret the test to determine whether the patient will require medication or home monitoring.

Retractions: The act of or condition of drawing back. A term used in relation to the neonate's chest wall drawing back during inhalation. A sign of respiratory distress.

Surfactant system: A surface-active phospholipid mixture secreted by the alveolar type 2 cells of the lungs. The surfactant reduces the surface tension of pulmonary fluid that contributes to the elastic property of pulmonary tissue.

Tachypnea: Excessively rapid respirations.

Common Abbreviations

BAER	Brain auditory evoked response
Bili.	Bilirubin
CPAP	Continuous positive airway pressure
DTP	Diphtheria, tetanus toxoid, and pertussis vaccine
ECMO	Extracorporeal membrane oxygenation
EDD	Expected delivery date
FOB	Father of birth
GCA	Gross Congenital Abnormalities
HBAg	Hepatitis B antigen
HMD	Hyaline membrane disease
HUS	Head ultrasound
ICH	Intracranial hemorrhage
LDRP	Labor, delivery, recovery, post partum
MOB	Mother of birth
NEC	Necrotizing enterocolitis
OCG	Oxycardiogram
OGT	Oral gastric tube
PALS	Pediatric advanced life support
PIV	Peripheral intravenous
PKU	Phenylketonuria
RDS	Respiratory distress syndrome
ROP	Retinopathy of prematurity
RSV	Respiratory syncytial virus
SAT	Saturation
SCN	Special Care Nursery
TTN	Transient tachypnea of the newborn
UAC	Umbilical arterial catheter
UAL	Umbilical arterial line
UVC	Umbilical venous catheter
Vit K	Vitamin K

Introduction

If you are a Health Unit Coordinator (HUC) considering a lateral move to a neonatal intensive care unit (NICU), you are destined for a unique challenge. This directional change will enlighten you with a new appreciation for the miracle of life and a greater understanding of the life cycle. Unlike the adult, the patients of the NICU are unable to verbally communicate their needs. The staff of this special care area is trained to interpret the signals of these tiny creatures in its charge. This section will attempt to help you understand the atmosphere of an NICU and the activities therein.

Description of the Unit

A NICU exists to care for sick newborns with special medical needs. Some infants may require only a little observation, whereas others may need closer individual attention. The patient populace includes medically ill and low birth weight infants. The majority of the infants experience respiratory distress, are at risk for infection, and/or are born prematurely.

Newborn nursery units vary in the level of care that they are capable of delivering. These range from a level 1, which represents the minimum amount of care given to patients, to a level 4, or tertiary center, which can provide the maximum amount of care required. Level 1 nurseries deliver normal postnatal care, which includes newborn assessment, initial inoculations, and circumcisions. Level 2 nurseries deliver the same care as a level 1 nursery plus treatment for hyperbilirubinemia, dehydration, and symptoms related to feeding or nursing problems. Level 3 nurseries deliver neonatal intensive care. Neonates or infants admitted to this level require close cardiac or respiratory monitoring, mechanical ventilation, chest tubes, and other lifesaving techniques. Finally, there is the level 4 or tertiary NICU. These units

The abbreviations listed for this chapter are those that a HUC working in this area would be expected to know. Only those in boldface type are used in the text and appear in boldface when they are used for the first time.

treat neonates or infants born with serious or life-threatening abnormalities and deliver the maximum level of care that the other levels cannot. Some examples of this level of care are extracorporeal membrane oxygenation (**ECMO**) for respiratory conditions not supported by regular mechanical ventilation, open heart surgery for cardiac abnormalities, renal dialysis for kidney disease or abnormalities, and any other condition not supported in the other levels.

The NICU team includes neonatologists, neonatal nurse practitioners, NICU nurses, respiratory care technicians, occupational and physical therapists, social workers, and the HUC. Larger facilities may employ NICU technicians.

The neonatologist is a physician who specializes in the health care and management of the newborn. In most cases, the neonatologist assumes the care of the neonate from the pediatrician. The treatment and daily examination are done by the neonatologist until such time as the care of the newborn is returned to the pediatrician or, in some instances, until discharge.

Neonatal nurse practitioners, under the tutelage of the neonatologist, function much like physician assistants. Their training consists of a degree in nursing followed by an intensive 2-year study and practicum in a level 4 NICU. There they are trained in neonatal intubation and ventilator maintenance, the insertion of an umbilical venous catheter (**UVC**) and umbilical arterial catheter (**UAC**), physical assessment and treatment, lumbar puncture, chest tube insertion, and several other diagnostic and treatment procedures. In most cases, the neonatal nurse practitioner has had several years' experience as a neonatal nurse prior to the advanced training.

NICU nurses are health care professionals who specialize in the care of sick or low birth weight newborns. They are trained in pediatric advanced life support (**PALS**) and provide the bedside care as well as continuous cardiac care. They educate the parents of newborns with special needs in CPR, car seat safety, tracheotomy care, apnea monitoring, and much more. The nurse will remain at the bedside in order to continually monitor and assess the neonate's condition.

The respiratory care practitioners, or respiratory therapists (RTs), are an important part of the NICU team. These professionals specialize in respiratory management and monitoring. They perform diagnostic tests and procedures that assist the neonatologist in the assessment and diagnosis of the sick infant.

Occupational and physical therapists are specialists in the developmental, behavioral, and feeding concerns and other physical needs of the premature or sick full-term infant. They assess the infant's physical abilities in the areas of muscle tone, reflex, movement pattern, and feeding skills. These therapists evaluate and recommend special programs tailored to the needs of the patient, during or after hospitalization.

Social workers help the patient's family work through the emotions of anxiety, fear, depression, guilt, and anger. All these can be a source of stress for the entire family unit. They assist the parents and other family members to deal with issues related to the hospitalization of the neonate. They often provide emotional support, financial advice, and community resource referrals.

The HUC is a valuable member of this health care team. He or she is responsible for telephone management, receptionist duties, maintaining of charts, ordering of supplies, and coordination of the activities of the nursing unit. Much of the unit's organization is the result of this individual's efforts and professional training. With cueing from the neonatologist, the HUC frequently initiates the emergency transport team to pick up or transfer a sick neonate.

A NICU technician functions in the same capacity as a certified nurse's aide. The technician is usually assigned to routine tasks such as bottle feeding, diaper changing, or consoling irritable low-risk infants. This position may also require the person to clean and maintain the equipment used in the neonatal setting.

Medical Terminology of the NICU

Upon entering the NICU, HUCs may feel as though they have arrived in a foreign land, with the inhabitants speaking a foreign language. Some of the medical terminology is generic to other areas of the hospital; however, the following are medical terms that you may come across in a typical NICU setting.

Acrocyanosis: A condition marked by symmetric **cyanosis** of the extremities
Caput succedaneum: Edema occurring in and under the fetal scalp during labor
Cephalhematoma: A hemorrhage of specialized connective tissue limited to the surface of one cranial bone, sometimes occurring during the birthing process
Circumoral: Around or near the mouth
Conjunctival hemorrhage: Bleeding of vessels into the delicate membranes that line the eyelids
Ecchymosis: A small hemorrhagic spot in the skin or mucous membrane, larger than a petechia, that forms a nonelevated, rounded or irregular, blue or purplish patch
Expiratory grunting: A grunting noise produced by the infant, usually accompanied by nasal flaring. Indicative of respiratory distress or cardiac anomalies
Fontanelles: A soft spot; membrane-covered spaces remaining in the incompletely ossified skull of a fetus or infant
Gluteal folds: The folds of the buttocks
Gravida: The number of pregnancies (gravida I is the first pregnancy; gravida II is the second pregnancy)
Hypertonic: A condition of the newborn or neonate characterized by excessive tone of the skeletal muscles
Hypotonic: A condition of the newborn or neonate characterized by decreased tone of the skeletal muscles
Intercostal retractions: The muscles in the area of the xiphoid and the ribs are retracting during inhalation. A sign of respiratory distress.
Mongolian spot: A birthmark typical of neonates born with Down syndrome
Nasal flaring: Exaggerated opening of the nasal passages indicative of respiratory distress
Nevi: Plural form of nevus; a birthmark
Para: Used with roman numerals to designate the number of pregnancies that have resulted in the birth of a viable offspring
Petechia: A pinpoint, nonraised, perfectly round, purplish red spot caused by intradermal or submucous hemorrhage
Plethoric: Characterized by the appearance of a red florid complexion or, specifically, an excessive amount of blood
Rooting: The normal response of the newborn to open the mouth at the slightest touch of either side of the cheek. It indicates that the infant can tolerate oral feedings.
Scaphoid: Boat-shaped, a term used to describe the shape of the abdomen
Seesaw retractions: The right and left sides of the chest wall retract opposite to each other, causing a seesaw effect. A sign of respiratory distress.
Stridor: A harsh, high-pitched respiratory sound, such as the inspiratory sound heard in acute laryngeal obstruction
Suprasternal retractions: The areas situated above the sternum are retracting during inhalation. A sign of respiratory distress.
Sutures: A type of fibrous joint or "seam" in which the opposed bony surfaces are so closely united by a very thin layer of fibrous connective tissue that movement can occur; found only in the skull
Turgor: The normal condition of being turgid; the normal consistency of living tissue
Xiphoid retractions: The xiphoid process retracting during inhalation, indicative of respiratory distress.

Terminology Related to the Sick Newborn

Health problems of the neonate are abundant. They vary from genetic factors to pathologic or physiologic conditions to congenital malformations. This section discusses the most common of these problems.

Respiratory Distress

The most common admitting diagnoses for the newborn are those related to respiratory disorders.

Respiratory distress syndrome (RDS), also

known as hyaline membrane disease (HMD), is one of the most frequent diagnoses. RDS is a severe lung disorder that is responsible for most deaths in the preterm infant. It is seen almost exclusively in infants of diabetic mothers, infants born by cesarean section, and infants born prematurely.

The premature neonate usually presents at birth with low **Apgar scores.** The Apgar scoring system was developed by Dr. Virginia Apgar in 1952. The score is based on assessment of the heart rate, respiratory effort, muscle tone, reflexes, and color. Each parameter is given a score from 0 to 2. These evaluations are done at 1 and 5 minutes after birth.

Shortly after birth, the infant is at risk to develop symptoms of respiratory distress due to immature lungs. The underdeveloped lungs are inefficient for proper gas exchange. Typical symptoms exhibited are hypoventilation, tachypnea, tachycardia, and cyanosis.

Transient tachypnea of the newborn (TTN), also known as respiratory distress syndrome type 2, is a respiratory disorder seen in some full-term or slightly premature infants. It is characterized by symptoms of tachypnea and cyanosis. Most neonatologists believe that the primary cause is the interruption of the normal development of the **surfactant system.** Surfactant is a mixture secreted by the alveolar cells of the lungs that contributes to the elastic property of pulmonary tissue. Premature infants may not be prepared for satisfactory gas exchange because of their incomplete lung maturity.

Apnea, or periodic breathing, is another complication seen in premature infants. The infant will experience periods of rapid respiration accompanied by intervals of very slow, and sometimes short, cycles of no discernible signs of breathing. The deficiency of automatic breathing is usually accompanied by bradycardia and color changes. In most cases, a simple touch of the nurse's hand is sufficient management of the apneic episode. Apnea monitors, which monitor the preterm infant's respirations and heart rate, will sound an alarm to alert the NICU staff of a potential problem. If the problem persists, an **oxycardiogram** (OCG) may be ordered.

Hyperbilirubinemia

Hyperbilirubinemia means increased levels of bilirubin in the blood. This causes a yellowish discoloration of the infant's skin and other organs. The discoloration is also known as jaundice, or **icterus.** In the normal newborn, jaundice may appear within the first 24 hours. Physiologic jaundice is the result of underdeveloped liver function.

Kernicterus

Whatever the cause of hyperbilirubinemia, once the concentration of bilirubin reaches a toxic level, the infant is at risk of developing kernicterus. Kernicterus is severe brain damage due to the deposits of unconjugated bilirubin in the brain cells. The neonatologist orders daily total and direct bilirubin levels whenever jaundice is present.

Sepsis

Sepsis, also known as septicemia, is a bacterial infection in the bloodstream. Susceptibility in neonates is primarily due to a compromised immune system. Infections can occur:

From the mother during the prenatal period.
During labor from infected amniotic fluid.
By direct contact with infected material during the passage through the birth canal.

Septicemia is treated with antibiotics, fluid regulation, and careful monitoring of electrolytes. It is important that the HUC processes the requisition orders for daily electrolyte testing as requested by the neonatologist. Equally important is posting of the test results in the patient's chart as soon as possible. Abnormal results should be brought to the nurse's attention immediately.

Necrotizing Enterocolitis

Necrotizing enterocolitis (NEC) is a dangerous condition in the premature infant. Decreased oxygen and/or blood to the intestines causes inflammation of the bowel. If undetected, necrosis or death of the tissue will follow, requiring surgery to fashion an ileostomy or colostomy. Research has shown significant decrease of NEC in breast-fed animals. This may be because breast milk contains elements that protect the intestines from damage.

Neonatal Treatments and Procedures

Although many of the treatments and procedures are the same from unit to unit, the NICU has some that are unique to the care of the neonate.

Kangaroo Care

Kangarooing is also known as skin-to-skin contact. It provides the premature infant the opportunity to recover from the effects of interrupted intrauterine growth and development. This is achieved once the infant is stabilized and free of any complications. The theory of skin-to-skin contact and its benefits originates from a marsupial mammal, the kangaroo. The female of the species carries the premature young in an abdominal pouch. The young are born after a short gestational period, usually from 27 to 40 days. Once born, they climb into the abdominal pouch to complete their growth and development. This period may be as long as 8 months.

The procedure of kangarooing is simple. Clad only in a diaper and in some cases a skullcap, the infant is removed from the incubator and placed on the mother's bare chest. Mother and child are covered with a blanket. The room is kept dark and the noise level reduced, thus simulating the womb. The hospital facility usually provides the NICU with comfortable overstuffed glider rockers or recliners. Electrodes and cables remain attached to the infant for uninterrupted monitoring by the nursing staff.

The benefits of kangaroo care are outstanding. According to the book *Kangaroo Care, The Best You Can Do To Help Your Preterm Infant*, by Susan M. Ludington-Hoe with Susan K. Golant, international scientific studies have shown that skin-to-skin contact offers the preterm infant many physical and emotional benefits. These include:

- A stable heart rate
- More regular breathing
- Improved oxygenation throughout the body
- Prevention of cold stress. (When a preemie becomes too cold, he or she burns up much-needed oxygen and calories to stay warm.)
- Longer periods of sleep (allows for brain maturity)
- More rapid weight gain
- Reduction of purposeless activity, which simply burns calories at the expense of the infant's growth and health
- Decreased crying
- Longer periods of alertness
- Opportunities to breast feed and enjoy the benefits of breast milk
- Earlier bonding
- Increased likelihood of an earlier discharge from the hospital.

Both parents benefit from kangaroo care. Studies show that those who have practiced the skin-to-skin contact have felt more positive about the difficult birth experience. They gain confidence in the handling of their baby and are more eager to take the baby home.

Although there are no supplies for the HUC to maintain with this treatment, he or she may be responsible for restricting noise so that the procedure can be fully effective.

Phototherapy

Phototherapy is a treatment for hyperbilirubinemia. The infant is placed under an intense fluorescent light, also known as a bili light. A bili blanket (Fig. 14–13 can also be used. The bili blanket is placed on the bottom of the isolette or incubator; a receiving blanket is placed over it; and the infant is placed on the blanket. If the bilirubin levels are high, the neonatologist may order both treatments at the same time. In either case, the infant's eyes are covered to prevent direct exposure to the bright light. The blue range of the light causes photo-oxidation of the elevated

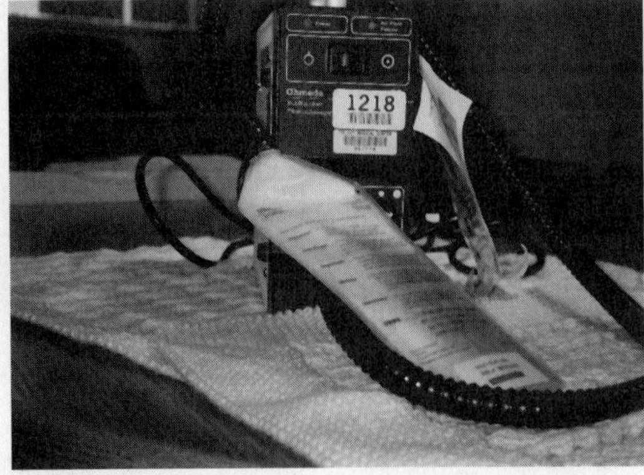

Figure 14–13
Bili blanket for phototherapy. (Courtesy of Tri-City Medical Center, Vista, CA.)

bilirubin. In some facilities the HUC is responsible for the upkeep and inventory of this equipment. Broken or malfunctioning equipment should be reported as soon as possible so that it can be repaired. An inventory of such equipment should be included in the day's routine so that treatment of the patient is not delayed until rental equipment arrives. The frequent use of this treatment dictates that a sufficient number of eye shields be available at all times.

Exchange Transfusion

An exchange transfusion is performed on an infant with hyperbilirubinemia due to ABO or Rh factor incompatibility. Small amounts of the infant's blood are removed and replaced with compatible blood. The exchange removes sensitized erythrocytes and lowers the serum bilirubin. The exchange transfusion is a sterile surgical procedure, and the proper sterile equipment should be on hand at all times. Although this procedure is not an everyday event, the HUC must maintain supplies to ensure that inventory is sufficient and that supplies are within the expiration date.

Mechanical Ventilation

As in any ICU, mechanical ventilation is a routine affair. In most facilities, it is the responsibility of the respiratory therapy department to maintain this equipment. The NICU staff is always prepared for admissions that might utilize such equipment.

Surfactant Therapy

Surfactant is a surface-active phospholipid mixture secreted by the epithelium of the alveoli in the lungs. This mixture reduces the surface force of pulmonary fluids that add to the elasticity of pulmonary tissue. The neonate who is delivered before the lungs have completely matured will not be prepared for satisfactory gas exchange. Surfactant therapy is the administration of a synthetic surfactant substance. This is done using sterile technique. Depending on hospital policy, either the NICU nurse or the respiratory therapist, or both, administers the medication directly into the endotracheal tube while maintaining mechanical ventilation. Synthetic surfactant is a medication that promotes normal growth and development of immature lungs.

Umbilical Arterial and Venous Catheters

The insertion of an UAC or UVC is done under sterile surgical technique. A catheter is inserted into a blood vessel in the umbilicus of the newborn. Each umbilical cord has venous and arterial access. The UVC is used for intravenous fluid therapy, venous access for blood drawing, or an exchange transfusion. The insertion of a UAC is done principally for continuous cardiac pressure monitoring in high-risk neonates or for arterial access for blood gases.

Lumbar Puncture and Blood Cultures

Although lumbar puncture and blood culture are not unique to a NICU, they are done frequently. An abundant supply of infant lumbar puncture trays is required to maintain continuity of care. The same is true for aerobic and anaerobic culture medium bottles for blood cultures.

Brain Auditory Evoked Response

The brain auditory evoked response test (BAER) is a routine hearing test done on premature infants. Because of the interruption of intrauterine growth and maturity, the preemie is susceptible to hearing impairment. Early intervention can benefit the child's speech patterns in later years. The neonatologist will frequently order the test at a specific gestational age. It will be the responsibility of the HUC to make the necessary arrangements at the proper time.

Retinopathy of Prematurity (ROP) Ophthalmic Examination

In premature births, the infant's eyes may be affected by interrupted development. The neonatologist routinely orders an ophthalmology consult. The HUC will make the necessary arrangements. During consultation, the ophthalmologist examines the infant's eyes for signs of retinal detachment, dilation of posterior vessels, iris vessel dilation, pupil rigidity, hemorrhages, and other signs of abnormality that may need early intervention or treatment.

Equipment and Supplies Used in the NICU

The NICU is supplied with highly sophisticated equipment to monitor newborns and neonates during their stay. This equipment is designed to promote the growth and development of the patient as well as to treat emergencies as they arise.

Thermoregulated Environments

Thermoregulation, or regulation of external body temperature, is crucial to the premature and newborn infant. The infant's ability to maintain body heat enables him or her to burn less calories. If the infant does not need to generate his or her own heat, the energy will be devoted to development. Heat conservation is achieved by placing the naked infant in a temperature-regulated environment. The initial assessment is carried out while the newborn is placed on a radiant warmer (Fig. 14–14). Because all four sides can be lowered, the surface of the radiant warmer allows the neonatologist the space to perform diagnostic or lifesaving procedures.

Incubator and Isolette

Once stabilized, the patient may be placed in an incubator (Fig. 14–15) or an isolette (Fig. 14–16). The incubator has a Plexiglas top that allows a clear view of the infant from all angles. Access is through six portholes, two each on the front and back and one on each side. Access can also be gained by pushing back the cover or rolling back the Plexiglas top. Both incubator and isolette

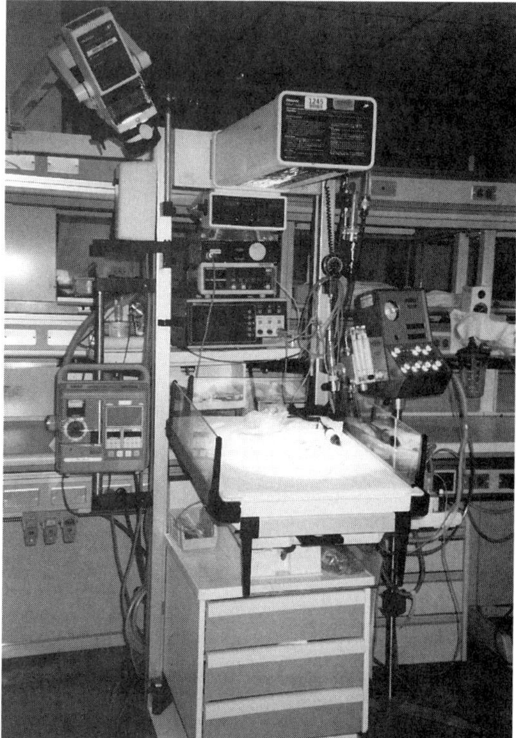

Figure 14–14
Fully equipped radiant warmer. To the right is a Bear Ventilator. In the center are oximetry and cardiac monitors. (Courtesy of Tri-City Medical Center, Vista, CA.)

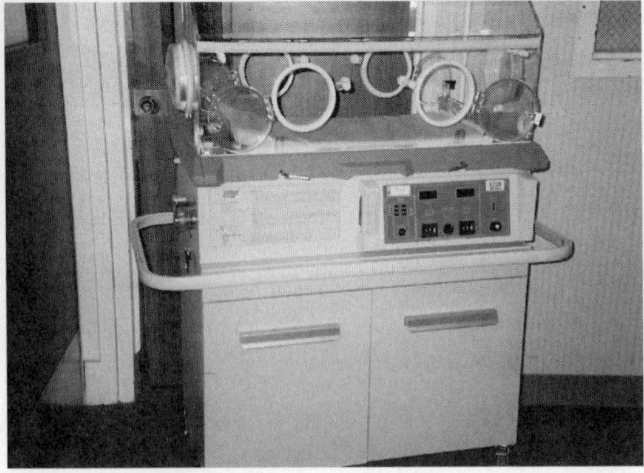

Figure 14–15
Incubator with six access portholes. (Courtesy of Tri-City Medical Center, Vista, CA.)

can provide the patient with an oxygenated environment with controlled humidity and temperature.

The Emergency Transporter

The emergency transporter (Fig. 14–17) is a mobile incubator equipped with a ventilator, oxygen, a cardiac monitor, and an oximetry monitor; it is also capable of temperature and humidity regulation. Most NICUs maintain a transport bag equipped with medications, IV supplies, umbilical catheters, and endotracheal tubes of various sizes that is stored with and will accompany the transporter. This ensures that the team will be prepared for any emergency.

Arterial Blood Gas Analyzer

An arterial blood gas analyzer machine (Fig. 14–18) is vital to any NICU. Because mechanically ventilated patients require constant gas exchange monitoring, most NICUs are equipped with one. The respiratory therapy department is responsible for the daily maintenance and cleaning of the analyzer. The machine is a computerized tool capable of interpreting arterial blood gas results in minutes.

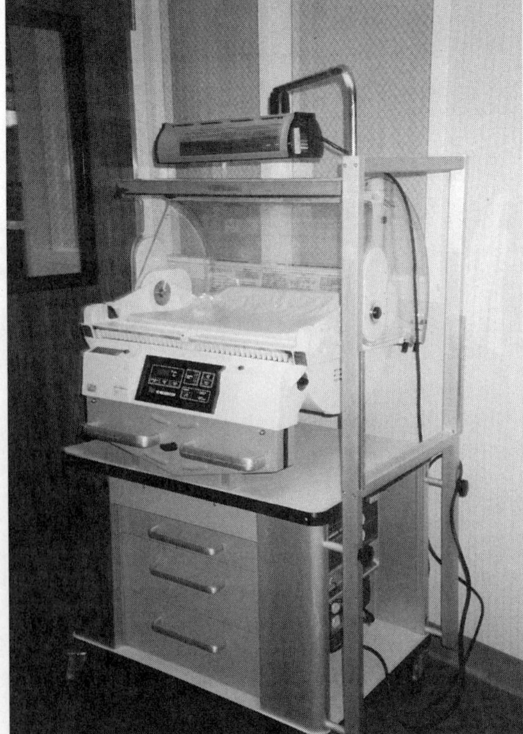

Figure 14–16
Isolette with Bili light. (Courtesy of Tri-City Medical Center, Vista, CA.)

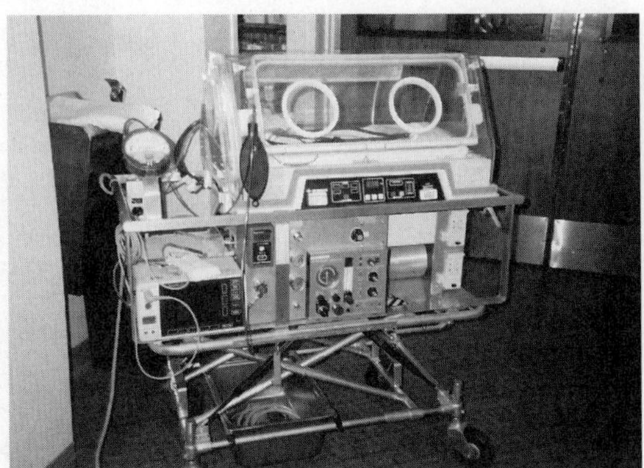

Figure 14–17
Fully equipped emergency transporter. (Courtesy of Tri-City Medical Center, Vista, CA.)

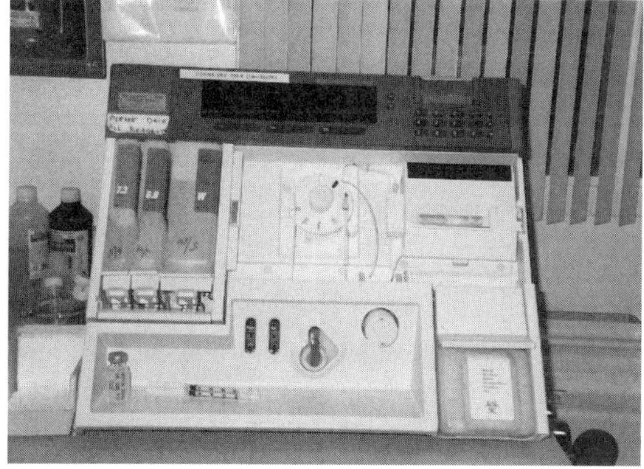

Figure 14–18
Arterial blood gas machine. (Courtesy of Tri-City Medical Center, Vista, CA.)

Communication Within the NICU

Communication is the key to a successful operation. It is vital that there be an open line of communication between the staff of the NICU, the staff of the labor and delivery departments, and the HUC. Daily shift change reports between the two units are usually established in order to be prepared for high-risk deliveries. This is also true of other facilities with lower or higher levels of care capabilities. The HUC plays an important role in the preparation for potential admissions or transfers. The well-trained HUC will be aware of the needs of the staff and will ensure that all equipment and supplies are available when an emergency arises.

The Role of the HUC During a Neonatal Emergency Transport

The chances for survival of the neonate born with complications lie within the first 30 to 60 minutes. It is vital that the NICU transport team be prepared for that primary call. The neonate's pediatrician will notify the facility's neonatologist. A complete history of the infant's condition is relayed. This alerts the team to assemble the equipment and staff needed to complete the transport. The transport team usually consists of a neonatologist, a neonatal nurse practitioner, a NICU nurse, and a respiratory therapist. The HUC is responsible for mobilizing the Emergency Medical Service (EMS) system by calling the local ambulance service. The next step is to contact the transferring facility to obtain demographic information on the patient. This information is immediately called in to the admissions department. For the necessary documents to be expedited, good communication between the NICU HUC and the admitting department is essential. Any documentation or chart preparation that can feasibly be accomplished prior to the arrival of the patient should be done and placed at the bedside for the nurses to use. The transportation of a high-risk infant is very stressful. However, the turmoil of the incident can be transformed into an uneventful episode with anticipation, coordination, open communication, and teamwork.

Medication in the NICU

Medications ordered for patients in the NICU are similar to those ordered for any other unit in a hospital. The same is true for drug classifications, except that the dosage will differ because of the patient's weight. There are, however, two medications that are unique to the NICU. These are Exosurf and Survanta. Both medications are used to treat RDS neonates who are being mechanically ventilated. Both are synthetically created surfactant substitutes with some chemical variations. These agents are extremely costly, at approximately 1000 dollars per 10 ml vial.

Stock Drugs

Cost containment of stock drugs is the responsibility of the HUC in the NICU. To prevent lost revenue from missing stock drug charges, a counting system is implemented and maintained. This is easily accomplished by working the task into the daily HUC routine of each shift. A careful inventory of all stock drugs should be cataloged. The nursing staff is alerted if medications are missing. The HUC and the nurse can investigate the situation as a team.

Closing Thoughts

Working in the neonatal intensive care unit can be a very a rewarding experience. It can also be a stressful one. If you are considering such a professional move, it is wise to be prepared to handle the additional anxiety by attending workshops or seminars in "how to deal with stress" and "death and dying." A new emergency arises with every admission; your composure during those times will produce a more favorable atmosphere for the staff, the patient's family, and yourself.

The organization of the unit is dependent on the skills of the health unit coordinator. A check-off list of the routine daily tasks is suggested. The tasks can be checked off as you complete each one. This is the best way to stay on track in high-pressure situations.

The neonatal intensive care unit is a genuine challenge to one's abilities. It offers the HUC the opportunity for professional growth and a true sense of fulfillment.

Review Questions

1. Differentiate between the four levels of neonatal care.
2. Describe the treatment for RDS.
3. Name and describe two procedures that are unique to neonatal care.
4. List the duties of the HUC role in the emergency transport scenario.

Bibliography

Dorland's Illustrated Medical Dictionary, 27th ed. Philadelphia, WB Saunders, 1988.

Grolier Encyclopedia of Knowledge, Vol 11 Danbury, CT, Grolier, 1995.

Jorgensen KM: Developmental Care of the Preterm Infant, A Concise Overview. Published as an educational service by the Developmental Care Division of Children's Medical Ventures, Inc., 1993.

Ludington-Hoe SM, Golant SK: Kangaroo Care: The Best You Can Do To Help Your Preterm Infant. New York, Bantam Books, 1993.

Whaley LF, Wong DL: Essentials of Pediatric Nursing. St. Louis, CV Mosby, 1992.

Whitelaw A: Kangaroo baby care: Just a nice experience or an important advance for preterm infants? Pediatrics 1990;85:4.

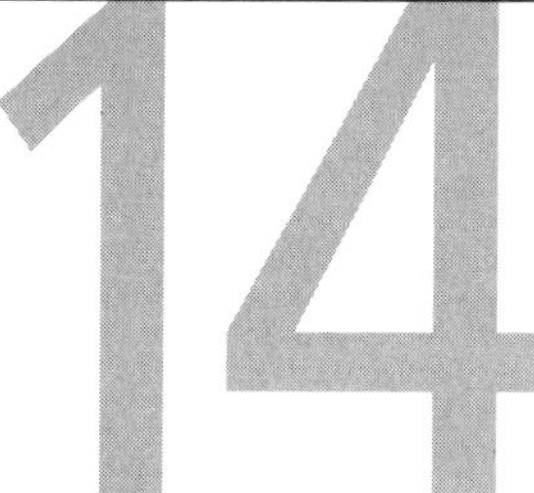

Special Care Units

PART 3: OPEN HEART RECOVERY

Linda Black/Christina Washington

Objectives

At the completion of this chapter, the reader should be able to:

1. List the reasons for the development of open heart recovery units.
2. List four basic open heart surgical procedures.
3. Identify the blood vessels that are used as grafts in the CABG procedure.
4. Name five different types of equipment that are used for the patient in the open heart recovery unit.
5. Briefly describe the role of the health unit coordinator in the open heart recovery unit.

Vocabulary

Allograft: Transplantation of tissue or organs from members of the same species

Annuloplasty: A procedure that reduces an enlarged annulus

Annulus: The fibrous ring surrounding a valve

Commissurotomy: Surgical separation of stenosed valve leaflets

Dysrhythmia: Any abnormal heartbeat or deviation from the normal pattern of heartbeat

Hemodynamic: Relating to the forces involved in circulating blood through the body

Homeostasis: The state of dynamic equilibrium of the internal environment of the body

Thermistor: A form of resistor that is capable of determining very small changes in temperature

Valsalva sinuses: Three dilated areas in the wall of the aorta just behind the three flaps of the aortic valve

Valvuloplasty: Surgical repair of torn leaflets of a valve

Xenograft: Transplantation of tissue from species other than human

Common Abbreviations

ABG Arterial blood gas
AS Aortic stenosis
ASD Atrial septal defect
AVR Aortic valve repair or replacement
CABG Coronary artery bypass graft
CAD Coronary artery disease
CBP Cardiac bypass pump
CI Cardiac index
CO Cardiac output
CP Chest pain
CPAP Continuous positive airway pressure
CT Chest tubes
CVP Central venous pressure
Cx Circumflex artery
DP Dorsalis pedis
DTA Dissecting thoracic aneurysm
ET Tube Endotracheal tube
IABP Intra-aortic balloon pump
IMA Internal mammary artery
IMV Intermittent mandatory ventilation
LAD Left anterior descending
LCA Left coronary artery
LIMA Left internal mammary artery
LVAD Left ventricular assist device
MIDCAB Minimally invasive direct coronary artery bypass
MV Mixed venous
MVR Mitral valve repair or replacement
OHRU Open heart recovery unit
PAP Pulmonary artery pressure
PCWP Pulmonary capillary wedge pressure
PEEP Positive expirator-end pressure
RCA Right coronary artery
SaO_2 Oxygen saturation
SVG Saphenous vein graft
SVR Systemic vascular resistance
TEDS Thromboembolic deterrent stockings
TR Tricuspid regurgitation
VSD Ventricular septal defect

History

In the third decade of the 20th century, the first recorded heart surgery was performed on a human patient. The procedure was the repair of a stenosed mitral valve (MVR). The procedure came to be known as a **commissurotomy.** Since that time, amazing progress has been made in the variety of heart procedures that have become available. These include valve repairs and replacements, repairs of structural defects, coronary artery bypass grafts (CABG), and total heart transplants. In 1994 the following statistics were reported by the American Heart Association:

Procedure	Number Performed
CABG	501,000
Heart transplants	2,340
Other open heart surgery	67,000
Valve replacements	60,000

Although it is common practice to refer to any heart surgery as open heart surgery, technically only those procedures in which the heart is cut into qualify as "open heart surgery."

The abbreviations listed for this chapter are those that a HUC working in this area would be expected to know. Only those in boldface type are used in the text and appear in boldface when they are used for the first time.

Introduction

The increasing number of heart surgical procedures made it obvious that the time was coming to have units devoted to the immediate postoperative care of the patients undergoing them. The patients required diligent monitoring of many parameters, and they were ventilated. The amount of equipment alone made it difficult for recovery and other care to take place in a unit such as the PACU, SICU, PICU, or CCU. If hospitals have PICUs, the infant and pediatric heart surgical patients may be sent directly to that unit.

A major advantage to having the postoperative heart surgery patients in one area is that the physician specialists involved in their care can be immediately available to several patients who may need their attention. Another advantage is skill retention by the members of the staff of the unit.

Open heart recovery receives its patients directly from the operating room. The transport team consists of an anesthesiologist, a nurse anesthetist, and two operating room registered nurses. A patient typically spends an average of 18 to 48 hours in the unit, depending on how well he or she has tolerated the surgical procedure and how long it takes to fully recover from anesthesia.

Design of the Unit

The number of beds in the open heart recovery unit (OHRU) depends on the size of the heart center that it serves and the volume of heart surgical cases that it handles. The OHRUs are among the latest in the series of specialty units.

A configuration that seems to work well is one of "open concept." There are a number of bays that can be a single size or, left open, up to twice the size, if necessary to accommodate the extra equipment required by some patients. Each patient is separated from the others by curtains, when necessary for privacy. At the head of the stretcher or bed in each bay is wall oxygen, suction, and monitoring equipment. There is an alarm bell for the caregivers to use in the event of a cardiac arrest or other life-threatening emergency as well as a large wall clock with a second hand.

Another design involves large private rooms with half-glass walls. This type of area provides more privacy, yet allows visibility by essential personnel. This design is more expensive than the first.

The desk is located so that all patient care areas can be seen. The central bank of monitors is sometime off to the side, away from trafficked areas. In large units there may be several pods of patient care areas, each of which has a central desk.

Staffing of the Unit

The OHRU is usually attended by a combination of physicians, led by the board-certified cardiovascular surgeons. There are cardiologists, pulmonologists, and anesthesiologists, also board-certified, immediately available on a rotating on-call schedule. In teaching hospitals there are residents and fellows on the medical team as well.

The nurses working in OHRU are usually Bachelor-prepared, have completed ACLS certification, and preferably have had either PACU or CCU training and certification, or both.

A respiratory therapist is usually assigned to the unit, because every patient comes back from the operating room on a ventilator. There are monitor technicians, who watch the bank of monitors to troubleshoot for problems with heart rhythm. In some institutions, health unit coordinators are trained into this position and alternate between coordinating and monitoring. The HUCs are centrally located so that they can provide support to any of the staff who needs it. They are the heart of the communication system.

Related Anatomy

The heart is the cornerstone of the circulatory system. It is a hollow muscular organ, a bit larger than a man's closed fist. It is about 12 cm long,

9 cm wide, and 6 cm thick and weighs about 300 gm (10 oz). The heart rests on the diaphragm and to the left of the sternum, between the second and fifth ribs. It is surrounded by the lungs, each of which has a notch called the cardiac impression into which the heart fits.

The heart beats over 240 billion times in an average lifetime, beating over 100,000 times a day. It pumps over 7000 liters (1835 gallons) of blood through 60,000 miles of blood vessels daily. The blood vessels form a network of tubes that carry blood from the heart to the body tissues and then return it to the heart.

The heart is divided into two halves by a muscular wall, the septum. Each half has two chambers: the upper (atrium), a collecting chamber, and the lower (ventricle), a pumping chamber. As each chamber contracts, blood is pushed into the ventricles or out of the heart through an artery. The heart contains structures known as valves to prevent the backflow of blood.

Blood returning to the heart enters the right atrium from the coronary sinus, which collects circulated blood from the walls of the heart and two veins:

- The superior vena cava returns blood from the upper torso and limbs.
- The inferior vena cava carries blood from the lower torso and limbs.

The blood is pumped from the right atrium through the tricuspid valve into the right ventricle. From there it goes into the pulmonary artery (the only artery in the body to carry unoxygenated blood) to be distributed to the lungs, where the blood exchanges carbon dioxide for oxygen. The enriched blood leaves the lungs via the pulmonary veins and is carried to the left atrium. It passes through the mitral valve into the left ventricle. The blood leaves the heart through the aortic semilunar valves and into the aorta itself for distribution throughout the body.

The heart, like any other tissue in the body, must have its own blood vessels. Coming directly off the aorta are the two main coronary arteries: the left coronary artery (**LCA**) and the right coronary artery (**RCA**). The LCA divides into two branches, the left anterior descending artery (**LAD**) and the circumflex coronary artery (**CX** or CCA). The LAD supplies the left ventricle, myocardium, septum, and portions of the right ventricle with nourishment. The CX and its branches supply most of the left atrium, the lateral wall of the left ventricle, and part of the posterior wall of the left ventricle. Diagonal branches that arise between the LAD and CX are distributed along the free wall of the left ventricle. The RCA arises from the right **Valsalva's sinus** of the aorta and has branches that supply the right ventricle, a portion of the septum, and, in 50 percent of the population, the sinoatrial node, which is known as the natural pacemaker of the heart.

There can be many variations in the branching patterns of the coronary arteries. The myocardium contains many collateral circulation paths (alternative routes) that increase in number with age. These collaterals help keep the heart muscle alive when the main vessels become obstructed. When a major coronary vessel is about 90 percent obstructed, blood will flow through the collaterals (Fig. 14–19).

The flow of blood through the coronary circulation provides adequate blood supply and oxygen to the heart muscle. Despite scientific advances, coronary artery disease (**CAD**) and its complications remain the leading cause of death in the United States.

The Surgical Experience

There are four basic cardiac surgical procedures: coronary artery bypass grafts (**CABG**), septal repairs, valvular surgery, and aneurysm repairs.

Coronary Artery Bypass Grafts

Traditional CABG

CABG surgery is performed when coronary arteries have been critically stenosed. The patient will typically undergo diagnostic testing consisting of echocardiogram, stress testing, and cardiac catheterization with coronary arteriography before treatment is undertaken. Less invasive proce-

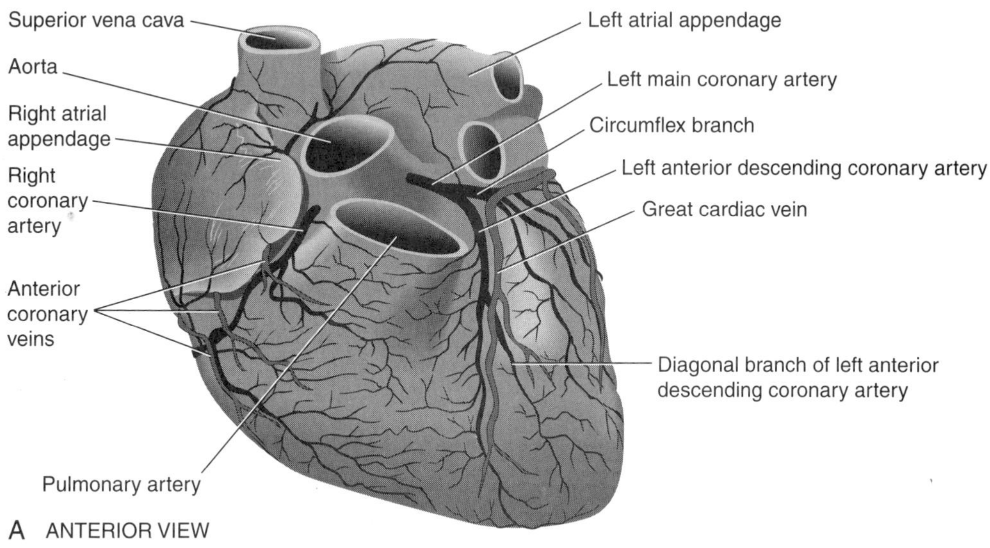

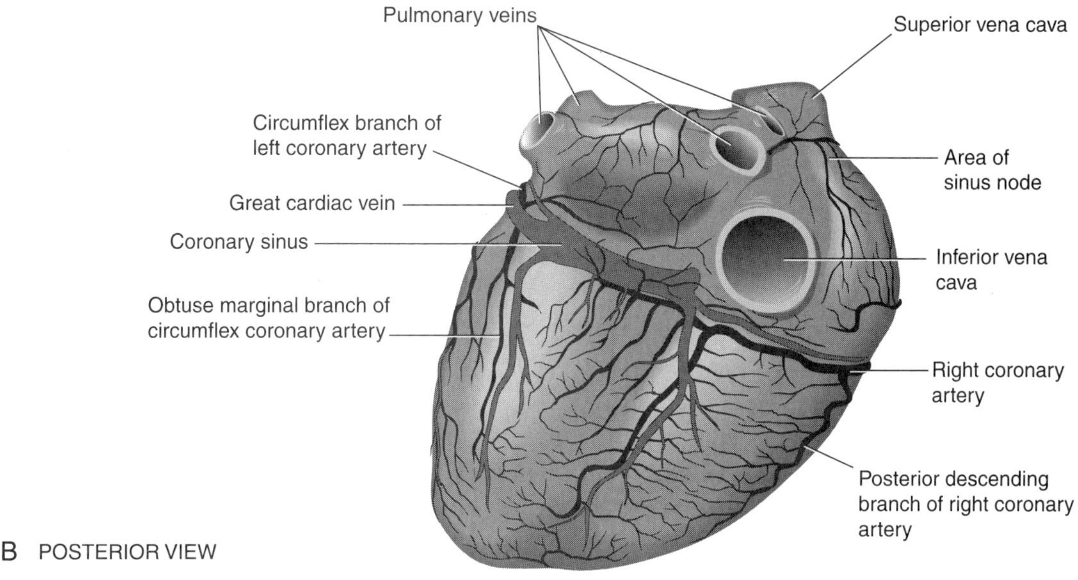

Figure 14–19
Views of the heart.

dures, such as angioplasty, stent procedures, and ablations, are considered first; only if they are found inappropriate for the situation does CABG become the treatment of choice.

Favaloro and his colleagues first perfected the CABG procedure in 1969. The procedure that they developed used saphenous vein grafts (SVG). It soon became one of the most widely performed surgical procedures in the United States. Studies done in 1982 and 1983 influenced the choice of vessel used for the graft. It was demonstrated that using the internal mammary artery (**IMA**) improved long-term patency and minimized atherosclerosis, so now that procedure has come into favor.

The CABG procedure begins with harvesting a segment of healthy vessel from the saphenous vein (**SVG**). This is then sutured from the site of a small hole made in the aorta to an area in the affected coronary artery that is relatively disease-free (Fig. 14–20). The alternative procedure utilizes the IMA.

The saphenous veins are typically obtained by removing them through an uninterrupted longitudinal incision. James H. Khan, M.D., and Kathy Mannion, P.A., of Charleston, West Virginia, have pioneered a technique that minimizes the incision to harvest the saphenous vein. Small incisions

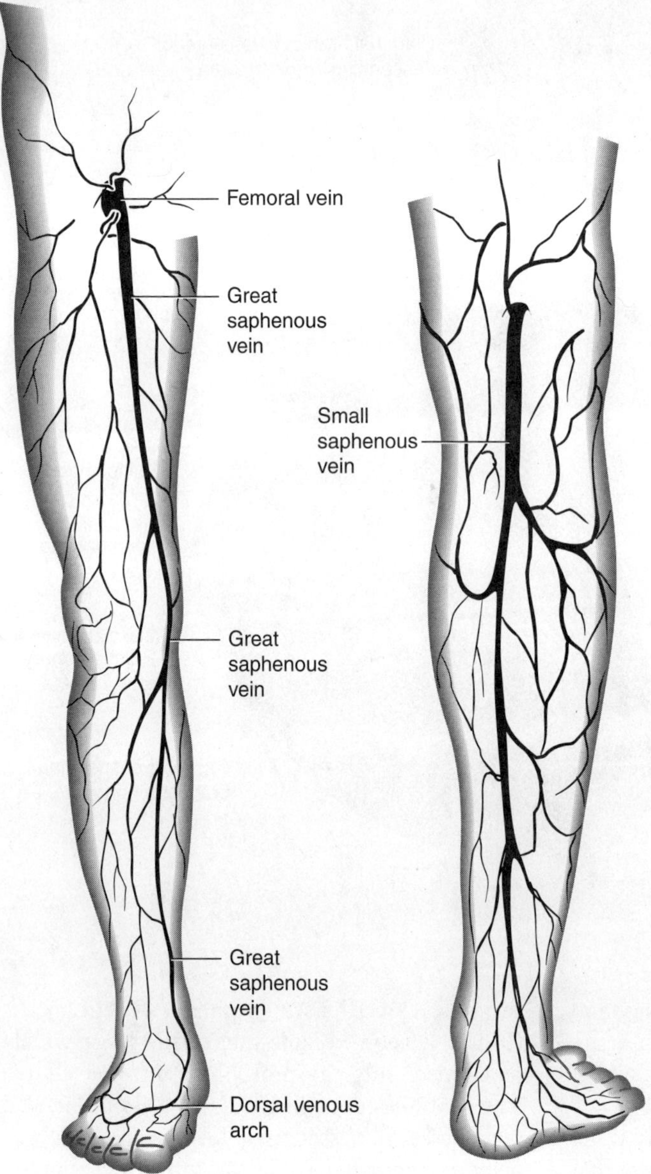

Figure 14–20
Saphenous veins.

are made in the leg, and the vein is visualized microscopically and removed. This technique limits the potential for infection. The IMA is retrieved by retracting the sternum and entering the pleural space. The adjacent tissue is dissected to expose the artery (Fig. 14–21).

Although the SVG and IMA are the vessels of choice, there are situations that preclude their use. Examples of such situations are trauma, burns, patients having had previous vein strippings, patients having had previous CABG, and amputees. In these cases, alternative venous and arterial **allografts** have been used:

- Cephalic vein
- Basilic vein
- Radial artery
- Right gastroepiploic artery (GEA)
- Inferior epigastric artery
- Umbilical vein

In some cases, the patient's vessels are damaged to the extent that frozen donor veins are used, when available. Synthetic grafts are used as a last resort. Dacron or polytetrafluoroethylene (PTFE) is the most common material used in the manufacture of artificial grafts.

A cardiopulmonary bypass machine **(CBP)** with a pump oxygenator (heart-lung machine) is used in nearly all coronary bypass procedures. The use of this machine dictates that a perfusionist be on the surgical team in addition to the cardiovascular surgeons, anesthesia personnel, and operating room nurses.

The blood is drained from the left atrium and ventricle and is passed through this pulsatile pump or roller mechanism. The blood is heparinized, oxygenated, and even anesthetized and returned to the circulation (Fig. 14–22). Advances in CBP have been such that it is possible to accomplish the entire procedure without the use of banked blood, using the patient's blood and a device known as a cell saver.

Minimally Invasive Direct Coronary Artery Bypass

MIDCAB is also known as limited access coronary artery surgery. Like the CABG, its purpose is

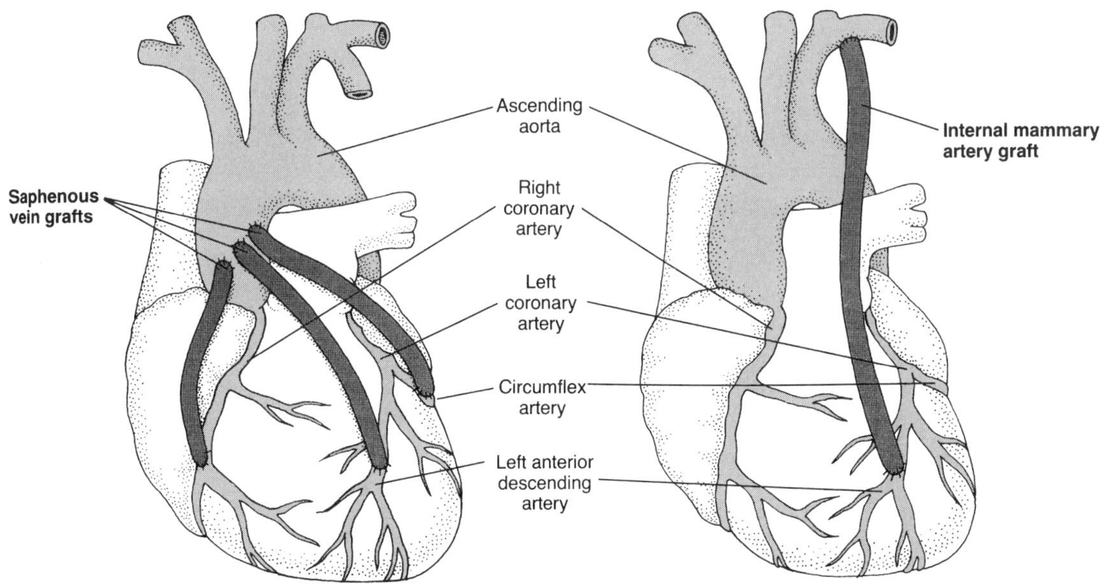

Figure 14–21
CABG, two methods. (From Ignatavicius DD, Workman ML, Mishler MA [eds]: Medical-Surgical Nursing: A Process Approach, 2nd ed. Philadelphia, WB Saunders, 1995.)

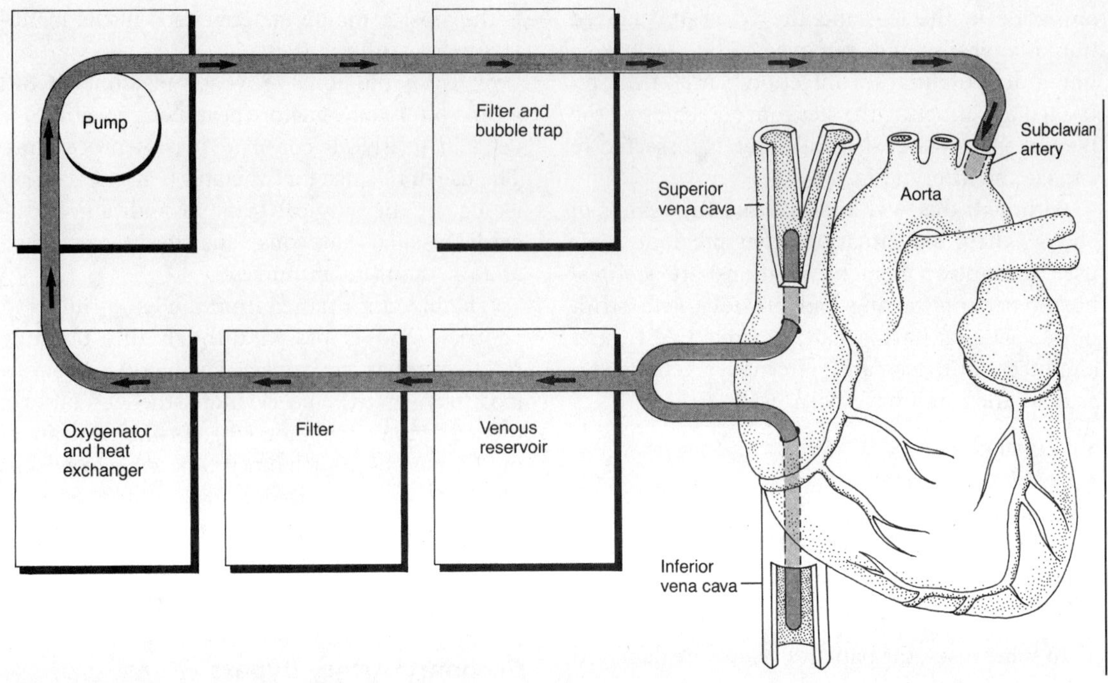

Figure 14–22
Cardiac bypass pump. (From Ignatavicius DD, Workman ML, Mishler MA [eds]: Medical-Surgical Nursing: A Process Approach, 2nd ed. Philadelphia, WB Saunders, 1995.)

to reroute blood around the blocked areas in the coronary arteries. The main advantage of the MIDCAB is that in many cases the use of the heart-lung machine can be avoided. It is therefore performed on the beating heart. It is best used when only one or two arteries need to be bypassed. A series of small ports (holes) are made in the chest through which the cardiac surgeon can insert instruments. An incision is made directly over the artery to be bypassed. The IMA is detached inside the chest wall under direct vision through a scope and is reattached to the coronary artery in question. In case of complications, the open chest procedure may need to be done.

Another procedure that does use the CBP machine but is easier on the patient than the traditional CABG is the port access CABG (PACABG). Several small ports are made in the chest. This procedure uses the IMA to attach to the heart. A second choice is the femoral vessel from the leg. The surgical team passes instruments through the ports to accomplish the bypass. With the use of a special scope, the surgeon can view the manipulations on video monitors.

Statistics are still being gathered on both these procedures. The results have been promising thus far. The ultimate goal is to develop a procedure for grafting the arteries that is no more invasive than coronary angioplasty. If this can be accomplished, the savings will be tremendous.

Septal Repairs

Ventricular Septal Defect Surgery. VSD surgery is performed when there is a large opening between the ventricles. Oxygen-enriched blood from the left ventricle flows through the defect into the right ventricle, where it is pumped back into the lungs. This is an ineffective use of the system. The pump is asked to pump extra to no avail, since it is merely recirculating volumes of oxygenated blood through the lungs. This extra work causes the heart to enlarge. Small defects often close on their own, but the larger ones become symptomatic and require surgical correction. Determination of the best time to operate on infants with this problem depends on the exhibition of associated problems. If these infants have hypertension in the lungs, correction must be immediate. In some other cases it can be delayed.

The corrective surgery may be as simple as suturing the defect. More often, it requires a patch. The patch is of synthetic material that is covered by normal heart lining and sewn into place, where it becomes a permanent part of the heart. In facilities where there is no PICU, the infant will be seen in the OHRU.

Atrial Septal Defect Surgery. During intrauterine development, the fetus has a naturally occurring opening in the membranes between the atria. Problems occur when the opening does not spontaneously close after birth. The results are very good when surgical procedures for this defect (**ASD**) are performed before the infant is 1 year of age.

The exact procedure performed is determined by the nature and location of the defect. When there is simply a failure of the opening to close, a patch graft is sufficient to correct the problem. If the opening is near the top of the atria, there is also a malpositioning of the pulmonary veins. When the defect is repaired, an additional step must be taken to direct the oxygenated blood into the left atrium. This is done by use of a "baffle patch." When the defect occurs very low in the atrial septum, there frequently are associated abnormalities in the mitral and tricuspid valves and occasionally a ventricular defect as well. The repair in these cases involves procedures to correct all those problems.

Occasionally the smaller, simple defects are not discovered until later in life, because they have not been symptomatic. It is recommended that once discovered they be repaired, because the opening raises the risk of a clot traveling into the circulation and causing a stroke. The repair in adults is very safe and effective. In most centers the operative mortality rate is less than 1 percent.

Valve Surgery

The valves can be considered the doorways of the heart. Open doorways allow the blood to flow only in one direction. When the doorways are closed, a strong seal is created to prevent the backflow of blood. Although there are four valves, problems serious enough to require surgery generally occur in the two on the left side of the heart—the mitral valve and the aortic valve. When they become damaged, it may be in either of two ways:

Leaky valves regurgitate and allow reverse blood flow. Stenotic valves restrict the blood flow forward by not opening fully.

These problems may be caused by aging, infection with scarring, heart attacks, or congenital defects. Valves can be repaired or replaced, depending on the extent and location of the damage.

Valvuloplasty is the repair of a valve. It is usually reserved for incompetent mitral or tricuspid valves, which are the valves that separate the atria and ventricles.

Commissurotomy is a surgical procedure done to treat mitral stenosis. The adhesions that cause the leaves of the valve to stick together are incised, and the size of the mitral orifice is increased.

Annuloplasty involves surgically tightening the natural ring (**annulus**) in which the valve is seated.

Valve Replacements. The material used for the replacement valves varies. Tissue valves are usually **xenografts** from pig aortic valves or from the pericardium of cows. Human grafts (allografts) are rarely available. Tissue valves have a tendency to wear out in 10 to 15 years, which limits their use. One of their major advantages is that they do not require the postoperative use of anticoagulants.

Mechanical valves are of space age technology. The same material is used for them as is used for the space shuttle tiles. The valves have a long life span. They are more typically used in patients under 65 years of age. The disadvantage is that the patient is anticoagulant-dependent for the rest of his or her life.

Pericardial bioprosthesis valves are a mix of natural materials and modern technology. Cow pericardium, used to create the leaflets, is imposed on a structure of man-made polyester and plastic. Studies have shown these valves lasting over 14 years.

Mitral valve replacement (MVR) is accomplished through a lateral thoracotomy incision if it is done as a single procedure, or through a sternal incision if it is combined with another procedure. The surgeon approaches the valve with a gloved finger to feel the competence of the valve or lack of it. Often the choice of replacement type is made at this time.

Aortic valve replacement (AVR) is open heart surgery utilizing the CBP, cooling techniques, and heart-preserving solution while the heart is stopped. The valve is accessed and excess calcium cleaned from the area, and then the valve is removed. The new valve is sutured into place. The heart is restarted; mechanical assistance is stopped; and the chest is closed.

Minimally invasive aortic valve surgery requires use of the CBP. The location of the aortic valve in the chest is what allows this surgical procedure to be done through a 4-inch incision. Based on the results of a cardiac catheterization, a decision will have been made as to whether the valve should be repaired or replaced. If the valve is damaged, it is removed and replaced. The type of valve chosen is dependent on the factors mentioned previously. The valve is tested for function; the patient is taken off the CBP; and the incision is closed. The scar rests over the breastbone and fades quickly as healing takes place.

Aneurysm Surgery

The following discussion of aortic aneurysm surgery is limited to those procedures performed on the thoracic aorta, which begins at the aortic valve as the aortic root and becomes the ascending aorta. The aortic arch is the section that travels over the heart and branches into the innominate artery. After passing through the diaphragm the descending aorta becomes known as the abdominal aorta.

There are two main causes for aortic aneurysm surgery—an aneurysm itself and aortic dissection (DTA). The terms are often used interchangeably but have distinct medical meanings.

An aneurysm is an enlargement of the blood vessel caused by weakening of the vessel walls and a lack of elasticity. The blood no longer rushes through the vessel but pools. Aneurysms are most common in Marfan's syndrome.

Aortic dissection occurs when an aneurysm tears in the layers of the weakened section, causing a breach through which the blood leaks and becomes trapped. Dissections are typically seen in persons with hypertension or those who have a pre-existing aneurysm. Dissections of the ascending aorta are known as type A dissections and those in the descending aorta as type B (Fig. 14–23).

The type of surgical procedure done depends on the location of the aneurysm. In many cases of aneurysms of the ascending aorta, there is also damage to the aortic valve. If the valve cannot be repaired, it is replaced at the same time as the aneurysm is repaired, using a Gore-Tex or Dacron tube graft with a valve attachment. If the aortic valve is undamaged, a plain Gore-Tex or Dacron tube graft is used.

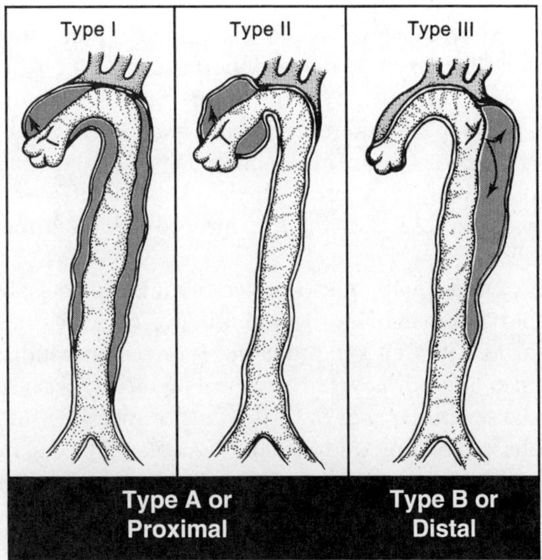

Figure 14–23
Common sites of aortic aneurysms. (From Braunwald E [ed]: Heart Disease: A Textbook of Cardiovascular Medicine, 5th ed. Philadelphia, WB Saunders, 1997.)

The procedure is performed on CBP. The blood is diverted through cannulation of the femoral artery, freeing the aorta of blood flow during the operation. Procedures on the aortic arch may require extending the graft to the ascending aorta. The aortic arch procedure is more complex and requires suspension of circulation while the surgeon replaces the section of the aorta attached to the innominate, left common carotid, and left subclavian arteries. The repair is accomplished with a single Dacron graft.

Usually there is a medical nonoperative approach to aneurysms of the descending aorta, which are usually small. With effective blood pressure control, they may never become problematic. Surgical correction is reserved for those patients in whom medical treatment has failed and whose aneurysm has enlarged. The aneurysm, which may technically extend into the abdomen, is removed and replaced with a simple Gore-Tex or Dacron tube graft. CBP is required only to support circulation in the lower half of the body.

In relatively few patients the entire length of the thoracic aorta is enlarged. This condition is corrected by a procedure known as the elephant trunk procedure, so called because the graft resembles an elephant's trunk. Usually the ascending aorta and aortic arch are approached and repaired, followed by the descending aorta.

Other Heart Surgical Procedures

Heart transplantation will be mentioned only briefly because it is done only at specific transplant centers. Heart transplants are usually performed on individuals with severe heart failure due to weak heart muscles. The weakening may be of viral or, in some cases, unknown origin. These individuals have no other treatment options available to them. Transplants are occasionally performed when all treatment alternatives have been exhausted, including heart failure medication combinations. This group of patients includes those who have failed previous CABG or valve surgery with persistence of symptoms that prevent the tissues, including the heart muscle, from being sufficiently oxygenated.

The supply of donor hearts falls far short of the demand, necessitating criteria that heart transplant candidates must meet. Generally, the procedure is not performed on the elderly (over 65 to 70 years of age), on those whose other medical conditions threaten to limit the life span, or on those whose compliance with a demanding medical regimen is suspect. A priority list is established based on how sick the patient is.

Some individuals on the wait list are compromised to the extent that they require implantation of a left ventricular assist device (**LVAD**). The LVAD is a pump type mechanical device that helps maintain the pumping ability of the heart on a temporary basis to provide a "bridge to transplant."

A tube is placed into the left ventricle that pulls the blood into a pump. The pump sends the blood into the aorta, effectively bypassing the weakened ventricle. The pump is placed in the upper abdomen. Another tube is attached from the pump to the control system outside the body. LVADs may be used for weeks to months.

The goals after the transplant are to prevent rejection of the foreign tissue, avoid infection, and prevent narrowing of the coronary arteries. These goals are achieved with the use of medications and close monitoring.

Alternative Heart Surgery

Alternative heart surgery being performed at this time includes procedures such as the following:

Cardiomyoplasty. *Cardiomyoplasty* is a procedure using skeletal muscle from the patient's abdomen or back to wrap around the heart. It is believed that this additional strength will assist the pumping action of the heart. Cardiomyoplasty is usually accompanied by the implantation of an electrical stimulating device similar to a pacemaker. The long-term potential of this procedure has not yet been established.

Batista Heart Failure Procedure. The Batista heart failure procedure is being studied by some medical centers in the United States. It was developed by a Brazilian surgeon, Dr. Rrandas J. V. Batiste, primarily as a treatment for heart failure. It is also being studied for effectiveness by heart surgeons in Great Britain and Italy.

The procedure is used for patients whose heart muscles have been weakened or stretched by disease, including any of those that produce inflammation, usually from infection. The result of the stretching and weakening is congestive heart failure. These hearts cannot pump enough blood to sustain themselves and the body. Thus far it appears that heart failure resulting from myocardial infarction does not respond as well.

In the Batista procedure, a triangular or elliptical piece of living heart tissue about the size of a golf ball is sliced from the left ventricle. The heart is then stitched back together. The ventricle is made smaller and can contract more effectively so that the main pumping chamber of the heart can pump more blood. Many centers and surgeons are awaiting the final reports on the success of the procedure The testimonies to date have been promising.

Maze Procedure. The **Maze procedure** is performed to cure atrial fibrillation. It is an open heart procedure, so it is generally reserved for situations in which a patient who has chronic atrial fibrillation is undergoing another procedure requiring use of the CBP. The procedure entails a series of small incisions in the walls of the atria. The incisions create a mazelike path that helps organize the electrical activity to prevent recurrence of the atrial fibrillation.

Monitoring in the OHRU

Arterial blood gas testing (ABG) is performed to determine the amount of oxygen in the arterial blood and to indicate when it is appropriate to change ventilator settings or to extubate a ventilated patient.

Hemodynamic monitoring is a general term used to describe procedures to evaluate cardiovascular function. Included in the catchall term are procedures ranging from very simple to very sophisticated:

Arterial blood pressure
Pulses, carotid and peripheral, including **DP**
CVP monitoring
Swan-Ganz monitoring
Peripheral Doppler studies

Heart monitoring through the use of 12-lead EKGs to determine heart damage and continuous cardiac monitors to identify **dysrhythmias**.

Laboratory monitoring: **Homeostasis** is monitored by the use of laboratory tests such as

Hemoglobin and hematocrit
Electrolytes
BUN and creatine
Cardiac enzymes
Other chemistries as indicated
White blood cell count and differential
Urinalysis
APTT and PT

Radiography is used to detect alterations in lung function as well as to determine proper placement of tubes and catheters.

Equipment Used in the OHRU

Chest Tube Drainage

All patients come from the OR with chest tubes (CT) in place to facilitate mediastinal and/or thoracic drainage and to assist in maintaining lung pressures as they should be. The amount and character of what is collected are indications of whether excessive bleeding or drainage is present. There are a variety of chest tube drainage collection devices on the market. They range from a simple gravity drainage apparatus to complex two- and three-chamber units that can be attached to suction. The type used depends upon what is available at a particular facility and the surgeon's preference (Fig. 14–24).

Pacemakers

Temporary pacemakers are used on most open heart surgery patients to prevent the heart from

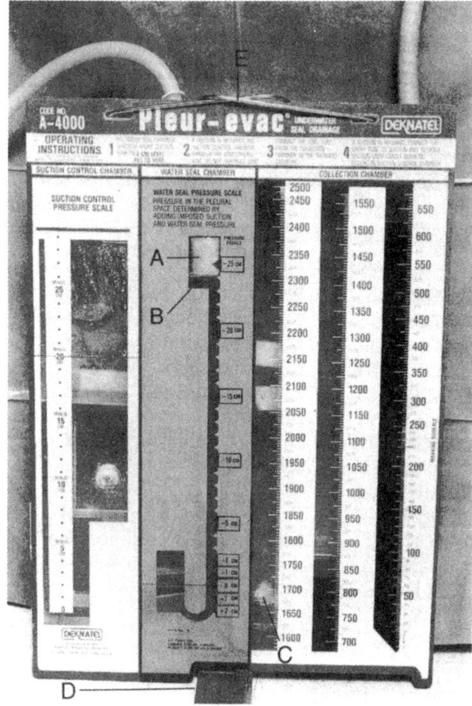

A

B

Figure 14–24
A and *B*, Chest tube drainage system. (From Ignatavicius DD, Workman ML, Mishler MA [eds]: Medical-Surgical Nursing: A Process Approach. Philadelphia, WB Saunders, 1995.)

beating too slowly or too quickly. Both DDD and AV sequential types might be used. Ultimately the pacemakers augment cardiac output (**CO**) by maintaining a prescribed rate (Fig. 14–25).

Ventilators

Following surgery, every patient has an **ET tube** in place and is attached to a mechanical ventilator (**IMV**) that provides sufficient volume of oxygenated air for transport to the tissues. The ventilators are set to maintain alveolar airways until the effects of the anesthetic drugs are out of the system.

Warming Devices

Heat lamps and BAIR Huggers are the usual heating devices used to raise the body temperature.

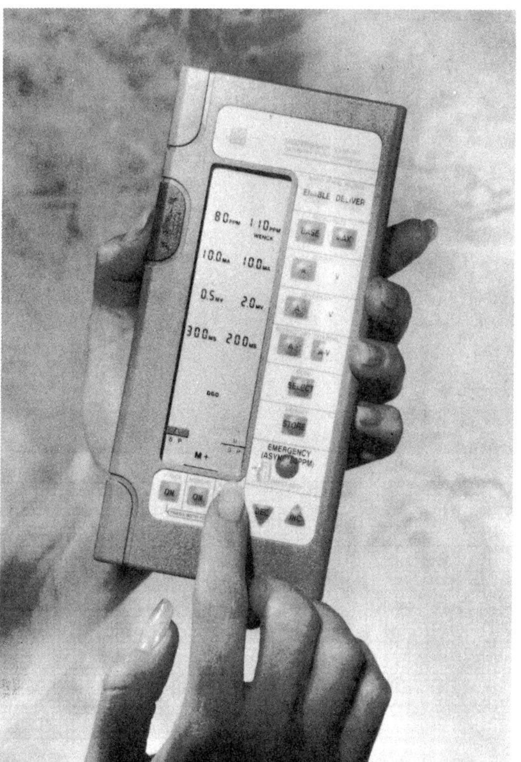

Figure 14–25
Temporary sequential AV pacemaker. (From Ignatavicius DD, Workman ML, Mishler MA [eds]: Medical-Surgical Nursing: A Process Approach. Philadelphia, WB Saunders, 1995.)

The reheating is done slowly to prevent shivering, which increases the workload on the heart.

Infusion Pumps

Automated infusion pumps are used on all open heart surgery patients to monitor the rate of all IV fluids and medications. It is not unusual to see as many as three or four of these pumps if the patient requires several types of medication.

Arterial Monitoring Devices

A catheter is placed in an artery, usually the radial or femoral artery. It is then connected to a high-pressure flush system that is heparinized. This apparatus is hooked up to an electronic transducer that creates a waveform that is displayed on a monitor (Fig. 14–26). The waveforms represent fluctuations in the blood pressure in the catheterized artery. The waveforms are converted to a numerical display on the monitor. In most patients the arterial blood pressure obtained in this manner correlates closely with that obtained with an external cuff. The parameters displayed are watched closely to ensure patency of the bypass grafts and adequate tissue perfusion.

Swan-Ganz Catheter

The venous system is monitored through the use of a Swan-Ganz catheter, which is used as indicator of cardiovascular function. The catheter, which has several openings along its length, is inserted into the superior vena cava via the subclavian or internal jugular vein and advanced into the right side of the heart. The system can be connected to a transducer monitoring system similar to that used in arterial monitoring. The **CVP** measurements are used to provide information about changes in the right ventricle. Low readings usually indicate insufficient blood volume and a need for fluid replacement.

There is a port for measuring pulmonary artery pressure (**PAP**) and pulmonary capillary wedge pressure (**PWCP**). Elevated readings indicate increased pressure in the pulmonary bed and are an indication of left-sided heart failure.

A third port contains a **thermistor**. This is used to measure CO by the thermodilution method and to monitor internal body temperature (Fig. 14–27).

The Swan-Ganz catheter is a valuable tool for obtaining data about right and left heart functioning and for evaluating the response to vasopressors. It can also be used for the infusion of fluids as a central venous line.

Other Monitoring Devices

Pulse oximeters are used to continuously measure oxygen saturation (SaO_2) to indicate blood oxygen levels and proper tissue oxygenation.

Merlin monitors are sophisticated devices that enable the monitoring of arterial blood pressure, right and left heart function, EKG, temperature, calculation of drugs, CO, and SaO_2 levels.

Medications Used in the OHRU

Most of the medications used in the OHRU are administered intravenously; some others are given intramuscularly. The types of drugs most commonly used are for the following purposes:

Analgesia (pain control)
Antirejection (used in heart transplants)
Antibiotics
Anticoagulant reversers
Anticoagulants
Assistance in tolerating the ventilator
Blood pressure control
Cardiac medications
Nausea and vomiting control

The Health Unit Coordinator in the OHRU

The OHRU demands on the HUC are high. No two days or even hours are the same. There is a constant turnover of patients. Some are arriving

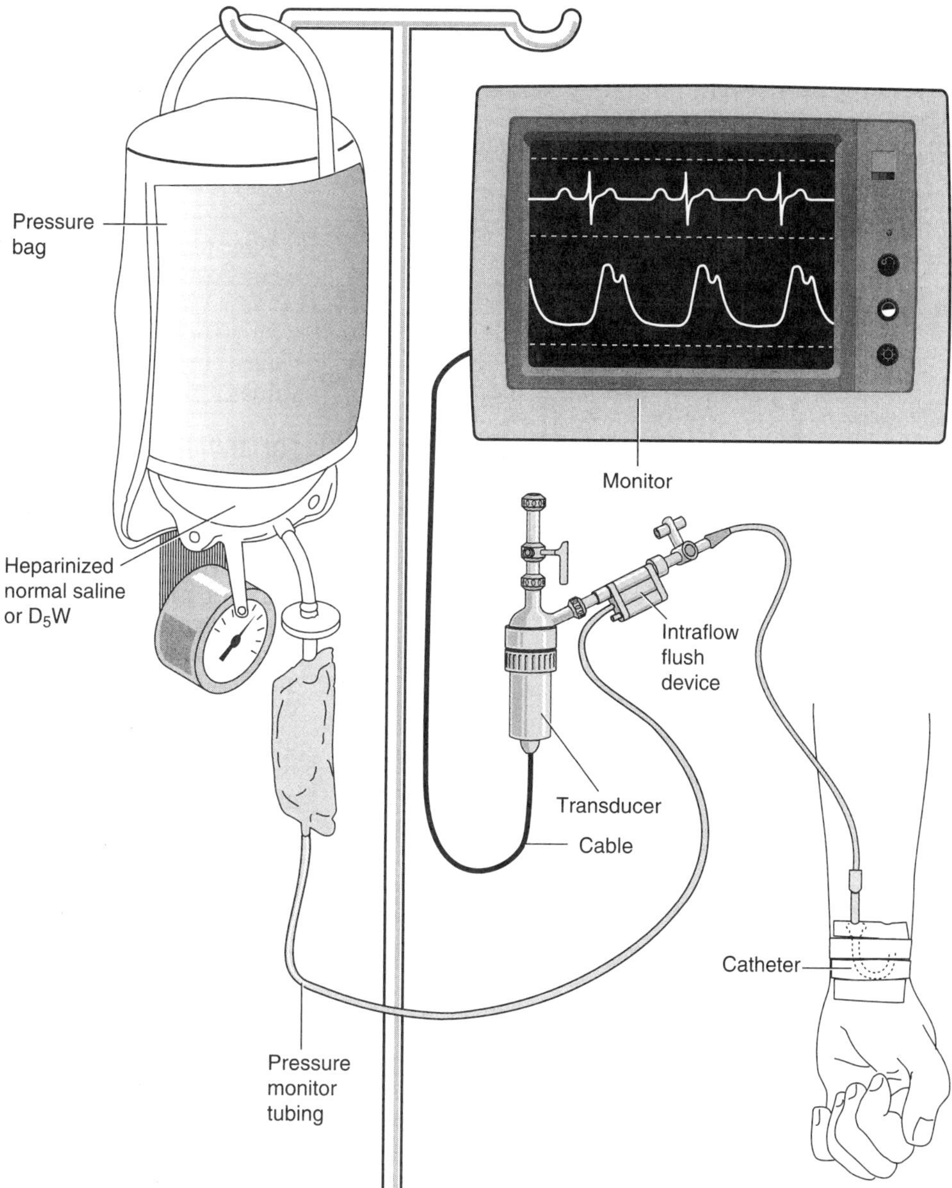

Figure 14–26
Arterial pressure monitoring. (From Ignatavicius DD, Workman ML, Mishler MA [eds]: Medical-Surgical Nursing: A Process Approach, 2nd ed. Philadelphia, WB Saunders, 1995.)

from the operating room, whereas others are being transferred to other units. The orderly transfer of records must be accomplished for all patients.

When a patient is brought from the OR, there are many orders to process, including ventilator settings, STAT lab work, x-rays, and medications. When the reports are available, the information must be given to the appropriate professional staff. If a patient's condition is critical, consultants may be called in and the family must be notified

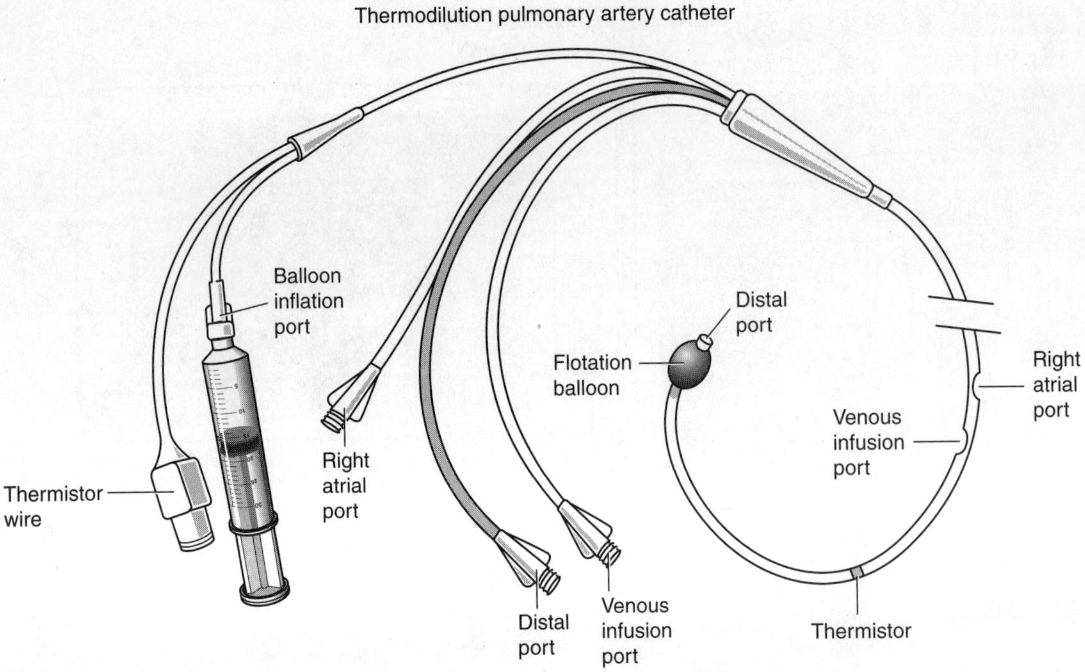

Figure 14–27
Swan-Ganz catheter.

and spiritual care provided—all in the midst of an emergency situation.

The HUC may be in charge of ensuring that all the equipment needed for patient care is available on the unit. This will include inventory, tracking, and ordering.

The HUC must be aware of the location of key personnel in the unit as well as visiting professionals. Often the consultants are not aware of where the items that they need can be found, and the HUC is the person available to direct and assist them.

The HUC's ability to be organized and to prioritize is a valuable asset in this unit, especially when combined with flexibility and the ability to be accurate in carrying out duties. Knowledge of medical terms, the procedures done on patients, and the needs of this highly specialized unit are also a plus (Fig. 14–28).

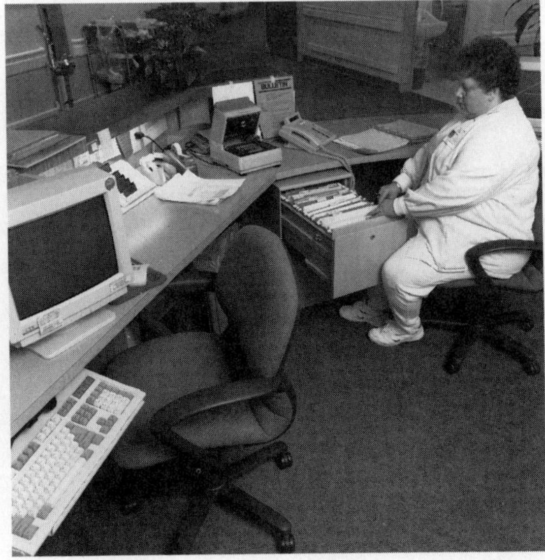

Figure 14–28
HUC in OHRU.

Communication With and About Patients in the OHRU

Communicating with patients who are on ventilators is a subject that deserves special consideration. Many of them can hear what is going on but cannot respond verbally because they are intubated. The preoperative teaching must include preparation for this situation. When able to move, the patient can communicate with hand or finger signals. It is important that patients be asked only close-ended questions that can be answered by a "yes" or "no" signal. For example, the question and response to "Do you have pain?" cannot be followed by a question such as "Where is it?" Rather, it requires the time and patience to ask if the pain is "in your chest?" or another site. As the patient becomes more alert, a writing tablet and pencil or pen is an option.

The most critical communication with the patient is in the preparation phase with respect to postoperative expectations. The need for changes in lifestyle, eating habits, exercise, and stress levels cannot be repeated too often. Most cardiac rehabilitation teaching starts at this point as well. Patients are taught the type of regimen that they will be following after discharge, including medications, activities, and follow-up medical appointments.

When the HUC receives inquiries about a patient's condition, he or she should identify the caller and transfer the call to the appropriate nurse. When HUCs are required to make calls about patients, they must have accurate information and pass it on succinctly, for it is often a crisis or emergency call for additional help.

Quality Assurance

Most of the heart centers keep statistics on morbidity and mortality as well as relative success rates. Educational and technical meetings are held constantly to present new information on available procedures. As with any hospital unit, JCAHO standards must be maintained. Special attention is paid to infection control.

Most units have a committee to do peer review. HUCs may be involved in data gathering for any of the QA processes.

Logs are required to demonstrate that monitoring equipment is checked and maintained. Special records must be kept on implantable devices, such as pacemakers and artificial valves.

Closing Thoughts

If a health unit coordinator is interested in being a member of a team in a dynamic area, the OHRU may be a good choice. The professional team is always learning and sharing educational experiences with the support staff. Seeing patients brought to the unit in an almost bionic state, with tubes and machines of all sorts, and knowing that within less than a week many of them will be home, is amazing.

The rapport among all team players is a decided plus. After a hectic day, which the HUC made better for everyone by using his or her skills, it is a comfort to go home knowing that you made a difference and are appreciated for that.

Review Questions

1. Explain the reasons for the development of open heart recovery units.
2. List four basic open heart surgical procedures.
3. Identify the blood vessels that are used as grafts in the CABG procedure.
4. Name five different types of equipment that would be used on the patient in the open heart recovery unit.
5. Briefly describe the role of the health unit coordinator in the open heart recovery unit.

Bibliography

Ignatavicius DD, Workman ML, Mishler MA: Medical-Surgical Nursing. Philadelphia, WB Saunders, 1989.

Merck Manual, 14th ed. Rahway, NJ, Merck, Sharp & Dohme, 1900.

New England Heart Institute: Understanding Your Cardiac Surgery (booklet).

Taber's Medical Dictionary. Philadelphia, FA Davis, 1998.

www.aha.org

www.cardiac consults.com

www.heart surgeons.com

www.Marfans.org/cardiac.htm

Special Care Units

PART 4: PEDIATRIC INTENSIVE CARE UNIT (PICU)

Mary Andrew Stirrup

Objectives

At the completion of this chapter, the reader should be able to:

1. Identify five members of the health care team who may be involved in the care of a PICU patient.
2. Name the most common cause of death in children.
3. Explain what is meant by ECMO and why it is used.
4. Discuss the purpose of a MICU.
5. List three other hospital departments that may be involved in the care of a PICU patient.

Vocabulary

Anastomosis: Creation of a union between two anatomic parts

Anesthesiologist: A physician who is trained in the specialty of anesthesia, including pain control and airway management

Atresia: Ending in a blind pouch where there should have been an opening

Barotrauma: Pressure trauma, seen in mechanically ventilated children

Congenital: Existing from the time of birth

Dextrocardia: Congenital condition where the heart is positioned to the right

Dialysate: The solution which attracts the impurities in dialysis procedures

Immunologist: A physician trained in the diagnosis and treatment of disorders of the immune system

Nephrologist: A physician with specialized training in diseases and disorders of the kidney

Continued

Vocabulary *Continued*

Oscillating: Swinging back and forth in a regular motion

Pediatric intensivist: A pediatrician who has additional training in the diagnosis and treatment of the patient with the acute and life threatening problems seen in a PICU

Percutaneous: Access through the skin

Pulmonologist: A physician trained and specializing in disease of the respiratory tract

Stenosis: Narrowing of a duct or canal in the body

Transposition: Reversal in the order of placement

Common Abbreviations

ABG Arterial blood gas

ACLS Advanced cardiac life support

Ao Aorta

ARDS Acute respiratory distress syndrome

AV Aortic valve

CDH Congenital diaphragmatic hernia

CHD Congenital heart defect

CHF Congestive heart failure

COR Corrective

CP Cerebral palsy

ECMO Extracorporeal membrane oxygenation

FDA Food and Drug Administration

GA Great arteries

HFOV High-frequency oscillating ventilator

JAMA Journal of the American Medical Association

LA Left atrium

LV Left ventricle

MICU Mobile intensive care unit

NICHD National Institute of Child Health and Human Development

PA Pulmonary artery

PAL Palliative

PALS Pediatric advanced life support

PDA Patent ductus arteriosus

Pharm. D. Educational degree of Doctor of Pharmacy

PPRU (Network of) Pediatric Pharmacology Research Units

PTLS Pediatric trauma life support

PV Pulmonary vein

RA Right atrium

RV Right ventricle

SVC Superior vena cava

TGA Transposition of great arteries

VA Venoarterial

VSD Ventricular septal defect

VV Venovenous

Introduction

Nancy Felsing, a **pediatric intensivist** at the Children's Hospital of Austin, was quoted on an Internet Web site as having said: "Critically ill children are not like critically ill adults. You assess them differently and you treat them differently." This type of thinking brought about the advent of the PICU. Diseases and injuries can manifest themselves very differently in children because their physiology is not the same as that of the adult. They are undergoing constant growth and development, which necessitates a unique mindset in decision-making regarding their diagnosis and treatment. Who would not prefer to have their critically ill child cared for in a specifically designated PICU than in an adult ICU? *Children are not merely miniature adults.*

The PICU patient mix varies from unit to unit. It often reflects the area of specialization of the institution. If the hospital is a major trauma center, there will be a higher percentage of pediatric trauma cases, whereas in a pediatric hospital, there may be more general surgical patients. The patient age may range from neonatal to late teens. Some facilities even accept patients over 20 years of age who have had repeated admissions over the long term. The mean length of stay in a PICU is 4.6 days, which reflects a balance between the short-term surgical patients and those with complicated congenital problems.

Design of the Unit

The PICU must be designed to accommodate advanced monitoring equipment and other technologies to care for critically ill children suffering from single- and multiorgan system failure. The physical layout varies from facility to facility; it is usually dictated by availability of space and whether the PICU is in an existing building or of

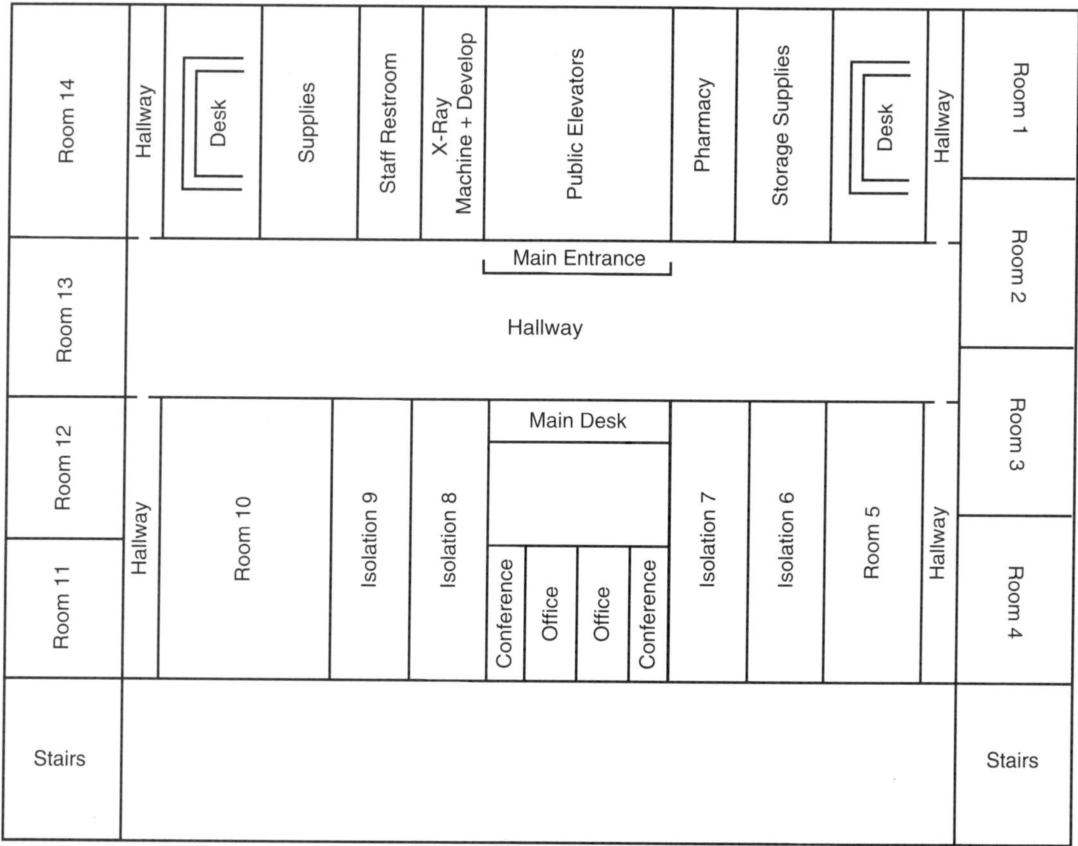

Figure 14–29
Layout of typical PICU unit.

new construction. Many units are long halls with a desk in the middle and rooms in both directions off the hall (Fig. 14–29).

Another common design is one large room fitted with curtains and dividers, with a single main desk off to the side. This arrangement has the advantage of flexible space that can be utilized according to the individual's needs; however, the unavailability of a closed isolation space is a disadvantage. The latest concept is the arena style (Fig. 14–30). This layout, featuring one or two desks in the middle with any number of rooms around the central area, affords good visibility of all the patients.

Staffing of the PICU

The medical director of the PICU will be a pediatric intensivist, a specialist trained in the care of the critically ill child. JAMA published a study demonstrating that the odds of survival in critically ill children cared for by pediatric intensivists is 1.54 times higher than for those who are not. There will typically be at least two other such specialists on the staff—perhaps more in larger facilities. Other physicians available to PICU will be pediatric surgeons, **nephrologists**, **pulmonologists**, **anesthesiologists**, infectious disease spe-

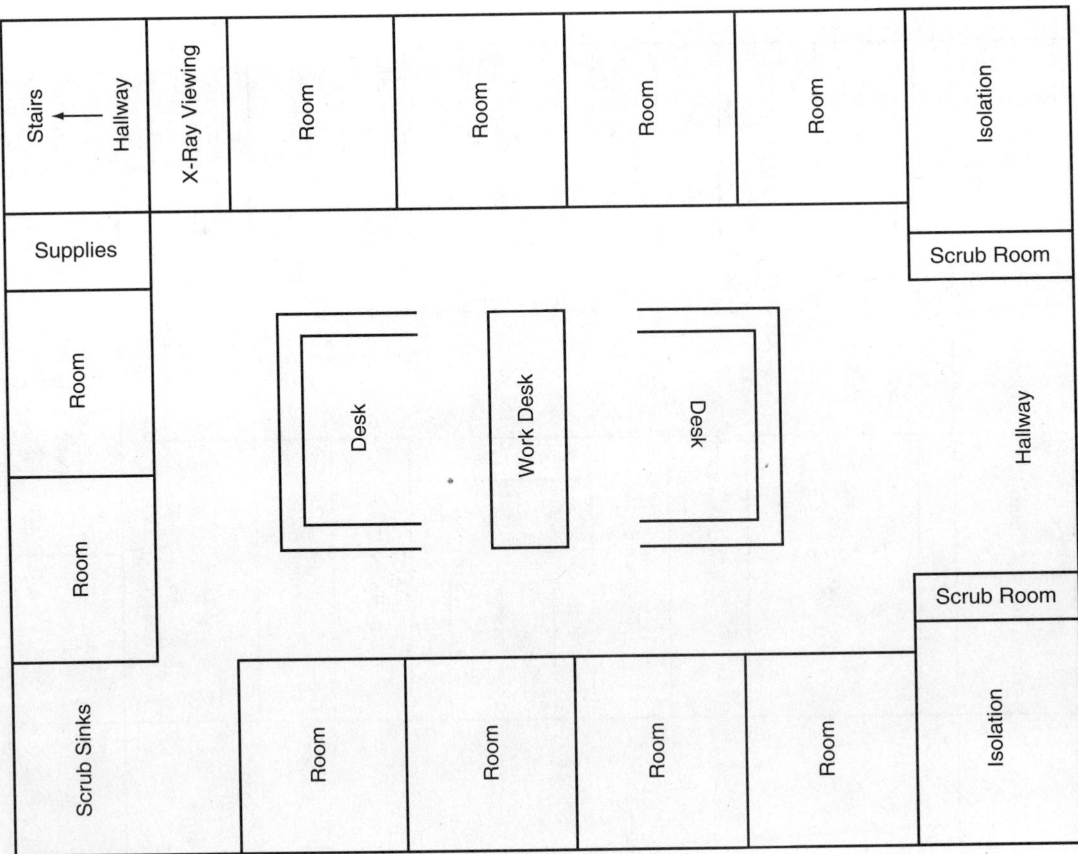

Figure 14–30
Arena style layout.

cialists, and **immunologists.** The physicians typically work in teams, and it is not unusual to see as many as 20 physicians, including residents, interns, and fellows on morning rounds (Fig. 14–31).

The nurses have additional training in pediatric advanced life support **(PALS)** and trauma life support **(PTLS)** certification. The usual ratio is one nurse to one patient, but in emergency situations this ratio can be as high as two or three to one. Some PICUs offer programs for training as pediatric intensive care nurse practitioners.

The nurses can be seen routinely administering medications by all methods, watching monitors of all sorts, and checking ventilators. They also provide the routine but important care that is needed to prevent skin breakdown in the immobilized patient. On occasion they may assist the operating room nurses at a bedside surgical procedure. They assist with family consultations, giving as well as receiving information from families in times of difficulty.

There are respiratory therapists with special training in pediatrics and the special equipment used in the PICU. They must be sure that appropriate ventilators and related equipment are available and in working order. They hook up the vents and change settings as ordered by the physicians. The respiratory therapists draw **ABGs,** assist physicians with endotracheal intubation, and perform breathing treatments, chest physiotherapy, and spirometry tests.

Another crucial member of the team is the pharmacist. The pharmacist attends rounds to provide concise patient-specific drug information when called on to do so and will research items on an as-needed basis. Among these are therapeutic drug monitors and MedLine searches as well as recommended doses, including maximum dosages, strengths, and dosage forms.

Diseases and Disorders Seen in the PICU

This team collectively offers care to patients whose survival is dependent on life support equipment, including mechanical ventilation, dialysis, and pacemakers; patients dependent on titrated drugs to maintain vital functions; patients requiring sophisticated hemodynamic monitoring; and patients with respiratory and/or circulatory failure, airway obstruction, acute alterations of con-

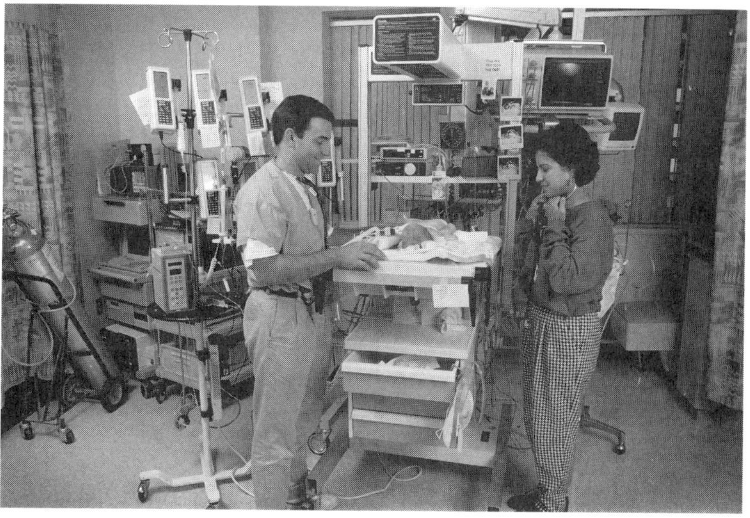

Figure 14–31
Team evaluating patient. (Courtesy of Children's Hospital of Wisconsin, Milwaukee.)

sciousness, severe fluid or electrolyte imbalance, multiple organ system failure, or multiple trauma.

Neurologic problems may be the result of closed or open head trauma, often requiring surgery. Unrelenting seizures are also a cause for admission to the PICU. One consideration in seizure disorders is the need to diagnose the underlying cause before effective treatment can begin. It is sometimes the case that seizures are caused by an infectious process, so it is not unusual to see these patients in the isolation room until an infectious process can be ruled out.

Kidney problems, including congenital anomalies, are occasionally seen in the PICU. In renal failure that has followed untreated hydronephrosis, surgery must be undertaken promptly. If the child is too ill, **percutaneous** drainage can be done on a temporizing basis.

Of the *congenital problems* seen in the PICU the most common are **congenital** cardiac problems. Among the patients are children who are either preoperative or postoperative for cardiac surgery to correct the condition (Tables 14–5 and 14–6).

Respiratory problems include severe asthma, particularly status asthmaticus. The complications seen in children with cystic fibrosis also are reason for admission. A respiratory emergency, acute epiglottitis, has become more prevalent in recent years. The child must be intubated and ventilated until the inflammation has dissipated.

Postsurgical patients who have had major surgical procedures are also cared for in the PICU (Fig. 14–32).

Accidents are the most common cause of death in children. Accidents are responsible for more childhood mortality than poliomyelitis, congenital malformations, heart disease, meningitis, and cancer combined. The natural curiosity of a child is usually the catalyst for accidents, most of which are preventable. Accidents occur more often when the child is hungry or tired, is in new surroundings, or is being cared for by a mother substitute. Accidents leading to an admission to the PICU are near-drowning, accidental amputations, trauma from automobile accidents, falls, or gunshots.

Poisonings are the most common cause of nonfatal accidents in childhood. The ingestion of aspirin is the type of poisoning seen most often in children. The aspirin causes CNS stimulation with initial vomiting, hyperpnea, and hyperactivity. The hyperpnea leads to lowered carbon dioxide levels and respiratory alkalosis. The kidneys respond by excreting base and creating metabolic acidosis. Convulsions, high fever, collapse, and respiratory failure can ensue. In older children, this process can be more easily reversed than in toddlers.

Ingesting strong acids and caustics can happen when children go into storage areas where detergents and other cleaning and household aids are kept. Although it is a convenience to have many cleaning products in a liquid form, it is potentially more dangerous for the child who ingests them. In a solid form, the caustics cause immediate burning, and the amount is limited by the discom-

Table 14–5 INCIDENCE OF CHD

Type of Lesion	Per 1000 Liveborn Children
Patent ductus arteriosus (as single lesion)	0.60
Ventricular septal defect	1.71
Atrial septal defect	0.36
Aortic atresia or stenosis	0.41
Coarctation of the aorta	0.62
Pulmonary stenosis	0.28
Tetralogy of Fallot	0.26
Truncus arteriosus communis	0.09
Transposition of great vessels	0.38
Dextrocardia (isolated)	0.05
Dextrocardia with situs inversus	6.35

Table 14–6 EXAMPLES OF CHD AND SURGICAL PROCEDURES

Problem	Surgical Procedure	Classification
Obstructed valve	Valvotomy	Cor
Obstructed PV	Valvectomy	Pal
Transposition of GA	Valved conduit from RV to PA VSD closure	Cor
Valve regurgitation	Valvuloplasty	Cor
Transposition of GA (TGA)	Surgical removal of atrial septum	Pal
Decreased pulmonary flow	Anastomosis between Ao and PA	Pal
Patent ductus arteriosus	PDA ligation	Cor

fort. The liquid forms, however, are easily swallowed, causing destruction of the entire esophagus.

Every year products such as gasoline, kerosene, paint thinners, furniture polish, and cleaning fluid are responsible for over 25,000 poisonings in children under the age of 5 years. The adverse signs and symptoms are related to the respiratory system, although the ones that the patients usually complain about more are those related to the GI tract. Death may occur from related pneumonitis within 24 hours of the ingestion.

Procedures and Treatments

Hemodialysis

A hemodialysis system is sometime referred to as an artificial kidney. In the simplest form, it consists of a tubing system designed to take the blood from the patient to the machine; a membrane unit for the blood to come in contact with; and a system to supply the dialysate to the other side of the membrane. The type of dialysate depends on the clinical requirements. The dialysate attracts the impurities through the membrane, thus cleansing the blood. The blood is then returned to the patient.

Most hemodialysis is accomplished using arteriovenous shunts that are surgically placed in the patient. The procedure takes about 4 to 6 hours to accomplish. Side effects are hypotension, hemorrhage due to the heparinization that is required, air emboli, and infection.

Venovenous Hemofiltration

Hemofiltration, which works similarly but on a different principle than hemodialysis, is sometimes preferable for the child in distress. It causes fewer problems with blood pressure and is thought by some to be a gentler way to achieve the same end. This form of filtration runs continuously, processing smaller amounts of blood over a longer period of time than in hemodialysis. It is, however, more expensive than hemodialysis.

Extracorporeal Membrane Oxygenation (ECMO)

ECMO is a type of modified heart-lung machine. It offers unique therapy in that it supplies an artificial lung outside the body to place needed oxygen into the blood while the diseased lungs of the child heal. The machine can also act as an artificial heart to provide support for infants and children who have a failing heart, either during or after heart surgery.

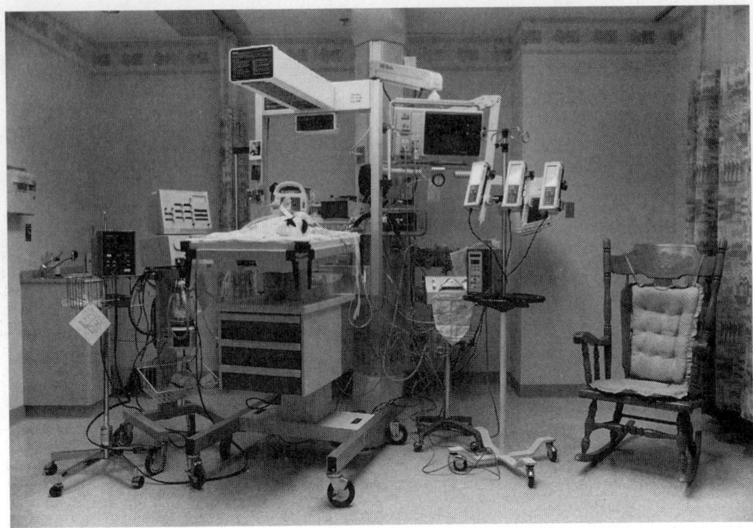

Figure 14–32
Infant returned from OR with equipment and monitors in place. (Courtesy of Children's Hospital of Wisconsin, Milwaukee.)

Since the inception of ECMO in 1975, many children have survived who would have otherwise died. As experience with its use has advanced, so have the figures for its success rate. In 1993, this was reported as 84 percent. ECMO is offered only to children whose heart and/or lung disease is thought to be reversible.

Poorly oxygenated blood drains by gravity from a venous catheter into the ECMO pump, which acts as an artificial heart. The blood is pumped into the oxygenation component of the machine, which acts as the artificial lung. It is cleansed of carbon dioxide, and appropriate amounts of oxygen are added. The blood is warmed and returned to the child via an arterial catheter or second venous catheter. The venoarterial (**VA**) technique is utilized when a child also has blood pressure problems and will benefit from the added support to the heart. The venovenous (**VV**) technique is used when the blood pressure is stable. It is possible to convert from VV to VA if a child develops further problems while on ECMO.

The draining out of the blood and the return are programmed to occur at the same rate in order to cause as little disruption to the body as possible. The catheters are placed by a surgical team, at the bedside, under general anesthesia using sterile technique. In the VA technique the carotid artery and internal jugular or subclavian veins are used. In VV the same neck veins and the femoral vein are used. X-rays are performed to confirm correct placement before the catheters are connected to the ECMO machine (Fig. 14–33).

As long as the child is on ECMO, a mechanical ventilator at very low settings will be used. This provides a mechanism for the removal of secretions and keeps the lungs well inflated.

Heparin infusions are utilized to prevent the blood from clotting when it goes through the machine. If the child bleeds excessively or does not respond well to heparin, ECMO may have to be discontinued before bleeding into the brain occurs.

The risks associated with ECMO are as follows:

1. The VA ECMO technique involves tying off the carotid artery for the duration of the therapy. No information is yet available as to whether this will contribute to stroke in adulthood.
2. Whenever a catheter is inserted into a blood vessel, there is a risk for infection. IV antibiotics are generally administered prophylactically.
3. A child on ECMO will require frequent

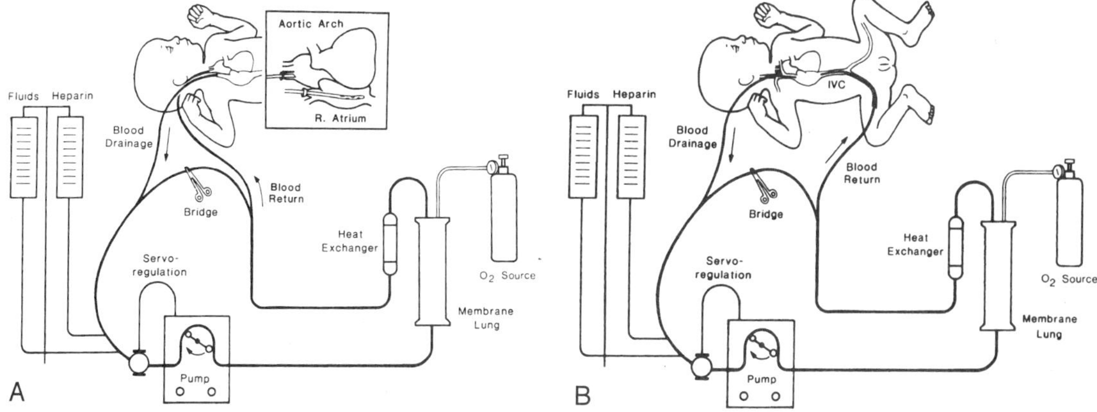

Figure 14–33
Diagrams of VA (*A*) and VV (*B*) for ECMO. (J LA State Med Soc 1986; 138:40. Copyright © 1986 and published by The Journal of the Louisiana State Medical Society, Inc., New Orleans, LA.)

blood transfusions. As with any transfusion, there is a risk of blood reactions, AIDS, and hepatitis.

4. Despite every available safety measure, the circuit can malfunction or fail.

5. Small clots or air emboli may enter the circuit.

The average duration of ECMO therapy is 10 to 30 days. Since each child is unique and each disease is different, there cannot be a precise prediction of the length of time that will be needed when the therapy is initiated. Frequent evaluation and monitoring will track improvement so the child can be slowly weaned off the machine in a controlled situation (Fig. 14–34).

There are always two members of the professional care staff with the child on ECMO, one to monitor the patient and the other to monitor the pump.

The HUC will be involved in calling the right

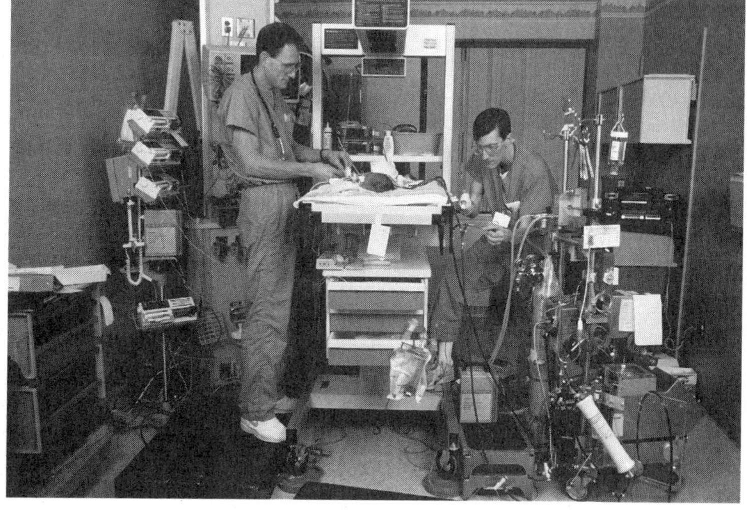

Figure 14–34
Infant on ECMO. (Courtesy of Children's Hospital of Wisconsin, Milwaukee.)

parties to have ECMO initiated when the decision is made to use it. The HUC is responsible for seeing that the informed consent form is available (Fig. 14–35). The laboratory and X-ray and respiratory therapy departments must be notified to be prepared to assume their roles in the procedure.

High-frequency Oscillatory Ventilation

This procedure was initially used exclusively for neonates with a gestational age of 24 to 43 weeks who weighed between 0.54 and 4.6 kg. In 1995, the FDA approved the use of the high-frequency oscillating ventilator (**HFOV**) in children with severe respiratory failure who, in the opinion of their physicians, are failing on conventional ventilation. The decision was based on a study showing that there were fewer complications in children on the HFOV as well as a higher survival rate. There is no upper weight limit, and the children demonstrate better oxygenation, less **barotrauma**, and less chronic lung disease than the survivors treated by other means.

This ventilator is designed to employ higher mean lung pressures than the conventional ventilators but without the high peak pressures that lead to lung injury. The tidal volumes are delivered at supraphysiologic ventilatory frequencies. The ventilator utilizes a humidified gas source.

The most common indications for its use in children are pneumonia, acute respiratory distress syndrome (**ARDS**), and congenital diaphragmatic hernia (**CDH**).

Pharmacology-Related Topics

The medications given in a PICU cover the spectrum from acetaminophen to potent chemotherapeutics. Antibiotics are often given by the IV route as are drugs to produce relaxation and sedation when a child is being mechanically ventilated.

Nowhere in treatment is it more important to recognize that the child is not just a miniature adult than it is in the use of pharmaceuticals and IV fluids. Most of the medication and fluid doses are calculated by one of several formulas based on the child's weight in kilograms. Pharmacists are available to advise on drugs that are appropriate for use in the various stages of development. They also provide information on the speed with which a drug should be given, frequency of dosing, and compatibility with other substances being administered. Information must be readily available so the unit staff can monitor the child for effects and side effects of the drugs.

It is interesting to note that three quarters of all medications marketed today do not carry **FDA**-approved labeling for use in neonates, infants, children, and adolescents. A mere 5 of the 80 most frequently used drugs for newborns and infants are labeled for pediatric use. In 1994 a pediatric plan was published by the FDA section on drug evaluation and research. This plan encouraged studies on pediatric patients during the drug development process. Many PICUs are in a position to contribute information to these studies by virtue of the close involvement of pharmacists in their care planning.

Most studies have shown that most pediatric drug-related mishaps occur because the recommended dosages are based on adult studies. The **NICHD** has established a network of pediatric research units (**PPRUs**) to facilitate and promote pediatric labeling of drugs already on the market as well as new ones. The overall goal of the PPRU network is the safe and effective use of drugs in children.

It is not unusual for the PICU to be part of a pharmacy training program. **Pharm.D.** students participate extensively in the management of patients in the PICU. This increases their awareness of factors influencing drug delivery to the critically ill child and affords them the opportunity to develop effective communication skills within a multidisciplinary team.

The internships, which are monitored by a preceptor, include:

Attendance at PICU rounds for providing concise patient-specific drug information

ECMO CONSENT FORM

Most children respond to ECMO within 10 days. If your child does not respond, this will be discussed with you and the decision to discontinue ECMO will be made with you.

The ECMO procedure has been explained to me by ______________________________. I understand the risks and the benefits of the ECMO therapy and agree to have my child, ______________________, receive this therapy. I understand that routine therapy can be started at any time if I wish to remove my child from ECMO therapy. I also understand if I have any questions or concerns, I can ask anyone on the ECMO team.

____________________ Witness	____________________ Parent/Guardian Relationship
____________________ Date	____________________ Date
	____________________ Parent/Guardian Relationship
	____________________ Date

I have explained the ECMO procedure, its potential benefits and known risks. I have given the above a copy of the ECMO information booklet.

____
ECMO Physician

Figure 14–35
ECMO consent form.

Attendance at radiographic rounds to contribute information to dye and other drug dosing
Attendance at pharmacy minirounds
Attendance at PICU educational offerings by house staff
Monitoring and assessing drug therapy on all unit patients on a daily basis.

The student is asked to:

Prepare educational projects to present to the pharmacy staff
Prepare in-services based on new information that he or she has learned
Accomplish MedLine searches on a selected PICU topic
Research recommended doses, strengths, and frequency on a specific number of pediatric drugs given IV, IM, or p.o.

These students often interact with the HUC as they become oriented to the unit and may enlist their help in locating information needed for their projects.

Monitoring and Equipment in the PICU

The monitoring done in the PICU is essentially the same as in the other special care units. The difference is in the size of the equipment that is used. Hemodynamic monitors, IV monitoring pumps, and ventilators are all adapted to the size of the child on whom they are used. Patients are closely monitored for 24 hours after surgical procedures. It is not unusual to see a patient returned directly from surgery with all monitoring equipment in place (see Fig. 14–32). The endotracheal tubes, IV line, and urinary catheters are available in very small sizes and must be stocked in sufficient quantities at all times.

MICU

The PICU is such a specialized unit that it is usually a designated tertiary center, receiving patients from a large geographic area. To facilitate the safe transport of those critically ill individuals for whom time is so important, PICUs have their own transport teams or have trained a specialized outside team to transport patients.

The mobile intensive care units (**MICUs**) are usually ambulances that have been outfitted with all the equipment necessary to accomplish the safest possible transfer. Other transport units used are helicopters and fixed-wing aircraft, depending on the distance to be covered and the weather conditions of the day. The team, which is either hospital-based or employed by the transport service, consists of highly trained individuals. The core team includes a pediatric critical care nurse or nurse practitioner and a pediatric respiratory therapist. Other specialists, including a pediatric intensivist, may be called upon to accompany the team if the situation warrants it. A pediatric intensivist is always available to consult by telephone with the referring physician to assist in preparing for a safe transport.

The team, by its training, is acutely aware of the differences between transporting children and transporting adults. They continuously monitor the following functions during transport:

Cardiovascular
Pulmonary
Neurologic
Fluid and electrolyte balance
Gastrointestinal
Metabolic
Immunologic

If there is not a physician on board the transport vehicle, constant communication is maintained by radio.

Transport team specialists usually must have 2 years of PICU experience as well as and training in pediatric trauma, toxicology, pain management, and pediatric transport medicine. They must be certified in pediatric advanced life support (**PALS**) and advanced cardiac life support (ACLS).

When the call comes and it is determined that the transport team must be mobilized, the HUC is instrumental in placing the appropriate calls to initiate this. The HUC will often be the one to request the necessary information from the referring facility as well.

Communication With and About the Child

Communicating with the Patient and Family

If the child is old enough to understand what is happening, the staff will talk directly to him or her. Explanations of procedures are made in terminology that is geared to the child's age and level of understanding. This simple process will go a long way in allaying the child's fears. In conversation with children, especially young ones, it is important to give them answers to questions as they ask them. Often all that they want is a simple answer, and adults have a tendency to complicate this. Children have the amazing capacity to understand and accept information when it is presented appropriately.

The most critical communication in the PICU is with the parents of the children who are admitted. There is, understandably, a high stress level in the parents of a seriously ill child; keeping them constantly updated on what is happening helps alleviate it.

The staff of a PICU must be very sensitive to the heart-wrenching agony of a parent whose child is critically ill. The parents will have many questions and will present them to anyone available. In many PICUs, by design of the unit, that person will be the HUC. HUCs should tactfully respond to those questions that they are allowed to answer and promptly refer the rest to the appropriate individual. The HUC is in a unique position to offer support to parents who are waiting for condition reports on a gravely ill child. If the family can communicate only in a foreign language, an interpreter must be made available to assist. The HUC maintains a list of interpreters for the PICU.

One time when the HUC is certain to become involved in communicating with parents is in the case of an MICU transport. The transportation arrangements are shared with the parents, and historical information can often be obtained at this time. If the family is unable to accompany the patient to the receiving facility, the HUC can ensure that they have good directions to reach it as well as instructions to locate the unit. The parents may call in for updates while they are en route.

Generally, information is given only to the immediate family. In some cases in which major decisions have to be made, the physicians will, with the parents' concurrence, involve other family members, particularly grandparents.

Communicating About the Patient

Most of the communication about the child will be to request tests from other hospital departments and obtain consults from outside physicians. The HUC may be asked to pass on general information about the child's condition to other departments to have them decide which method of testing would be best as well as where the testing should be carried out. When calls are made to other departments or physicians about the children in a PICU, the messages must be 100 percent accurate and concise. Time and accuracy are of the essence in this unit.

The HUC must tactful in referring calls from distraught extended family members. When the call is referred to a member of the nursing staff, the HUC should be prepared to identify the caller and his or her relationship to or interest in the patient.

Support Teams

Some units have volunteer support staff who have been specially trained to deal with the critically ill child. These people are nonthreatening to the child and will often be found sitting with a child. If the children's condition allows, they will play with them, read to them, or listen to music with them. All this helps the child remain calm. The availability of these volunteers makes it easier for family members to allow themselves some respite time, knowing that the child will be receiving care and attention.

The pastoral counseling personnel are available at all hours. They are particularly helpful in assisting the family during times when difficult decisions have to be made. Volunteers from the department will often spend time with the families while a child is undergoing a surgical procedure. They provide support and are a source of comfort to the family.

The public relations department comes into play when the hospital admission is the result of an accident, trauma, or other medically newsworthy event. All media contact are dealt with by this department, allowing the family to deal with the immediate problem.

The patient relations department assists families in making arrangement to stay with or close to the child. They also see to it that the family members are fed. Many hospitals with PICUs have associated buildings or areas on the campus that are designated as temporary living facilities for the families of the critically ill pediatric patient.

The social service department becomes involved when there are circumstances of hardship, whether emotional or financial, for the family. This department is also a part of the discharge planning team from the day of admission. The plans developed for discharge from the unit or the facility are very comprehensive and often involve several community resources, such as a home health agency, financial support agencies, and services providing special transportation and educational support.

Quality Assurance

PICUs by their nature must have very stringent standards. Those facilities utilizing ECMO and HFOV must report in detail each time these modalities are used. There is an ECMO registry that publishes statistics on its use nationally. Peer review and case conferences are held on a frequent basis, and outcome monitors are used for many of the procedures performed in the unit. Close monitoring of the staff members' educational and technical competence is conducted on an ongoing basis.

Closing Thoughts

If you are a certified health unit coordinator looking for a challenge in life, the pediatric intensive care unit is the place for you. You will receive an amazing education in many areas of medicine, especially if the facility is a research and teaching hospital.

Be willing to be an extra set of hands when needed—maybe just by getting a clean blanket for a busy nurse. In some facilities, it will be beneficial to take the monitor technician course that is offered by educational services.

Stress levels can run high at times, but if you are strong enough to use it to help you rather than letting it distract you, the PICU may be for you. The duties are varied, and at times you may be needed to do six different things at the same time. If you can stay focused, however, the job will get done. The PICU HUC is regarded by doctors as a valuable resource and as a person who can get things done in a competent manner. If you are up to the challenge of keeping the unit running smoothly and efficiently, you should consider a career in PICU.

Review Questions

1. Identify five members of the health care team who may be involved in the care of a PICU patient.
2. Name the most common cause of death in children.
3. Explain what is meant by ECMO and why it is used.
4. Discuss the purpose of a MICU.
5. List three other hospital departments that may be involved in the care of a PICU patient.

Bibliography

Chabner D-E: The Language of Medicine, 4th ed. Philadelphia, WB Saunders, 1991.

Webster's II New Riverside Dictionary. Revised edition. Boston, Houghton Mifflin, 1996.

Extending the Reach of Critical Care Services for Children. Goodhealth Magazine July/August 1996 (Internet). www.peds-criticare@uokhsc.edu

Pediatrics Intensive Care Children's Hosp of WI (Internet)

VisNiranjan MD: Treating a Child Like a Child. University Health Quarterly.

Special Care Units

14

PART 5: THE POSTANESTHESIA CARE UNIT

Sandy Fisher

Objectives

Upon completion of this chapter, the reader will be able to:

1. Differentiate between different anesthesia techniques.
2. Explain the transcription of orders in PACU.
3. Describe the communication about the patient in PACU.
4. Describe the role of the HUC in a "Code" situation.

Vocabulary

Airway: The passage for oxygen to travel from the mouth or nose through the trachea into the lungs. General anesthesia and sedation relax the muscles and may cause a mechanical obstruction. The cough and gag reflexes that protect and clear the airway are suppressed under anesthesia.

Endotracheal tube: A tube introduced through the nose or mouth and advanced between the vocal cords into the trachea. The procedure can be carried out under direct laryngoscopy or by blind technique. The tube provides a patent airway for oxygen and gaseous anesthetic agents.

Hemodynamics: A study of the forces involved in circulating blood through the body.

Radioactive isotope: An isotope in which the nuclear composition is unstable. The implantable form is used in radiation therapy.

Common Abbreviations

CTU	Cardiothoracic unit	**ICU**	Intensive care unit	**PICU**	Pediatric intensive care unit
Dx	Diagnosis	JP	Jackson-Pratt	**SICU**	Surgical intensive care unit
EBL	Estimated blood loss	**LMA**	Laryngeal mask airway	TKO	To keep open
ETT	Endotracheal tube	med(s)	Medication(s)	TKVO	To keep vein open
FOB	Foot of bed	mEq	Milliequivalent (per liter)	TRA	To run at
HOB	Head of bed	N & V	Nausea and vomiting	WBAT	Weight bearing as tolerated
Hx	History	NGT	Nasogastric tube		

Introduction

Prior to World War II, anesthetized patients were transported directly back to their medical/surgical bed after surgery. A nurse was assigned to sit with the patient, take and record vital signs, and assist patients who were vomiting. The postanesthesia care unit (PACU) of today represents a centralized recovery area that offers the following advantages: (1) availability of skilled personnel; (2) increased patient safety due to closer observation; (3) centralization of like patients, personnel, and equipment; and (4) economy of resources.

Description of the Unit

The PACU is set up in a large open room. There are individual bays with monitoring equipment and supplies for each patient (Fig. 14–36). Privacy is provided by curtains that can be pulled around each individual patient area. The openness of the room enables the nurses to assist each other with patient care while closely observing each patient. There are closed isolation rooms for patients with medical problems such as TB or for those who have had radioactive isotopes implanted. Separate pediatric areas are designed to prevent the crying of infants and children from disturbing others.

A centrally located storage area affords easy access from it to patient care areas (Fig. 14–37). Here are stored IV solutions and administration supplies, medications, and syringes. The core of the unit is the HUC desk (Fig. 14–38), which can be easily accessed from any area. The computer, telephones, fax and copy machines, and pneumatic tube system are found here. Physicians and nurses can finish their charting in this area and still see all that is happening in the unit.

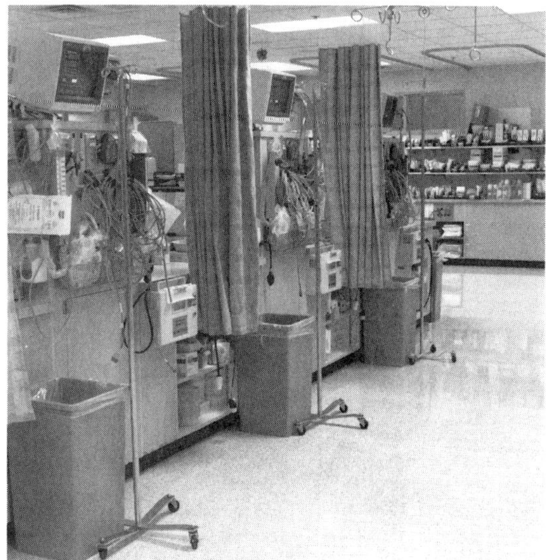

Figure 14–36
PACU.

The abbreviations listed for this chapter are those that a HUC working in this area would be expected to know. Only those in boldface type are used in the text and appear in boldface when they are used for the first time.

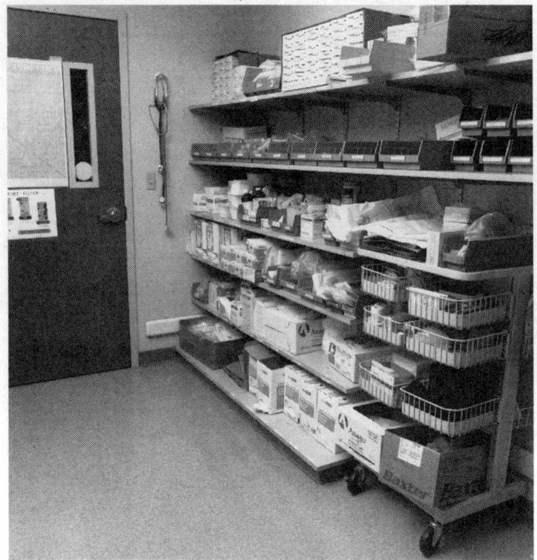

Figure 14–37
Storage area.

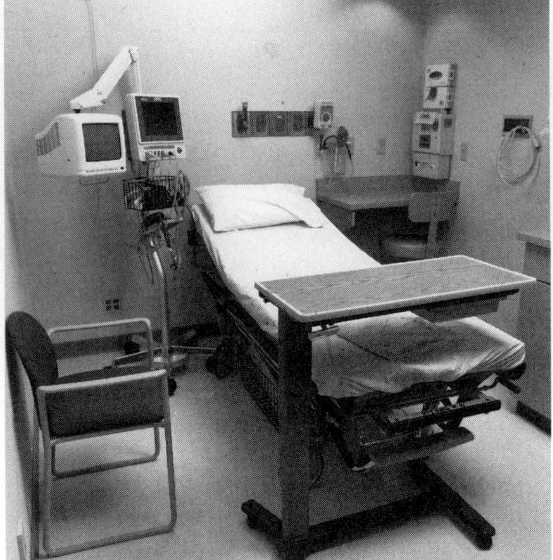

Figure 14–39
Preop area.

In facilities that require PACU personnel to be responsible for immediate preoperative care, a similar but smaller open area with open bays is set up for this purpose (Fig. 14–39).

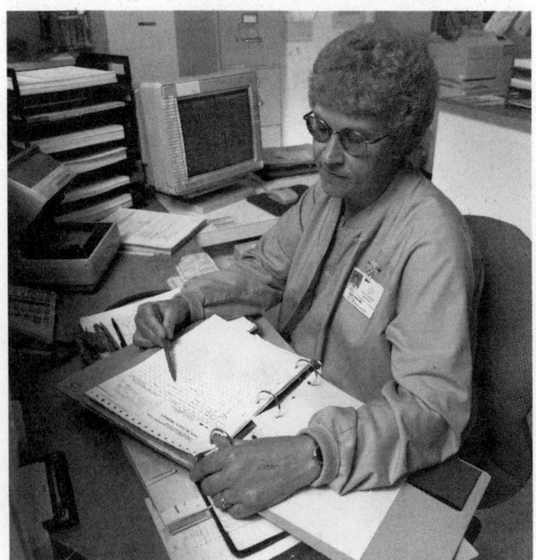

Figure 14–38
HUC desk area.

Staffing of the PACU

The PACU is staffed by registered nurses with additional training in **airway** management and advanced cardiac life support (ACLS). Anesthesiologists provide the majority of the medical care given in the PACU while the patient is returning to a normal physiologic state after receiving an anesthetic. The surgeon, primary physician, or consultants are contacted when problems arise in their area of expertise. The HUC employed in a PACU must be familiar with medical terminology, equipment, and procedures related to all body systems and age-appropriate care. Many HUCs in the PACU are CPR-trained.

Anesthesia Techniques

The following are the most commonly utilized anesthesia techniques:

General anesthesia (GA) is a reversible state of unconsciousness produced by intravenous and/or inhalation anesthetic agents. In this state, motor, sensory, mental, and reflex functions are decreased or absent.

Monitored anesthesia care (**MAC**) requires an anesthesiologist or nurse anesthetist to be present on standby during the surgical procedure to monitor the patient and administer sedation or anesthesia as the need arises.

Spinal anesthesia block (**SAB**) involves the injection of drugs into the arachnoid space, below the level where the spinal cord ends. The level of the drug in the space is controlled by volume and patient position to produce a loss of sensation in the operative area without a loss of consciousness.

Local anesthesia is the injection of an anesthetic drug or application of it topically to numb only the proposed operative area. Supplemental agents are available for analgesia, anesthesia, or the emergency treatment of adverse reactions.

Conscious sedation is a state achieved by the injection of intravenous medication. The term refers to a mildly to moderately depressed level of consciousness that allows the patient to maintain a patent airway. The patient will be able to respond to verbal instructions or physical stimulation.

Nerve block is accomplished by injecting local anesthetic drugs at a location remote to the surgical area. This will block the conduction of impulses to the operative site and render a defined area of anesthesia.

Bier block is also known as IV regional anesthesia. An IV catheter is introduced into the affected extremity distal to the surgical site. A special inflatable tourniquet is applied proximally to the surgical site, and the blood is drained from the area. The tourniquet can then be inflated. Injection of a local anesthetic drug through the venous access will result in loss of sensation. The extremity remains pain-free as long as the drug is effective and the tourniquet remains inflated.

Epidural analgesia is the administration of narcotic analgesics through a percutaneous indwelling epidural catheter. The catheter is introduced into the epidural space and fixed to the skin so that it will not dislodge. Attached to it are an infusion port, implantable device or pump, and reservoir for the administration of the medication. This technique is typically used for severe postoperative pain for up to 3 days and for long-term pain relief in the oncology patient. The epidural route may also be used for anesthesia during surgical procedures.

A special record is used by anesthesiologists and nurse anesthetists. It is designed to provide a sequence of information that can be used for the medical record as well as for data retreival (Fig. 14–40).

Activities in the PACU

Immediate Preoperative Phase

Preoperative preparation encompasses assessing and making the patient ready for the operative suite. It includes (1) determination of NPO status; (2) review of the record for signed surgical permit, completed history (**Hx**) and physical, and studies pertinent to the diagnosis (**Dx**); (Fig. 14–41); (3) skin preparation as ordered; (4) infusion of appropriate fluids through a peripheral IV (usually started in the preop area); (5) continuation of teaching; and (6) reduction of anxiety by sedation and reassurance.

The Recovery Phase

The main focus of the PACU is the management of patients recovering form anesthetic agents utilized during surgical procedures. All age groups and diverse surgical procedures are represented by the patient population cared for by the widely skilled PACU staff. Most of the activities center on the patient as he or she makes the transition from a totally anesthetized state to one requiring less acute intervention.

When a patient is admitted to the PACU, two or three nurses simultaneously take vital signs and perform a physical assessment, connect the patient to monitoring equipment, receive reports from the anesthesiologist, apply warming measures to the patient, and review the perioperative history.

The anesthesiologist leaves when the patient is considered to be hemodynamically stable. The

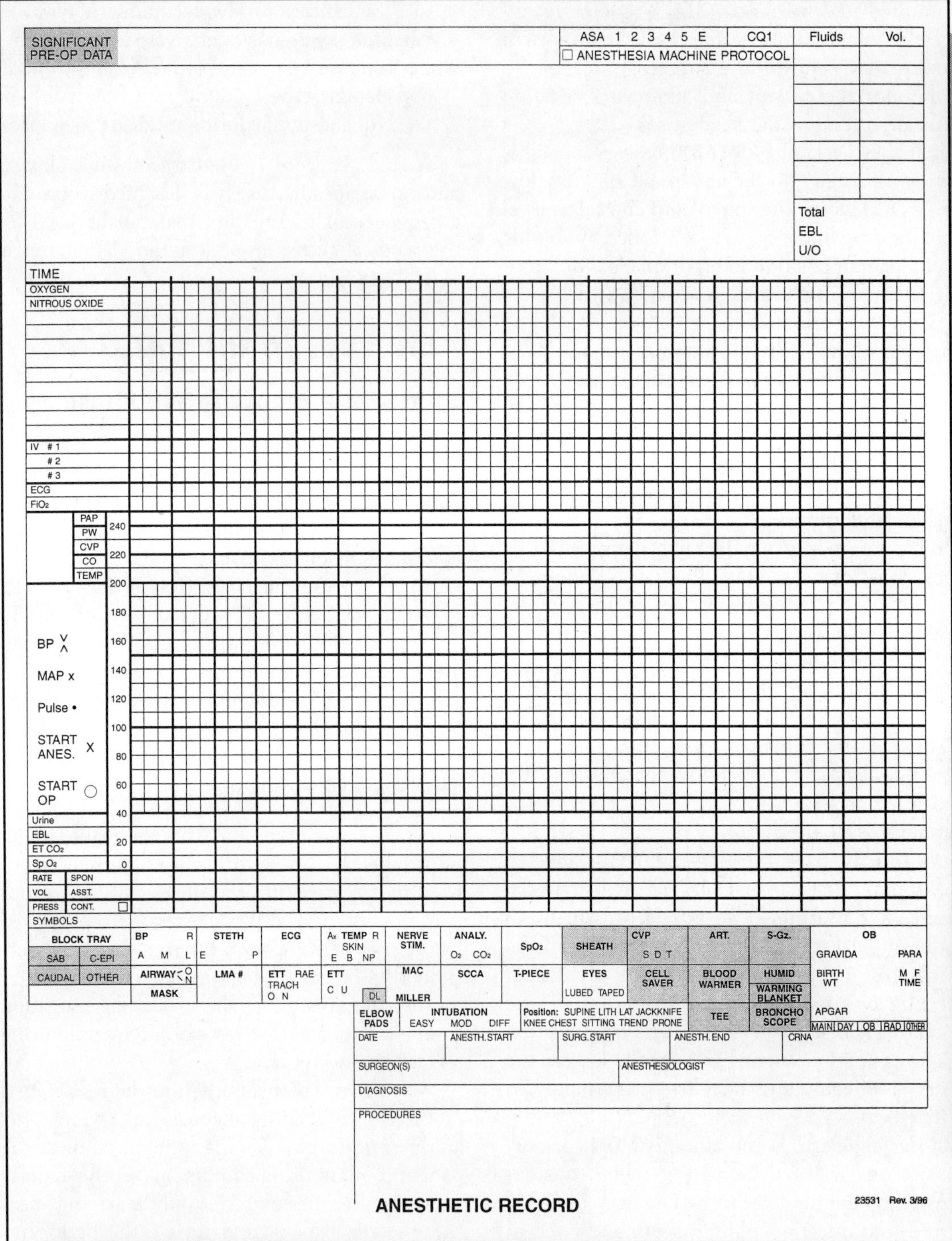

SIGNIFICANT PRE-OP DATA

ASA 1 2 3 4 5 E | CQ1 | Fluids | Vol.

☐ ANESTHESIA MACHINE PROTOCOL

Total
EBL
U/O

TIME
OXYGEN
NITROUS OXIDE
IV #1
#2
#3
ECG
FiO_2
PAP
PW
CVP
CO
TEMP

240 220 200 180 160 140 120 100 80 60 40 20 0

BP ˅˄
MAP x
Pulse •
START ANES. X
START OP ○

Urine
EBL
ET CO_2
Sp O_2
RATE | SPON
VOL | ASST.
PRESS | CONT. ☐
SYMBOLS

BLOCK TRAY
SAB | C-EPI
CAUDAL | OTHER
BP R
A M L
E
STETH
P
AIRWAY < O N
MASK
LMA #
ECG
ETT RAE TRACH O N
Ax TEMP R SKIN E B NP
ETT C U
DL
NERVE STIM.
MAC
MILLER
ANALY. O_2 CO_2
SCCA
SpO_2
T-PIECE
SHEATH
EYES LUBED TAPED
CVP S D T
CELL SAVER
ART.
BLOOD WARMER
S-Gz.
HUMID
WARMING BLANKET
OB
GRAVIDA PARA
BIRTH WT M F TIME
ELBOW PADS
INTUBATION EASY MOD DIFF
Position: SUPINE LITH LAT JACKKNIFE KNEE CHEST SITTING TREND PRONE
TEE
BRONCHO SCOPE
APGAR
MAIN | DAY | OB | RAD | OTHER

DATE | ANESTH. START | SURG. START | ANESTH. END | CRNA
SURGEON(S) | ANESTHESIOLOGIST
DIAGNOSIS
PROCEDURES

ANESTHETIC RECORD

23531 Rev. 3/96

Figure 14–40
Anesthetic record. (Courtesy of Deaconess Medical Center, Spokane, WA.)

HISTORY & PHYSICAL

DATE:__________ AGE:__________

CHIEF COMPLAINT:__________

PROPOSED PROCEDURE:__________

SYSTEM REVIEW: CARDIAC: _____ NEURO: _____ PULM. _____ EENT: _____ GI: _____ GU:_____

PERTINENT ROS:__________

PAST MEDICAL HISTORY:__________

MEDICATIONS:__________ **ALLERGIES:**__________

PERTINENT PHYSICAL FINDINGS: BP: P: HT: WT:

SYSTEM:	WNL	FINDINGS:
HEENT	☐	
HEART/LUNG	☐	
ABDOMEN	☐	
EXTREMITIES	☐	
REFLEXES	☐	
PELVIC/GU	☐	

PRE-OP ORDERS

PRE-OP ORDERS: LAB TO BE DONE: H & H ☐ CBC ☐ K+ ☐ NO LAB ☐ OTHER:__________

COMPLETED LAB:__________ Where Drawn:__________

☐ See Standing Orders__________

POST-OP ORDERS

PROCEDURE DONE:

DISCHARGE ORDERS FROM SURGEON:__________

MAY BE DISCHARGED TO__________ WITH ESCORT, WHEN DISCHARGE CRITERIA MET.

ADMIT TO HOSPITAL ROOM ☐ REASON:__________

24° OBSERVATION ☐ REASON:__________

POST-OP DIAGNOSIS: SURGEON SIGNATURE__________

ADDRESSOGRAPH

WHITE COPY – CHART
YELLOW COPY – PHARMACY – PRE-OP

DAY SURGERY CENTER - DEACONESS MEDICAL CENTER
SURGICAL HISTORY AND PHYSICAL
DOCTOR'S ORDER SHEET

01.12030-005 DMC 4/94

Figure 14–41
History, physical, and order sheet. (Courtesy of Deaconess Medical Center, Spokane, WA.)

nurses perform a more detailed assessment and record their findings on the PACU record. Patients are observed and monitored for hemodynamic or airway management problems. Vital signs are typically taken on admission, then every 5 minutes × 3, and then every 15 minutes until discharge from the unit

The RN constantly assesses for

Airway protection and maintenance—by closely monitoring the patient who has an artificial airway in place (**endotracheal tube** [ETT] or oropharyngeal airway) until it can be safely removed. It must be ensured that the patient's protective reflexes, which were obtunded under anesthesia, have returned.

Hemodynamic stability—by maintaining the blood pressure within a prescribed percentage of the patient's normal pressure. If it remains higher or lower, treatment for hypo- or hypertension is instituted.

Hemorrhage—by checking for signs and symptoms of bleeding. If bleeding occurs, the attending surgeon is notified, and the patient may need to return to the operating room.

Pain treatment—by providing individual pain therapy to achieve patient comfort. Each patient's pain must be objectively evaluated, since individuals respond uniquely to pain and pain medication.

Discharge from the PACU

The length of stay in the PACU varies with patient acuity, the severity and length of the operative procedure, physician preference, and the age of the patient. Other factors are the anesthetic agent used, the method of administration, and the patients's response to it. The average length of stay is 1 hour. The anesthesiologist is responsible for the discharge of the patient from the PACU. One procedure for discharge involves a standing order based on written criteria that are applied to each patient:

1. Level of consciousness: Patient is awake, alert, and oriented or has returned to preanesthetic state. *Exception*—the sedated patient returning to a specialty care unit such as **CTU**, **SICU**, **PICU**, or **ICU**.
2. Patient is able to move all extremities on command or has returned to preanesthetic state. *Exception*—regional block or spinal anesthetic block patients. Spinal anesthesia patients are discharged when they are able to identify sensation below the level of the umbilicus.
3. Respiratory rate and depth are normal for age. The patient is able to cough and deep-breathe and manage secretions or has returned to preanesthetic state. *Exception*—those patients going to a special care unit for ventilatory support.

3A. Oxygen saturation is 95 percent or greater or represents a return to preanesthetic recording.

4. Vital signs, including pulse, respirations, and blood pressure, are determined to be stable if they are consistent with the patient's age and are within 20 percent of the preanesthetic values.
5. Skin color is normal for the patient's skin tone.
6. The temperature is >95°F in adults, >96°F in children. Values based on oral or tympanic methods.
7. If invasive lines were inserted in the operating room, radiologic confirmation of proper placement is needed before discharge from the PACU.
8. Pain relief is adequate. Patient may be discharged from the PACU 25 minutes following the administration of IV sedation or narcotics. *Exception*—patients on PCA pump may be discharged within 10 minutes of maintenance dose. Patients on epidural or continuous PCA administration of narcotics may be discharged when criteria 1–7 have been met.
9. Pediatric patients may be sent to ambulatory care or pediatric unit when awake. *Exception*—Following tonsillectomy and adenoidectomy, patients must stay a minimum of 30 minutes.

If the patient does not meet the above criteria, discharge must be done on direct order from the anesthesiologist.

The PACU is considered phase I recovery.

Phase II, which is considered a progression to more independence and return to a normal physiologic state, takes place in the ambulatory care area for those patients who are going home the same day. It takes place in the in-patient units for those patients who require continued hospitalization.

Medications Used in the PACU

Some of the dugs given in the PACU are

Narcotics—fentanyl, morphine, Demerol
Oral pain medications—Vicodin, Tylenol No. 3
Antiemetics—Inapsine, Reglan, Zofran
Antibiotics—cefazolin, gentamicin, vancomycin
Narcotic antagonist—Narcan
Muscle relaxant reversal drugs—neostigmine, Tensilon, atropine
Neuromuscular blocking agents—Anectine, Pavulon
Antianxiety drugs—Versed, Valium

Treatments and Procedures Specific to the PACU

Many of the procedures done in the PACU involve the maintenance of a clear airway. Suctioning is used if a patient is unable to cough and the airway is blocked with secretions. A patient may develop complications and have an ETT inserted and attached to a ventilator. A laryngeal mask airway (**LMA**) is a flexible tube with an inflatable silicone ring and cuff. When the device is inserted and the cuff inflated, it fills the space around and behind the larynx, forming a seal between the tube and the trachea. Oxygen saturation monitoring is carried out on these as on all patients.

A blood patch is a procedure used in the treatment of spinal headache. Five to eight milliliters of the individual's blood is administered at the spinal puncture site by the anesthesiologist.

Hemodynamic monitoring includes the use of the invasive techniques of arterial, central venous, and pulmonary artery pressure monitoring to indicate the blood pressure and volume status. If invasive monitoring lines are not present, the hemodynamic monitoring is accomplished by closely observing the blood pressure, level of consciousness, skin temperature, and urine output. Postprocedural x-rays and laboratory tests are done in the PACU, and blood is administered in addition to IV fluids.

Equipment and Supplies Used in the PACU

All patients are connected to monitors for heart rate and rhythm, blood pressure, and oxygen saturation. The electrodes, leads, and lines needed to accomplish the monitoring are kept in the individual bays. There are tissues and emesis basins in each bay as well as oral airways. Bair Huggers are used to warm the patients to near-normal temperatures after surgery. Tympanic or oral thermometers and thermometer sheaths and covers are made available. Ventilators are readily available for use when needed. There is a crash cart with defibrillator, drugs, IV solutions, and endotracheal intubation equipment on the unit.

Role of the Health Unit Coordinator in the PACU

Immediate Responsibilities

Physician Order Transcription

Most patients are in the PACU for only an hour. Charts must be reviewed in a quick and efficient manner to maintain smooth patient flow. X-rays, laboratory studies, and EKGs that are to be done in the PACU are ordered STAT. This is a cost-containment measure taken to avoid prolonged patient waiting time in the PACU.

The physician's orders are reviewed immediately. The HUC highlights those that need to be carried out in the PACU. This alerts the nurses to medications and procedures that are marked "now" or "give in PACU." The orders that are carried out while the patient is in the PACU are noted on the order sheet as completed. This prevents their being duplicated at a later time. The anesthesia standing order form (Fig. 14–42) is checked for special orders written by the anesthesiologist.

Some medications are ordered to be given in PACU. The HUC checks the anesthetic record, the intraoperative record (Fig. 14–43), and the preop information form (Fig. 14–44) for prior doses of the medication. The HUC then notes the time of any previous doses next to the order.

When blood is to be administered in PACU, it may be a new order or it may have been ordered preoperatively. If the former, it must be submitted to the blood bank of the lab ASAP for processing. If the latter, the patient will already have been typed and crossmatched. In many facilities, the blood is available in a special refrigerator in the operating suite. Occasionally, medications are ordered that are not routinely stocked in the PACU. The HUC will send a highlighted copy of the order to the pharmacy, utilizing the pneumatic tube system if the facility is so equipped. The order will be immediately filled and returned to the PACU.

Processing Charts

The charts of ambulatory care patients will remain in the binder or folder that they came in. The forms are placed in the order that is most helpful to the nurses. This allows easy access to the forms that they use most frequently (Fig. 14–45). The ambulatory care charts contain a special form for patient discharge instructions. The PACU HUC will enter the MD phone number of the surgeon, the next MD appointment date and time, and instructions for dressing changes, diet, and bathing and showering on this form. Any prescriptions will be attached to this form.

If a patient is an AM admission, the PACU chart is disassembled. An in-patient chart is created by adding extra forms to it. It is reassembled into the recommended order for an in-patient chart. The HUC is responsible for adding special forms to the PACU record, such as diabetic care forms or anticoagulant therapy record.

Other Responsibilities

The day goes by quickly in the PACU because of the fast pace and quick turnover of patients. An efficient HUC must be focused and cannot be distracted. There are times, driven by the surgery schedule, that allow the HUC to accomplish other tasks that are his or her responsibility.

Directly Assisting the Nurses

The PACU HUC may obtain the IV solution bags for the nurses. The HUC must get the ordered fluid, label it correctly, and charge it to the patient. The HUCs assist by collecting the belongings of patients who are going to be in-patients. They may be asked to help transport patients to their rooms. Occasionally they may be asked to hold or sit with fully recovered infants or children while the nurse finishes charting.

Entering Patient Charges

Patient charges are entered into the computer by the PACU HUC. Charge systems vary from facility to facility. Some use charge cards and others a sticker system. It is important that the charges be entered accurately so that the patient is not overcharged and yet the hospital recoups what is due. The basic PACU charges are entered from a form used by the nurses that designates the length of stay and the extent of nursing need for each patient.

Ordering Equipment and Supplies

Some of the supplies are ordered to replace stock supplies. These include solutions, basins, tissues, forms, and desk supplies. This ordering is done by phone, computer, or requisition form. When the supplies arrive, the area is restocked, checking the supplies against what was ordered.

Other supplies are ordered for individual patients on an as-needed basis. These include such

Text continued on page 315

DATE:________ PATIENT STATES ALLERGIC TO: ____________________ ____________________

MEDICAL CENTER
PHYSICIAN'S ORDERS

Draw a line through orders that are not applicable and/or should not be implemented. Date and initial the deletion as well.

PRE-OPERATIVE

I. NPO Requirements: SEE SCHEDULE 1

II. Laboratory Requirements:
  A. Serum K+ within 7 days of surgery for all patients on diuretics or digitalis receiving anesthesiology services; otherwise, at surgeon's discretion.
  B. K+ must be repeated if there have been changes in the patient's health after the original laboratory values were obtained.
  C. An H/H should be drawn pre-operatively if there is a history of blood loss in the last month or if the scheduled surgery has a possibility of moderate or greater blood loss.

III. Intravenous Fluids:
  A. IV or male adaptor plugs in all patients can be waived only via written order from the surgeon.
  B. Adults - Plasma-Lyte 148
  C. Children - PL 148, soluset microdrip of child's weight is less than 80 lbs.

IV. Medication:

V. Special Circumstance:
  A. Diabetics - Insulin dependent patients - D5PL 148 with a dial-a-flow.
  B. Pregnancy - Contact Anesthesiologist.
  C. Dialysis Patients - Saline lock - consult attending physician for additional orders.
  D. Bier Block - #22g. Saline lock in hand of operative extremity (one attempt only).

POST-OPERATIVE

Nursing Care:
  A. Cardiac Monitor
  B. O_2 6-8 liters per mask/or 2-3 L per NC.
  C. Extubate when awake and Inspiratory Effort is -30cm H_2O or more.
  D. ABGs at 20 min if on Ventilator after changes or when placed on Briggs.
  E. PCXR for CVP, P.A. or E.T. placement.
  F. Ventilator Settings O_2 _____ Mode _____ Rate _____ T.V. _____ SV _____ Peep _____
  G. If O_2 SAT below _____ Add O_2 _____ per NC x _____ hrs.

Medications:

1. Bradycardia: Atropine 0.1 - 0.4 mg IV.
2. Adults: Pain
   a. Fentanyl 25 micrograms IV prn, not to exceed 100 micrograms
   b. Narcotic may be given IV or IM in small divided doses q 10 min. not to exceed maximum dose ordered.
   c. Acetaminophen or Tylenol #3, 1-2 tabs PO prn if tolerating fluids and solids.

   Epidural Analgesia
   a. RN may give up to a 5 cc Epidural Bolus x 1 in PACU only.

   Children: Pain
   a. Fentanyl IV: SEE SCHEDULE 2.
   b. Acetaminophen Elixir or tablets PO or Acetaminophen suppository rectally: SEE SCHEDULE 3.
3. Adults: Nausea/Emesis
   a. ☐ Metoclopramide 10 mg IV, may repeat x _________prn
   b. ☐ Droperidol 0.25 mg IV NOW and may repeat x 1 prn
   c. ☐ Ondansetron 4 mg IV x _________ prn
   d. ☐ Promethazine supp. 25 mg PR x 1 prn

   Children: Nausea/Emesis
   a. ☐ Metoclopramide 0.1 mg/kg IV x 1 - NOT TO EXCEED 10 mg prn
   b. ☐ Droperidol 0.25 mg IV x 1.
   c. ☐ Ondansetron 0.1 mg/kg for pts x _________ under 40 kg prn
   d. ☐ Trimethobenzamide 100 mg PR x 1 prn
4. May give 300 cc IV solution rapidly for hypotension in adults.
5. May add Plasma-Lyte 148.
6. Discontinue IV/male adaptor plug before discharge from DSC.
7. May Heparin Lock rather than DC IV. For patient going to ward flag chart front.
8. May be discharged when Discharge Criteria met for Phase I____________________ Phase II____________________

Dr. Signature: ____________________ Date: __________

ADDRESSOGRAPH:

ANESTHESIA PRE AND POST OP STANDING ORDERS

Figure 14–42
Anesthesia standing order form. (Courtesy of Deaconess Medical Center, Spokane, WA.)

PRE-OP: Date: ______ Time: ______ Pre-Op Assess. Reviewed ______

___ ID/Blood/Allergy bands on ___ H&P done

___ Surgery Consent Signed ___ EKG Overread

___ Sterilization/IOL/Video ___ Labs complete

___ Verbally verifies procedure ___ Seen by AA

___ NPO since ______ ___ Surgeon ID time

___ X-Ray done here

BLOOD PRODUCTS ORDERED:
T & S T & C
RBCs: ______
Platelets ______
FFP: ______
Cryo: ______
Auto: ______

Dentures Contacts Glasses Hearing Aids Rings

w/Family ______ To O.R. ______

Meds: ______

Allergies: ______

Comments: ______

Signature: ______

INTRA OP: O.R. RM. # ______ PreOp Dx: ______

AA ______ **CRNA** ______

ANES: Gen. Spinal Epid. MAC Local Other: ______

SURGEON ID TIME: **TIME IN:** **TIME OUT:**

PROCEDURE	Start	End	Class
1.			
2.			
3.			

SURGEON: #1 ______
#2 ______
#3 ______

ASSISTANT #1 ______
#2 ______
#3 ______

SCRUBS #1 ______
#2 ______
#3 ______
#4 ______

Scrub Relief ______

CIRCS. #1 ______
#2 ______

Circ. Relief: ______

NURSING DIAGNOSIS: Potential for injury
PATIENT OUTCOME/GOAL: Patient injury free

Position: Supine Prone Lith. Lat. Other: ______

Position Aids: Elbow pads Safety belt Stirrup Straps Pillows Donut Bath blanket Other: ______

K-Thermia: # ______ Temp. ______ Ordered by: ______ Policy

Bovie # ______ Pad Site ______ Bovie # ______ Pad Site ______

Tourniquet # ______ Insp. by ______ Appl. by ______ Site: ______

Pressure Up ______ Down ______ Up ______ Down ______ Setting: ______

SKIN INTEGRITY P.O. Satisfactory Unsatisfactory See Comments

DEACONESS MEDICAL CENTER
SURGICAL SERVICES INTRA OP RECORD
Plan & Implementation

NURSING DIAGNOSIS: Potential for infection
PATIENT OUTCOME/GOAL: No wound infection

Shave: N/A By ______ Area ______

Prep Site: ______

w/: Betadine Scrub Sol. Iodine 1% 3½% Gel Alcohol 70%

Other: ______

Meds/Irrigations: ______

Implants Intra-Op: ______

Specimens: ______

Cultures: ______

Urinary Cath: No Type ______ to D.D. Uri. Other ______

Amt. Emptied in OR: ______ by ______

Tubes & Drains: ______

Packing/Dressings: ______

X-Rays: ______

CELL SAVER: # ______ Returned cc's ______

COUNTS: Sharps: Correct Incorrect N/A
Sponges: Correct Incorrect Deferred

Signature (if appl): ______

Inst.s sterility checked by: Indicator Graph

Inst.s disinfected w: ______ x ______ Min.

COMMENTS: ______

Transferred to: PACU CICU ICU PDR Unit Other: ______

w/Dentures Contacts Glasses Hearing Aids Rings I.D. Band

Other: ______ Received by: ______

w/Airway O2 Mask ET Tube Ambu Monitor Other: ______

Report by: AA Other: ______ To: Unit Staff Other: ______

Signatures: ______

ADDRESSOGRAPH

01-12020-061 8/93

Figure 14–43
Intraoperative record. (Courtesy of Deaconess Medical Center, Spokane, WA.)

PERIOPERATIVE DATA COLLECTION AND ASSESSMENT

Page 1

ADMISSION ASSESSMENT

Pre-Reg. Visit Date:
Pre-Op Call Made Date:
Busy X ___ No Answer X ___ Other ___
PROCEDURE: Per Pt.

Information Given For:
☐ General ☐ Local ☐ MAC ☐ Block
Previous Surgeries:

Anesthesia Problems:

SENSITIVITIES/ALLERGIES: ☐ No known allergies

Drugs	Reaction	Drugs	Reaction

Food/sulfiting agents

Iodine: ☐ No ☐ Yes Latex: ☐ No ☐ Yes Tape: ☐ No ☐ Yes

Current Medications:

	Medication	Dose	Freq	Time last dose taken
1)				
2)				
3)				
4)				
5)				
6)				
7)				
8)				
9)				
10)				

If patient or family is unsure of above information, note by / (slash) in appropriate box

Y N
Pre-Admission information given
Instructed to arrive @
Reminded to bring consent
Reminded of NPO
Instructed to bring own meds.
ASA taken within 72 hours
Transportation home arranged

Y N
BELIEFS/VALUES:
Spiritual, personal or cultural beliefs that will affect your care
A specific concern to discuss with Chaplaincy Services
Concerned about your safety or violence or abuse at home

NURSING COMMENTS:

HISTORY OF MEDICAL CONDITION:

Y N
Heart/chest pain/Pacemaker
BP Problems
Stroke/Seizures
Respiratory/TB
Diabetes
Kidney
Gastrointestinal
Liver/Hepatitis
Back/neck problems
Arthritis
Implants/Prosthesis
Bleeding tendency
Pregnant
Motion sickness
Loose/Capped Teeth
Dentures/Partials
Alcohol use: Amt:
Tobacco ☐smoke ___ pk/day/___ yrs ☐chew tobacco/___ years
Recreational drugs ☐ quit ___ years ago
Auto blood given ___ units
Units of Blood ordered
Previous Blood Transfusions
Reactions: If yes, describe
Any Objections ___ Refusal signed

POTENTIAL FOR INJURY

MOBILITY ASSESSMENT:
Steady on feet ☐ Unsteady on feet ☐ Recent falls: ☐
Aids to mobility: NA ☐ Cane ☐ Walker ☐
Crutches ☐ Wheelchair ☐ Prosthesis ☐

POTENTIAL FOR IMPAIRED COMMUNICATION

IMPAIRMENTS:
Hearing: Adequate ☐ Decreased Rt ☐ Lt ☐
Deaf Rt ☐ LT ☐ Hearing Aid Rt ☐ Lt ☐
Vision: Adequate ☐ Decreased Rt ☐ Lt ☐
Glasses ☐ Contacts ☐ Prosthesis ☐
Communication: English ☐ Other ☐
Interpreter

Discharge Planning
Lives: Alone ___ With ___
No known Residence
Intended destination post-discharge
Home ___ Other ___ Undetermined ___
Previous utilization of community resources
Home care ___ Home health aide ___ Hospice ___
Meals/Wheels ___ Chore services ___ Church Group ___
Comm. Mental Health ___ Comm. support group ___
Other

VITAL STATISTICS
DATE: TIME: AGE: HT: WT: lbs. Kgs. P: Radial ___ Apical ___ Regular☐ Irregular☐
NPO since ___ FHT: Temp: PO/REC/AX/TYMP R: BP: Room Air O_2 Sat Level ___

DATE IF PRE-REG:
UA
CBC
H & H
K+
C-Pop
SMA12
PT
PTT
Type/Cross/Screen/ Auto Blood

Lytes
Acid P'Tase
Rh Factor
Bleeding Time
Creatinine
HCG
Other:
Lab Sent @

Chest X-Ray done
EKG done
EKG Monitor On
No abnormalities
See Progress Notes
Chem Stick: Results:
X-ray Requisition sent
To X-ray via WC/Stretcher @
From X-ray via WC/Stretcher @

INSTRUCTIONS GIVEN TO PT:
Douche
Enema
Shower
Incentive Spirometer

TED Hose Measurements:

INI	SIGNATURE

ADDRESSOGRAPH

DEACONESS MEDICAL CENTER - SPOKANE
PRE-OP INFORMATION & CARE
01.12030-001 7/94 pg.1

Page 2

ADMISSION DATA

1% Lidocaine 0.1cc subdermal for local anesthesia
Peripheral cath
MAP lock c̄ Saline flush
PL 148 1,000cc
PL 148 D5W 1,000cc
D5W 500cc
Soluset
Other:
1" 1¼" 2"
22ga. 20ga. 18ga. 16ga.
Rt. Lt. Hand Wrist Forearm Antecubital Basilic

Additional IV's:
Attempted X
Attempt Site(s):
Treat. unsuccessful Site(s):
☐ Hot Pack ☐ Pressure Dressing
☐ Elevated ☐ Cold Pack
SIGNATURE:

PRE-OP MEDS
☐ Pts. condition stable after pre-op medication.
If not, describe: B/P P R
☐ Side Rails Up

EYE LOCAL PER DR.
Time:
Wydase amp. i
___ % Xylo.
___ % Xylo c̄ Epi. 1:200,000
___ % Marcaine
___ % Marcaine c̄ Epi. 1:200,000
Other:

SURGICAL PREP:
SIG:

NURSING CARE PLAN
NURSING DIAGNOSIS: Knowledge Deficit
PATIENT GOAL: Understands Pre-op teaching

Y N
Explain treatment/procedure and expected outcome
Orient patient to surgical/recovery environment
Instructions for post-op extremity exercises/activity/cough & deep breathing
Orient patient to discharge criteria/alternative admission if applicable
Explain oral intake/IV intake
Explain urinary output/foley catheter if applicable
Instructions for pain control/PCA pump if applicable

Y N
PARTICIPATION OF SIGNIFICANT OTHER:
Orient significant other to hospital surroundings.
Explain anticipated time schedule
Significant other's questions/concerns addressed
Pt. receptive to instruction and education

Comments:

NURSING NOTES
YES NO Authorizes Posting of Name

DSC PRE-OP CHECKLIST
INITIAL ALL ITEMS CHECKED
Yes No
ID/Allergy/Blood band on (circle)
Surgical Consent signed & on chart
Sterilization AB/IOL/Video Consent signed
Voided
Seen by AA
ID by Surgeon
Labs Complete
EKG Overread
H & P done
Verbal verification of proc./site

Disposition to Family/OR/Locker #
Clothes
Contacts
Glasses
Dentures
Hearing Aids
Prosthesis

Admission Assessment Reviewed: ☐ Agree ☐ Disagree ☐ Comments:
Circled items to OR: Dentures / Hearing Aids / Contacts / Glasses
☐ To OR @ via stretcher c rails up / WC / Amb / Carried SIG:

OBSERVATIONS
Emotional Status
Relaxed/Cooperative ___ Uncoop.
Openly anxious ___
Other (explain)
Respiratory
Dyspnea Yes ___ No ___
Precipated by
Cough Yes ___ No ___
Productive? ___ Nonproductive? ___
Sputum
Breath Sounds ☐ Clear to bases
Other
Circulatory
Edema Yes ___ No ___
Describe
Calf Tenderness Yes ___ No ___
Pedal Pulses Palpable Bilat. Yes ___ No ___
Extremity Sensation WNL ___
If Not, Describe
Neurological
Awake & Oriented Yes ___ No ___
If Not, Describe
Speech Clear/Appropriate Yes ___ No ___
If Not, Describe
Pupils PERRLA Yes ___ No ___
If Not, Describe
Grips equal bil. Yes ___ No ___
Abdomen
Distention Yes ___ No ___
If so, describe
Bowel tones in 4 quadrants Yes ___ No ___
If not, describe
Nutritional Assessment
Appetite WNL ___ Time of last meal ___
Special diet Yes ___ No ___
If special diet, describe
Weight fluctuations, last 6 mos Yes ___ No ___
If yes, describe
Skin *Color WNL* Yes ___ No ___
Hot ___ Cold ___ Dry ___ Diaphoretic ___
If not WNL, describe

Describe and Mark Diagram *No Abnormalities*
1. Incision
2. Bruise/Contusion
3. Laceration
4. Decubiti
5. Burn
6. Rash
7. Petechiae
8. Other

R L L R

Comments:

INI	SIGNATURE

ADDRESSOGRAPH

DEACONESS MEDICAL CENTER - SPOKANE
PRE-OP INFORMATION & CARE
01.12030-001 7/94 pg.2

Figure 14–44
Preop info and care form. (Courtesy of Deaconess Medical Center, Spokane, WA.)

POST ANESTHESIA

DAY SURGERY CENTER
DEACONESS MEDICAL CENTER

DATE__________

ANESTHESIOLOGIST__________ PRE-OP V.S.__________

SURGEON__________ MEDICAL PROBLEMS:__________

PROCEDURE:__________ ALLERGIES:__________

STRETCHER ☐ Both siderails up ☐ PACU 4 W.______

PER CRIB ☐ Safety strap on above knees ☐ PACU I______

W/C ☐ Elbow Protected Rt. ☐ Lt. ☐ PACU II______

AMBULATION ☐ Chair #______

ANESTHESIA: General ☐ Local ☐ Regional ☐ MAC ☐

SCORE	AD	DC
Color		
LOC		
Circ.		
Resp.		
Act.		

LEVELS OF ANESTHESIA: Legs ☐ Rt. Arm ☐ Lt. Arm ☐

	Y	N
Warm, Pink		
Sensation		
Pulses		
Motion		

AIRWAY____/____

Time DC'd______

O_2 1/min.______

Time DC'd______

O_2S______

Breath Sounds Clear ☐

T:

LOCATION: IV ☐ HL ☐ LT. ☐ RT. ☐ Hand ☐ Wrist ☐ Forearm ☐ Anticubital ☐

#	Time	Sol.	Inj.

SOLUTION #
1 L. PL 148
1 L. PL 148 w/D5W
Other:

SITE: Redness ☐ Swelling ☐ Tender ☐ Asympt ☐

IV DC'd By:
Inj.______ Time:______
Cath Intact ☐
Pressure dsg. ☐
Site Asympt. ☐

SITE HAS: Swelling ☐ Redness ☐ Tender ☐

Other:______

Total IV:______

☐ Pre-op Assessment, History & Physical Reviewed

☐ Report given to PACU-Phase II RN

The following protocols have been followed:

__Basic Monitoring in PACU
__General anesthesia
__Spinal anesthesia
__Local anesthesia

The following problem specific care protocols have been followed:

1. Inadequate ventilation related to anes.
2. Hemodynamic instability
3. Pain related
4. Hemorrhage related to surgery
5. Hypo-hyperthermia
6. Hyperactivity
7. Continued somnolence
8. Nausea/vomiting

Psychosocial Assessment
Emotional Status

Relaxed/Cooperative______
Openly anxious______
Uncooperative______
Other (explain)______

TIME	COMMENT

RECOVERY RECORD **EKG STRIP**

V Λ RESP. X PULSE •

190
170
150
130
110
90
70
50
30
10

TIME ACCOUNTABILITY

Level	Nrs	PT.
1	1	4
2	1	3
3	1	2
4	1	1
5	2	1

OUTPUT

Time	Amt	Source

TIME	MEDICATION	AMT.	ROUTE	SITE	INIT.

	Y	N
Discharge instructions and instruction sheet given to — States Understands		
Responsible adult to take home		
Take Home Medication (see home inst)		
Discharge criteria met		

Transported via: Ambulation ☐ W/C ☐ Carried ☐

Escorted by: Time

SIGNATURE	TIME	INIT.	SIGNATURE	TIME	INIT.

ADDRESSOGRAPH

01.12030-003 7/95

Figure 14–45
Postanesthesia care record. (Courtesy of Deaconess Medical Center, Spokane, WA.)

items as binders, braces, slings, compression devices, and cold therapy equipment. As soon as it is known that a ventilator is needed, the HUC notifies the respiratory therapy department of the type of ventilator and when it will be needed.

Collecting and Submitting Statistical Data

The HUC compiles the statistics for the unit. These are collected daily to record the number, length of stay, and types of patients cared for in the PACU each day. If there is a preoperative area, the same data must be retrieved. The statistics are critical to the budgeting process by demonstrating the productivity of the nursing staff and the use of supplies. The information is collated and submitted to the manager biweekly.

Cleaning of the Unit

HUCs utilize slack time to perform cleaning duties around the desk area. They may also work as a team player by assisting the nurses to clean around the patient care area.

Communication

Communication About the PACU Patient

Communication is a large part of the PACU HUC job. Triaging the many telephone calls coming into the unit frees the nursing staff to provide patient care. A call from the circulating nurse in the operating room gives an estimated time of arrival for a patient into the PACU. The HUC notifies the charge nurse that the patient is arriving and relays the information received, such as the patient's general condition and the need for drainage equipment, ventilator, or special monitoring equipment.

When the patient arrives in the unit, the HUC calls the waiting area to notify the family that the surgery is over and that someone will be out to speak to them. If the patient is going to a special care unit or other in-patient unit, a call is made to notify the staff that the patient is in the PACU. The receiving unit can anticipate the patient's transfer and free up staff accordingly. When the patient is about to be transferred out of the PACU, a call is made to the waiting area to instruct the family where the patient will be. A physician may order a patient to be transferred to a unit other than what was anticipated. The HUC must notify both units of this change in plans.

The HUC notifies the charge nurse of any add-on surgeries, cancellations of surgeries, or any patient who has been sent directly back to ambulatory care or a special care unit. The HUC must understand the jargon or short forms of terms used in the area to understand the surgical schedule (Table 14–7).

In an emergency or "Code" situation, the PACU HUC will move closer to the patient to hear orders, place telephone calls for needed personnel and equipment, and order diagnostic tests per computer. The assistance by the HUC during this hectic time once again frees the nursing staff to provide direct patient care. The HUC places calls to chaplains, physicians, and other departments as requested. The charge nurse, staff nurses, and HUC are focused on optimal patient care, and communication is coordinated to provide this.

Communicating with the Postanesthesia Patient

Patients are still asleep or just beginning to awake when they enter the PACU. The nurses ask questions to assess their level of consciousness. Statements are made to orient them. The patients are questioned about pain, and the pain is evaluated on a scale of 1 to 10. The greatest imaginable pain is 10, and 1 is the least. The patients are asked to move their extremities and squeeze the nurse's hands to assess their motor activity.

Anesthesia has unique effects on people. Some may awaken violently—crying, screaming, and shaking. Others awaken as they would from a night's sleep. Patients must be reassured that the

Table 14–7 LANGUAGE OF THE PACU: SURGICAL AND ANESTHESIA PROCEDURES

Term	Refers to
ACF	Anterior cervical fusion
AKA	Above-knee amputation
Anes	Anesthesia
AVR	Aortic valve replacement
BKA	Below-knee amputation
BMT	Bilateral myringotomy with tubes
BSO	Bilateral salpingo-oophorectomy
CABG	Coronary artery bypass graft
CBD Expl	Common bile duct exploration
Chole with Gram	Cholecystectomy with cholecystogram
Crani	Craniotomy
CRIF	Closed reduction internal fixation
CT	Carpal tunnel
D & C	Dilation and curettage
Disc	Discectomy
EUA	Exam under anesthesia
FEM-POP	Femoral popliteal
FME	Full-mouth extraction
FTSG	Full-thickness skin graft
Ing	Inguinal
Lap	Laparotomy
Lig	Ligament
LIH	Left inguinal herniorrhaphy
Loc	Local
MAC	Monitored anesthesia care

Table 14–7 LANGUAGE OF THE PACU: SURGICAL AND ANESTHESIA PROCEDURES *(Continued)*

Term	Refer to
MLT	MiniLap tubal
MMK	Marshall Marchetti Krantz procedure
MVR	Mitral valve replacement
ORIF	Open reduction internal fixation
PUL	Percutaneous ureteral lithotomy
RGP	Retrograde pyelogram
RIH	Right inguinal herniorrhaphy
SAB	Spinal anesthetic block
Scope	Laparoscopy
T & A	Tonsillectomy and adenoidectomy
TAH	Total abdominal hysterectomy
THR	Total hip replacement
TKR	Total knee replacement
TURB	Transurethral resection bladder tumor
TURP	Transurethral resection of prostate
TVH	Total vaginal hysterectomy
TVR	Triscuspid valve replacement

surgery is over and that they are well. The nurses repeat these reassurances often during the recovery period.

Quality/Risk Management

The PACU HUC must be 100 percent accurate in order transcription and communication. Anything unusual noted in the record, such as allergies, is communicated to the nurses. Safety is ensured for the patient in the unit by adjusting the nurse-to-patient ratio to meet the changing requirements of the patients.

Stretcher safety is very important in PACU. The stretchers are narrow, and some patients are restless. Side rails must be in use at all times in the unit. Seatbelts are used during transportation. Unusual occurrences are recorded and reported to the appropriate department.

Closing Thoughts

The specific duties of the HUC in the PACU may differ somewhat from the duties on a medical/surgical floor in the hospital, but the basic goals are the same—to coordinate communication, transcribe physician's orders, and help keep the unit running smoothly. The HUC in a PACU must be able to manage a fast-paced flow of patients in an efficient and logical manner. Flexibility and willingness to assist in a variety of situations are important characteristics. It is useful to be able to anticipate the contributions that are most helpful. The HUC should be willing to float to other areas during low patient census in the PACU.

Review Questions

1. List and describe two anesthesia techniques.
2. A postop patient comes into PACU with the following MD order: "H & H STAT, if HCT below 30 or HG below 10, transfuse with 2 units of packed cells." Explain the process that the HUC would use to see to it that this order is carried out.
3. Name three places outside the PACU that an HUC might be in communication with. Describe the possible reason for each communication.
4. What is the role of the HUC in a "Code" situation?

Bibliography

Atkinson LJ, Fortunate NM: Berry & Kohn's Operating Room Technique, 8th ed. St. Louis, CV Mosby, 1996.

Discharge Criteria. Spokane, WA, Deaconess Medical Center.

Post Anesthesia Care Record. Spokane, WA, Deaconess Medical Center.

Special Care Units

14

PART 6: THE SURGICAL INTENSIVE CARE UNIT

Janice Wyse/Nancy Mania

Common Abbreviations

BIPAP	Bi-positive airway pressure
CVAHD	Continuous arteriovenous hemofiltration
ECMO	Extracorporeal membrane oxygenator
IABP	Intra-aortic balloon pump
ICP	Intracranial pressure (monitoring)
IS	Incentive spirometry
JP	Jackson-Pratt (suction)
MAST	Medical antishock trousers
PEG	Percutaneous endoscopic gastrostomy (tube)
PNS	Peripheral nerve stimulator

Objectives

Upon completion of this chapter, the reader will be able to:

1. Explain the unique considerations of the design/decor of the SICU.
2. List and describe procedures that can be carried out in the SICU.
3. Identify the difference in process relative to ordering x-rays in the SICU.
4. Explain the role of the health unit coordinator in a "code" situation.

Vocabulary

Chest tube: A tube placed into the pleural cavity to drain fluid

Jejunal feeding tube: A long flexible feeding tube placed into jejunum via the endoscope

Percutaneous endoscopic gastrostomy tube: An access tube placed through the abdominal wall into the stomach for nutrition and/or medication

---

The abbreviations listed for this chapter are those that a HUC working in this area would be expected to know. Only those in boldface type are used in the text and appear in boldface when they are used for the first time.

Medical Terms

Antiembolic stocking: Apply external pressure to help prevent the formation of blood clots in the legs

Arrhythmia: Irregular cardiac activity

Axiom drain: A device for applying low suctioning of a wound or incision

Bi-positive airway pressure (BIPAP): Mechanically assisted breathing that applies pressure at both the inspiratory and the expiratory phases

Cyanosis: Bluish skin color resulting from the interference of oxygenated blood flow

Edema: Excessive fluid in the tissue

Foley catheter: An indwelling urinary catheter

Glasgow Coma Scale: Measures neurologic status. The nurse observes the patient's verbal response, motor response, reactions to pain, and whether the eyes open in response to sound or painful stimulus (Table 14–8).

Hemovac suctioning: A draining device with an antireflux valve

Hyperalimentation: A high-calorie intravenous solution

Incentive spirometry (IS): Technique utilizing a device to encourage deep breathing in a postoperative or bedridden patient (Fig. 14–46)

Intracranial pressure monitoring (ICP): Measures fluid pressure within the cranium

Jackson-Pratt (JP) suctioning: A bulb suction for wound drainage

Montgomery straps: Multiuse tape designed for use on large and/or long-term dressings

Nasogastric suction: Emptying of the stomach via a tube placed there through the nose. It may be continuous or intermittent suction.

Neurologic checks: Measure mental status, orientation, pupillary reaction, and whether the strength is equal in both hands

Pacemaker: An electrical device to stabilize the heart rate

Red Robinson drain: A catheter type drain placed surgically to promote drainage from a wound or incision without the use of a suction device

T-Tube drainage: Dependent drainage of bile from the common bile duct

Table 14–8 GLASCOW COMA SCALE

Eyes Open	
Never	1
To pain	2
To verbal stimuli	3
Spontaneously	4
Best Verbal Response	
No response	1
Incomprehensible sounds	2
Inappropriate words	3
Disoriented and converses	4
Oriented and converses	5
Best Motor Response	
No response	1
Extension (decerebrate rigidity)	2
Flexion abnormal (decorticate rigidity)	3
Flexion withdrawal	4
Localizes pain	5
Obeys	6
TOTAL	3–15

The medical terms are some that might be used in a SICU. They do not appear in the text, but they are terms that the reader who is interested in the SICU should be familiar with.

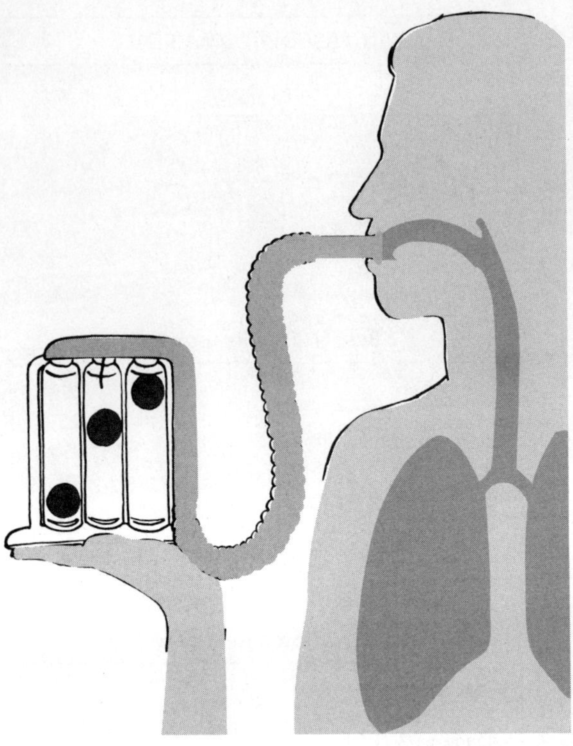

Figure 14–46
Incentive spirometer. (From Black JM, Matassarin-Jacobs E: Medical-Surgical Nursing: Clinical Management for Continuity of Care, 5th ed. Philadelphia, WB Saunders, 1997.)

Traction: Externally applied fixation devices used to stabilize fractures. Most commonly seen are Bucks, Crutchfield tongs, and halos.

Ventriculostomy: Placement of a drainage tube to decrease fluid in the brain.

Description of the Unit

The hospital intensive care unit can provide a picture of modern health care at its finest. Here, patients in their hours of greatest need receive the most skilled care that medical professionals can give. Lives are saved literally every day. This section will examine one such place, specifically the surgical intensive care unit, or SICU. It will describe the physical layout of the SICU, the type of patients found there, and the type of care that they might receive. Of course, our focus ultimately will be on the role of the health unit coordinator (HUC) in a typical SICU, including the unique opportunities and challenges.

For our purposes the SICU is defined as a unit that might accept the following cases postoperatively: radical neck surgery, craniotomies, radical nephrectomies, and carotid endarterectomies and certain other vascular surgeries. Also included are patients who have suffered severe physical trauma, such as some survivors of motor vehicle accidents (**MVAs**). We will not include patients who have undergone cardiac surgery, as they are dealt with in a separate part of this chapter.

Just as the way that each hospital organizes its ICUs varies, so does the unit's physical layout. Some are a series of private rooms arranged in a horseshoe around the HUC's desk or nurses' station. Other are rooms arranged in blocks surrounded by a corridor. Still others are wards of several beds divided by curtains. Where rooms are private, a large window usually provides visual access to the patient from the corridor. Some hospitals have installed collapsible walls between the patient room and corridor that can be completely removed. Excellent lighting is always essential.

More and more hospitals are realizing the benefits of decorating ICUs in soothing colors. Studies have been done to determine which colors are the most healing to the patients and most calming to their families.

Other areas of most ICUs include HUC's and nurses' desk with space for patient monitors, a pantry with at least a sink and refrigerator, waiting areas for patients' families, and at least one storage and equipment room. Many units have conference rooms for nurses and small private areas where doctors and families can confer.

What does not vary among SICUs? Basically, two things: (1) Each patient is monitored; and (2) each patient's condition is unstable enough that a nursing ratio of only one to two patients per nurse is required.

Laboratory Tests

An area where the HUC is sure to encounter many abbreviations is in the ordering of diagnostic laboratory work. The following are some common laboratory tests ordered for patients in the SICU.

SMA-17 or *Chem-17*—a profile of blood chemistry, including electrolytes
Electrolytes (lytes)—the measurement of sodium (Na^+), potassium (K^+), chloride (Cl^-), and carbon dioxide (CO_2) in the blood
Magnesium (Mg^{2+})—level
Blood urea nitrogen (BUN)—a blood urea level
Creatinine (Creat)—level
Hemoglobin and hematocrit (H&H)—a blood cell profile
Partial thrombin time (PTT)—a measurement of blood clotting

Frequently Used Medications

The role of the HUC in maintaining patients' medication records has changed greatly in recent years. Not long ago, many institutions kept such records by hand, and it often was the HUC's job to write out each medication as well as the times that it was to be given! Now, of course, most health care facilities generate medication records by computer. Still, it is necessary for the HUC to be familiar with commonly prescribed drugs.

The following are drugs that may be ordered for patients in an SICU. It should be kept in mind that medications frequently have a generic as well as a brand name, and physicians may use either when they write their orders. Here, we have divided the list into categories, briefly describing the function of each category. The generic name is given first, followed by the brand name, if given, in parentheses.

Vasopressors—increase blood pressure and cardiac output:

Epinephrine
Phenylephrine (Neo-Synephrine)
Dopamine
Norepinephrine (Levophed)

Vasodilators—increase blood flow within coronary vessels:

Nitroglycerin
Nitroprusside (Nipride)

Neuromuscular blockers—induce muscle relaxation and paralysis:
Pancuronim (Pavulon)
Vecuronium (Norcuron)

Analgesics—control pain:

Morphine
Meperidine (Demerol)
Ketorolac (Toradol)
Hydromorphone (Dilaudid)

Antianxiety agents—some are given preoperatively or to control psychosis:

Lorazepam (Ativan)
Diazepam (Valium)
Haloperidol (Haldol)
Midazolam (Versed)
Propofol (Diprivan)

GI drugs—may decrease gastric secretion or increase gastrointestinal motility:

Famotidine (Pepcid)
Sucralfate (Carafate)
Metoclopramide (Reglan)

Respiratory drugs—aid breathing by inducing bronchodilation or by relaxing smooth muscle:

Albuterol (Ventolin)
Theophylline

Anticonvulsants—control seizure activity:

Phenytoin (Dilantin)
Fosphenytoin

Diuretics—increase fluid excretion from the body along with chloride, sodium, and potassium:

Bumetanide (Bumex)
Furosemide (Lasix)

Antiemetics—control nausea and vomiting and may tranquilize or induce sleep:

Prochlorperazine (Compazine)
Droperidol

Electrolytes—are given to replace and maintain blood levels of the following:

Sodium
Potassium
Magnesium
Calcium

Antibiotics—fight bacterial infection:

Cephalosporins
Aminoglycosides
Vancomycin
Quinolones
Macrolides

Antifungal—fight fungal infections:

Amphotericin B (Fungizone)

Antivirals—combat viruses:

Acyclovir (Zovirax)

Diagnostic Procedures and Treatments

Many patients in the SICU require invasive monitoring that might not be done on a regular medical/surgical unit. Some types of invasive monitoring that an HUC might encounter in SICU include:

Swan-Ganz, which measures pulmonary arterial pressure.
Central venous pressure (CVP), which assesses the total fluid volume in the patient.
Arterial, which measures blood pressure (Figs. 14–47 and 14–48).

Patients in the setting of an intensive care unit are, needless to say, more acutely ill than those in other health care settings. Often, their physical condition is critical and unstable, making it difficult to move them off the unit should they require diagnostic testing or treatment procedures. Ironically, it is their critical condition that makes it imperative that they receive such testing and treatment. Fortunately, many test and procedures can be performed on the unit. These include ultrasounds, echocardiograms, EKGs, respiratory diagnostic testing, insertions of **PEG** tubes or **chest tubes** (Figs. 14–49 and 14–50 and placement of arterial lines. These last three procedures are performed by a physician, as are Swan-Ganz catheter insertions.

Also done by physicians in the SICU are some endoscopic procedures, such as **jejunal feeding tube** placement and gastroscopies or flexible sigmoidoscopies. In the latter two diagnostic tests, the upper gastric system or the sigmoid colon, respectively, is visually explored by the doctor through the insertion of a thin flexible tube.

Most hospitals can take portable x-rays in the patient's room, The HUC should keep in mind that not all x-ray views can be taken with the patient lying in bed. The x-ray technician or radiologist can inform the HUC who is uncertain if a certain x-ray can be done portably. Diagnostic tests that cannot be done in the patient's room are computed tomography (CT) scans and magnetic

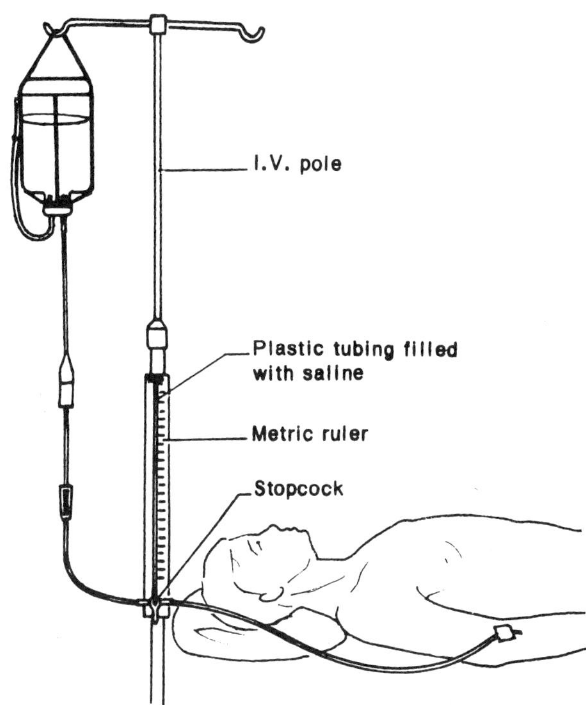

Figure 14–47
CVP monitor. (Adapted from Cyginski J, Tardieu B: The Essentials in Pressure Monitoring: Blood and Other Body Fluids. An Illustrated Guide. The Hague, Martinus-Nijhoff Publishing, 1980.)

resonance imaging (MRI). Both tests involve the noninvasive picturing of internal organs. The equipment needed is very large and obviously not portable.

Whenever patients must leave the SICU for a test or procedure they travel to the ancillary department in their bed. Monitors, IV pumps, and portable oxygen, if needed, go with them. The nurse assigned to the patient goes with them and stays with them throughout the procedure. As always, the patient's chart accompanies the patient whenever he or she travels off the unit.

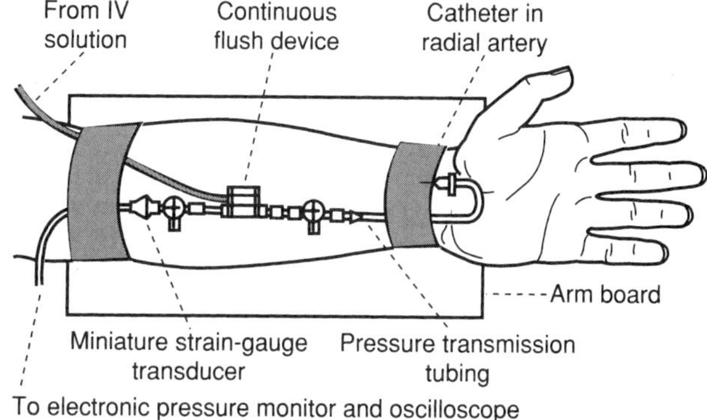

Figure 14–48
Arterial line. (From Black JM, Matassarin-Jacobs E: Medical-Surgical Nursing: Clinical Management for Continuity of Care, 5th ed. Philadelphia, WB Saunders, 1997.)

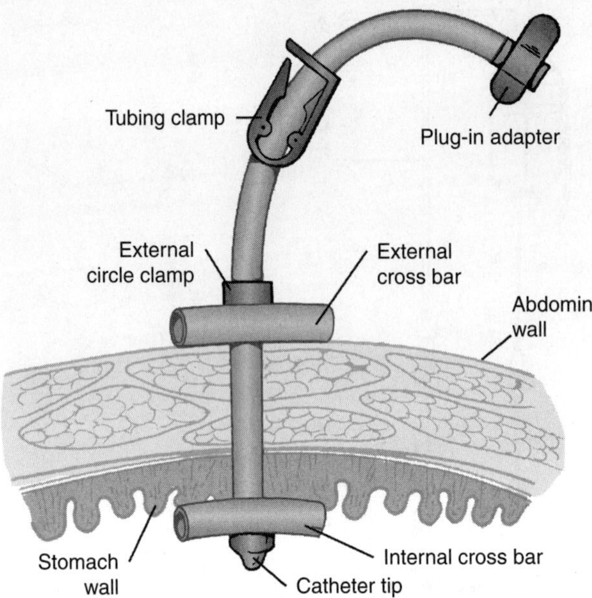

Figure 14–49
PEG tube. (From Black JM, Matassarin-Jacobs E: Medical-Surgical Nursing: Clinical Management for Continuity of Care, 5th ed. Philadelphia, WB Saunders, 1997.)

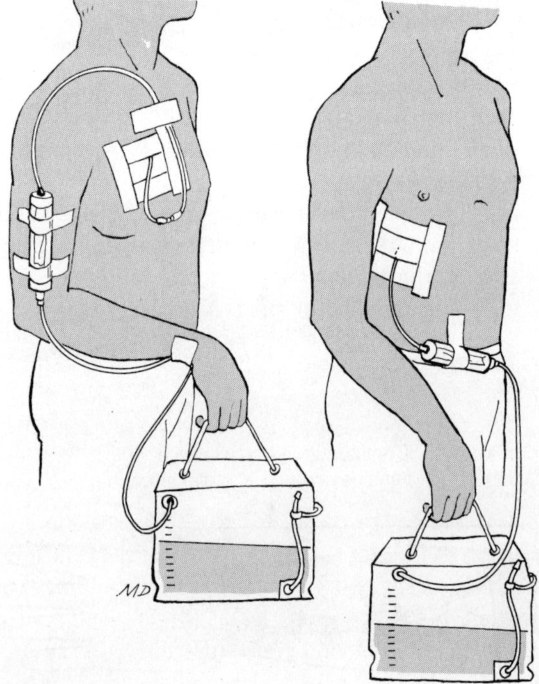

Figure 14–50
Chest tube drainage. (From Black JM, Matassarin-Jacobs E: Luckmann and Sorensen's Medical-Surgical Nursing: A Psycho-Physiologic Approach, 4th ed. Philadelphia, WB Saunders, 1993.)

The HUC's Role in a "Code" Situation

Cardiac and respiratory arrest are facts of life in the SICU; when they occur, there are moments that can mean life or death for the patient. When a patient's heart or breathing stops, the health care professionals on the unit (including doctors, nurses, respiratory therapists, and other technicians) become a team dedicated to reviving that patient. It is crucial that the HUC know his or her role as a member of that team so that the entire procedure runs smoothly.

Different hospitals have different terms for an episode of cardiac or respiratory arrest, such as "Red Code" or "Code Blue." It may be the HUC's responsibility to "call a code," that is, to initiate notification of the code team, either by overhead page or pocket pager system. However, a HUC never initiates a code unless instructed to do so by a doctor, nurse, or technician.

Some terminally ill patients have a "no code" status. This means that the patient and his or her family has expressed the wish that the patient not be revived in case of arrest. The instructions may include not intubating the patient, not placing the patient on a respirator, or not inducing the heart to resume beating through electrical stimulation. These instructions are documented in the patient's chart; if there are no instructions the patient is assumed to be a "full code," and all necessary measures are taken.

During a code the "crash cart" is taken immediately to the patient's bedside. This heavy metal cart on wheels contains equipment needed to revive the patient, such as heart defibrillator, portable oxygen, special medication, and intubation and suctioning supplies. It may be the HUC's responsibility to help take the cart to the patient's bedside and to call the appropriate department to restock or replace the cart when the code is completed. HUCs also may aid in documenting the patient's heart rhythm at the onset of arrest and whenever changes are noted. This is done by printing "rhythm strips." Some HUCs print such strips throughout the code.

Laboratory and medication orders during a code are, obviously, always ordered STAT. This is one situation in which orders may be given to an HUC verbally, as there may not be time to write them in the chart. Almost always, an HUC will need to order arterial blood gases, potassium and magnesium blood levels, and a portable chest x-ray. Other duties that may befall the HUC during a code include fetching equipment to the patient's room, notifying physicians or the nursing supervisor that a code is in progress, or comforting distressed family members.

The better the HUC knows his or her duties, the location of supplies and equipment, and the policies of the health care facility, the more valuable he or she will be during this crucial situation. And the time to learn these things is before, not during, a code.

Supplies and Equipment in the SICU

The role of the HUC in maintaining equipment and supplies varies from one health care institution to another. In some hospitals, the HUC may be primarily responsible for maintaining supplies. Other institutions may employ a supply specialist to do all ordering. At the least, many HUCs need to be able to do the following:

Maintain the supply of forms and papers used in the medical record, in ordering tests and procedures, or in carrying out any other aspect of the HUC's job. These forms may be obtained from the print shop, central supply department, or outside private company.

Call the proper hospital department for equipment and supplies not routinely stocked on the unit. The ancillary departments might include those mentioned above as well the sterile processing department, pharmacy, physical therapy department, and so forth.

Call outside companies for special equipment needed by a patient on an individual basis, usually as ordered by a physician. Examples include specialty beds or custom-fitted orthopedic braces.

Equipment Commonly Used to Treat Patients in the SICU

Air pressure stocking pump—applies intermittent pressure to lower limbs to prevent deep vein thrombosis.

Aqua K—heating pads that treat muscle spasm and promote patient comfort.

Bair Hugger—is a convection warmer.

Barrier-free gowns—protect staff from body fluids, as do face masks and gloves.

Blood warmers—warm blood products being infused into a patient.

Buck's traction—provides weighted traction to the lower extremities.

Chest tube—prevents air or fluid buildup in the pleural space to restore normal breathing.

CVAHD (continuous arteriovenous hemofiltration)—is renal replacement therapy that filters blood.

Defibrillator—terminates ventricular fibrillation and pulseless ventricular tachycardia.

Doppler—amplifies the sound of blood flow to assess circulatory impairment and blood pressure (Fig. 14–51).

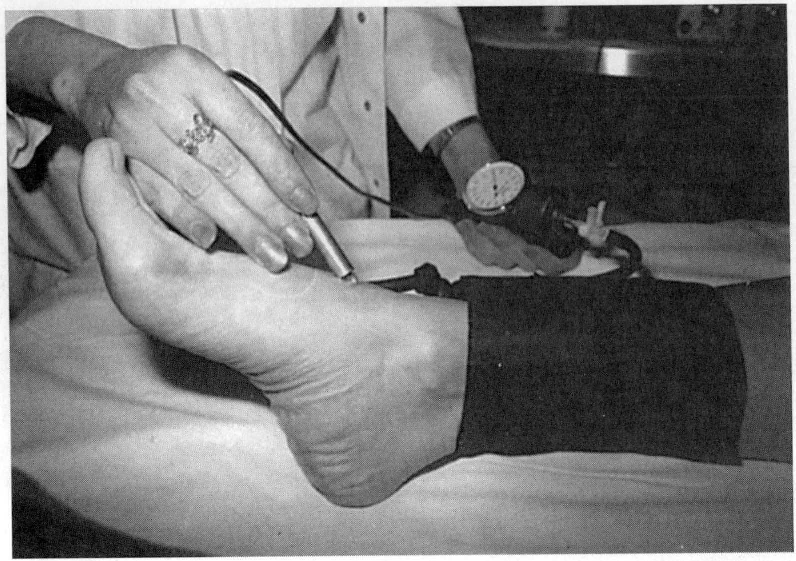

Figure 14–51
Doppler probe. (From Fahey V: Vascular Nursing. Philadelphia, WB Saunders, 1994.)

External transcutaneous pacing—provides emergent pacing for heart block/asystole.

ECMO (extracorporeal membrane oxygenator)—is an external device that oxygenates blood delivered from the body and then returns it to the body.

Feeding pumps—deliver enteral nutrition to the patient who cannot eat normally.

Flashlights—are used in neuro checks.

Foley catheter with urometer—measures urinary output.

Halo vests—immobilize the cervical spine to prevent further damage to the spinal cord (Fig. 14–52).

Hemodialysis machine—artificially filters blood using reverse osmosis.

Hyper/hypothermia machine—raises or lowers a patient's body temperature.

IABP (intra-aortic balloon pump)—increases coronary perfusion and decreases oxygen consumption.

ICP monitor—is an invasive monitor to diagnose and manage patients with increased intracranial pressure.

IS (incentive spirometer)—promotes removal of lung secretions.

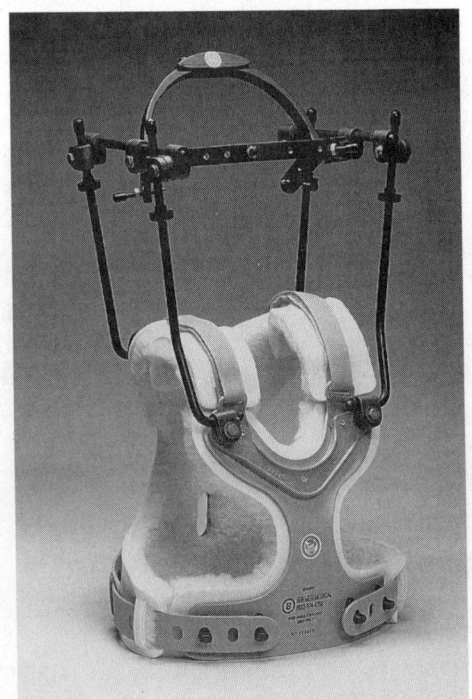

Figure 14–52
Halo traction. (Courtesy of Bremer Medical, Jacksonville, FL.)

IV infusion pumps—deliver IV fluid at a selected rate.

Low air loss beds—promote skin healing and prevent skin breakdown.

MAST trousers—are placed on patients in shock. They inflate, compressing the legs and preventing pooling of blood and fluid in tissue (Fig. 14–53).

Oximeter—measures oxygen saturation of blood.

Pacemaker generators—electronically pace heart rate.

PCA (patient-controlled analgesia) pumps—are operated by the patient to deliver pain medication.

Percussors—are mechanical vibrators used for sputum production.

PNS (peripheral nerve stimulator)—reduces the risk of prolonged paralysis related to the overdosing of paralytic drugs.

Protective eyewear—is used by staff whenever they are in contact with body fluid.

Pyxsis—is a computerized medication dispensing station used by nurses on the unit.

Skeletal traction—realigns and immobilizes fractured limbs.

Wright respirometer—measures respiratory volume.

Documentation

In the SICU, as in other units, HUCs are the keepers of the charts. That is, they are responsible for creating a chart for the patient upon admission and turning it over to medical records upon discharge. In between, the HUC places needed forms on the chart, making sure that doctors have space to write their orders and progress notes and nurses to record vital signs and patient activity.

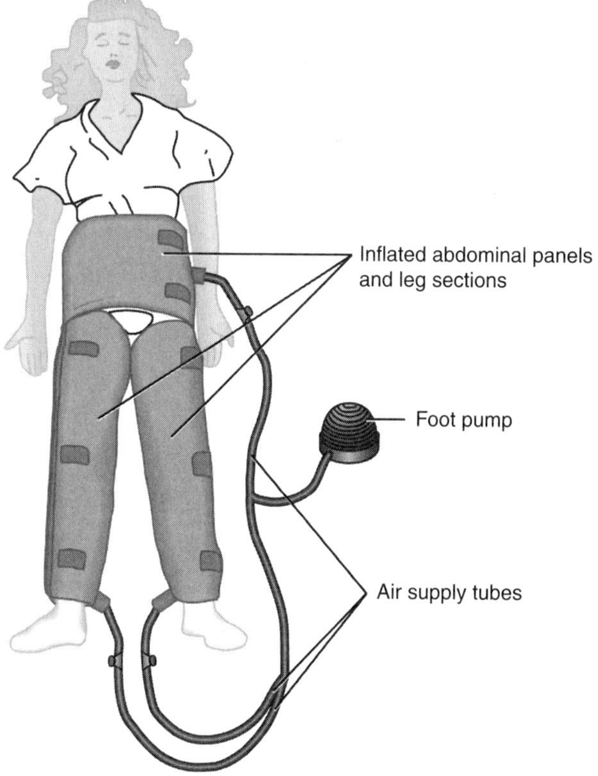

Figure 14–53
MAST (pneumatic antishock garment). (From Black JM, Matassarin-Jacobs E: Medical-Surgical Nursing: Clinical Management for Continuity of Care, 5th ed. Philadelphia: WB Saunders, 1997.)

In some health care institutions, HUCs are taking this process a step further, by actually registering the new patient. Traditionally done by a separate admitting department, registration may be done on the unit by the HUC, using a computer. What does this registration process entail? Simply, it means gathering information about the patient: name, address, birth date, social security number, next of kin, type of insurance, and so forth. These data are fed into the computer using the hospital's registration mode. When completed, the computer generates the new patient's unique registration number. This number is used to identify the patient throughout his or her hospitalization whenever a test is ordered. It appears on most chart documents. It is used to bill patients for all the services that they received. Obviously, the need for accuracy is great, both in gathering information for registration and in typing it into the computer. A wrong insurance policy number, for example, can delay reimbursement to the hospital.

But in the SICU, HUCs who perform patient registration face a special problem. That is, patients may be unconscious or simply too ill to answer questions. To solve this problem, the HUC may need to interview the patient's next of kin, either in person or, if need be, over the telephone. Who signs legal forms if the patient is unable to do so? If the HUC can answer that question, he or she will know who can provide needed registration information. It must be remembered that registration and the signing of all forms should be done as quickly as possible, especially in the SICU.

The patient's chart is perhaps a more familiar area of HUC expertise. Each health care institution's chart looks a little different and the order of the various documents may vary, but certain rules are fairly constant. The HUC writes only in black ink, except those areas (such as diet) where pencil is appropriate. Liquid "white-out" is never used. Errors are corrected by drawing a single line through them, followed by the HUC's initials.

The computer is the HUC's most important tool. Although it has not totally replaced the paper chart, it is used more and more in the noting of orders. Diets, diagnostic tests, and supplies are ordered on the computer. Communication with ancillary departments via e-mail is the norm.

Here the HUC in the SICU must take pause. Computers can crash, or shut down temporarily. SICU patients are often in critical condition and cannot tolerate delays in their treatment. Their care cannot be interrupted by computer downtime. The solution is to keep handy a supply of paper requisitions to use for ordering tests and supplies. It is essential to have a plan to revert to the old-fashioned system of carrying out orders during downtime. Such a plan can even be practiced in advance during mock downtime drills.

Risk Management

HUCs handle legal documents every day: the patient chart itself, living wills, consent for treatment, death certificates, and others. This is one reason why HUCs follow such strict policies and procedures. The proper handling of legal documents, the rights of the patient, the proper reporting of errors, and the issue of confidentiality all fall under the broad heading of risk management. HUCs in the SICU need to know and follow their hospital's policies regarding risk management.

Confidentiality cannot be emphasized enough. In the SICU are patients who are critically ill or injured, perhaps as the result of an auto accident. It is not unusual for HUCs to receive telephone calls from the news media asking for information about such patients. The HUC should never comply with such a request but instead politely refer the call to the hospital administration or public relations office. Similarly, the SICU HUC never gives information about a patient to anyone, referring all requests to the nursing supervisor. In any event, when they are off the unit HUCs do not discuss patients. Practicing strict confidentiality is important because patients expect and deserve it. There is one other very important reason: In almost all hospitals, violation of confidentiality is grounds for dismissal.

Closing Thoughts

Benjamin Franklin said that the only sure things in life are death and taxes. Health care workers can add a third sure thing to that list: change—constant and relentless. In recent years HUCs have seen incredible changes in their field. Examples include the advent of computerization; expanding roles in areas such as patient registration; increased emphasis on patient rights and confidentiality; greater opportunities for education in the form of seminars, classes, and in-services; the chance to become certified by passing an exam; and many other issues.

Change can cause stress for all health care workers, including the HUC. Flexibility is essential but not always easy. The wise HUC will learn to accept change and will try not to fear advancing technology. Such technology is not our enemy—it can make our jobs easier. Therefore, take every opportunity to learn. Read, attend seminars, participate in hospital and unit committees, and take part in decision-making as much as possible.

The atmosphere in the SICU can be hectic and intense. The HUC who is calm, competent, and cheerful can set the tone that allows everyone's day to go better. Realize that the doctor who is brusque may be overworked. The demanding nurse may be worried about his or her own job performance. Do not return rudeness with rudeness but with professional courtesy.

Similarly, family members of SICU patients may be greatly stressed. Their loved one's life may be in danger. They may not get enough sleep, drink too much coffee, and feel helpless in the face of what may seem an impersonal health care system. The SICU HUC needs to learn to deal with family members who may vent their feelings on them. Willingness to listen and help solve problems, if possible, are essential, as are patience and kindness. Some SICUs have support groups for family members, and HUCs can be an important part of such groups. After all, HUCs are a vital part of the SICU team.

Review Questions

1. Describe two possible layouts for the SICU.
2. List and describe three procedures that might be carried out in the SICU.
3. What consideration must be taken into account when ordering x-rays for a SICU patient?
4. List five tasks that a HUC might be expected to carry out in a "code" situation.

15 Transplant Unit

Wendy Bollinger

Common Medical Terms

Six-antigen match or zero mismatch—Term used in tissue typing compatibility testing

Cold agglutinins—An antibody that causes clumping of red blood cells at temperatures below 37°C

Fistula—A permanent vein access performed in the operating room, in which the surgeon connects a vein directly to an artery in the forearm

Gambro—A temporary catheter placed in a large vein in the chest, neck, or groin for temporary vein access

Haplotype—A term used in tissue typing compatibility testing

Leukopoor packed red blood cells—Packed red blood cells from which the white blood cells have been filtered out

Objectives

At the completion of this chapter, the reader should be able to:

1. Identify the organs that can be transplanted.
2. List five diagnostic procedures that may be performed on transplant patients.
3. Explain what is meant by rejection.
4. Describe two sources of kidney donation for transplant.
5. Name the organization that oversees the identification of potential organ recipients.

The abbreviations listed for this chapter are those that a HUC working in this area would be expected to know. Only those in boldface type are used in the text and appear in boldface when they are used for the first time.

Common Abbreviations

ATN	Acute tubular necrosis
BX	Biopsy
CMV	Cytomegalovirus
CsA	Cyclosporin A
ESLD	End-stage liver disease
ESRD	End-stage renal disease
GN	Glomerulonephritis
HAT	Hepatic artery thrombosis
HLA	Human leukocyte antigen
HCV	Hepatitis C virus
IDDM	Insulin-dependent diabetes mellitus
INR	International normalized ratio for prothrombin
LRRTX	Living related renal transplant
LTX	Liver transplant
P/RTX	Pancreas/renal transplant
PNT	Percutaneous nephrostomy tube
RAS	Renal artery stenosis
RTX	Renal transplant
TIPS	Transjugular intrahepatic portalsystemic shunt
TX	Transplant
VCUG	Voiding cystourethrogram
UNOS	Unity Network of Organ Sharing

Vocabulary

Biliary sclerosis: Hardening of the bile ducts

Cytomegalovirus infection: A viral infection that can affect organs; detected in blood and urine

Donor: The person who has donated organs (both living and cadaveric)

Enteric conversion: A surgical procedure to reroute the connection of the pancreas from the bladder to the bowel

Final crossmatch: A test performed in the tissue typing laboratory that determines if a recipient's antibodies are compatible with the donor's

Glomerulonephritis: Inflammation of the glomerulus of the kidney

Graft: Refers to the transplanted organ

Hepatic artery thrombosis: Constriction of an artery in the liver

HLA (human leukocyte antigen): Tissue typing test performed to determine compatibility between recipient and donor

Hydronephrosis: Urine collection in the transplanted kidney caused by an obstruction in the ureter

Hypertension: Increased arterial blood pressure

Immunosuppression: Suppression of the immune system

Liver cirrhosis: A chronic liver disease that interferes with liver function and circulation, eventually causing death

Lymphocele: A fluid mass

Obstruction: Blockage

Patency: Openness

Continued

Vocabulary *Continued*

Perfusion/Extraction/Excretion: Terms used to identify kidney and kidney/pancreas function

Polycystic kidney disease: Multiple cysts that result in kidney failure

Portal hypertension: Increased blood pressure in the portal vein

Recipient: The person who receives a donated organ

Rejection: Term used when a recipient's immune system is fighting off a transplanted organ

Renal artery stenosis: Constriction of an artery in the kidney

Sclerosing cholangitis: Inflammation and hardening of the bile ducts

T-tube: A tube placed in a liver transplant recipient's common bile duct that enables the bile duct to remain open

Introduction

One of the most remarkable achievements of modern surgery is the transplanting of vital organs from one human body to another. Since the first kidney transplant was accomplished at Peter Bent Brigham Hospital in Boston in 1951, many kidney transplants have been performed. Teeth, cornea, liver, heart, and pancreas transplants have also been successful. The first human heart transplant was performed in 1967 by Christiaan Barnard in Capetown, South Africa.

In most types of transplants the difficulties that arise are not ones of surgical technique. Instead they are due to **rejection** of the new organ by the **recipient**'s immune system. To prevent this immune attack and increase the patient's chances of a successful transplant, specialized nursing units were created. Health unit coordinators (HUCs) who work in these units are introduced to many new and advanced treatment modalities. New drugs, laboratory tests, diagnostic tests, and therapies all have to be learned.

Patient Population

The patient population on a transplant unit would typically include:

- Patients admitted for transplant
- Patients readmitted after transplant
- Patients who are awaiting transplant
- Donor nephrectomy patients.

The average length of stay for a transplant recipient is 7 to 10 days.

Patients Admitted for Transplant

Patients who are admitted for a transplant may include patients needing a liver transplant, kidney transplant, a pancreas/kidney transplant, and liver/kidney transplant.

Indications for a liver transplant may include end-stage liver disease due to hepatitis, **liver cirrhosis** (Fig. 15–1), drug overdose, alcohol abuse, **sclerosing cholangitis**, and **biliary sclerosis** (Fig. 15–2). A liver transplant work-up may include diagnostic tests such as an ultrasound examination of the hepatic vessels, echocardiogram, electrocardiogram (EKG), chest x-ray, abdominal CT scan, and hepatic arteriogram. A liver transplant work-up would also include laboratory tests such as liver enzymes, hematology survey, ammonia level, fibrinogen level, hepatitis panels (A,B,C), HIV testing, chemistry survey, amylase, electrolytes, prothrombin time (PT), activated partial thromboplastin time (APTT/PTT), ABO blood

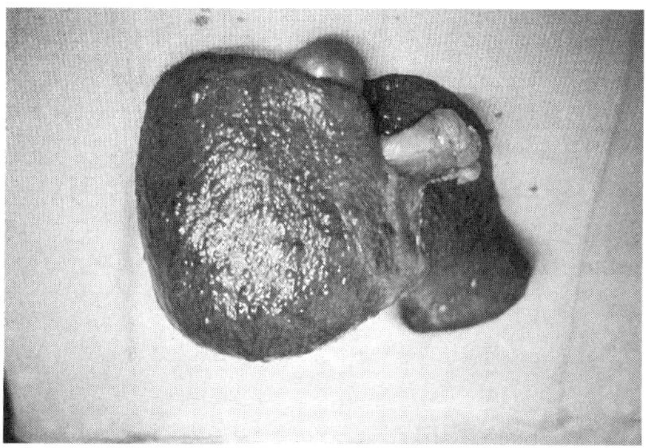

Figure 15–1
Cirrhotic liver.

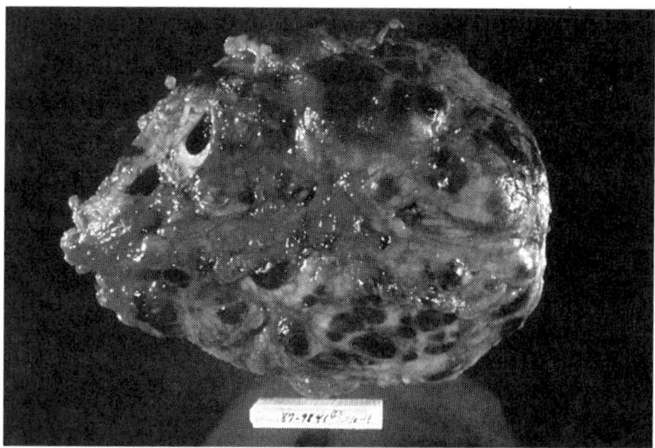

Figure 15–3
Polycystic kidney.

grouping, copper, ferritin, iron, tissue typing, carcinoembryonic antigen (CEA), alpha-fetoprotein, ceruloplasmin, antinuclear antibodies (ANA), and a urine culture.

Indications for a kidney transplant may include end-stage renal disease due to diabetes, **glomerulonephritis, polycystic kidney disease** (Fig. 15–3), **hypertension**, drug overdose, and trauma.

Indications for a kidney/pancreas transplant would include patients with end-stage renal disease and diabetes. Indications for a kidney/liver transplant would include patients with end-stage liver disease and end-stage kidney disease.

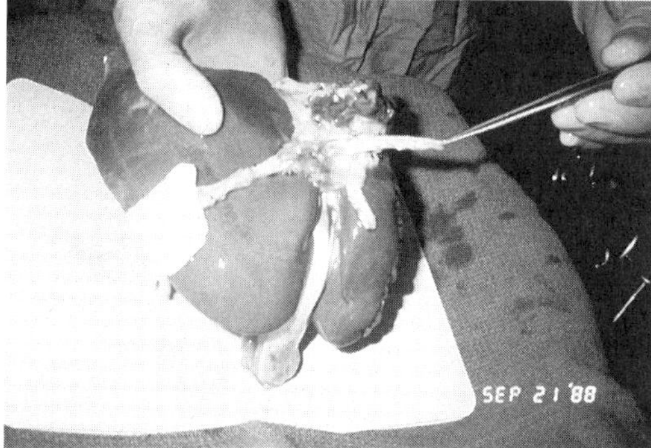

Figure 15–2
Healthy donor liver.

Patients Admitted After Transplant

Patients who have had a transplant may be admitted for the following reasons: an increased serum creatinine level (which may be due to dehydration, an **obstruction**, cyclosporine toxicity, or a rejection), increased liver enzymes, elevated temperature, a transplant-related infection, a surgical procedure related (or unrelated) to the transplant, and medical reasons related (or unrelated) to the transplant.

Patients admitted for an increased serum creatinine (Cr) level or increased liver enzymes would typically have an ultrasound examination to rule out an obstruction. An ultrasound-guided biopsy may be performed to rule out a rejection. If rejection is confirmed, drug therapy is initiated in an attempt to reverse the rejection process. If the biopsy rules out a rejection, further tests and treatments may be ordered to identify the reason for the increased serum Cr or increased liver enzymes.

Patients admitted with an elevated temperature may have a transplant-related infection. A common transplant-related infection is caused by **cytomegalovirus (CMV)**. When a patient has an increased temperature, blood cultures and CMV cultures are ordered.

Medical procedures performed post transplant that would require hospitalization may include nephrostomy tube placement, abscess drain placement, ureteral **stent** placement, and IV drug therapy. Surgical procedures performed post transplant and related to a transplant may include an **enteric conversion**, **lymphocele** repair, and exploratory laparotomy to determine a leak or blockage to a vessel. An enteric conversion is a surgical procedure that reroutes the connection of the pancreas from the bladder to the bowel. A lymphocele repair is a surgical procedure to drain the lymph tissue, which has formed a fluid collection.

Patients Awaiting Transplant

Patients awaiting transplant may be admitted for end-stage liver disease, transjugular intrahepatic portalsystemic shunt (**TIPS**) procedure, and liver transplant work-up evaluation.

Donor Nephrectomy Patients

There are two sources for kidney (nephrectomy) donation. One source is a kidney transplant using organs procured from a cadaver. The other is the use of a kidney from a living **donor**. Donor nephrectomy patients agree to donate one of their kidneys to someone in need of a transplant. When a relative donates a kidney for transplant, it is referred to as a living related kidney transplant. Sometimes a kidney is donated to a spouse or a friend. This is called a living unrelated kidney transplant. Cadaver transplants are chosen for individuals who are on a waiting list. The individuals are prioritized on the list based on blood type, tissue typing compatibility, and stage of disease.

Before a person can donate a kidney, a donor nephrectomy work-up must be completed. This work-up includes the following laboratory tests: ABO blood grouping, crossmatching, tissue typing, fasting blood sugar, hepatitis B testing, HIV testing, creatinine levels, blood urea nitrogen (BUN) level, and urine testing. A glucose tolerance test may also be ordered if there is a family history of diabetes. The work-up also includes diagnostic tests such as intravenous pyelogram (IVP), chest x-ray, EKG, and renal arteriogram.

Frequently Used Medications

Common medications prescribed for a transplant population include **immunosuppression** therapy (antirejection medication), infection treatment (antibiotics, antivirals, and antifungals), diuretics, and other drugs (Table 15–1). All transplant patients must take some kind of immunosuppressive drug daily. Immunosuppressive therapy helps to prevent rejection of a transplanted organ. When rejection of an organ occurs, an additional antirejection drug may be prescribed to reverse the rejection process. In some situations the dosage of the immunosuppressive drug may be temporarily increased in an attempt to prevent rejection of the transplanted organ.

Other Frequently Ordered Medications

Lasix and Bumex are common diuretics prescribed for transplant patients. These medications may be administered orally or intravenously. Diuretics are used to promote secretion of fluid overloads. Insulin is prescribed for patients with diabetes to stabilize blood sugar levels within normal limits. DDAVP (desmopressin acetate) is an antidiuretic hormone that helps prevent excessive bleeding during a procedure on a patient with a coagulation problem. Antacids such as Maalox and Tums are used to help with stomach upset, which may occur with most immunosuppressive drug therapy.

Diagnostic Procedures

Radiology

Radiology procedures performed on a transplant patient include a voiding cystourethrogram (VCUG) and a **T-tube** cholangiogram.

Table 15–1 COMMONLY PRESCRIBED IMMUNOSUPPRESSION AND ANTIREJECTION MEDICATIONS

Medication	Brand Name	Abbreviation	Route of Administration
Antithymocyte globulin	Atgam	ATG	IV
Azathioprine	Imuran	AZA	IV or p.o.
Basiliximab	Simuleet		IV
Cyclosporine	Neoral, Sandimmune	Cyclo, CSA	IV or p.o.
Daclizumab	Zenapax		IV
Methylprednisolone	Solu-Medrol	Methylpred	IV or p.o.
Muromonab-CD3	Orthoclone	OKT3	IV
Mycophenolate	CellCept	MMF, MM, RS61443	IV or p.o.
Prednisone	Deltasone	Pred	p.o.
Tacrolimus	Prograf	FK506	IV or p.o.
Commonly Prescribed Antibiotics			
Cephalosporins			IV or p.o.
Ciprofloxacin		Cipro	IV or p.o.
Gentamicin	Garamycin	Gent	IV
Tobramycin	Nebcin	Tobra	IV
Trimethoprim-sulfamethoxazole	Bactrim, Septra	TMP-SMX	IV or p.o.
Commonly Prescribed Antiviral Medications			
Acyclovir sodium	Zovirax	ACV	IV or p.o.
Ganciclovir sodium	Cytovene	DHPG	IV or p.o.
CMV hyperimmune globulin	CytoGam	CMV Ig	IV
Immunoglobulin	Gammagard, Gammaimmune, Sandoglobulin, Gamimune	Ig	IV
Commonly Prescribed Antifungal Medications			
Amphotericin B	Fungizone, Abelcet, Amphotec	Ampho	IV, p.o., or topical
Clotrimazole troche	Mycelex		p.o.
Fluconazole	Diflucan		IV or p.o.
Miconazole cream 2%	Monistat		Topical
Nystatin suspension	Mycostatin	Nystatin	p.o.

Voiding Cystourethrogram

A voiding cystourethrogram is a diagnostic procedure performed to determine if a kidney/pancreas transplant patient has a bladder leak.

T-Tube Cholangiogram

A T-tube cholangiogram is performed on a transplant patient to view the bile duct. Contrast medium is injected through the T-tube. This procedure can identify an obstruction in the bile duct. There are many other radiology procedures that might also be performed on transplant patients.

Intravenous Pyelogram

An IVP is a radiology procedure performed (on an outpatient basis) to outline the kidney, particularly the renal pelvis, ureters, and bladder.

Computerized Tomography

Computerized tomography (CT) scans of the abdomen or pelvic area are often performed on transplant patients. The patient is usually given an oral or intravenous contrast agent prior to the test. This enables the scanner to record and display selected cross-sectional images of the transplanted organ. CT scans are performed to rule out an abscess or tumor in a transplant patient.

Arteriograms

Renal and hepatic arteriograms are invasive radiology procedures often performed on transplant patients. A renal arteriogram is a procedure that provides information including the position of the kidneys and the number of renal veins and renal arteries in each kidney. A renal arteriogram visualizes the renal arteries and veins after injection of a contrast medium. This procedure is also used to determine if a patient has **renal artery stenosis.**

A hepatic arteriogram is a procedure that provides information such as the position of the liver and the number of hepatic arteries and hepatic veins and their patency. Preoperative arteriograms are used to provide the surgeon with a surgical road map.

Nuclear Medicine

Nuclear medicine studies performed on transplant patients include a renal perfusion transplant scan, a renal/pancreas transplant scan, and a cystogram leak study.

Renal Perfusion Transplant Scan

A renal perfusion transplant scan is performed by injecting a dye through a vein, after which a machine measures how the transplanted kidney is functioning. The scan provides information including the **perfusion, extraction, and excretion** capabilities of the transplanted kidney. A renal/pancreas perfusion transplant scan is similar to a renal perfusion transplant scan; however, it also provides an indication of the functionality of the transplanted pancreas.

Cystogram Leak Study

A cystogram leak study is performed to determine if a kidney/pancreas transplant patient has a bladder leak. If a leak is identified, an enteric conversion procedure may be performed.

Ultrasound

Ultrasound procedures performed on a transplant patient may include a renal transplant ultrasound, a hepatic or abdominal ultrasound, and an ultrasound-guided transplanted kidney or liver biopsy.

Renal Transplant Ultrasound

A renal transplant ultrasound is performed to determine if a kidney or kidney/pancreas transplant patient has an obstruction in the ureter causing

hydronephrosis. Ultrasound technology is also used to determine **patency** of the vessels affected by a transplant operation.

Hepatic or Abdominal Ultrasound

A hepatic or abdominal ultrasound may be performed to determine if a liver transplant patient has **hepatic artery thrombosis**, a blockage in the vessel going to the transplanted liver, or an abscess.

Ultrasound-Guided Liver or Kidney Biopsy

An ultrasound-guided liver or kidney transplant biopsy is performed to determine if a kidney or liver transplant patient is experiencing organ rejection. These biopsies are performed under the direction of the physician or radiologist using an ultrasound technique. The physician inserts a needle through the skin into the transplanted organ to obtain a piece of tissue. This tissue is sent to the pathology laboratory, where rejection can be diagnosed. This tissue can also be sent to the laboratory to determine if the patient has a CMV infection.

Shortly before a biopsy is performed, coagulation studies (such as a PT and platelet count) must be obtained to determine if a patient is at risk for excessive bleeding during the procedure. The patient is usually given medication prior to the procedure to help reduce anxiety and pain. A liver biopsy can also be performed at the bedside by a physician without ultrasound guidance.

Daily Laboratory Testing

Daily laboratory testing is an essential part of a successful organ transplant. All newly transplanted patients require daily laboratory testing. The results of these tests determines how the transplanted organ is functioning (Table 15–2).

All transplant patients participate in educational programs to understand the importance and meaning of laboratory tests. A laboratory flow chart is placed in the patient's room and identifies the important laboratory values (Fig. 15–4).

The laboratory tests monitored and recorded daily on a kidney flow chart may include: Hct, WBC, K^+, Cr, BUN, blood glucose, and a cyclosporine or tacrolimus level if the patient is on that medication. The laboratory tests monitored and recorded on a pancreas/kidney transplant flow chart would include all the kidney transplant lab studies in addition to serum amylase, urine amylase (if the pancreas is connected to the bladder and not the bowel), and blood glucose levels. The laboratory tests monitored and recorded on a liver transplant flow chart may include: Hct, WBC, BUN, Cr, K^+, BILI, AST, ALT, GGT, LDH, alkaline phosphatase, blood glucose, NH_3, and a cyclosporine or tacrolimus level if the patient is on that medication.

The laboratory flow chart also tracks other useful information, such as the patient's daily weight, blood pressure, and immunosuppressive therapy. The laboratory flow chart is not a permanent part of the patient's record. However, when a patient is readmitted to the hospital, the same flow chart is used for that individual. This helps the patient and the staff see the trends of the laboratory values at a glance.

Treatments

Surgical Procedures

Treatments and procedures specific to the transplant population are absess drain placement and removal, biliary drainage tube placements, a Whittaker procedure, transjugular intrahepatic portalsystemic shunt (TIPS), ureteral stent placement and removal, nephrostomy tube placement and removal, and hemodialysis.

Abcess Drain Placement and Removal

An abscess drain placement is a procedure usually performed in the interventional radiology depart-

Table 15–2 COMMONLY ORDERED TRANSPLANT LABORATORY TESTS

Test Name and Abbreviation	Approximate Normal Range	Description of Test
Hematocrit (Hct)	40–50 ml/dl	Measures volume of percent of red blood cells
White blood count (WBC)	3.5–8.5 k/μl	A count of the number of WBCs present in the blood; WBCs fight infection
Creatinine (Cr)	0.6–1.3 mg/dl	Waste product from muscle breakdown. Measures kidney function
Blood urea nitrogen (BUN)	7–20 mg/dl	Waste product from protein breakdown. Measures kidney function
Potassium (K^+)	3.5–4.8 mmol/l	An electrolyte that affects muscle contraction
Serum amylase	<100	Measures pancreas function
Urine amylase	20–100 μ/l	Measures pancreas function
Fasting blood sugar (FBS)	70–100 mg/dl	Determines the amount of sugar in the blood. Measures pancreas function and monitors diabetes
Aspartate aminotransferase (AST or SGOT)	40 μ/l	Enzyme released into the circulation from destroyed liver cells. Measures liver function
Alanine aminotransferase (ALT or SGPT)	65 μ/l	Enzyme released into the circulation from destroyed liver cells. Measures liver function
GGT	40 μ/l	Measures liver function
Alkaline phosphatase (Alk phos)	35–110	Measures liver function
Lactic dehydrogenase (LDH)	90–200 μ/l	Enzyme released into the circulation after tissue damage. Measures liver function
Bilirubin	0–1.4 mg/dl	Measures liver function
Ammonia (NH_3)	0–40 μmol/l	Measures liver function
Activated partial thromboplastin time (APTT, PTT)	25.0–35.0 sec	Coagulation study
Prothrombin time (PT) INR	10.9–12.9 sec	Coagulation study
Platelet count (Plt)	160–370 K/μl	Coagulation study
Beta$_2$ microglobulin (β_2M)	1.1–2.0 mg/l	Measures kidney function
Cyclosporine (CSA)	200–300 ng/ml	Measures the blood level of the medication cyclosporine
Tacrolimus (FK506)	10–20 ng/ml	Measures the blood level of the medication tacrolimus

UWH 466

INPATIENT "FLOW" SHEET FOR RENAL TRANSPLANT PAT

RECIPIENT NAME	HOSPITAL NAME	TRANSPLANT No. (1st, 2nd.)	STARTING DATE OF THIS FLOWSHEET (MONTH / DAY / YEAR)

DATE			TEMP.	WEIGHT	MAXIMUM BLOOD PRESSURE		URINE STUDIES									HEMATOLOGY							
											TOTAL EXCRETION 24 HOURS							DIFFERENTIAL					
MONTH	DAY	Post-Op Day Number Optional	High In 24 Hours Circle Unit Used C° or F°		SYSTOLIC	DIASTOLIC	URINE VOLUME	URINE OSMOLALITY	SODIUM	URINE SEDIMENT	GLUCOSE	PROTEIN	CREATININE	URINE CULTURE SPECIFY ORGANISIMS	OTHER URINE STUDIES	HCT	WBC	N	L	M	E	PLATELETS	RETICULOCYTE COUNT
							ml/24 HOURS	MOsm/L	mEq/L		gm	gm	gm			%	10³/mm³	%	%	%	%	10³/mm³	%RBC

Continued

PATIENTS / UNIVERSITY HOSPITALS

RECIPIENT'S HOSPITAL RECORD No.	DATE OF TRANSPLANT (MONTH / DAY / YEAR)	DATE OF TRANSPLANT REMOVAL (MONTH / DAY / YEAR)	RESPONSIBLE PHYSICIAN

	BLOOD CHEMISTRIES											OTHER LAB STUDIES		IMMUNOSUPPRESSIVE THERAPY					OTHER THERAPY				OTHER
														24 HOUR TOTAL DOSE								CHECK IF DONE	
RETICULOCYTE COUNT	Na	K	Cl	HCO_3	Ca	P	GLUCOSE	ALBUMIN	GLOBULIN	BLOOD UREA N	CREATININE		ALG	Azathioprine	Steroids	Steroid Bolus	CYCLO DOSE	CYCLO LEVEL	B_2M		Other Medications	HEMODIALYSIS	
%RBC	mEq/L	mEq/L	mEq/L	mEq/L		mg/100ml	mg/100ml	mg/100ml	mg/100ml	mg/100ml	mg/100ml			mg	mg				Sr	Urine			

Figure 15–4
Laboratory flow chart.

ment. The radiologist inserts a tube into the abscessed area to drain the fluid. The fluid is usually ascites fluid or peritoneal fluid. The patient will require regular tube checks and tube changes while the tube remains in place.

Biliary Drainage Tube Placement

This procedure is performed in the interventional radiology department. A small needle is placed through the patient's liver and into the bile ducts to drain the bile. The tube is attached to a drainage bag. Placement of a biliary drainage tube is done to relieve a blockage of the bile ducts.

Whittaker Procedure

A Whittaker test measures the pressures in the ureter to determine if an obstructive hydronephrosis is present. If the test is positive, a nephrostomy tube is usually placed.

Percutaneous Nephrostomy Tube (PNT) Placement

A **PNT** is a plastic tube that enters the skin in the flank area to drain urine from the kidney. This tube placement can be permanent or short-term. The patient will require regular PNT checks while the tube is in place. If the tube is permanent, the patient will require PNT changes every 4 to 6 weeks. A patient with a PNT may require a ureteral stent placement.

Ureteral Stent Placement

A ureteral stent placement is done in the interventional radiology department. A stent (which is like a flexible plastic wire) is placed in the ureter. This allows the ureter to remain open to prevent obstructive hydronephrosis. The PNT may or may not be removed when the stent is placed.

Transjugular Intrahepatic Portalsystemic Shunt

A transjugular intrahepatic portalsystemic shunt (TIPS) is a metal stent placed in a newly made opening in the liver between the hepatic vein and the portal vein. This stent is permanent. The purpose of a TIPS procedure is to decrease recurrent bleeding by lowering **portal hypertension.** TIPS procedures are usually done on patients who have liver disease and are waiting for a liver transplant. Patients who have liver disease and are not liver transplant candidates may also require a TIPS procedure to help maintain a better quality of life.

Hemodialysis

Hemodialysis is a procedure used on patients who have poor or no kidney function. The patient is connected to a machine called a hemodialyzer, which acts as an artificial kidney. It cleans and filters the blood and removes extra salts, fluid, and harmful wastes from the body. The patient is disconnected from the hemodialyzer when the procedure is completed, usually after 2 to 4 hours. Patients who have just received a kidney transplant may have acute tubular necrosis (ATN), a condition in which the kidney does not work efficiently. Patients with ATN may require hemodialysis until their newly transplanted kidney starts to function.

Transplant Coordinator

A transplant coordinator is a registered nurse who has clinical experience with the transplant population. The coordinator is responsible for the evaluation and preparation of patients for organ transplantation. In addition, this person acts as the patient's representative in the coordination of care before, during, and after the organ transplant in order to ensure continuity of care across settings.

The transplant coordinator arranges for and conducts pretransplant interviews with patients, families, and the transplant surgeon. During these interviews, eligibility for organ transplantation is determined, and clinical information about the patient's health is obtained. If initial eligibility is determined, the patient undergoes a pretransplant work-up to further ascertain eligibility for a transplant. This work-up is the final stage in identifying a patient as an eligible transplant recipient.

From this point on, the coordinator is involved in planning and organizing the patient's care related to receiving a transplanted organ. This includes coordinating outpatient clinic appointments, monitoring laboratory tests, notifying potential recipients when an organ becomes available, and ensuring post-transplant lab testing.

The transplant coordinator maintains an open line of communication with patients after discharge from the hospital and provides general supervision and direction to patients and their families. He or she oversees the long-term health care management of the transplant patient. The coordinator works with both transplant recipients and individuals who are interested in kidney donation. All transplant recipients have an assigned transplant coordinator.

Organ Donation and Procurement

There are two ways in which kidneys can be donated for transplant. The first is called living related or living unrelated kidney donation. The kidney is the only organ that can be transplanted from a live donor. Living related kidney donors are volunteering donation of a kidney to a relative. Living nonrelated kidney donors are volunteering donation of a kidney to someone in need, usually a spouse or friend. In order to be eligible for kidney donation, the donor must undergo a pre-donation work-up. This is usually done in an outpatient setting. Kidney transplants by living related or unrelated donors are planned and scheduled in advance.

Kidney transplants can also be performed using organs procured from a cadaver. In this type of transplant, a procurement team is sent to the hospital to recover transplantable organs after brain death has been determined. Kidneys as well as the pancreas and liver are usually procured from the cadaver. A cadaver kidney transplant is done within 72 hours after removal of the organ. Because of the limited time between procurement and transplant, potential kidney recipients must be available to come to the hospital on an emergent basis.

Liver and pancreas transplants are usually performed using cadaver organs. A liver transplant must be performed within 24 hours after the liver is obtained. A pancreas transplant must be performed within 36 hours after harvesting of the organ. In order to procure a cadaver organ for transplant, consent must be obtained from the family of the potential donor.

Donation of an organ begins with the identification of a potential donor and referral to the procurement office of a hospital that performs transplant services. An organ procurement specialist completes an evaluation to determine donor eligibility. Important factors that are considered include cause of death, age, sex, blood type, medical history, and brain death declaration by a physician. Consent from the family of the organ donor must be obtained before any further steps can be taken. Once consent is obtained, the donor is hemodynamically stabilized in order to maintain the viable organs.

Organ recipients are identified using guidelines established by the transplant facility and **UNOS**. (UNOS is the abbreviation for United Network of Organ Sharing. This private, nonprofit organization functions under a federal government contract to oversee the National Organ Procurement and Transplant Network.) The organ recipients are notified by the transplant coordinator that a donor organ is available. The procurement team is responsible for reporting recipient information to the UNOS program. The procurement team is also responsible for recovering donor organs from a cadaver. This occurs at the facility where brain death was declared. The organs are then transported to the facility where the transplant operation is to be performed.

The procurement organization also follows up with the donor family. They offer support and provide general information about the organ recipient, such as age, sex, occupation, marital status, and the number and ages of children and grandchildren. The procurement organization also provides public education pertaining to organ donation in an effort to convey the urgent need for transplant organs.

Testing and Tissue Typing to Determine Organ Compatibility

The histocompatibility laboratory is responsible for various testing done on a potential organ recipient's blood and a donor's blood and organ tissue to determine compatibility. The first test is ABO blood grouping, which determines the blood type. Blood type O is the universal donor, and blood type AB is the universal recipient. After ABO compatibility testing is done, a crossmatch is performed. A **final crossmatch** between the recipient's white blood cells and the donor's white blood cells is done to rule out organs to which the recipient has antibodies.

The testing done to identify antigens is called tissue typing. Antigens identified by tissue typing are called **human leukocyte antigens (HLAs)**.

Antigen testing determines the compatibility between the donor's body and the recipient's body.

Surgical pathology is a division of the laboratory that does diagnostic studies on tissue samples. The pathologists diagnose such things as rejection of a transplanted organ, cancer, or other disease process. Tissue samples are usually sent to the surgical pathology department in formaldehyde solution.

Documentation

A critical pathway (Fig. 15–5) is a preprinted form used by the multidisciplinary team, including nurses, HUCs, physicians, PT, respiratory therapists, and others, for documentation and reference. This document contains a variety of information such as the patient's plan of care, diagnosis, allergies, treatments, activities, procedures, laboratory tests, diet orders, and discharge planning. The HUC may transcribe physician's orders onto this document.

In many instances the physician will have prepared a preprinted set of orders (Fig. 15–6) related to the type of transplant that the patient will receive; these will correspond to the information found on the critical pathway.

The transplant service has several different pathways available, which include:

- Donor nephrectomy
- Liver disease with TIPS
- Liver shunt
- Liver transplant work-up
- Liver transplant
- Medical admit post transplant
- Pancreas/renal tx enteric conversion
- Pancreas/renal transplant
- Post-transplant surgical
- Readmit liver transplant
- Renal transplant with OKT3/ATG
- Renal transplant without OKT3/ATG
- Renal transplant: r/o rejection

When a patient is admitted to the hospital, the HUC or registered nurse chooses the appropriate pathway for the patient based on the symptoms and diagnosis.

Consents

Patients who are to receive an organ transplant must sign a consent for the procedure; this is explained to them by a physician prior to the operation (Fig. 15–7). There are several different consents used in organ transplant, such as a consent for kidney transplant, pancreas transplant, liver transplant, and kidney transplant from a HCV-positive donor. In addition to a special organ transplant consent, a regular surgical consent must be obtained.

Follow-up Care

Transplant recipients may require home care upon discharge from the hospital. Some of the common services provided by a visiting nurse are home IV drug therapy and dressing changes. Discharge planning is an important part of a successful transplant **graft** survival. Once patients are discharged from the hospital, it is their responsibility to follow the discharge instructions. Nursing staff provides the teaching necessary for recipients to take care of their newly transplanted organ.

Closing Thoughts

Health unit coordinating on the transplant unit is unique and exciting. Procedures and protocols are constantly changing and improving. Your ability as a HUC will always be challenged by the complex situations that can arise. A good understanding of transplant and its terminology will prove helpful in your ability to perform with confidence and accuracy. The reward of seeing patients being given a second lease on life makes the job fulfilling.

RENAL TRANSPLANT CRITICAL PATHWAY

Addressograph

Admitting MD/Service Transplant
Primary Nurse ______________ Associate Nurse ______________
Allergies ______________ Religion ______________
Case Manager Transplant Coordinator
Admitting Diagnosis: ______________

History:

Pt/family support systems; special considerations include: ______________

Significant Other (*Name & Phone*): ______________

CODES:
√ = Within Parameter
* = Variance (does not meet parameter) AIR Note required for variances in the outcomes section
= Variance in patient condition unchanged
NR = Not Required

Daily Tx labs: Creat, BUN, Hct, K$^+$, FBS, B$_2$M, cyclo or FK level, WBC c diff, send central line tips if pt febrile
Wed: Chem Lytes, plts
If on OKT3: Flow cytometry 1 week p̄ Tx

Date	*Time*	*Initial & Signature*	*Date*	*Time*	*Initial & Signature*

WORKING DIAGNOSIS							
DATE/TIME INTERVAL	Pre-op/ ______ (N D E)	Post-op/ ______ (N D E)	POD #1/ ______ (N D E)	POD #2/ (N D E)	POD #3, 4/ (N D E N D E)	POD #5/ (N D E)	POD #6, 7/ (N D E N D E)
UNIT SETTING	B4/6	B4/6	B4/6	B4/6	B4/6	B4/6	B4/6
CONSULTS	Anesthesia (possible) Hemodialysis		*Dr. Redwood *Diabetic Nurse	*Dr. Redwood *Diabetic Nurse	Dietary		
LABS	CBC c̄ diff, plt, lytes, BUN, Creat, glu, PT, PTT, hep panel, T&C + cold agglutinins, SMA$_{12}$, B$_2$M, ELDL, CMV antibody, tissue typing, HgbA, C. Tx Hematology	6^0 post-op: Hct, lytes (___) Recheck labs per RN discretion	Daily Tx labs Q Wed. SMA$_{12}$ & Mg CBC, lytes Repeat labs per RN discretion	Daily Tx labs Q Wed. SMA$_{12}$ & Mg Lytes Repeat labs per RN discretion	Tx labs Recheck labs per RN discretion	Tx labs Recheck labs per RN discretion	Daily Tx labs Recheck labs per RN discretion POD #7: Chem, Heme c̄ diff, plt
SPECIMENS (RN)	UA, C&S Stool for c̄ diff PRN watery diarhea Pan/cx PRN for temp>38^0	Stool for c̄ diff PRN watery diarhea Pan/cx PRN for temp>38^0	Stool for c̄ diff PRN watery diarhea Pan/cx PRN for temp>38^0	Stool for c̄ diff PRN watery diarhea Pan/cx PRN for temp>38^0	Urine cx q̄ Tues. Stool for c̄ diff PRN watery diarhea Pan/cx PRN for temp >38^0	Urine cx q̄ Tues Stool for c̄ diff PRN watery diarhea Pan/cx PRN for temp >38^0	POD #7 urine cx (2 days p̄ foley d/c'd) Stool for c̄ diff PRN watery diarhea Pan/cx PRN for temp >38^0
TESTS	CXR EKG	CXR in PAR	Renal Scan PRN				
ACTIVITY I = Independent A = Assist (indicate amount needed) D = Dependent Indicate assistive devices	Bathing:I Transfer:I Chair___ x/d:___ I Amb ___ x/d: ___ I Toileting:I	Reposition q̄ 2^0 while in bed Bathing:A Transfer:A Dangle c̄ in 8^0 post-op Chair/amb c̄ in 16^0 post-op	Reposition q̄ 2^0 while Feeding:I Bathing:A Transfer:A Amb 2x/d 2x/pm 2x/noc	Feeding:I Bathing:A Transfer:A Amb 2x/d 2x/pm 2x/noc Tuileting:A	Feeding:I Bathing:A Transfer:A Chair___x/d:___ I Amb ___ x/day, 2x, pm, 1x/noc Tuileting:A	Feeding:I Bathing:I Transfer:I Chair: ad lib Amb: ad lib Toileting:I	Feeding:I Bathing:I Transfer:I Chair: ad lib Amb: ad lib Toileting:I
TREATMENTS *Call H.O. for:* T___ P___ R___ BP___ U.O.___	VS q 4^0 & PRN I & O Weight *One touch QID Tap H$_2$O enemas X2 Hibiclens scrub Prep abdomen shave TEDS Wrap fistula c̄ Kerlix IV-	VS q̄ 15 min till stable then q̄ 4^0 I & O Weight √ orthostatics prior to amb UO q̄ 1^0 CD&B q̄ 2^0 while awake IS q̄ 1^0 while awake *One touch QID CVP q̄ 4^0 & PRN Foley to DD Irrigate foley c̄ sterile NS PRN Hickman care Pulse ox PRN IV-D5.45NS @ (UO+30) max 200cc/^{0}, min 30cc/^{0}	*Post OKT3 or ATG VS:* q̄ 15'x4, q 30'x2, routine Remain in room for 1^0 Have emergency cart available I & O Weight √ orthostatics PRN UO q̄ 1^0 C&DB q̄ 2^0 while IS q̄ 1^0 while awake *One touch QID CVP q̄ 4^0 Foley to DD Irrigate foley c̄ sterile NS PRN Hickman care Pulse ox PRN Suture line care IV-D5.45NS @ (UO+30) max 200cc/^{0}, min 30cc/^{0}	*Post OKT3 or ATG VS:* q̄ 15'x4, q̄ 30'x2, routine I & O Weight √ orthostatics PRN UO q̄ 1^0 *One touch QID CVP PRN Foley to DD Routine foley care Irrigate foley c̄ sterile NS PRN Hickman care Pulse ox PRN Suture line care IV-D5.45NS @ (UO+30) max 200cc/^{0}, min 30cc/^{0}	*Post OKT3 or ATG VS:* q̄ 30'x1 q̄ 2^{0}x2 I & O Weight *One touch QID Foley to DD Routine foley care Suture line care IV-	*Post OKT3 or ATG VS:* q̄ 30'x1 q̄ 2^{0}x2 I & O Weight *One touch QID Foley & stent d/c'd Hickman care Suture line care Straight cath PRN IV-H.W.	VS q̄ 8^0 I & O Weight *One touch QID Hickman care Suture line care IV-H.W.
DIET	NPO	NPO	NPO	Diet_______	*ADA (_____ K/cal)	General	General *ADA (_____ K/cal)
MEDICATIONS							

Pt Name: ______________ MR# ______________ Pt Name: ______________ MR# ______________

Figure 15–5
Critical pathway.

MR ______________ A ________
Name ______________
BD ______________ Sex ________
Serv ______________

University Hospital & Clinics
PHYSICIAN'S ORDERS

Patient Name

DATE & TIME	ph	RN	ORDERS
			SHOULD THIS PATIENT BE IN ANY TYPE OF ISOLATION? YES ☐ NO ☐
			IF YES, WHAT DISEASE IS SUSPECTED?
			ADMISSION ORDERS--LIVING RELATED RENAL TRANSPLANT
			1) Admit to B4/6
			2) Activity: Up ad lib.
			3) Diet: Clear liquids day before surgery, then NPO after midnight
			4) Labs on admission: CBC with diff, Plts., HbA1c, Chem survey and Lytes, Hepatitis, A, B, C
			panels, ELDL, P.T., P.T.T., CMV antibody screen, B2M, and Tx. hematology.
			Send urine for U.A. and Cx.
			5) Draw 10cc red top for tissue typing if needed and keep on unit for pickup. (Call 3-8815)
			6) Type and Cross for 4 units of leukopoor packed red blood cells to be kept on hold for
			surgery. Order cold agglutinins to be done with crossmatch.
			7) Obtain pre-op CXR, pa and lateral, and EKG.
			8) Assure op permits are signed.
			9) Make sure final tissue crossmatch between donor and recipient is negative.
			10) Pre-op prep: a. Tapwater enema night before surgery.
			b. Hibiclens shower night before surgery.
			c. Knee high Ted stockings on to O.R. if nondiabetic. Order Stryker
			boots and sheepskin for diabetics.
			d. Wrap fistula or dialysis graft lightly with Kerlix and label.
			e. Have weight and vital signs, final x-match report, blood typing and cold
			agglutinins, CXR and EKG results on chart for O.R. Send old chart with
			current chart to O.R.
			Known Allergies: ________
			11) Medications a. If O mismatch (HLA identical) give prednisone 120mg. po and azathioprine
			150 mg. po day prior to surgery. On A.M. of surgery give prednisone 120mg.
			po and azathioprine 300mg. (may adjust for W.B.C.)
			b. Cefazolin 1 gm I.V. to be sent to O.R. on chart.
			c. Send 500mg. of methylprednisolone on chart to O.R.
			d. Mag & Al & Simeth. Concen.15ml and Alum. Hydrox. Conc. 20ml alternate po
			qid if receiving prednisone pre-op.
			e. 300mg. aspirin suppository p.r. pre-op.
			f. Pharmacy to send *bladder irrigation soln.*, gentamicin 50 mg. in 500mls NaCl
			0.9%, *wound irrigation soln*, gentamicin 20mg. and bacitracin 50,000 u in
			200mls NaCl 0.9% both solns in pour bottles. Also send *perfusion soln.*,
			(MUST BE ICE COLD) heparin 10,000 u, procaine 50mg. (5ml of 1%) sodium
			bicarbonate 22.3 mEq. and mannitol 25gm. in L.R. 1L.
			g. Temazepam 15mg. po q h.s. prn insomnia.
			h. Tylenol 650mg. po prn q 4hr.
			i. Nifedipine 10mg. sl/po q 2 hr prn SBP>17 0 or dbp>100.
			M.D. ________

PHYSICIAN'S ORDERS

Figure 15–6
Preprinted doctor's orders.

RENAL TRANSPLANTATION
Consent Form

In order for you to understand the significance of renal transplantation, we have prepared the following discussion for your information.

Although renal transplantation is no longer an experimental procedure and is now an accepted form of therapy, the results cannot be predicted. At the present time, approximately 80% of all cadaver kidneys are still functioning after two years, and the survival rate of kidneys from living related donors is 90 to 95% at two years, depending on the relationship of the donor to the recipient.

Rejection is the major problem with transplants (except those from an identical sibling), but rejection is most common in recipients of cadaver kidneys. To prevent rejection--a process whereby your body destroys the transplant--immunosuppressive drugs are used. Seven standard drugs, (Neoral cyclosporine or Tacrolimus, ATG or Muromonab, Mycophenolate mofetil or Imuran, and prednisone) are used routinely in varying combinations and amounts of suppress the immune system of the recipient of a transplant. These are not experimental drugs, but they may have severe side effects. These side effects include lowering of the body's defenses so that the changes of contracting viral, bacterial, and fungal infections are greatly increased. If these drugs are used in large doses, severe infections, bleeding from the gastrointestinal tract, or skin and lung infections may develop. Prednisone can produce bone problems especially deterioration of the hips. It can cause cataracts, and diabetes. Mycophenolate mofetil and Imuran can cause bone marrow depression and gastrointestinal distress. Neoral cyclosporine and Tacrolimus can produce kidney damage, cause tremors, nausea, and increase blood pressure. The long term side effects of Neoral, Tacrolimus and Mycophenolate mofetil are not yet known. All patients on any immunosuppressive drugs are at a greater risk for malignancies. To minimize these complications, our policy is to accept loss of the kidney if dangerous doses of drugs are required to prevent rejection. Should this occur, the transplanted kidney may be removed and if necessary you will be returned to chronic dialysis. It is possible that you will require dialysis after your transplant surgery until the transplant kidney is functioning well, or during a period of rejection until the transplant kidney recovers.

You, of course, understand that there is an alternative to transplantation, which is chronic dialysis. The fact that you are signing this consent form means that you have chosen to receive a renal transplant rather than continue chronic dialysis.

We ask that you sign the following statement to indicate (1) that you have read and understand the discussion; (2) that any questions you have had have been satisfactorily answered and explained; and (3) that you wish to take part in this procedure.

I, ______________________________ have read and understand the foregoing discussion. A copy of which has been furnished to me for my information, I hereby agree to receive a kidney transplant as treatment for my renal failure. I understand that success cannot be guaranteed and that the kidney may be rejected or may be removed if large doses of immunosuppressive drugs are required to prevent rejection. I understand the hazards of these drugs.

____
(Signature of Subject)

____
(Signature of Witness)

Figure 15–7
Transplant patient consent form.

Review Questions

1. Identify the organs that can be transplanted.
2. List five diagnostic procedures that may be performed on transplant patients.
3. Explain what is meant by rejection.
4. Describe two sources of kidney donation for transplant.
5. Name the organization that oversees the identification of potential organ recipients.

Bibliography

Division of Laboratory Medicine Handbook. Madison, University of Wisconsin Hospital, 1994.

Dorland's Illustrated Medical Dictionary, 28th ed. Philadelphia, WB Saunders, 1994.

Morris J: Kidney Transplantation: Principals and Practice, 3rd ed. Philadelphia, WB Saunders, 1988.

Oberley ET, Glass NR: Understanding Kidney Transplantation. Springfield, IL, Charles C Thomas, 1987.

Sollinger H: Transplantation Drug Pocket Reference Guide, Austin, TX, RG Landes, 1994.

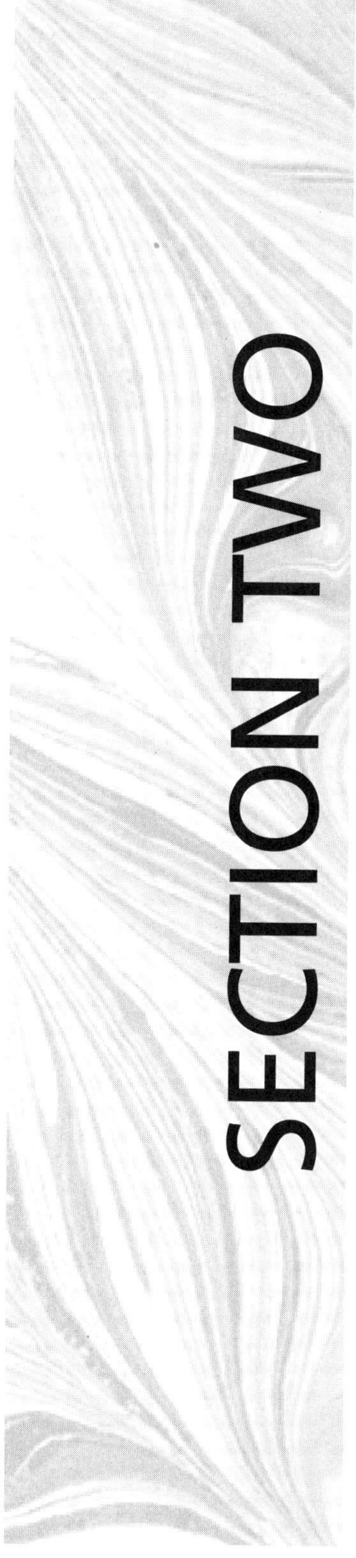

SECTION TWO

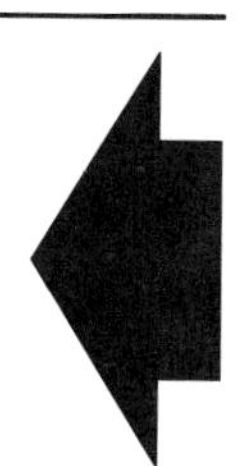

THE HEALTH UNIT COORDINATOR IN EXPANDED HOSPITAL ROLES

16 Administrative Assistant to Nurse Manager

Roylene Galbraith

Common Abbreviations

PCA Patient-controlled analgesia

QA Quality assurance

Objectives

At the completion of this chapter, the reader should be able to:

1. List the major areas of responsibility for an administrative assistant.
2. Explain the purpose of a "critical pathway."
3. Describe the role of the administrative assistant in quality assurance.

Vocabulary

Braden Scale: A method to assess risk for pressure ulcer development

Critical pathway: A plan outlining the usual care needs of patients with a specific diagnosis

Pain scale: A rating tool that uses a scale of 0–10 to help the patient indicate severity of pain

Point of care: Laboratory tests that are performed by the staff on the nursing unit

History

The administrative assistant position is a relatively new job position in hospitals. Many hospitals are "downsizing" in-patient units to save money. Downsizing is taking place because more out-patient surgeries are being performed and in-patients are spending less time on the units. As a result of this downsizing, nurse managers are being asked to manage two in-patient units instead of one. The administrative assistant takes on many of the jobs that the nurse manager no longer has time to do while managing two units.

Position Responsibilities and Duties

The administrative assistant works under the direction of the person who has overall responsibility for management on an in-patient nursing unit. This person may be referred to as the nurse manager, clinical nurse manager, unit manager, head nurse, or other titles. Job responsibilities include administrative support, effective management of fiscal records, data collection, maintenance of personnel records and schedules, and staff orientation and training.

Administrative Support

Administrative support on the nursing unit is a multifaceted task encompassing a variety of responsibilities. Duties may include maintaining appointment calendars for the nurse manager and other staff members, coordinating and scheduling meetings, submitting seminar and travel requests, drafting letters and memos, and compiling QA (quality assurance) and other reports. Maintaining unit manuals and bulletin boards, chart audits, photocopying, and filing are additional responsibilities of this position.

The administrative assistant must prioritize the daily duties in a manner that allows for unexpected and unplanned duties to be completed in a timely manner. Organization and good communication are important skills to develop, as well as an open relationship with the nurse manager.

Appointment Calendars

Some administrative assistants may keep the appointment calendar for the manager. The calendar may be in the computer, an appointment book, or posted on the unit for the staff to see the availability of the nurse manager's time. The manager and administrative assistant should have a daily routine for communicating and exchanging information on ongoing projects and assignments.

Scheduling Meetings

Scheduling meetings can be taken from a complicated chore to a simple task with the right organizational tool. On obtaining the list of people needed at the meeting, the administrative assistant might want to use a grid (Fig. 16–1) to help keep track of the participants' dates and times of availability. Once the date and time of the meeting have been established, a room needs to be reserved. The number of people expected, the date and time requested, and the approximate length of the meeting need to be communicated to the person in charge of room scheduling. Once a room number is assigned, the administrative assistant sends a memo to all expected attendees with the date, time, and place of the meeting. In addition, it may be necessary to arrange for special equipment: overhead projectors, video equipment, flip charts, and anything else needed for a

Name of Meeting: ______________________

Rm# *362* Length of meeting *1 hour*	Date *1/27*	Date *1/28*	Date *2/3*	Date *2/4*	Date *2/7*	Date	Date
Dolores Lenehan	*9-10, 2-3*		*9-12*		*9-10*		
Frank Dern	*10-2*		*9-11, 4-5*		*11-2, 4-5*		
Sarah Flynn		*10-12*	*9-11*	*9-11*			
Jenny Bergman		*1-2*	*10-12*	*3-4*			

Figure 16–1
Meeting time grid.

successful outcome. For some meetings, it may be necessary to make special arrangements for food or beverage service.

Submitting Seminar and Travel Requests

Another area of record keeping assigned to the administrative assistant is submitting seminar and travel requests. In a typical hospital, the employee fills out a "Request for Education/Travel Money" form and turns it in to the nurse manager along with a copy of the seminar brochure. After the nurse manager approves the expense, the clinical director of nursing also needs to give written approval. If all is acceptable, the administrative assistant submits the request for payment. If hotel, parking, or airline expenses are incurred, the administrative assistant needs to submit a travel expense report as well. These reports are necessary for reimbursement of any costs that the employee may have paid up front.

Drafting Memos and Letters

The administrative assistant may be required to draft memos and letters from standards developed and approved by the nurse manager. Memos, letters, reports, QA studies, staff meeting minutes, and other documents need to be completed in an accurate and appropriately formatted manner, and the final copy should be typed. Many times, these items need to be posted for staff to read or distributed to the appropriate mailboxes.

Compiling Quality Assurance and Other Data

Compiling QA and other data needed for monthly/quarterly/yearly reports is an important part of the job. The administrative assistant is assigned to distribute and collect staff members' annual safety and infection control examinations, glucose one-touch testing, and radiation safety tests (where applicable). Proof of cardiopulmonary resuscitation recertification is due yearly, and the administrative assistant verifies that each employee's certification is current. The administrative assistant follows up on staff attendance at mandatory training programs, such as tuberculosis mask fitting, assault and abuse education programs, and patient restraint programs. Often, this includes distributing a memo to each employee about these programs and signing up employees for dates and times they are available to attend. Should they need to complete a self-study packet, the administrative assistant would be responsible for distributing these to the employees and seeing that each employee turns in the packet by the deadline established.

Maintaining Unit Manuals

Periodically, sections of the administrative and nursing policy and procedure manuals need to be replaced. Other manuals that need to be updated might include safety manuals, health unit coordinator manuals, radiology policy and procedure manuals, and any other manuals specific to the unit. The old sections need to be discarded and replaced with updated information.

Photocopying

Xeroxing and distributing materials to staff members are significant parts of the role of the administrative assistant. Larger photocopying projects, such as manuals, or anything needing over 25 copies may be sent out to the hospital's professional duplicating source in order to be cost effective.

Filing

The administrative assistant is responsible for maintaining an efficient, orderly filing system. Color-coded, alphabetical file folders can be used as well as a separate "forms" file cabinet in which a "duplicated materials master file" is kept. Budget materials, travel records, and financial management data sheets might be kept in three-ring binders. Personnel evaluation records and other confidential employee information should be kept in a locked file cabinet in the office. If separate offices on two different units are being used by the nurse manager and administrative assistant, it is helpful to keep them organized in the same way. It is important to be able to find things easily and feel comfortable when working in either office.

Additional Responsibilities

In the event of the nurse manager's absence, the administrative assistant should be able to coordinate activities during this time. It would be up to the administrative assistant to gather and sort mail and respond as indicated, take telephone messages, redirect communications appropriately, and use resources when needed.

Effective Management of Fiscal Records

Ordering

It is essential that the administrative assistant order supplies, basing need on usage. It is also important to maintain an active ongoing file for ordering supplies and provide regular follow-up until supplies are received. Creation and maintenance of a record system for tracking office expenditures and ordered supplies are vital. The administrative assistant also prepares purchase orders and capital equipment requests, following hospital regulations.

Budget Reports

The nurse manager is required to submit quarterly budget reports. Information needed for these reports may be taken from the unit's "Operating Statement," "Statistics by Nursing Unit" report (which includes admission, discharge, and transfer information for the unit), and the "Human Resources Management" report. The administrative assistant compiles the information that the nurse manager has collected from these reports and inserts that data into a standardized budget report form. The completed report is then submitted to the clinical director of nursing.

Cost Containment

Maintaining a cost-effective approach in activities and assisting the nurse manager in defining cost-containment strategies are also responsibilities of the administrative assistant. Along with this is the preparation and dissemination of cost-containment reports. One example of a cost-containment strategy is to follow up on the "issues report" that is prepared for each in-patient unit every month. The issues report is a computer-generated document that tracks unit supplies used for each unit. The items listed on this report are stocked either on the linen carts or the back-up supply cart. This report shows a description of each charge item, the date the item was ordered, the quantity ordered, and the price charged to the unit. It also shows the *monthly* quantity of each individual item ordered and the *monthly* charge for each item. One tool that is used to track cost containment is an issues report grid (Fig. 16–2). On the grid, each item to be tracked is written in the box on the left. Every month, the total number of items ordered for that month is inserted as well as the total amount charged to the unit. This grid is used primarily to alert the administrative assistant to any obvious overcharging of supplies. By comparing the data month after month, discrepancies become noticeable.

Payroll

Hours are calculated for each employee on a biweekly time sheet. Included in the book with the biweekly time sheets is a comment sheet on which the employees may indicate what they would like done with extra time earned or other variances in their work time. For example, should employees come to work an hour early for a meeting, they may designate the extra hour to be calculated as comp time earned or paid time. Or, if they need to leave work early, they may indicate the type of time they would like to use to make up for the time missed. The administrative assistant needs to verify the accuracy of paid work time, vacation time, and sick leave when doing the payroll.

Department of Nursing
F4/6 – Issues Report

Year ____________

Expense Class		July	Aug.	Sept.	Oct.	Nov.	Dec.	Jan.	Feb.	Mar.	April	May	June
Patient gowns	#	215	240	315	233								
	$	50	55	72	(153)								
Sheet, fitted	#	600	770	535	725								
	$	260	322	224	303								
PJ bottom adult large	#	30	60	65	30								
	$	5	11	12	5								
Pillowcases	#	1,335	1,550	1,217	1,289								
	$	143	166	131	138								
Water Pitcher	#	153	158	152	169								
	$	39	41	40	44								
Mouthwash	#	28	30	43	40								
	$	5	6	8	7								
	#												

Figure 16–2
Issues report.

It is necessary to have a tracking system to determine exactly what type of time the employees have available to use when they are off work. The tracking system used is a report generated from the payroll office. This report indicates the amount of sick leave, comp time, vacation time, personal and legal holiday time that each employee has left to use. These reports are updated biweekly.

Payroll sheets need to be submitted by a predetermined deadline to ensure that employees receive their paychecks on time.

Data Collection Related to Quality Improvement/ Assurance

The administrative assistant needs to document quality controls and maintain reports related to quality improvement efforts. Examples of different quality controls include glucose monitoring, crash cart checks, and **point of care** laboratory tests. These may vary from one institution to another. An example of point of care laboratory testing would be the routine quality-control testing of the Gastrocult slide and developer and the Hemocult fecal blood slide and developer. (The Gastrocult test accurately screens gastric aspirate for occult blood and pH; the fecal occult blood Hemocult test accurately screens fecal samples for occult blood.) In many hospitals, point of care quality-control testing is performed weekly.

Collecting data and information as directed by the nurse manager is a vital part of the administrative assistant's job. Data collection includes tallying monthly chart documentation audits and quarterly patient satisfaction questionnaires, collecting sick leave data for each staff member, ordering patient charts for QA studies, and any other data collection requested by the nurse manager.

Quality Assurance Studies

Quality assurance studies such as **Pain Scale** and **Braden Scale** documentation results need to be graphed and posted for the units to see each month. Pain Scale audit results track how well RNs are assessing and documenting pain. For example, a large Pain Scale poster is placed on the wall in each patient's room. The Pain Scale is a rating tool that uses a scale of 0 to 10 to help the patient indicate to the nurse how severe his or her pain is. "Zero" indicates no pain, "3" indicates some pain, but tolerable, "5" indicates moderate pain, "7" severe pain, and "10" the worst pain possible. The patient's pain ratings are documented on the flow sheet at least once every 24 hours, but more frequently for those with an epidural, **patient-controlled analgesia (PCA)** device or those receiving oral or intravenous pain medications.

Pain Scale audits are done every month by selecting a random number of charts and reporting whether the patient's pain was properly assessed and documented, and if the patient's pain relief goal was met.

Skin assessment is performed on all patients entering the hospital. This includes the assessment of risk for pressure ulcer development using the Braden Scale. The first step in pressure ulcer prevention is determining in which patients ulcers are likely to develop. Once at-risk patients are identified, intervention can be taken to try to prevent those patients from acquiring pressure ulcers. The Braden Pressure Ulcer Risk Assessment Scale (Braden Scale) is a tool used on admission to identify those at-risk patients. The Braden Scale score rates the patient's level of risk for pressure ulcers.

The Braden Scale audit results are compiled monthly by auditing nursing admission forms to look for documentation of a Braden Scale score for each patient. The percentage of patients with or without a Braden score is documented each month and posted for the unit to see.

Development and Maintenance of a Personnel Evaluation Tracking System

Employee evaluations are spread out over a 12-month period. Using a monthly work plan, the nurse manager is scheduled to do a given number of evaluations each month. These could be scheduled throughout the month by doing two evaluations per week, or by doing several evaluations on a given day of the month, and so forth.

Development and Maintenance of Staff Schedule

Vacation requests are submitted annually, by a specified date, to the nurse manager. Requests are granted on a seniority basis. All requests for time off are recorded in a log book on the unit. This information is then transferred to a master schedule. The master schedule is used to determine staffing availability for a 4-week period. Requests for supplemental staff are submitted to the scheduling office before the start of the 4-week scheduling period.

Training

At times, it is necessary to provide cross-coverage to the administrative assistants in the in-patient clinical area during vacations or absences, or to provide back-up support during times of heavy workloads.

The administrative assistant is always available to be a preceptor for other health unit coordinators. Even after taking on this new position, the administrative assistant may be called on to answer questions and offer guidance to the health unit coordinators. Occasionally, the administrative assistant may be asked to fill in on the unit if one of the health unit coordinators is absent and there is no replacement available.

Health Unit Coordinator Skills

Health unit coordinators who move to the administrative assistant position in the same facility have a smooth transition. As a health unit coordinator, a person has an enormous understanding of how the hospital operates. Awareness of the many different in-patient units and departments in the hospital, knowledge of numerous phone numbers, and familiarity with many of the physicians is very beneficial. Because health unit coordinators and administrative assistants are required to solve problems, being acquainted with names of people to contact is a must. Last, but not least, there is the advantage of already having mastered the hospital computer system. However, it is not a requirement to have worked in the facility to be an applicant for this position.

In the position of administrative assistant, it will be necessary to keep the office organized, not only for the administrative assistant's sake, but also for the nurse manager. The experienced health unit coordinator will have developed good organizational skills, not to mention many other important skills needed in the role of administrative assistant, such as problem-solving techniques, telephone etiquette, good filing skills, knowledge of ordering supplies, and the ability to prioritize.

The capability to work without direct supervision and to meet deadlines is a fundamental part of the health unit coordinator position, as it is also for the administrative assistant.

Related Terminology

The importance of a good understanding of medical terminology cannot be overemphasized. Medical terminology is encountered every day in the job as an administrative assistant, just as it is in the health unit coordinator position.

For example, the administrative assistant could have a project to do involving patient critical pathways. A **critical pathway** (Fig. 16–3) is a map of care outlining the usual needs for patients/families in a certain case type during an episode of illness. The purpose of the critical pathway is to provide a method to coordinate the care delivered to patients/families across geographic settings, to standardize the process of care delivered to patients/families in a specific case type, and to iden-

Figure 16–3
Critical pathway.

CRITICAL PATHWAY

SERVICE	DAY 1	DAY 2	DAY 3
NURSING	Weigh Pt Vitals QID Sit side of bed Bed Bath Dressing change	Vitals TID Sit in chair Pt Assist with bath Dressing change	Weigh Pt Vitals BID Walk to door Assist Pt with bath Drain Removed
DIET	Clear Liquid	Soft	Reg as tolerated
RESP TX	O2 @ 2 liters	DC O2	
PHY TX	In-Bed Exercise	Chair Exercise	Walk in Room
LAB	CBC, Glucose		Hgb/Hct
X-RAY	Portable Chest		

tify benchmark outcomes to be demonstrated by the patient/family as health maintenance, convalescence, and wellness are facilitated.

A particular pathway is chosen for each patient on admission to match the diagnosis. A "pathway" is just as it says, a path of care to be followed during the patient's stay. Each day of care on the pathway is outlined so that the patient and family generally know what to expect on any given day of the hospital stay. Some of the things it includes are the different services consulted on a routine basis (Physical/Occupational Therapy, Respiratory Therapy, Anesthesiology, Infectious Disease); a list of lab work/specimens needed on a specific date (admission labs, urinalysis, timed specimens); tests the patient will undergo (e.g., chest x-ray, electrocardiogram, magnetic resonance imaging, computerized tomography scan); and the activity level of the patient, to include positioning parameters or exercise regime. Other items listed on the pathway are treatments/tasks to be performed by caregivers (e.g., drain removal, dressing changes, Accuchecks, daily weights), diet plan, routine medications ordered in this type of case, and supplies/equipment used to manage the care for patients in this type of case. Of course, these paths may change if a patient has an unexpected health problem. The discharge planning is also incorporated into the plan of care, as is the nursing activity and teaching, and the patient outcomes desired. The pathways are kept at the patient's bedside so they may be referred to by the patient/family whenever desired.

Preprinted standing admission orders (which match the contents of the critical pathway's admission day) are often available for most of the critical pathways. In addition, "patient recovery" pathways may be available for the patients to use in conjunction with the permanent critical pathways that the nursing staff uses to chart. These would be written in simplified language to make it easier for the average patient to understand what will be happening each day. Information devised to send home with the patient on discharge will answer any questions the patient may have and ensure the continuity of the patient's care.

The administrative assistant's job may be to type the preprinted order sheets, patient recovery pathways, or "take-home" information, in which case the correct spelling of diagnoses and a familiarity with medical phrases on the pathway as well as symbols used on pathways should be general knowledge for the administrative assistant. The administrative assistant will also be corresponding with doctors, nurses, and other professionals.

Knowing the terminology used throughout the hospital is also helpful. When corresponding with many different departments in the hospital, use of correct terminology is a must. Equipment and supplies need to be ordered for the unit. For example, blood pressure cuffs need to be ordered. The correct medical term is "sphygmomanometer." Placing orders for equipment and supplies could be a real challenge without the proper background in terminology.

Terminology also extends into abbreviations for different areas of the hospital. "DVI" might be called "interventional radiology," or "C.S."/"central supply" could be used interchangeably with "materials management," and "environmental services" referred to as "housekeeping." Some hospitals may have a "personnel office," and others may refer to it as "human resources." There might be two parts to the "engineering department," with part of it being called "plant engineering" (which would take care of problems such as beds not working, equipment safety checks, repairing blinds in patient rooms, or hanging items on the walls), whereas "clinical engineering" would take care of electrical problems such as call light or console malfunctions. At each place of employment, it is important to have accurate knowledge of names and locations of departments throughout the hospital.

Additional Training Required

The major part of the administrative assistant's job actually consists of various secretarial skills, including answering phones, typing, computer skills, record keeping, and filing. A formal medical terminology class would be a beneficial course in which to enroll.

As more hospitals are using personal computers, it would be appropriate training to attend a computer class. If there is E-mail through the hospital computer system, it is essential to master this system. A course in time management would also be very helpful for this position.

Procedures and Functions Specific to Position

One of the first things to be done at the start of each working day is to check the voice mail (and possibly the nurse manager's voice mail). It is therefore necessary to create a personal message for the administrative assistant position and learn the functions of the voice mail system.

The nurse manager will most likely have a mailbox on each of the units. It is the administrative assistant's job to collect and sort the mail and respond as indicated. It is beneficial to touch base with the nurse manager each morning to discuss the general plan for the day, review times of meetings, and the like.

Part of the work day is usually devoted to some type of problem solving, whether it be questions from the staff regarding their payroll or work schedules, ordering new name pins, or checking on broken supplies/equipment and the status of their repair. Many times the administrative assistant is asked to send malfunctioning equipment to plant engineering to be repaired. It is also the administrative assistant's responsibility to order new medical supplies or equipment to replace any that may have worn out. Sometimes special-order items need to be reordered. Incorrectly ordered medical or office supplies may need to be returned for credit.

When new employees are hired to a unit, it is the administrative assistant's responsibility to see that they get a locker and mailbox assigned to them. It is necessary to obtain a current phone number from each person to keep at the unit desk. The administrative assistant also needs to show new employees where to sign in and sees that they get a computer sign-on and a name pin.

A daily emergency cart check needs to be documented on each unit. This is usually done by the nurse who works the night shift. The administrative assistant may be responsible for doing a double check first thing in the morning to ensure that this was done. The weekly point of care laboratory testing (as explained in the section on data collection) might also be assigned to the administrative assistant. Payroll duties are carried out on the same day each week, and staff scheduling, which may be computerized or written, is done at the same time each month. Deadlines need to be met for each of these tasks. Aside from duties performed on specific days of the week, each day tends to be different and interesting.

Closing Thoughts

My nurse manager was the first person in our hospital to have two 29-bed surgical units combined, and therefore she needed secretarial support. I was the first person to be brought into the new position of the "administrative assistant." Since I was hired, a few more positions have opened throughout the hospital, and I imagine that this will be the continuing trend.

I have been employed at the University of Wisconsin Hospital and Clinics for 10 years. I was selected for the administrative assistant position because of my familiarity with both of the surgical units that were combined and with the hospital as a whole.

When I started my position as a health unit coordinator, I was in the float pool and got to know each of the units very well. After that, I had worked as a health unit coordinator specifically on each of the two surgical units that were combined. At times, when there was overlapping health unit coordinator coverage on the general surgery unit, I was asked to help out with various tasks for my nurse manager, many of which ended up being the same tasks that I now do as her administrative assistant.

The administrative assistant position is a great advancement opportunity for health unit coordinators. The knowledge and experience of the health unit coordinator is undoubtedly helpful when progressing to the administrative assistant role. Advancing to this position allows the health unit coordinator to stay active on in-patient units in a different capacity. After working many years as a health unit coordinator, this is a welcome advancement because it offers many new learning opportunities and less stress on the job.

Review Questions

1. List the major areas of responsibility for an administrative assistant and briefly describe each.
2. Explain the purpose of a "critical pathway."
3. Describe the role of the administrative assistant in quality assurance.

17

Centralized Staffing/ Scheduling Coordinator

Jan Bumgarner

Common Abbreviations

ACLS	Advanced cardiac life support
ADC	Average daily census
CPR	Cardiopulmonary resuscitation
FTE	Full-time employee
JCAHO	Joint Commission on Accreditation of Health Care Organizations
NE	Nurse extern
NHPPD	Nursing hours per patient day
NLN	National League of Nursing
OA	Office automation
OJI	On-the-job injury
OPS	Outpatient services
PAF	Personnel Action Form
PC	Personal computer
PCA	Patient care assistant
PCS	Patient care services
PTO	Paid time off
SNF	Skilled nursing facility
TBI	Time bank interface

Objectives

At the completion of this chapter, the reader should be able to:

1. List three sources the staffing coordinator might use to obtain needed staff.
2. Explain the importance of collaboration with the nursing supervisors.
3. List the communication devices a staffing coordinator would be expected to use.

Vocabulary

Back-up: Saving computer information on a diskette or floppy disk

Interface: A method of connecting two (or more) computer systems together

Office automation: Computer or electronic mail (E-mail)

The abbreviations listed for this chapter are those that a HUC working in this area would be expected to know. Only those in **boldface** type are used in the text and appear in boldface when they are used for the first time.

Overview

Accommodating the staffing needs of all nursing units (which may also include ancillary departments) is the main responsibility of the staffing coordinator. In many parts of the country, hospitals have more than one facility or service area to staff as well as the hospital. This may include off-site clinics or outpatient surgical centers. It may require more than one staffing coordinator to cover all areas. Some facilities have staffing coordinator coverage 24 hours a day, whereas others may staff this position only for one or two shifts a day. Administrative registered nurse (RN) supervisors may cover staffing on nights or weekends, or for last-minute staffing adjustments. However the coverage is maintained, the staffing coordinator must be well organized and detail oriented with regard to the changing demands this position makes.

Position Responsibilities and Duties

Staffing Office

The staffing office requires nursing personnel to submit all requests for time off well in advance of the printed schedule. Requests may be for vacation, military leave, jury duty, or family leave. Illness and disability usually are handled as they happen. Requests for time off are entered into the computer and honored whenever possible. Most hospitals have rules that dictate how many people may be on vacation from each unit at any one time and still maintain unit integrity.

Each unit has a recipe for the ratio and type of staff needed on average census days. For example, a Medical–Surgical unit with an average census of 30 patients may require at least 3 RNs, 6 patient care assistants (**PCA**), and 1 health unit coordinator (HUC), whereas an intensive care unit with an average census of 10 patients may require 5 RNs, 2 PCAs and 1 HUC. Unit schedules are made in advance using the unit recipe for average census. Anytime the unit census changes, the staffing office makes adjustments. This could mean moving staff from low-census units to areas with a high patient census. There are many methods used to meet the daily staffing needs, and facilities must use all the resources available to provide adequate staff for quality patient care. This may include contacting existing staff members who have requested extra work time or using other special resources.

Staffing Sources

Float Pools

Float pools are one method of meeting the needs of a fluctuating patient census. Staff working from a float pool are a multitalented group who are able to adapt to a different unit each shift. The pool may consist of RNs, licensed practical nurses (LPNs), PCAs, HUCs, and any other clinical or nonclinical staff required to cover a unit. Float pool members report to the staffing office and are given their assignments for the day. On days of low census throughout the hospital, float pool members may be asked to stay home before other workers or all workers may go into a rotating pool so that some workers are not asked more than others. Each hospital has its own method of dealing with low-census days.

Private Agencies/Registries

Private agencies or registries provide a service to hospitals when staffing needs become critical. The agency will have a prearranged contract with the hospital stating the type of staff it can provide and the fees involved. Agency staff is paid by the agency and the hospital is billed for the workers' salary plus a service fee. This makes agency staffing very expensive, and thus it is used only when other staffing is unavailable. The staffing coordinator must know which agencies or registries the hospitals has contracts with and when it is appropriate to call for this service.

Traveling Staff

Traveling staff members may be provided by a special agency that brings in staff from other parts of the United States to make up for nursing shortages. The agency often provides the staff with housing and transportation allowances. Each assignment may last from a few weeks to a year in one city or town. The staffing coordinator will be aware if this is an option that may be used during peak vacation times or during a nursing shortage.

Call-In Absences

Call-ins are something the staffing coordinator must deal with on a daily basis. These calls may be due to personal or family illness as well as many other unexpected contingencies. Although the hospital may have a policy requiring the staff to call hours in advance of their shift start time, many calls may come in minutes before the beginning of the shift. The staffing coordinator must deal with the challenge and stress involved with this last-minute, difficult situation.

Inclement weather and disasters may provide the most challenging call-ins for the staffing coordinator. In these situations, hospitals may have a policy or special plan worked out in advance to deal with the crisis. They may offer bonus packages for working extra shifts or provide existing staff with a place to sleep between shifts as an alternative to going home. Whatever the plan, the staffing coordinator will be at the heart of dealing with the crisis.

Communication Skills

Communication skills are the key to being successful in this position. The telephone, computer, fax, and mail are all part of the daily routine.

Receiving Call-Ins

When receiving a call-in, it is important to maintain a calm level of voice control. If there are required questions that must be answered by the caller, the staffing coordinator gets this done quickly because the caller will be stressed from either illness or personal emergency. After recording the staff member's absence, the staffing coordinator works toward filling the vacancy as quickly as possible using standard hospital policies. The vacancy is communicated to the nursing unit by telephone. As soon as replacement staff has been arranged, the nursing unit is called and given the information. At any given moment, the staffing coordinator may be handling several call-in and replacement situations at the same time, and must remain calm and collected in this stressful time.

Collaboration

Collaboration with the nursing supervisor takes place several times each shift. The staffing coordinator uses the supervisor's report log, sends computer **office automation** (OA) messages, and has direct contact with the supervisor. The report log notes staff changes, patient changes, and census per shift. Supervisors need to be kept informed so that they know which units are short staffed, who has been called in to work, if any staff members will be arriving late, and any additional call-ins since report at the beginning of the shift. This line of communication goes both ways, from the staffing coordinator to the Supervisor and back. Each unit's budget requires effective utilization and assignment of personnel. Because of call-ins and changes in census and acuity, collaboration must be a top priority.

Computer Responsibilities

Maintenance of the staffing/scheduling computer system is vital to achieve maximum productivity for all users. The staffing coordinator's computer responsibilities include:

Back-up—Saving information onto diskettes that can be used in the event that the hard drive or network fails.

Printer upkeep—Keeping the printers clean, on line, and stocked with paper.

Error messages—Error messages must be dealt with immediately so that the users do not get locked out of the system. This may require calling the software company for assistance.

The staffing/scheduling computer system is the backbone of the staffing coordinator's position.

Reports

Reports are generated by the staffing coordinator both routinely and by special request. The staffing office is the information center for the nursing division. All employee information is keyed into the staffing/scheduling computer system and includes demographics, salary, credentials, transfers, time off, and terminations. Reports available might concern productivity, attendance, individual or unit activity, agency usage, unit acuity, new hires, transfers, terminations, and many other topics. Providing reports for the nursing division and other departments is sandwiched between staffing issues.

Customer Service

Customer service is essential, requiring excellent communication skills and knowledge of community activities. This applies regardless of whether the customer is a unit in the hospital, an off-site center, an agency, or a member of the staff. It is part of nearly every staffing function.

Nursing Office Activities

Nursing office activities may be handled by the staffing coordinator when the space is shared with the nursing office and may also include some patient bed control issues. Regardless of where the office is located, the staffing coordinator should have knowledge of maintenance and use of fax and copy machines; distribution of interoffice mail; answering coworkers' telephones; proper message taking; and other skills, such as verifying time sheets.

Related Terminology

The staffing coordinator must understand the staffing requests to make the proper assignment, and that may require a knowledge of medical terminology. Additional staff may be required for higher patient acuity, a one-on-one heart patient, suicide precautions, or out-patient chemotherapy. The level of skill needed may range from an RN with dialysis experience to a PCA who can sit with a patient until a crisis is over. All of these situations require an understanding of and background in medical terminology.

Other terminology the staffing coordinator needs to know may center around the computer and software used in the department. It is essential to be able to communicate to the software vendor when problems arise or new software is introduced.

Procedures and Functions Specific to the Position

This section describes how a typical staffing coordinator position functions. Actual responsibilities may vary from one hospital to another.

Scheduling of the float pool is done centrally in the staffing office. The pool consists of RNs, LPNs, PCAs, HUCs, and any other staff necessary for the nursing unit. Pool members send in their availability in writing, which is put into the computer and on a planning sheet. If the computer is down, the planning sheet can be used. The documented availability should be filed alphabetically per schedule period to help prevent misunderstanding. The unit requests are then matched by skill and shift to the pool availability. For example, a day-shift RN is not placed into a PCA slot, and an RN with intensive care unit skills is not placed into a medical–surgical slot over an RN with medical–surgical skills. The units may make a first- and second-choice request—for example, first choice would be for an LPN, second choice would be for a PCA. The nursing unit request form is returned to the unit after every request possible is filled. Float pool staff members not chosen are asked if they would like to change their availability. If they cannot change, they will be used to cover call-ins and other high-census needs. If there is a low census, they may be canceled just before the shift.

Many float pool personnel may not want to work full time, but may be willing to cover full-time shifts during vacation or high-census times.

Sometimes two float pool people may cover one regular staff member's vacation time. If a unit member needs to change shifts for a short period of time, someone in the float pool may wish to "switch" with them. People who work in a float pool usually are flexible. The staffing coordinator may spend many hours looking at all the possibilities for matching requests to the float pool staff.

The staffing coordinator must know the guidelines for the float pool staff as well as the holiday and weekend requirements. The coordinator maintains a file for the float pool containing competencies and evaluations. Competencies are required for each area where the pool member works, and must be updated annually. Evaluations are done after 90 days for new hires, annually after that, and as needed for anyone on a disciplinary plan. Copies of license verification, cardiopulmonary resuscitation (CPR) certification, and other certifications are maintained by the staffing office. Float pool staff members are provided an area to view memos and collect hospital mail.

Contract Nurses

Contract nurses may be used when a need arises that is consistently difficult to fill. The nurse directors request special needs as far in advance as possible for vacations, educational classes, jury duty, and family or medical leave. The director and staffing coordinator review all the possibilities before agency coverage is considered. Overtime may be used to cover some situations, but as a last resort a contract nurse may be used for a long-term need. This is done only with prior approval from both the director of the unit making the request and the patient care services (PCS) administrator. The staffing coordinator must be familiar with the agencies with whom the hospital has contracts, the current rates, and the skill level of available staff. When the agency is called, the following information is given: length of service needed, type of unit, and shift and skill level needed. If the need is for an extended period of time, the hospital may want prior approval of the agency nurse. This may require a telephone interview with the agency nurse. Joint Commission on Accreditation of Health Care Organizations (JCAHO) standards require that all staff working in a hospital meet the same requirements. Therefore, if the hospital requires drug screens and an orientation of hired staff, the same is true for agency staff. All certifications and licenses must be on file and recorded in the staffing office. These details usually are worked out in the contract between the agency and the hospital.

Reports are run on a regular basis showing how many contract nurses are being used, on which units, and the length of service. These reports are distributed to all directors and PCS administrators. In addition, the cost of agency use is entered into the financial computer system. This report is compiled, printed, and distributed to the PCS vice president and accounting office every week. The agency invoices are reviewed and the correct unit cost center number is added for proper accounting before they are forwarded to the PCS administrator for signature.

Staffing Review

Staffing review for the needs of the next 24 hours is done at a staffing issues meeting, held daily Monday through Friday. At the Friday meeting, the weekend and Monday's 7 A.M.–3 P.M. shift are reviewed. The meeting is attended by the staffing coordinator and the nursing unit directors. Any director with a staffing need who cannot attend may call the staffing office with specific requests. To prepare for this daily meeting, the staffing coordinator enters the staffing and acuity of each unit into the computer. The computer compiles the information and then creates projections for the next three shifts. These are printed out on a worksheet that includes all units by shift for the next three shifts. Copies are made for each unit and handed out at the beginning of the meeting. Each director states the needs of his or her unit and, if possible, these needs are filled with available float pool personnel based on skill level. At that time, the code blue team is also designated for the next three shifts.

Any remaining needs are discussed as to possible solutions that meet budget needs and still accommodate acuity and skill level needs. Calls are made to fill the needs by both the staffing coordinator and directors. On low-census shifts, float pool staff and overtime shifts are canceled. If any unit has a low census, the excess staff may be reassigned to a high-census unit with the director's approval. Notes are made on the staffing worksheets for the incoming supervisors. After all phone calls have been made, needs have been met, and the meeting is over, any changes are entered into the computer by the staffing coordinator.

Credentials

Credentials for staff, including licenses and certifications, are maintained by the staffing coordinator. A reminder is sent to each director 5 days before the end of the month for any staff member with a pending expiration. As the renewed credentials come in, they are recorded in the computer, marked off the list (Fig. 17–1), and filed in the unit binder, and a copy is sent to human resources. The human resources department is responsible for suspensions or terminations due to expired licenses.

Reports

Reports can be generated from the information entered and maintained in the staffing office computer system. Productivity can by printed as needed by each director. Every 2 weeks, routine reports are printed and sent to directors and the PCS vice president on productivity, unit census/acuity, call-ins, and full-time employee (FTE) use. The staffing coordinator may be asked for lists (Fig. 17–2) that can be used by the directors for budget reports, JCAHO requirements, staff attendance at in-services, or any other purpose that assists management.

Computer System Use and Maintenance

Computer system use and maintenance requires being aware of what is normal for the system and what requires expert assistance. Other users call

9-15-98 PAGE 1

MEDICAL CENTER

6/W RNS AND LPNS TO RECERTIFY

FALL 1998

NAME:	S	CPREXP	SHIFTS
ABBOT,KERRI	R	093098	D E N
BASS,RHONDA	L	093098	E N
BROWN,JUDY	R	100198	E
CARMEN,IOLA	L	102398	D E
CARPENTER,HILLARY	L	103198	E
CARR,MARSHA	R	112398	D
GILLIS,HELEN	R	113098	A
HARVEY,THOMAS	R	120198	A D
HENRY,LILI	L	121298	P

Figure 17–1
CPR recertification list.

MEDICAL CENTER					9-15-98 PAGE 1
SEPTEMBER 15, 1998					
FULLTIME BSN NURSES HIRED					
BETWEEN JANUARY 1, 1997 AND DECEMBER 31, 1997					
U	POS	NAME	C	FTE	HIREDATE
B	202	ABBOT,KERRI	C	1.0	091297
N	222	BASS,RHONDA	C	1.0	081197
C	110	BROWN,JUDY	S	1.0	030997
E	113	CARMEN,IOLA	S	1.0	091897
H	220	CARPENTER,HILLARY	T	1.0	010597
G	111	CARR,MARSHA	T	1.0	031297
G	104	GILLIS,HELEN	S	1.0	001397
N	112	HARVEY,THOMAS	S	1.0	021397
B	213	HENRY,LILI	C	1.0	123097
B	302	HOLT,JANICE	S	1.0	010697
D	102	KELLY,TERRY	T	1.0	071297
I	115	MASON,FRANCIS	S	1.0	100197
A	107	MCGUIRE,ERIN	C	1.0	060897
K	311	PENDERGRAST,NELL	C	1.0	091097
N	310	PERTERSON,CLARA	S	1.0	022297
A	127	RICHARDS,JULIE	S	1.0	090897
F	101	VANCE,TRRI	H	1.0	022297
H	310	WEST,MARGIE	C	1.0	060297
H	115	YOUNGBLOOD,TERRY	S	1.0	010997

Figure 17–2
New BSN nurses list.

the staffing coordinator for assistance to find the right schedule code or how to print.

Back-up of the system should be run every day, if possible. It requires diskettes labeled for every day, and blank diskettes need to be on hand as more information is added into the computer. If using a network system, all users must be *off the system* during the back-up process. This is usually done either very early in the day, late in the evening, or during the night shift. Supervisors may run the back-up process at night and on weekends or in the absence of the staffing coordinator.

There may be an interface between the scheduling system and the payroll system. This sends paid time off (**PTO**) data to payroll so it does not have to be written or keyed into another system. On payday, the payroll system sends the actual time scheduling to the scheduling system. This process also requires all users to be off the computer system.

The staffing coordinator adds new units and creates new schedule codes as needed. Codes are used to make reading and modifying the schedule easier, for example:

A = 7A–3P
B = 7A–7P
C = 3P–11P
D = 7P–7A.

Codes may also be used to signify the skill level of an employee:

RN = 1
LPN = 2

PCA = 3
HUC = 4
CHUC = 5

These codes must be used any time a unit hires, fires, or transfers staff members.

In addition to maintaining the software, the staffing coordinator must maintain the computer hardware used by the staffing office. The printers used by the scheduling system must be on line and filled with paper. Color printers must have a color ribbon or cassette. Before adding paper, the printer should be vacuumed to get out any dust or paper particles. The coordinator also must be knowledgeable about when to troubleshoot problems, like paper jams, and when to call for repairs.

Information Management

Information management, both computerized and on paper, is a requirement for the staffing office. All employees must be entered into the computer (Fig. 17–3) as well as on a Rolodex card, so data are available if the computer system is down.

When an employee transfers, receives a pay increase, or resigns, the change must be made in the computer system. This is done after receiving a form called the Personnel Action Form (**PAF**) that is generated by the director and forwarded to the staffing office. After the changes are made in the computer, the staffing coordinator forwards the form to the PCS vice president for signature and then to the human resources department. This process may vary in each institution.

Communication

Computer

Communication begins with reading all messages in the computer that are sent to all PCS employees. These messages are printed out and filed for future references. The distribution lists used for computerized messages and notices that are located in the office automation section of the hospital computer system are maintained by the staffing coordinator. These lists are used to make sure the sender is sending the message to the right group of staff. For example, one distribution list may include only directors and supervisors, whereas another may include all float pool staff.

Telephone

The telephone is used constantly during the staffing coordinator's shift. Use of a headset leaves hands free for the computer keyboard or to write notes. Telephone courtesy is a must in this position, as is knowledge of staff members' names and

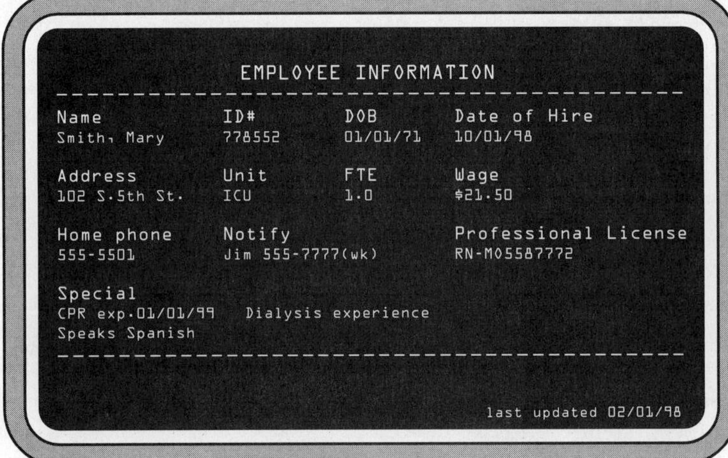

EMPLOYEE INFORMATION

Name	ID#	DOB	Date of Hire
Smith, Mary	778552	01/01/71	10/01/98
Address	**Unit**	**FTE**	**Wage**
102 S.5th St.	ICU	1.0	$21.50
Home phone	**Notify**		**Professional License**
555-5501	Jim 555-7777(wk)		RN-M05587772

Special
CPR exp.01/01/99 Dialysis experience
Speaks Spanish

last updated 02/01/98

Figure 17–3
Employee information card.

locations so that calls can be transferred to them quickly and accurately. Keeping a printed list of frequently called numbers along with the list of beepers used by the directors and supervisors is another duty of the staffing coordinator. Communication with the units regarding census, acuity, and staffing needs is done by telephone when the computer is down.

Fax

The fax is useful for communication between internal units as well as external contacts such as off-site units. The fax is also used to communicate with some of the nursing agencies for the purpose of sending resumés and time sheets back and forth. The unit staff may fax a copy of a recertification to the staffing office to be placed on file.

Interfacing

Communication with other computer systems may also be necessary for the staffing coordinator. This may be done by computer **interfaces** such as the one between the staffing office and payroll, or through the Internet. Internet access may require approval from the hospital computer service department or management.

Training and Orientation

Training and orientation are part of the duties of the staffing coordinator. New unit directors must be orientated and trained to use the software for staffing/scheduling. The amount of time needed for training depends on their computer experience and background. Providing printed instructions with training gives them a reference to use at a later time. After orientation, a password is issued and the proper form provided to the information services so the new director may be added to the network. After the training period, the coordinator schedules some time with the director for review with the **live** system to ensure proper understanding and use. In some cases, a director may have an assistant who may need computer access and training as well. The staffing coordinator assists them also, but they may be given a different level of access to the information in the system. A director may have full access, whereas an assistant may be given access only to specific units and functions, depending on his or her need. Staff confidentiality is as important as patient confidentiality.

Accuracy

Accuracy is extremely important in the position of staffing coordinator. One area where this might be critical is entering the payroll information into the computer. Benefits, such as overtime, may be different for groups within the hospital. Float pool staff may not receive vacation or sick pay, but may receive overtime pay. Supervisors may not qualify for overtime, but receive vacation and sick pay. Time sheets are verified weekly with the work schedules. Paychecks are issued every 2 weeks and employees must pick up and sign for their check in the staffing office.

Additional Training Required

The software used in the staffing/scheduling computer system requires increased knowledge and skill. It may be the responsibility of the coordinator to maintain and upgrade the computer software. If so, special classes on software maintenance will be necessary. Even if the software is maintained by others, it is necessary for the coordinator to take some classes on the usage of the software. Some systems operate from a single personal computer (**PC**) in the scheduling office, meaning anyone needing information or a printed schedule must use that computer. Others may use a network system so that the information can be obtained from any computer connected to the network. The network may be set up so others may view or print a schedule, but not have access to any other information. Regardless of how it is set up, all software must be upgraded on a regular basis, and the coordinator needs to keep informed of all new upgrades or changes in the system.

Attending regional and national workshops for the staffing system users is essential for maintaining and using this specialized software. Here experts explain software programs and how they operate. Networking with other users answers many questions.

Staffing coordinators must attend continuing education classes to keep informed of changes in acuity and productivity trends. Reading all available articles regarding staffing/scheduling and other trends in the health care field is very valuable. Stress management classes are always a good choice.

A computer keyboarding course increases typing speed and confidence in using the keyboard. Many high schools offer this course for Adult Education, as well as junior colleges. Other classes that may be helpful are in the areas of DOS, word processing, spreadsheets, or Windows.

Closing Thoughts

In my situation, the staffing coordinator position began as a paper-and-pencil job normally done by nurse directors and supervisors. As the PRN nurse pool began, someone was needed to do additional paperwork and scheduling. I began just assisting the responsible RN. When she left, another RN was hired, with me as her assistant. I was still doing some HUC duties, such as orienting and scheduling new HUCs. I also occasionally filled in on a unit if there was a shortage of HUCs. When my coworker (RN) retired, the budget did not allow for two staffing positions. I was offered the position and have been busy ever since. Slowly, the HUC responsibilities were given to others because staffing took all of my time.

When the staffing/scheduling computer system was purchased, I was very happy (it even prints in color!). It took a lot of work to get it started, but it is so much easier and I really enjoy the computer work. In my hospital, staffing and scheduling are no longer centralized. All directors have their own PCs, and make and print their own unit's schedule. Requests are sent to the staffing office for float pool staff. We review staffing needs for the next 24 hours each day to look at census and acuity changes. I spend a lot of time compiling data for reports and processing employee changes in the computer system. I am learning something new every day. Can an HUC do this job?—of course, HUCs have worked in an ever-changing world for many years.

Review Questions

1. List three sources the staffing coordinator might use to obtain needed staff.
2. Explain the importance of collaboration with the nursing supervisors.
3. List the communication devices a staffing coordinator would be expected to use.

18 Community Relations

Madeline A. Clark

Common Abbreviations

AA Alcoholics Anonymous

AHA American Heart Association

AIDS Acquired immunodeficiency syndrome

CPR Cardiopulmonary resuscitation

EMS Emergency medical services

HOSA Health Occupation Students of America

MADD Mothers Against Drunk Driving

SADD Students Against Drunk Driving

SIDS Sudden infant death syndrome

Objectives

Upon completion of this chapter, the reader should be able to:

1. Identify the typical functions of the community relations department in a health care facility.
2. List some of the educational programs offered by the community relations department in a health care facility.
3. Describe the duties of a notary public in the community relations department of a health care facility.

Vocabulary

Advocate: One who argues for a cause

Facilitator: One who assists or makes things easier

Lamaze: A method of teaching mothers-to-be to prepare for natural childbirth

History

A few years ago, it would not have been unusual to see a department in most hospitals bearing the title "Community Relations." As a result of increased competition for health care dollars and development of partnerships with community businesses, community relations in many facilities has become a part of larger departments such as marketing and public relations. Lately, some catchy terms have been concocted to name these departments. In some of the smaller hospitals, the department continues to be known as it was earlier. In any form, the importance of the function of "Community Relations" is greater than ever as facilities showcase themselves to potential and active clients (Fig. 18–1).

Functions

The typical functions of the community relations department may be described in the following categories.

Community Service

Community service consists of activities in which the facility may participate for the betterment of the community. Examples of such activities are:

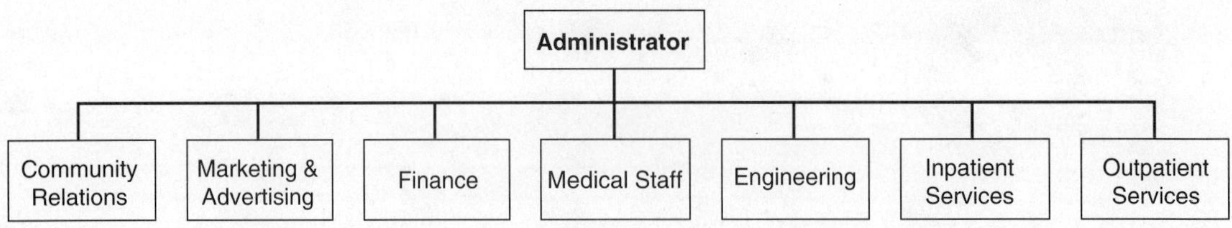

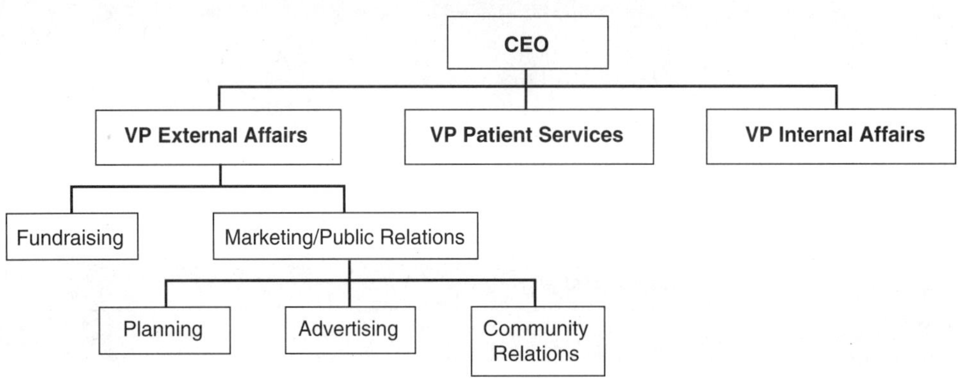

Figure 18–1
Organizational charts.

- Involvement in community fund-raising activities such as becoming the lead agency for United Way.
- Sponsoring or participating in health fairs where cursory screenings are performed and health information is distributed.
- Inviting the public to an open house at the facility to demonstrate new changes in equipment or services offered.
- Providing personnel for community events such as podiatrists and nurses for road races or first aid personnel for county fairs (Figs. 18–2 and 18–3).
- Presenting health care–related scholarship awards.
- Interacting with the emergency medical services (EMS) organizations in the community.
- Providing shelter and food in disasters and emergencies.

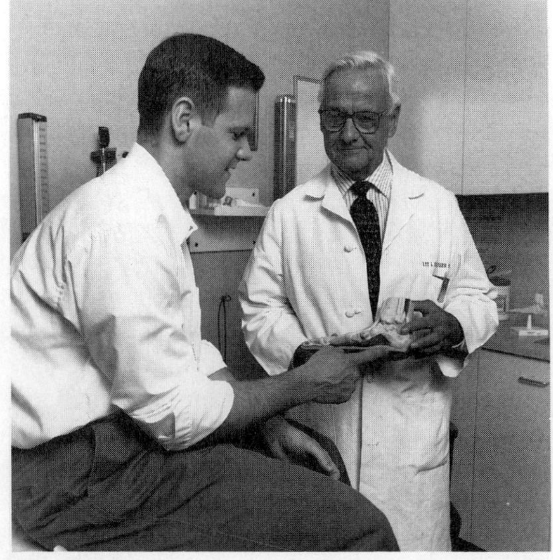

Figure 18–2
Podiatrist consulting with a runner before a race.

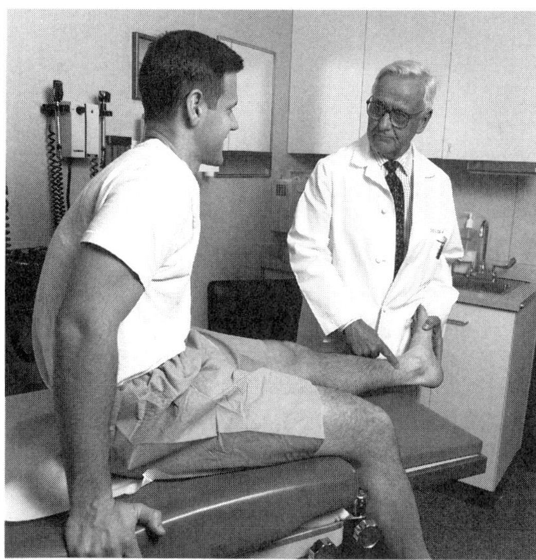

Figure 18–3
Post-race check.

- Providing support and manpower for Health Occupation Students of America (**HOSA**) activities.

Community Support

Community support usually takes the form of support groups sponsored by the hospital, using members of its staff as **facilitators**. The following are groups that may be included:

- Senior citizens
- Single parents
- Hospice
- Families of Alzheimer's disease victims
- Families of sudden infant death syndrome (**SIDS**) victims
- New mothers
- Survivors of a "near-death" experience

Hospitals may offer to serve as meeting places for local chapters of professional organizations such as:

- Medical societies
- Nursing specialty groups
- Hospice organizations
- Health unit coordinators

Many facilities offer space and support for organizations such as:

- Alcoholics Anonymous (**AA**)
- Mothers Against Drunk Driving (**MADD**)
- Students Against Drunk Driving (**SADD**)

Education

Education provides the opportunity for valuable community exposure through courses offered on a variety of topics:

- Cardiopulmonary resuscitation (**CPR**)
- **Lamaze** training
- Symptoms of impending heart attack
- Living with diabetes
- Alzheimer's and related dementias
- Accessing the Emergency Response System
- Appropriate use of the emergency department
- The Poison Control Center and how to access it
- Organ donation and transplantation
- Hepatitis
- Acquired immunodeficiency syndrome (**AIDS**)
- Cessation of smoking
- Nutrition
- Exercise

Booklets, pamphlets, and video or audio tapes can be produced to explain procedures and processes involved in:

- Hospital admission
- Surgical procedures
- Children in the hospital
- Infection control
- Anesthesia
- Protocols for visiting a patient in the hospital

Consumer Relations

Consumer relations involves several activities surrounding community members who have elected to use the services of the facility:

- Conduct, collect, collate, and retrieve data from patient satisfaction surveys, then follow up on the results.
- Investigate patient complaints and act on them.

- Provide support to the in-patients who cannot access peripheral services that would otherwise be available to them.

The Health Unit Coordinator in the Community Relations Department

Several of the aforementioned functions could use the talents of an experienced health unit coordinator (HUC) to be carried out properly. The known organizational and communications skills developed in health unit coordinating are the basis for this assumption.

In smaller facilities, the HUC could easily serve as the general coordinator for all of the activities, being responsible for most of the duties mentioned in the following sections.

Scheduling

The HUC is well equipped to maintain a calendar of events and to schedule the personnel necessary to participate in them. This includes sending reminders with all the necessary information about the date, time, and location. Directions to off-site events are also necessary. The equipment needed for the presentations is requested and arrangements made for its use.

Survey Work

The survey tools used by the department must be developed and produced. The HUC could easily participate in the tracking and collection of the tools, as well as retrieving and collating the data and providing them to the appropriate people.

Trainer

Learning to be a trainer in some of the subjects offered in the educational programs is a way HUCs can expand their role. They could serve as instructors in topics of interest or assist a lead instructor. Facilitators are always needed for the various support groups.

Consumer Advocate

Very interesting duties are required of consumer **advocates.** They investigate patient complaints, which may range from disliking a roommate to complaints about the service or, in some instances, serious breaches of care. The advocates often are the ones who take the time to explain advance directives and encourage the reluctant consumer to arrange them.

Finding Opportunities in Community Relations

In interviews held with HUCs who have found placement in community relations departments, they seemed to have one factor in common. They showcased their talents as volunteers and were invited to transfer to community relations.

One HUC had a history of volunteering in the community. She became involved with the Explorer Scouts. She arranged programs in the hospital where she was employed for the scouts to gain experience for their merit badges. She went through the appropriate channels to arrange the experiences, which ranged from volunteer work to observation in the operating room. She also served as mentor for these experiences (Fig. 18–4). She also had several ideas for projects that would further involve the hospital in community activities and ultimately was invited to and became a full-time member of the community relations department.

Another HUC was interested in organ transplantation, and with the assistance of her peers, began what became a successful eye donation awareness program at her hospital. She then developed a community awareness program that soon branched off into interest in other types of organ donation. Through these programs, a considerable number of people were recruited as organ donors. Her efforts were not only acknowledged by officials of the regional organ transplant

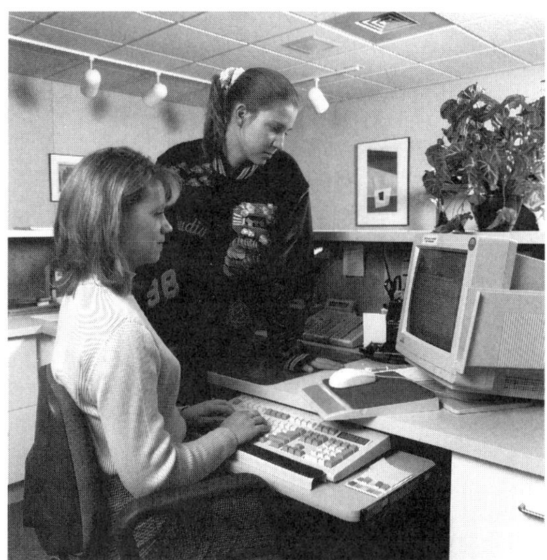

Figure 18–4
Working with an Explorer Scout.

group, but she was invited to apply for a position in the community relations department as well.

These are two examples of how HUCs can use their knowledge of communication, organizational skills, and interest in health care to create new opportunities for themselves.

To enhance further their success when considering a transfer to such a department, it is recommended that HUCs study the department and its philosophy, organization, and mission. They should also keep portfolios detailing their education, certification, continuing education, awards, and accomplishments. Reviewing the portfolios can assist in using the appropriate experiences as key points in the resume. The resume should be structured to match the person's skills, experience, and interests to the needs of the community relations department.

Additional Training

It could also be advantageous for the HUC to become a notary public to be available to patients who might have a need for such services. Depending on the jurisdiction in which a notary is commissioned, the duties may include some or all of the following: witnessing or attesting signatures, executing deeds and other instruments, taking acknowledgments, administering oaths and affirmations, witnessing affidavits, taking verifications, and making certified copies of documents.

The eligibility and requirements for becoming a notary vary from jurisdiction to jurisdiction. Typically, a person is required to be 18 years of age and a resident of the jurisdiction, usually a state (although in some states, such as Georgia, one can be commissioned by a county). The application process includes a statement of all criminal convictions, with the exception of minor traffic violations.

The educational requirements vary from state to state. Some states require none, whereas others, such as North Carolina, require a notary to complete a 3- to 6-hour course offered in the community college system, followed by an examination for initial appointment. There are courses available nationally that vary in length from 3 to 24 hours. Florida has a special section to educate and assist notaries, which is entirely separate from the department that issues the commissions. The section for education distributes educational materials and a newsletter for notaries, as well as presenting seminars on notary law and providing information and advice by telephone.

Although notary law varies some from state to state, there are certain steps that usually are taken for correctly notarizing a document and preparing a specific type of certificate required for various notarial acts.

- Screen the signer and the document
- Require personal appearance
  - Make a careful identification
  - Determine willingness and competence
  - Check the document for blank spaces
  - Scan the document for content
  - Check the date
- Complete the certificate
  - Read the certificate carefully before stamping and signing
  - Identify the signer
  - Affix the notary seal and your signature
  - Keep blank certificates secure
  - Keep a journal of details of activities.

SAMPLE RESUME
Clara Hazel Una Carson
127 Nowhere St.
Anywhere, USA

Objective: To pursue an opportunity in a health-related Community Relations Department, in order to utilize my communication and organizational skills in a creative manner.

Education: Six-month Health Unit Coordinator Program at Anywhere Community Hospital (completed 1989).

Evening courses, Nowhere Community College, 1994 to present.
Variations in Adult Education
Dynamics of Organizational Behavior
Nutrition for Health

Employment: 1988 to 1990—Nowhere Clinic, receptionist for Surgical Division.
1990 to present—Anywhere Community Hospital, Health Unit Coordinator ICU and Float. Additional duties included:
Precepting new Health Unit Coordinators
Organizing and maintaining schedule for unit
Communicating with representatives of all levels of health care personnel, families, and clients.
Training new physicians and nurses to computer system on Unit.

Licenses and Certification:
1993 Certified as Health Unit Coordinator
1997 Recertified as Health Unit Coordinator
1995 Commissioned as Notary Public
1998 Certified as AHA CPR Instructor

Other Pertinent Training:
Eight-hour Notary training program
Continuing Education
High-Impact Communication Skills (video)
Internet for Health Care Professionals (8 hr workshop)
Dealing with Difficult People (video series)
AHA CPR Instructor course

Other Pertinent Experience:
Volunteer chairperson for church building fund
Mentor for Explorer Scout group
Set up computer program for nonprofit educational group
Participated on committee choosing computer system for Anywhere Community Hospital

References available upon request.

Corrections may not be made using white-out. They should be crossed out using a single line in ink, and the correct information printed immediately above and initialed and dated. If the seal has been smeared, reapply it. If a correction is requested later to a certificate, compare the information on the certificate to the journal and then record the changes in the journal.

The term of commission may be from 3 to 5 years, depending on the state, and the fees also vary. Specific information about applying to become a notary can usually be obtained from the office of the Secretary of State (Fig. 18–5).

Equipment

The communication equipment the HUC has always used in day-to-day unit operations is the same in the community relations department (i.e.,

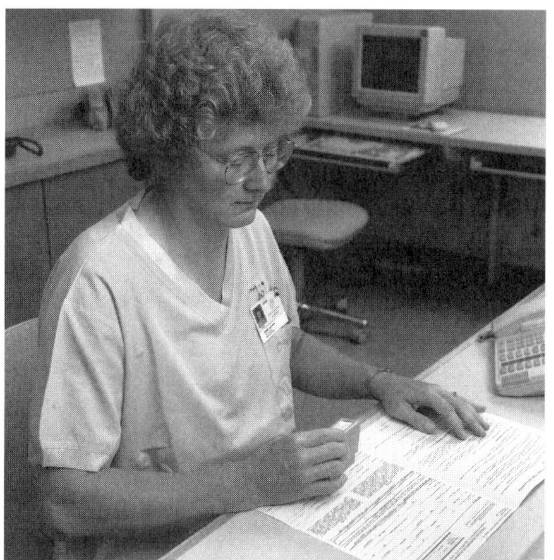

Figure 18–5
HUC notarizing a document.

computers, telephone, and fax machines). The other equipment with which a person working in community relations would have to become familiar is the audiovisual equipment. More often than not, when there is a problem during a presentation, it is not the speaker who fixes it. The equipment that HUCs will need to be oriented to includes:

VCRs
Display monitors
Overhead projectors
Screens
Slide projectors
Movie projectors
Microphone and sound systems

Many a doomed presentation has been saved by the person who is a "fix-it."

Closing Thoughts

The community relations department, by whatever name it is known, offers a unique opportunity for the HUC who is interested in the community and enjoys an opportunity for creativity. Relationships will grow with the many people with whom one will come in contact.

The special HUC who is creative can rise to any heights that he or she aspires. The community relations department offers many different learning opportunities. The sky is the limit, once you open the door.

Review Questions

1. Identify the typical functions of a community relations department in a health care facility.
2. List some of the educational programs offered by a community relations department in a health care facility.
3. Describe the duties of a notary public in the community relations department of a health care facility.

Bibliography

Kennedy J: Mission Success. Boulder, CO, Career Track Publications,1995 (video).

Rockhurst Continuing Education Center, Inc: Career Success Set. Shawnee Mission, KS, The National Press Publications, 1991.

Solomon M: What DO I Say When—. Englewood Cliffs, NJ, Prentice-Hall, 1988.

19 Computer Specialist

Nancy Charley

Common Abbreviations

IS Information system

LAN Local area network

PC Personal computer

WAN Wide area network

Objectives

At the completion of this chapter, the reader should be able to:

1. Identify five positions to which a health unit coordinator who is seeking opportunities as a computer specialist might aspire.
2. Briefly describe each position.
3. Briefly explain the data collection process and why it is important in the health care setting.
4. Explain the difference between TEST and LIVE in a hospital computer system and why there is a TEST system.

Vocabulary

Analyst: A person who observes a system for functionality and potential use

Fax: A piece of equipment connected by phone lines that accepts or sends images

Hardware: The monitor (TV screen), keyboard, printers, modem, and the like

Interface: A program that allows one computer to communicate with another computer even if they do not speak the same language.

Network: A group of computers all operating from the same server, allowing them to share software and printers

Scanner: A device attached to the computer that allows hard copy to be entered into the computer system

Software: The program (or computer language) that operates the computer

Vendor: Outside company that sell supplies and equipment.

The abbreviations listed for this chapter are those that a HUC working in this area would be expected to know. Only those in **boldface** type are used in the text and appear in boldface when they are used for the first time.

Related Terminology

Although the following terms are not found in the chapter text, they are terms a computer specialist might be expected to know.

Attributes: Options for printers. These are things the printer can do, such as printing a line, special characters, or bold lettering.

Cable: An electrical wiring system that encases the data lines that connect the hardware to the circuitry (usually plugged into the wall plates) of the system.

Data processing: A function of entering information into the automated system.

Diskette: A small, flat, plastic rectangle that holds programming information that can be inserted into a personal computer (**PC**). Diskettes have magnetic properties and should not be exposed to magnetic fields for any extended period of time (the magnetic field may erase the information on the diskette). Much larger disks (with greater data storage capacities) are found permanently installed in PCs or local area network (**LAN**) servers or mainframes.

Drop: Printing an order or request on a printer.

Dumb terminal: A piece of hardware that functions off of a larger system and cannot be programmed on its own. These pieces of hardware accept information and access a larger database for processing and storage.

End user: A person who enters data into the system.

Hard copy: A tangible piece of paper that holds data that have been generated from a computer.

Hub: A localized area for equipment storage that centralizes the wires, cables, and terminal servers along with any other electronic equipment that is necessary for the computer system to work away from the end user. There may be any number of hubs within an area or work environment.

Keyboard: A piece of hardware that allows data entry to occur. It usually has alphanumeric characters.

Keystroke: A depression of a key on a keyboard that enters the meaning of that key into the system.

Laptop: A small, self-contained computer that can be part of another computer system.

Mainframe: Principal part of the communication system. It usually is housed in a large building because of the large amount of information stored, sorted, and retrieved from its database.

Microwave: A type of wireless data transmission.

Modem: A device that allows access to a computer system through a telephone line.

Monitor: A screen used to visualize data. It can be multicolored or monochrome, and comes in various sizes.

Mouse: A peripheral device used for selecting and occasionally entering information into a computer.

Optical disk: Data stored digitally and read by laser.

Pen light: A peripheral device that activates a command through a light that connects with a monitor.

Peripheral: A separate device that usually plugs into the main unit of a computer. A peripheral assists the end user, but it is not usually a necessary part of the unit.

Personal computer: A self-contained unit consisting of a central processing unit, keyboard, and monitor that processes data independently.

Pin: A technical part of programming the computer. The pin configuration allows correct flow within the data lines.

Port: A position where cables can connect hardware. Ports accept the plug at the end of the cable.

Program: A method of communication using computer languages that allows specific functions to occur within the computer.

Overview

As the health care industry continues to meet the challenges in finding a balance between medical care and medical cost, the health unit coordinator (HUC) role will also continue to change. Fortunately, HUCs possess the skills that blend with the needs and desired outcomes of health care facilities. Problem solving, communication, and processing are just three of the skills that HUCs use daily. These skills, along with the hundreds of others that HUCs acquire, make them the perfect people to look toward when new trails need to be blazed. One could venture to say that if there is not a conventional method to accomplish a task, an experienced HUC will find a way to get the job done. It is this type of person who might look into a computer specialist job opening: a person who can anticipate future needs yet understand the nature of a critical request, a person who knows how to accomplish a number of tasks at the same time—in other words, a problem solver.

Department Summary

The hospital information systems (**IS**) department consists of a group of people with many talents and skill levels. There may be computer programmers, **network** experts, systems **analysts**, installation and repair staff, educators, trainers, help desk specialists, and many other positions. As few as 10 years ago, it was unusual to find anyone in this department with any medical background, but today many nurses and HUCs have found their way into the IS department. It is not unusual to see help-wanted ads for IS positions that **require** a hospital background.

The **software** the hospital purchases usually sets the pace for basic operation of the department and the number of employees it takes to support the software system. The people working in the IS department may be assigned to work with the same departments all the time, or may be assigned as department needs are assessed and prioritized. The primary function of the IS staff is to keep the computer on and functioning to meet the needs of the hospital staff, medical staff, and patients. Nobody is happy when the computer is DOWN!

Computer Specialist

As a computer specialist, some of the opportunities that a HUC could anticipate might be working as a system analyst, program analyst, technical support person, or perhaps in research and development. Computer specialists may not always work in a hospital setting. Opportunities may be available in free-standing clinics, physician offices, independent billing offices, home health agencies, insurance companies, and many positions that have not yet been created.

Systems Analyst

The systems analyst has broad opportunities and a very exciting career as long as the person placed in this position likes working with people, has a creative flair, and can concentrate in a sometimes confusing work environment. This person must be able to communicate with a wide variety of skilled people, practice active listening skills, and be flexible enough to contribute information to be considered for better functionality of the system to support the end user. It can be difficult to find the person with the right personality and work experience to fill a systems analyst position. However, if a health care facility is willing to train, a HUC is the optimum choice. The HUC has an understanding of the importance of automation of patient orders and charges and is tuned in to the needs of the nursing staff, medical staff, supporting departments, visitors, and patients. There may be several skill levels (or job descriptions) for the position of systems analyst, but basically this is the person who reviews the software and applies it to the appropriate departments.

Program Analyst

The program analyst position deals more with the actual software and how it operates in the background. The person holding this position may be working directly with a programmer and assisting with trouble-shooting or testing. A HUC who is interested in this position must be someone who has the ability to be able to think forward and work backward. Many processes in the computer world are built from the end to the beginning; if you want the computer to ask a question, first you must build in the possible answers. The program analyst also must think ahead to see how any new programs or changes to old ones will affect the data that have already been collected or may be collected in the future.

Technical Support

Technical support may come in different forms and be as varied as the number of hospitals. A HUC going into technical support may find a position that supports the **hardware** throughout the hospital.

Hospitals may have hundreds of computer users, and it is difficult to keep all users informed on the care and maintenance of computer hardware. For this reason, the hospital may employ a few experts who have been trained to take care of the expensive computer hardware. This could include minor service, such as installing and cleaning of printers, **fax** machines, computers, and keyboards. The person interested in this position must be someone who can work with a variety of people, be flexible, have good listening skills, and be able to change priorities from minute to minute.

Help Desk

This form of technical support may consist of manning the phone at the help desk. If the user cannot use the computer, then it is worthless to the entire hospital. Most hospitals have training programs to ensure that users are qualified to use the computer. However, situations still arise that may require additional assistance, and these are the responsibility of the help desk personnel. Workers at the help desk must be familiar with all the working programs and be able to troubleshoot over the phone. This can be a very difficult position, and patience is a key factor to success. This person must be able to recognize when the problem may be a "user" problem or a "system" problem. If it is a system problem, the information must be passed along to an analyst before some damage is done to the whole system. If the problem is a user problem, the help desk person must have the communication skills necessary to walk the caller through the problem and then talk them through the fix, if possible. In general, it is a matter of the user not understanding how the system works and needing further instructions.

Educator

To whom in the hospital do people go when they want to know how to use the computer? They go to the expert, the HUC. HUCs have been using computers in their duties longer than other health care workers, so it stands to reason that the IS department would look to this group of people to assist with the education and training of new employees or when introducing new software. Some IS departments may have permanent positions available for training new employees, updating current employees when new processes are added, and writing and updating training manuals. This position is a perfect transition for any experienced HUC trying to work into a computer-related position (Fig. 19–1).

Job Duties and Responsibilities

Every time a patient comes in for the emergency room, out-patient service, admission, or any other reason, a registration process must take place. Hospitals want a computer software system that finds the patient information, allows for verification and changes, and then allows for all information related to that registration to go into a computer file. That file is then considered part of the patient's historical data record and can be accessed in the future.

On the surface, this may sound easy, but there are many things that must be considered in the beginning of the process. The people working in the IS department are all working toward the same goal: to collect and maintain accurate information

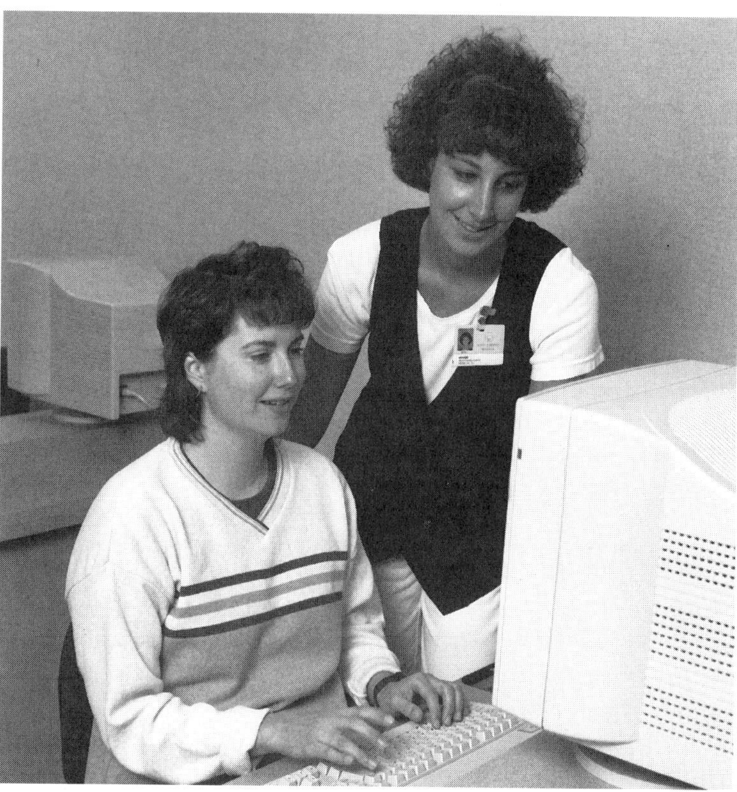

Figure 19–1
The computer specialist as an educator.

for the purposes of medical treatment, statistical reporting, and financial reimbursement.

Every hospital operates differently, and so does each IS department, including position titles and job responsibilities; therefore, it is difficult to describe the individual responsibilities of each person. For the purposes of this chapter, the general title of "computer specialist" is used. Unless indicated, these are all duties and responsibilities that an experienced HUC could move into with training and, sometimes, additional education. Using registration/admitting as an example, it will be easy to follow the process from beginning to end.

Data Collection

After the software is purchased and installed, the first step in building the system is to determine the data collection process. What data need to be collected? A review is done on the data that are currently being collected, and they are analyzed to see if they are meeting the needs of the department and the hospital. It could be that data questions will need to be added, deleted, or reworded. An example that comes to mind is adding data questions to the registration screen that will make it possible to preregister patients over the phone.

It is common to ask the usual questions about name, address, phone numbers, Social Security number, employer, and insurance information. The Americans with Disabilities Act requires that hospitals provide easy access for people with disabilities. By adding the question to the preregistration process, "Will the patient need any special assistance getting into the building?" the hospital would know in advance that this patient might need some additional assistance. A report could be printed out at the registration desk each day with a list of people who need special help, and the appropriate equipment could be ready and waiting. In addition, because this information has been entered into the patient computer record, it will be saved and can be used the next time this patient registers, without having to ask the same questions. This information would also print on all requisitions that are entered for services in the laboratory, radiology department, physical therapy department, or any other area in the hospital. So by adding one question that requests one piece of information, the entire hospital obtains valuable information that aids in the care and treatment of this patient.

The computer specialist works closely with specified individuals in the department to evaluate the data collection process and quizzes them about information they may need in the future. At the same time, other areas may be consulted as to their needs from the registration process. The business office, for example, may need information that is not being collected. The same could be true for the medical records department. Both of these departments deal with patients with the same or similar names, and it may be important to get the maiden names of all female patients, allowing for the combination of old records when a name changes. Maintaining all patient records under one file number is very important.

Once the decisions are made about *what* data should be collected, the next step is to decide *how* and *when* the data will be collected, and *who* will collect it. These decisions may seem simple, but if not planned correctly, the process can be confusing and complicated. How the data are going to be collected may determine some of the other steps. If the data will be collected in advance over the telephone, the computer specialist may want to build in some instructions on the computer screen that will help the user. For example, if the patient is elderly, disabled, or a child, it may be necessary to speak with someone other than the patient, and this information could be entered into the computer so that future users will know from whom to obtain information. If the data are being collected in person at the time of registration, this would be a moot point because it would be obvious.

The type of information gathered depends on who is gathering it. If a clerk is gathering preregistration information, it may be that only demographic information is gathered. If a nurse is making the preregistration call, the information gathered could include medical history and any current medications the patient is taking. It could also mean that some detailed patient instructions and education might be given to the patient before arrival at the hospital. Patients would have the opportunity to ask some questions about the procedure for which they are being registered.

When the preregistration process takes place also makes some differences to the computer. If the call is placed the night before and part of the instructions given to the patient are to eat a low-fat lunch, the call is too late. If instructions are to be given to patients during the preregistration process, then the best time for each patient would have to be determined. The computer could be programmed to print out a report of all patients who need instructions *today* for the next three working days.

The basic responsibility of the computer specialist is not to make these decisions, but to make sure the people working in the department understand their options and to guide them to improve the service. If they plan simply to computerize the exact process currently in use in the department, they probably are cheating themselves. Listening to what the current and future needs of the department and hospital are is the most important skill the IS person should acquire. The computer is a tool, like everything else, but if it does not work for us, then we will end up working for it . . . and that is not the plan. Just because a computer comes with impressive "bells and whistles" does not mean that we should use them. If we do not need one, we have wasted our time using one.

Testing the System

Building a computer that collects data is easy in the beginning: create a method for collecting the data and a method for reporting the data. It sounds easy enough, until you begin to test the system.

You may find that the simple data collected during the registration phase are not printing out in the laboratory. The more data you collect, the more outputs for the data, the more reports from the data collected, the greater the potential for problems. For these reasons, and hundreds of more complicated reasons, the computer specialist spends a large amount of time testing the system.

Most hospital software systems are in two separate areas of the computer. One is called TEST and the other is LIVE. The LIVE system is what is used on a daily basis. The TEST system is identical to LIVE, except it is not accessible to the general hospital population. It is what the IS people use when testing a new report or data trail. Information is entered into TEST to test the outcome without interfering with the LIVE data. For example, if IS wants to see how a new billing process is going to work, they put the information into TEST and follow it as if it were in LIVE. Thus, if it does not work correctly, the patient is not affected. Most "patients" in the TEST system are fictitious names created by IS just for testing.

Software is updated and improved on a routine schedule depending on the software **vendor**. In general, IS departments can expect one or two major enhancements each year. Each time there are enhancements, they *must be tested*. This could take weeks or months depending on the number of changes. If these changes are not tested before they are put into the LIVE system, there could be serious problems. A change in the system that is claimed to make the system faster may actually slow the system down until some minor modifications are made. Testing the change gives the IS department the opportunity to make all modifications before entering the changes in the LIVE system.

Any time enhancements or changes are made to the LIVE system, users need to be informed of and educated about the changes. One day they come to work, sign on to the computer, and find all the screens have changed. This is not productive; people must be educated and trained before that change occurs. The computer specialist will want to keep the users informed, educated, and up to date on all computer operations.

Statistical Analysis and Reports

Once the data have been collected, what happens to them next is the business of the computer specialist. Once again, listening to your customer is the key component of the position. Do the data need to be routed to another computer system? Should the data be shared with people from another department? Are the data to be reported out as statistical analysis only? The answers to these questions direct the actions of the computer specialist. Data that are to be shared with another computer system require an **interface**, or link to the other system. The computer specialist may not be the person who creates this link, but he or she will need to pass correct information to the people creating or providing the interface. This is generally performed by programmers.

Data that will be shared with other departments or used as statistical analysis can be handled by creating reports. Any data that are collected can be reported. Some computer software already has some report formats built into the system. The computer specialist may have to create some additional reports based on the data collected and the needs of the department or hospital.

Report writing can be very time consuming and detailed. The detail may be a direct result of the expertise and talent of the IS person. Some software companies offer special training for this purpose. Anytime an offer is made for additional training, it is wise to accept, particularly in computers. Report writing is in demand, and this is a skill that can be modified in any computer situation. Reports may be in the form of charts and graphs or written reports.

Data that are collected can be used as for purposes of comparison, to prove a point, or reach a conclusion, or they may just be informational. Figure 19–2 provides examples of three reports using the same data.

Regardless of how the report looks or of the information contained in the report, creating the format for the report is the work of someone in the

REPORT A (COMPARATIVE)

Medicare Update

	BLUE CROSS	MEDICARE
1980	80%	35%
1985	72%	44%
1990	70%	48%

REPORT B (CONCLUSIVE)

Fiscal Report

In 1980 the XYZ Hospital Board of Directors projected there would be a 27% increase of Medicare patients for the next five (5) calendar years. In 1980 the hospital treated 100 Medicare In-Patients. By the year 1985 the number of In-Patients with Medicare had increased to 144, a 44% increase.

REPORT C (INFORMATIVE)

Monthly In-Patient Report

Sex		Male			Female	
Age	0–35	36–64	>65	0–35	36–64	>65
Zip code						
66611	26	35	51	21	46	49
66614	14	44	68	09	41	76
66622	07	21	70	08	17	81

Figure 19–2
Different types of reports using the same data.

IS department, usually the computer specialist. In addition to reports, the data can be put into schedules—appointment schedules, surgery schedules, staff schedules, or any kind of schedule for which the data are collected in the computer. The possibilities are endless.

Security

Computer security is a growing issue in hospitals and has been a topic of discussion in the U.S. Congress. Patient confidentiality must be maintained and protected. People are given computer access to patient records and information based on their job responsibilities. Health care workers need to have information about the patient so that they can provide care and treatment for the patient. But this does *not apply to all* patients! Depending on the type of computer system used in the hospital, the IS department should be able to set up security codes so that workers have the access needed to care for their patients, but are not able to access all patients. The same is true for physicians; they should have access only to their own patients. The computer specialist may assist with menu planning for workers to make sure that all users have the tools they need to do their duties without jeopardizing patient confidentially.

Hardware

Who gets a computer? Where will it be placed? How many printers are needed? These are questions that must be decided at the beginning of the computerization process. Many decisions are based on these first few questions, and the computer specialist may be the person asking them and making the final decisions. Who gets computers may be decided based on job responsibilities and budget limitations. The person scheduling tests and services must have a computer all the time, but several nurses could share a terminal because part of their time is taken up with hands-on patient care. The person responsible for inputting patient charges must have a computer all the time, but several social workers might take turns making rounds and using the computer. A general rule would be if the person's job responsibilities are found at a desk, then that person probably needs a separate computer, but if the worker is in a direct patient care situation, he or she might be sharing with another worker. Budgets usually demand a conservative mix.

If a department has 10 computers and 15 workers, does that mean they need 10 printers? NO! Again, the computer specialist needs to review the needs of the department. What will the printers be used for and how often will they be needed? The intensive care unit may print more than the rehabilitation unit; accounting may print more than dietary. After determining the volume that will be printed, the computer specialist needs to determine the acuity of what is printed. This is necessary so that the size of the printer can be determined. Does the department need a printer that will print ten pages a minute, or will the slower five-page-per-minute printer work just as well? It might be that the department should have two slower (cheaper) printers over one fast (expensive) printer. Because, in general, there may be only a few printers for each department, their location should be as central as possible. The computer specialist needs to work closely with the technical support/installation people in IS to make sure all the proper wiring and outlets are in place before hardware delivery.

Other hardware the computer specialist may work with could include fax machines (both internal and external), **network** servers, **scanners**, and any other piece of equipment that could interface with a computer.

Training

Hundreds of thousands of dollars are spent on computer software, equipment, and installation. Hundreds of thousands of hours are spent on configuration of the software. This will all be wasted if the proper people are not trained to use the system correctly. Training begins the day a decision is made that a new computer or a current system upgrade is necessary. Training should begin with the needs of the department or user. If the system does not meet those needs, then a lot of time and money will be wasted.

Once the needs of the department have been assessed and the system has been directed to meet those needs, the hands-on training phase in put into action. As mentioned earlier, training starts during the information-gathering period of determining needs. The hands-on training should begin while the system is still in the testing phase. The everyday user is more likely to "see" problems than the occasional user. The computer specialist works closely with the users during this testing/training phase to make sure the system is operating in the most efficient manner. During this time, the computer specialist may want to work on the training manual. Once the system is operational and ready to go LIVE, all users will need to be trained at the same time.

The software **vendor** may provide the hospital with a training or user's manual that is easy to read and understand. When that is the case, it makes the computer specialist's job easier. Generally speaking, the software companies do provide the hospital with a training or user's manual, but it is written for the IS user and not the general hospital worker. The computer specialist can take the more technical manual and convert it to convey the information that will help the daily computer user.

Training all users at the same time can be a challenge, but it can also be very rewarding. There were some key people in the beginning of the process who helped to determine the needs of the department. These people were given some basic training so they could understand how the needs would be met. Along the entire process, these same people were contacted with questions to determine the direction to go with data collection and reporting. This same group helped with the testing and review of the written manual. So it is only natural that this group becomes the first group to receive formal training for the conversion to LIVE.

The computer specialist puts together a formal lesson plan with objectives and expected outcomes and presents it to the key group of initial helpers. During their training process, the lesson plan is revised and reformed to meet the needs of the other users. Depending on how many users need to be trained, additional trainers may be selected from the key group. The computer specialist maintains a list of people who need to go through training and a list of those who have completed the training. Depending on the scope of the training, there may be a user testing phase; several weeks after training, each user may be required to test on the information before being given access to the LIVE data system.

Once all the users are trained and using the system on a daily basis, the computer specialist may want to keep the training duty or pass it off to one of the key users. Someone must be available to train new employees or existing employees who have been out on leave. The computer specialist maintains the upkeep of the official training manual so that it is always up to date.

Additional Education Required

Education levels in the IS department range from high school graduate to master's and doctorate degrees, depending on the position held and the job responsibilities. There are several areas that a HUC could explore. Many IS departments may be willing to train the right person with a high school diploma and background as a HUC. If a HUC is lucky enough to be present at the beginning of a new system, a lot of knowledge can be acquired and the scope of training could be very broad. On-the-job training is very valuable and takes the HUC a long way in IS.

There are associate degrees available from community colleges in IS that are very valuable to HUCs. These are often obtainable while continuing to work as a HUC. Once working in IS, many HUCs may want to continue in school and get a higher degree. Many hospitals are willing to pay all or part of the tuition if the employee plans to remain at the hospital; an employee who remains with the hospital saves them money over hiring someone new. Orientation is expensive, and long-term employees are a much better investment. The most important thing to remember when applying for a new position is that the employer is looking for the right person to fill a position. They may list educational qualifications as guidelines, but if you feel you are the right person, apply for that position and prove to them you are worth training.

Closing Thoughts

Working with computers at any level can be an invigorating career choice. A health unit coordinator can be on the cutting edge by taking that experience and developing a computer background. The use of computerized information systems in health care is a growing field that few people can grasp and do well in without medical exposure. One who possesses the combination of health care and computer systems background is in demand to fill a unique position within a vital, thriving team environment.

Hopefully, some of the basics of this chapter have stimulated you enough that you realize this tremendous field has a great deal of opportunity limited only by your willingness to present excellence in your own career path.

Review Questions

1. Identify five positions to which a health unit coordinator who is seeking opportunities as a computer specialist might aspire.
2. Briefly describe each position.
3. Briefly explain the data collection process and why it is important in the health care setting.
4. Explain the difference between TEST and LIVE in a hospital computer system and why there is a TEST system.

Bibliography

Burns J: Opportunities in Computer Systems Careers (Software). Lincolnwood, Illinois, UGM Career Horizons, 1996.

Byte MK: How to Make Love to a Computer. New York, Pocket Books, 1984.

Eberts M, Gisler M: Careers for Computer Buffs and Other Technological Types. Lincolnwood, Illinois, UGM Career Horizons, 1993.

Gookin D, Rathbone A: PC's for Dummies. San Mateo, CA, IDG Books, 1992.

20 Diagnostic Laboratory

Jackie Perkins

Objectives

Upon completion of this chapter, the reader should be able to:

1. Describe the laboratory information system.
2. List the duties of the laboratory health unit coordinator.
3. Describe the procedure for handling specimens.
4. List the diagnostic tests that require fasting as a preparation.

Vocabulary

Axial: Along a line around which a turning body rotates

Barium: Silvery white to yellow element used as contrast medium

Cholecystogram: X-ray of the gallbladder

Electrolyte: A chemical that when in solution conducts electricity

Polycythemia: Excessive number of red blood cells

Pyelogram: X-ray of the pelvis or the kidney

Transducer: A device that converts energy of one system to another system

Common Abbreviations

APTT	Activated partial thromboplastin time
BUN	Blood urea nitrogen
Ca^{2+}	Calcium ions
CAT	Computed axial tomography
CBC	Complete blood count
CEA	Carcinoembryonic antigen
CK	Creatine kinase
Cl^{-}	Chloride
Diff	Differential
ESR	Erythrocyte sedimentation rate
FBS	Fasting blood sugar
HDL	High-density lipoprotein
IVP	Intravenous pyelogram
K^{+}	Potassium
KUB	Kidneys, ureters, and bladder
LDH	Lactate dehydrogenase
LDL	Low-density lipoprotein
LIS	Laboratory information system
MRI	Magnetic resonance imaging
MS	Multiple sclerosis
Na	Sodium
PET	Positron emission tomography
PSA	Prostate-specific antigen
PT	Prothrombin time
RBC	Red blood cell
RBS	Random blood sugar
RUQ	Right upper quadrant
SST	Serum separator tube
TSH	Thyroid-stimulating hormone
UA	Urinalysis
WBC	White blood cell

History

Outpatient diagnostic laboratories came into existence for several reasons. One is that the emphasis on outpatient care as a cost saver has continued to grow in popularity with insurance companies. Very few patients today are admitted for testing only.

As the outpatient population grew, hospitals found that it was more economical to have a centralized area for staffing purposes. Another reason for the diagnostic lab is to offer patients a centralized place to perform all their testing, rather than having them wander all over the hospital trying to find the right department.

Introduction

The diagnostic laboratory is a centralized area in a hospital that makes it easy for patients to receive a variety of outpatient testing, including labs, x-ray, electrocardiography, and Holter monitoring. Most patients have been sent by their private physicians, but in some facilities, a few services are "patient pay", and available without a doctor's order, such as complete blood count (CBC), cholesterol screening, pregnancy testing, and premarital rubella testing. It is the responsibility of the health unit coordinator (HUC) to make sure the patient gets to the correct area, with the correct orders, at the correct time. This can be a challenge to the HUC because often the patient does not have the necessary paperwork or understanding of the process.

Position Responsibilities and Duties

It is the HUC's responsibility to meet and greet the patients as they arrive into the area. Patients coming into the lab are taken care of in the order they arrive unless they have STAT orders, are scheduled for surgery that day, or have a timed appointment. If the patient is expected and orders have been received from the doctor, the HUC begins the routine processing needed to get the patient on to the area of testing. This procedure includes registration of the patient into the computer system, followed by entering the orders into the computer system. New patients are asked to provide detailed information on demographics, employment, and insurance coverage. Once the paperwork is complete, the patient is either directed to the appropriate area for testing or asked to have a seat if the testing is done in the current location. It is the HUC's responsibility to see that patients are not kept waiting or overlooked in the testing process. The goal is to get the patient in and out as quickly as possible.

Patients may arrive in the area unexpectedly or without orders. This may happen for several reasons. The patient may have come straight from the doctor's office and the orders have not been received by fax or phone. Sometimes patients arrive on the wrong date or time. It is the HUC's responsibility to locate the orders for the patient. This may require calling the doctor's office and getting the orders or instructions. During this time, the HUC keeps the patients informed on the progress and assures them they will not have to wait long before someone will be taking care of them. Whenever the HUC is waiting for a call back, it is important to document (even on a piece of scratch paper) the times the calls were made. It is easy to lose track of time when the workload is heavy. As soon as the orders have been obtained, the HUC can register the patient and enter the orders into the computer system. When patients have arrived on the wrong date or time, the situation is evaluated for the possibility of testing them while they are at the lab. If it is a simple blood test, the lab will usually go ahead and process the patient. If it is a test that must wait for the appointed time, the patient will be instructed to return at the scheduled date or time.

The diagnostic lab also serves as the area where patients and families can come to find out where they need to go for other services within the hospital. These may include outpatient surgery, gastrointestinal (GI) lab, cardiovascular lab, rehabilitation services, and other outpatient clinics in the hospital. The HUC must be knowledgeable about the physical layout of the hospital as well the services provided by all departments (Fig. 20–1).

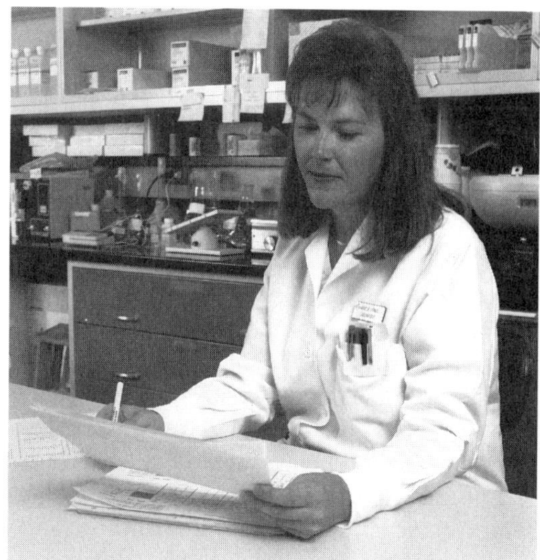

Figure 20–1
HUC at central lab desk.

Diagnostic Testing

The following descriptions are written to assist the HUC to answer questions about the tests when asked by consumers. Basic information about many of the tests performed on an outpatient basis is presented. Outpatient diagnostic tests usually require that an informed consent form be signed.

Special X-Ray Procedures

Several of the x-ray procedures involve more than a simple picture being taken or have special preparations required for them. Some of these preparations are the following:

Barium enema is also known as a lower GI series and involves an examination of the large intestines. Barium sulfate is administered through a rectal tube into the colon. In special studies, air is also introduced as a second contrast. The double contrast best demonstrates polyps and subtle bleeding from ulceration.

The barium enema helps in the diagnosis of colon cancer, rectal cancer, and inflammatory disease. It is also useful in the detection of polyps and diverticula.

A liquid diet, free of milk products, is required for 24 hours before the exam. It is recommended that five 8-ounce glasses of water be consumed 12 to 24 hours before the test to reduce dehydration. In some facilities, physicians order strong laxatives for a day or two before the exam. The morning of the test, the patient must have cleansing enemas until the bowels are clear. The test takes about 30 to 45 minutes. The patient is placed on a tilting x-ray table and secured. Barium or air is introduced through a rectal tube. The patient may complain of discomfort. The patient is told to breathe deeply and close the anus tightly around the rectal tube. Films are taken from several views and angles. After the patient expels as much of the barium as possible in the bathroom, a final x-ray is taken. A cleansing enema is usually given to remove any residual barium.

Barium swallow is a test devised to examine the uppermost portion of the GI tract. Barium sulfate is mixed into a liquid similar in consistency to a milkshake. The barium can be followed as it is swallowed. The test is done on a person who has a history of difficulty swallowing or persistent vomiting. It is used to diagnose hiatal hernia, polyps, and several esophageal disorders, including diverticula, varices, and stenosis.

The patient must fast from midnight the night before the exam. The test lasts about 30 minutes. Initially, thick barium liquid is swallowed at intervals indicated by the radiologist. Later, the test involves swallowing a thin mixture. At some point, a piece of bread soaked in barium is consumed. X-rays are taken on a tilting table and from many angles. After the test, the patient may have chalky stools for 2 to 3 days. Patients should contact the physician if no stool occurs after 2 to 3 days. Some doctors order a mild laxative to avoid problems.

Upper GI series examines the upper and middle portion of the GI tract. The ingestion of barium in liquid is required so it can be followed as it passes down through the digestive tract. It is performed when a patient exhibits symptoms such as gnawing upper abdominal pain, vomiting of bright blood, passing of dark, tarry stools, and unexplained diarrhea or weight loss. It is useful in a work-up for ulcers, malabsorption syndrome, and regional enteritis.

The patient is on a low-fiber diet for 2 or 3 days before the test, and fasts from midnight the night before the exam. A complete upper GI test includes the entire small bowel and takes about 6 hours to complete. An exam limited to the stomach and duodenum takes about 30 to 40 minutes. The patient ingests about 20 ounces of liquid barium. X-rays are taken from many angles and views. The patient must change position as often as directed. As the barium passes through the length of the small intestine, further films are taken at 30- to 60-minute intervals. It is recommended that the patient take a cathartic or enema after the test.

Gallbladder x-rays are known as **cholecystograms**. Pills containing a special dye are dispensed to be taken as directed. The test is typically performed when a patient presents with right upper quadrant (**RUQ**) pain, intolerance of fatty foods, and jaundice. The exam is done to detect gallstones and to diagnose tumors and inflammation of the gallbladder.

The patient is told to eat a fatty meal at noon the day before the test is to be performed. This is followed by a fat-free evening meal. After the evening meal, water is the only thing allowed by mouth. The tablets containing the dye are taken at 5-minute intervals the evening before the test. They may cause some discomfort from cramping and diarrhea. The test takes about 30 to 45 minutes to complete. X-rays are taken from various angles. A fatty meal may have to be ingested during the test. Some facilities have replaced the fatty meal with a synthetic fat–containing agent. X-rays of the gallbladder emptying are taken at intervals. Unless there are symptoms of fat intolerance, the patient can resume a regular diet after the exam.

One type of urinary tract examination is referred to as an intravenous **pyelogram** (**IVP**). In this test, a dye is injected into a vein in the arm. The dye is followed on its path from the kidneys, down the ureters, and into the bladder. The test is used to evaluate the size and position of the kidney, ureters and bladder. It is useful in the diagnosis of calculi, injuries, and anomalies present from birth. It can also be used to assist in the diagnosis of hypertension caused by kidney problems.

The patient increases oral fluids the day before the exam. There is usually a laxative given the night before. The patient fasts after midnight. The test takes a little over an hour. A set of x-rays known as a **KUB** (kidneys, ureter, and bladder) is taken initially. The dye is then injected. It may cause burning or warmth, a metallic taste in the mouth, and possibly increased salivation. These symptoms disappear quickly. A minute after the dye is injected, x-rays are taken. Additional films are taken 5, 10, and 15 or 20 minutes after the injection. After the 5-minute film, soft rubber devices are placed on the abdomen to hold the urine and dye in the ureters. They cause no discomfort and are removed at the 10-minute film. At the end of the test, the patient is asked to urinate and a postvoid film is taken.

Bladder exam or voiding cystourethrogram is performed after dye is injected into the bladder through a catheter. The test is used to detect reflux, neurogenic bladder, enlarged prostate, and other diseases that might obstruct the lower urinary tract. It is sometimes used to investigate urinary tract infections.

The test takes about 30 to 45 minutes. The doctor instills dye into a catheter that has been inserted into the bladder. It is instilled until the bladder is full, which may cause discomfort and an urge to void. Next the catheter is clamped while x-rays are taken in various positions as ordered by the radiologist. The doctor removes the catheter, repositions the patient, and asks the patient to urinate on the x-ray table. Many patients are embarrassed by this part of the procedure and find it difficult to accomplish despite the bladder being full. After the test the patient should drink a lot of fluid to flush the dye from the bladder.

Computed Axial Tomography Scans

Computed **axial** tomography (CAT) scans can study the areas of the body in much greater detail than the ordinary x-ray is capable of doing. An x-ray beam is aimed at the target area. Directly opposite the source of the beam, there is a radiation detector known as a scintillation counter that measures the amount of unabsorbed radiation. The information is fed into a computer that converts the information into a three-dimensional image displayed on a monitor. The images can be converted to photographs for study and documentation.

Brain CAT scans are performed to discover tumors and other abnormalities in the brain, to check the function of the brain, and to detect blood clots. These disorders show up as areas of abnormal density on the scan.

There are no dietary restrictions unless it is planned to use contrast dye. In that case, a fast of 10 hours is required. The exam involves a series of x-rays from many different angles. Some patients are bothered by the fact that they are strapped onto a table that moves into the scanner. The scanner rotates around the table to get the pictures at all possible angles. People with claustrophobia do not do well with this test. It usually takes 15 to 30 minutes and causes little to no physical discomfort.

Liver and biliary CAT scans are performed to assist in the differentiation of the causes of jaundice, to detect blood clots and any other abnormalities in the biliary tract and liver, and to aid in the diagnosis of liver tumors and disease.

A contrast dye is given by mouth, so a fast after midnight is required. An initial scan is taken and a second one is performed after the dye is ingested. The test takes about 60 minutes to complete.

Pancreatic CAT scans are done to provide a series of cross-sectional views of the pancreas to distinguish it and surrounding organs. The exam is useful in the diagnosis of pancreatic cancer and pseudocyst. It is also done as part of the evaluation of pancreatitis.

The contrast medium is either given by injection or ingested orally. A fast from midnight is required. A series of x-rays is taken before the medium is administered, followed by another series after the administration. The test is painless and takes about 60 minutes.

Skeletal CAT scans taken with contrast dye can provide hundreds of thousands of clear readings that can be combined into three-dimensional images by the computer. The exam can demonstrate problems undetectable by other methods. It is used in the diagnosis of soft tissue and bone tumors and for the spread of cancer into the bone.

If dye is used, a 4-hour fast is necessary. The test takes 30 to 60 minutes, depending how much of the skeleton is involved.

Spine CAT scans are performed to obtain views of the spine from various angles that would be impossible to see otherwise. The test is performed to diagnose spinal lesions and tissue damage after an injury, and to monitor progress after spinal surgery.

If contrast dye is ordered, a 4-hour fast is required. If not, no dietary restrictions are imposed. The test takes 40 to 60 minutes. The procedure is essentially without pain, but having to lie still for a prolonged period may cause discomfort for some. If dye is used, a regular scan is taken first, and then the dye is injected and another series of scans is taken.

Positron Emission Tomography

Positron emission tomography (**PET**) scans produce highly detailed images of brain structure and function. This procedure uses the radioactive forms of oxygen, fluorine, carbon, and nitrogen that give off minute particles known as positrons. The scanner detects the radiation and transmits the information to a computer, which translates the information into an image.

Various substances can be tagged with the positron-emitting elements. Armed with the information from the PET scan, researchers have been able to diagnose disorders such as Parkinson's disease, multiple sclerosis (**MS**), and Alzheimer's disease as well as psychiatric and seizures.

The PET scan is a very expensive test, so it is not widely done except in major medical centers and research centers.

Magnetic Resonance Imaging

Magnetic resonance imaging (**MRI**) scans differ radically from CAT scans in that they do not involve the use of x-rays. Instead, magnetic fields and radio waves are used to produce computerized images. The magnetic fields and radio waves are reported to be harmless.

Magnetic resonance imaging of the brain and spine is used to diagnose brain tumors, abscesses, swelling, and bleeding. It can also indicate areas of irregularity in the spinal cord.

The scan takes about 90 minutes to complete. The area for the head is small and deep and causes problems for patients with claustrophobia. Sedation may be required. The newer machines are transparent, and this seems to help. The patient must lie still during the exam. The scanner makes several sounds—whirring, clicking and thumping—from moving inside its housing. Earphones and music are offered to relieve the annoyance. A two-way communication system is provided so the patient can be in verbal contact with the technician at all times.

Magnetic resonance imaging scan of the skeleton allows the production of clear images of areas that cannot be visualized by x-ray or CAT scan. It eliminates the risks involved with exposure to radiation. The test is done to check the soft tissue and bones for evidence of tumors and irregularities. Changes in bone marrow composition can be perceived. Spinal disorders can also easily be viewed in three dimensions.

The test takes about 90 minutes. The patient is placed on a narrow table and passed into the scanner. The patient has to remain still for this MRI, as for any other. Fans are provided to improve the circulation of air inside the device.

Nuclear Scans

Nuclear scans involve the administration of substances that have an affinity for certain body tissues. The substances contain (are tagged with) tiny amounts of radioactive material. These combined substances are generally known as "radiopharmaceuticals." The presence of radioactivity in the target organs is measured by a radioactivity detector similar to a Geiger counter.

Bone scans have the capability of demonstrating cancer in the bones long before it is detectable by x-ray. Bone scans are also done to detect fractures that are hard to determine, bone infections, and degenerative bone disease. Bone pain of unknown origin can be evaluated with bone scans.

A small amount of radioactive substance is injected into an arm vein. In the next 1 to 3 hours, the patient is instructed to drink four to six 8-ounce glasses of water. A camera-type scanner is passed over the body and pinpoints "hot spots" of radioactivity. These areas are converted into images. The actual test takes about an hour. The patient must stay still during the various phases of the scanning. Several position changes are necessary during the procedure.

A thyroid test (iodine scan) is used to diagnose hyperthyroidism with a great deal of accuracy. It seems to be far less accurate in the diagnosis of hypothyroidism. It is also useful in differentiating between Graves' disease and thyroid hormone-releasing tumors.

Fasting after midnight is required. A capsule or liquid containing radioactive iodine is administered. Six hours later, a scan is done. A second scan is done 18 hours after the first. A light diet is allowed 2 hours after the iodine is taken. Normal diet may be resumed after the scan is completed. The test is painless and involves exposure only to a small, harmless amount of radiation. Test results are usually available 24 hours after the scan is completed.

Ultrasound

In an ultrasound, a **transducer** is used to direct sound waves of a very high pitch at the target area. These sound waves cannot be heard by the human ear. The echo created by the waves hitting the targets is converted to an image that is displayed on a monitor and recorded on a paper strip or videotape.

Blood vessel ultrasound is referred to as Doppler ultrasonography. It is used to evaluate blood flow in the arms, legs, or neck. The test is done for venous insufficiency and to diagnose venous thrombosis, arterial blockage, and changes secondary to aortic stenosis. The transducer is aimed along the course of the vessel in question. The sound waves strike the blood cells as they pass through the vessel. The frequency of the waves varies with changes in the turbulence of the blood flow. The results are recorded as waveforms on a paper strip.

The test takes about 20 minutes to accomplish and requires no special preparation. The patient may be asked to change position and breathing patterns during the procedure.

Heart ultrasound is known as an echocardiogram. It is used to evaluate abnormalities of the heart. It can measure the size of the atria and ventricles. It is helpful in the diagnosis of cardiomyopathy, tumors of the atria, and pericardial effusion. After a heart attack, the function of the heart wall can be evaluated.

There are no dietary restrictions. The test takes 20 to 30 minutes. The room is typically darkened to assist the technician in visualizing the images on the oscilloscope screen. The patient lies on an examination table for the test. Cold conductive gel is applied to the chest. The technician angles the transducer in different directions to get views of all of the areas of the heart. If it is necessary to evaluate the heart under various conditions, the patient may be told to breathe quickly or slowly or to hold his or her breath.

A medication called amyl nitrate may be administered by inhalation to produce stress similar to that seen in exercise conditions.

Pelvic ultrasound is used most frequently to perform an evaluation of a fetus in utero. It is also used to examine the pelvic organs of reproduction and the bladder. The test is particularly useful in distinguishing between cysts and tumors. In pregnancy, it affords a noninvasive way to evaluate fetal strength, heart rate, position, gestational age, and the presence of multiple pregnancy. When amniocentesis is necessary, ultrasound is used to guide the operator by locating the position of the fetus and the placenta.

This test requires that the bladder be used as a reference point. To accomplish this, the bladder must be full. Large quantities of water are consumed and the patient is asked not to void before the exam. The abdomen is lathered with mineral oil or gel before the exam. The transducer is moved gently over the entire abdomen. The test takes from a few minutes to several hours, depending on what is to be determined. The test causes no harm to mother or fetus.

Laboratory Tests

Laboratory diagnostic tests are usually performed in specialty areas of the main laboratory. Most blood tests require a venipuncture, although some can be done on capillary sticks. Many of the laboratory tests do not require special dietary restrictions.

ABO blood typing is performed to ascertain a person's blood type, typically before a transfusion is going to be given. The test is carried out in the blood bank. The blood is drawn into plain red-topped tubes.

Acid phosphatase is a group of enzymes that are found in greatest quantities in the prostate gland and in semen. The test is used to indicate problems in the prostate gland. The test is performed in the chemistry section of the lab. Blood is drawn in a serum separator tube (**SST**). The reference range is 0.5 to 1.9 International Units (IU)/l.

Activated partial thromboplastin time (**APTT**) evaluates the factors that go into clotting, with the exception of platelets. The test is done to monitor heparin therapy. A normal fibrin clot forms in 25 to 36 seconds after adding reagents to the sample. The test is performed in the hematology section, and blood is drawn in a blue-topped tube.

Alanine aminotransferase is an enzyme that is associated with the liver and, to a lesser extent, with the heart, skeletal muscles, and kidneys. The test is an indicator of the amount of the enzyme released into the bloodstream as a result of liver damage. The test is carried out in the chemistry section of the lab. The blood is drawn in an SST, which has either a yellow or marbleized top. The reference range is 8 to 20 IU/l.

Albumin is a protein component of the blood. The levels are abnormal in malnutrition, kidney disorders, liver disease, and certain tumor-causing conditions. The test is usually done as part of the total protein (with globulin levels). The test is carried out in the chemistry section of the lab. The blood is drawn into an SST. The normal values are 3.3 to 4.5 g/dl.

Alkaline phosphatase is an enzyme involved in the calcification of bone. The test is done to identify bone or liver disease. An 8-hour fast is required. The test is carried out in the chemistry section of the lab, and the blood is drawn in an SST. The reference ranges are:

90–239 IU/l in men
76–196 IU/l in women younger than 45 years
87–250 IU/l in women 45 years of age and older

Amylase is an enzyme formed in saliva and in the pancreas. It is instrumental in changing starch into sugar. High levels of amylase are indicative of pancreatitis. The test is done in the chemistry section of the lab. The blood is drawn in an SST. The normal range is difficult to ascertain because there are several methods to determine the levels. Less than 300 IU/l is considered the general average.

Antibody screening is also known as "indirect Coombs' testing." It screens for and detects up to 96 percent of circulating antibodies. It is used to detect antibodies before transfusion and to determine Rh-positive antibodies in a pregnant mother's blood. The test is done in the blood bank section of the lab. The blood is drawn into a plain red-topped tube.

Aspartate aminotransferase is an enzyme found in the heart, liver, pancreas, kidneys, and skeletal muscle. In the presence of heart or liver problems, it is released into the bloodstream in amounts indicative of cell damage. The test is carried out in the chemistry section of the lab. The specimen is collected in an SST. The reference range is 8 to 20 IU/l.

Bilirubin is produced by the destruction of red blood cells. It is a component of bile. The results may be reported in three elements: (1) indirect bilirubin, which indicates liver damage; (2) direct bilirubin, which indicates obstruction in the biliary tract; and (3) total bilirubin, which is a general indication of the level of jaundice or icterus.

A fast of at least 4 hours is required. The test is performed in the chemistry section of the lab.

The blood is drawn in an SST. The reference ranges are as follows:

Indirect bilirubin: 1.1 mg/dl
Direct bilirubin: ≤0.5 mg/dl
Total bilirubin: <2.0 mg/dl

Blood cultures are done in the presence of fevers over 103°F and higher. Blood is drawn into special tubes or vials. The blood is transferred to culture media and incubated, then examined for identification of organisms and for sensitivity to various antibiotics.

Blood urea nitrogen (**BUN**) testing measures the amount of nitrogen found in the end product of protein destruction by the body. The level of the results reflects the effectiveness of kidney function. It is advisable to avoid a diet high in meat the day before the test. The test is performed in the chemistry section of the lab. The blood is drawn into an SST. The reference range is 8 to 20 mg nitrogen per deciliter of blood.

Calcium ion (**Ca^{2+}**) testing measures the levels of calcium in the blood. Calcium plays an important role in the regulation of many other activities in the body. The test is done in the chemistry section of the lab and blood is drawn in an SST. The reference range is narrow, from 8.9 to 10.1 mg/dl of blood.

Carcinoembryonic antigen test (**CEA**) detects and measures the presence of a protein substance that is not normally found in the adult. The test is used for cancer screening and for monitoring cancer treatment. The test is done in the chemistry section of the lab. The normal results are less than 5 ng/ml of blood.

Carbon dioxide content (venous sample) testing is done to determine the balance in a total **electrolyte** block or as indication of the acid-base balance. The blood is drawn in an SST and done in the chemistry section of the lab. The reference range is 22 to 34 mEq/l of blood.

Chloride (**Cl^-**) is part of the electrolyte block. It is a useful in helping to determine a patient's fluid status. Testing is done in the chemistry section of the lab and blood is drawn in an SST. The reference range is from 100 to 108 mEq/l of serum.

Cholesterol is a component of certain structures in the blood and of cell membranes. Levels of cholesterol help provide information relative to risk for heart disease. Fasting for 12 hours is required before the test. The test is performed in the chemistry section of the lab. The blood is drawn into an SST. The normal range is considered to be less than 200 mg/dl of blood. The levels vary with sex and age.

Creatine kinase (**CK**) is an enzyme that has a major role in the metabolism of muscle cells. Total CK and three types of it known as isoenzymes are measured to detect muscle damage, particularly heart muscle damage. Alcoholic beverages should be avoided before the test. The test is done in the chemistry section of the lab and blood is drawn in an SST. The reference ranges for total CK are 25 to 130 IU for men and 10 to 150 IU for women. The isoenzyme reference ranges are:

CK-BB: undetectable
CK-MB: undetectable to 7 IU
CK-MM: 5–70 IU

Creatinine testing provides a more sensitive measurement of kidney function than the BUN does. In some facilities, a 1-hour food and fluid restriction is required. The test is performed in the chemistry section of the lab and blood is drawn in an SST. The normal ranges are 0.8 to 1.2 mg/l of blood in men and 0.6 to 0.9 mg/dl of blood in women.

Crossmatching is done to establish the compatibility of blood intended for transfusion. It is done in the blood bank section of the lab. The blood is drawn in a plain red-topped tube and a lavender-topped tube. The absence of clumping indicates compatibility with the blood to be transfused and that of the recipient.

Erythrocyte sedimentation rate (**ESR**) measures the rate at which red blood cells settle out of a sample in a given period of time. The rate is usually increased in inflammatory disease. The specimen is drawn in a lavender-topped tube. The normal range is from 0 to 20 mm/hour.

Fasting blood sugar (**FBS**) is used to measure the levels of glucose in the blood after a 12-hour fast. The test is used to screen for diabetes and other disorders in glucose metabolism. The test is performed in the chemistry section of the lab. Blood is drawn in an SST. The reference range is 70 to 100 mg of true glucose per deciliter of blood. The range may very from lab to lab.

Glycosylated hemoglobin is a test used to monitor the effects of diabetes therapy. The results indicate average blood sugar levels during the past 2 to 3 months. The test is done in the hematology section of the lab, and the blood is drawn into a lavender-topped tube. The results are reported as a percentage of total hemoglobin and are usually compared with each other in a series every 6 to 8 weeks.

Hematocrit measures the percentage of red blood cells; it is part of a CBC. Blood is collected in a lavender-topped tube. The normal range may vary from lab to lab and with age and sex. A rough guide in adults is 35 to 50 percent in men and 33 to 45 percent in women.

Hemoglobin is also part of a CBC. It is a measurement of the oxygen-carrying protein in the blood, and is useful in detecting anemia and **polycythemia**. The normal values in adults vary with age and sex. The following are the norms:

Men younger than age 45 years: 14–18 g/dl
Men 45 years of age and older: 12.4–14.9 g/dl
Women younger than age 45 years: 12–16 g/dl
Women 45 years of age and older: 11.7–13.8 g/dl

Lactate dehydrogenase (**LDH**) is an isoenzyme involved in the body's energy production. If cells become damaged, LDH in the blood becomes elevated. The test is used to detect general tissue damage. It is not as specific as some of the other tests available. The test is performed in the chemistry section of the lab, and the blood is drawn in an SST. The normal range for total LDH is 45 to 90 IU/l. Further breakdowns into five types can be done to try to identify the specific tissue that is damaged. The norms for these are:

LD-1: 14–26% of total LDH
LD-2: 29–39% of total LDH
LD-3: 20–26% of total LDH
LD-4: 8–16% of total LDH
LD-5: 6–16% of total LDH

Lipoprotein-cholesterol fractions (high-density lipoprotein [**HDL**] and low-density lipoprotein [**LDL**]) testing measures the "good" cholesterol (HDL) and the "bad" cholesterol (LDL) to indicate their relative effects on heart disease.

A normal diet should be maintained for 2 weeks before the test. Alcohol should be avoided for 24 hours before the test. The patient should fast and avoid exercise for 12 to 16 hours before the test is performed. The test is done in the chemistry section of the lab. Blood is drawn in an SST. The normal results are as follows:

HDL: 29–77 mg/dl of blood
LDL: 62–185 mg/dl of blood

The normal values may change with age, sex, ethnicity, and region of the country.

Phospholipids are forms of fat in the body that contain phosphorus. The test is done to evaluate how the body metabolizes fats. Abstinence from alcohol for 24 hours and fasting from food and fluids is required from midnight the night before the test. The test is done in the chemistry section of the lab and blood is drawn in an SST. The reference range is 180 to 320 mg/dl of blood. Results vary in men and women, and pregnant women may have unusually high results.

Platelet count is a measurement of the smallest formed elements in the blood, thrombocytes (platelets). It provides insight into clotting by evaluating platelet production. It can be ordered as part of the CBC. The test is done in the hematology section of the lab. The blood is drawn into a purple-topped tube. The normal platelet count ranges from 130,000 to 370,000 per cubic millimeter of whole blood.

Potassium (**K^+**) is part of the electrolyte block. The test determines the potassium content of the blood. It is used to evaluate the role in disease played by hyperkalemia or hypokalemia. The test is done in the chemistry section of the lab and blood is drawn in an SST. The reference range is narrow 3.5 to 5.0 mEq/l of serum.

Prostate-specific antigen (**PSA**) testing measures antigens in the immune system to determine the presence and stage of prostate cancer. The test is done in the chemistry section of the lab.

Blood is drawn in an SST. The results should not be in excess of 2.7 ng/ml of blood in men younger than 40 years or 4 ng/ml in those age 40 years and older.

Prothrombin time (**PT**) measures the time it takes a fibrin clot to form in a specially treated blood sample. The test is performed in the hematology section of the lab; the specimen is drawn in a blue-topped tube. It is used to monitor the effects of oral anticoagulants. The normal range for the results in an untreated person is from 10 to 14 seconds. An acceptable range for someone taking oral anticoagulants is from 1.5 to 2 times the normal time.

Random blood sugar (**RBS**) refers to testing blood sugar without respect to fasting or mealtime. The test is performed in the chemistry section of the lab. The blood is drawn into an SST. A result of less than 145 mg of true glucose per deciliter of blood is considered in the normal range. If it is elevated beyond this, a follow-up fasting sugar is usually ordered.

Red blood cell (**RBC**) count is usually done as part of a CBC. The test is done in the hematology section of the lab. The blood is drawn in a lavender-topped tube. The reference ranges are 4.2 to 5.4 million per microliter in men, and 3.6 to 5.0 million per microliter in women. Normal counts may be higher in people living at high altitudes.

Reticulocyte count is a measurement of the number of immature red blood cells expressed as a percentage. This test can assist in differentiating between different types of anemias. On its own, it is somewhat imprecise and is compared with RBC count and hematocrit results. Normally, blood is composed of 0.5 to 2 percent reticulocytes.

Sodium (**Na**) is part of the electrolyte block. A certain proportion of this element with carbon dioxide, potassium, and chloride must be present in the full electrolyte panel. Sodium measurements are useful in the evaluation of kidney functions. The test is done in the chemistry section of the lab. Blood is drawn in an SST. The reference range is from 135 to 145 mEq/l of serum.

T- and B-cell counts measure the number of certain lymphocytes that can recognize antigens. The test is useful in the diagnosis of immunodeficiency diseases. The test is performed in the hematology section of the lab. The blood is drawn in a lavender-topped and a green-topped tube, both of which must be left at room temperature.

Abnormal counts suggest but do not confirm specific disease entities. Values of normal may vary from lab to lab, but an effort is being made to standardize them. Their measurement as a percentage of the total WBC count is as follows:

T cells: 68–75%
B cells: 10–20%
Null cells: 5–20%

Thyroid-stimulating hormone (**TSH**) measures the activity of the hormone that dictates the action of the thyroid gland. The analysis takes 2 days to accomplish. The test is done in the chemistry section of the lab and blood is collected in an SST. The results should not exceed 15 micro-IU/ml of blood.

Two-hour postprandial blood sugar gives an indication of the levels of glucose in the blood 2 hours after the ingestion of a normal meal. The test is done in the chemistry section of the lab. Blood is drawn into an SST. The result is considered normal if the value is less than 145 mg sugar per deciliter of blood.

Uric acid is, at the end point, a component of urine, but it appears in the bloodstream before being excreted. Elevated levels are indicative of gout. An 8-hour fast is required. The test is done in the chemistry section of the lab and the blood is drawn into an SST. The normal ranges for results are 4.3–8.0 mg/dl in men and 2.3 to 6.0 mg/dl in women.

The WBC differential (**diff**) is based on the fact that WBCs are classified into five types: neutrophils, basophils, eosinophils, monocytes, and lymphocytes. Levels of each of these players in the immune system are higher in various disease processes. In adults, the normal ranges are:

Neutrophils: 47.6–76.8%
Lymphocytes: 16.2–43%
Eosinophils: 0.3–7%
Basophils: 0.3–2%
Monocytes: 0.6–9.6%.

White blood cell (WBC) count is also known as a leukocyte count. It is part of the CBC. It measures the total number of WBCs in a small sample of blood. There are influences that may alter the number by as many as 2000. These factors are strenuous exercise, digestion, and stress. The test assists in the detection of inflammation and infection. The reference range is from 4000 to 10,000 WBC/ml of blood. This may vary a little from lab to lab (Figs. 20–2 and 20–3).

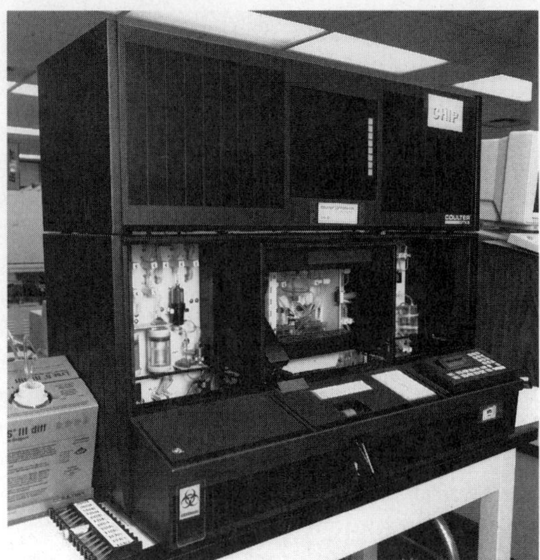

Figure 20–3
Coulter counter for hematology studies.

Urine Tests

Routine urinalysis (UA) is used to screen the urine for urinary tract disorders. A clean container is used to collect the specimen. Only a half ounce of urine is needed. The specimen is studied for the following normal values:

Color: straw
Odor: slight aroma
Appearance: clear
Specific gravity: 1.005–1.035
pH: 4.5–7.0
Sugar: none
Epithelial cells: none to few
Casts: none to occasional translucent
Crystals: present
Yeast cells: none

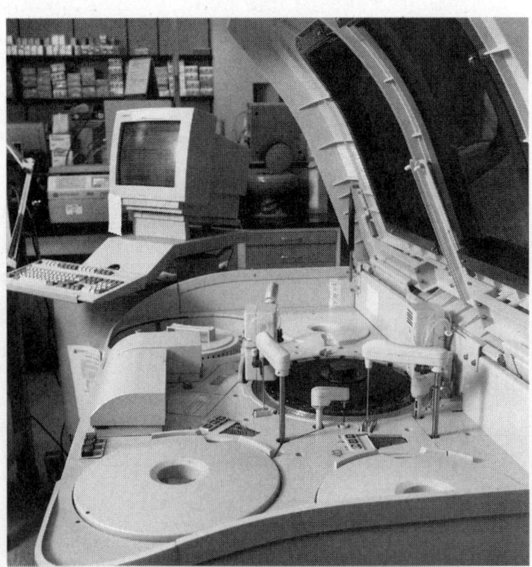

Figure 20–2
Autoanalyzer for blood chemistries.

Bence Jones protein testing can detect an abnormal protein in the urine, the presence of which is an indicator of the presence of multiple tumors. The test requires that an early-morning, clean-catch specimen be taken. The urine should contain no Bence Jones protein.

Creatinine clearance is an evaluation of the efficiency of the kidneys. The test involves a timed urine specimen and at least one blood sample. The first voiding is discarded. Subsequent voidings are made into a special container to which the patient must add preservatives that are provided. At the completion of the urine collection (usually 24 hours), a blood sample is drawn, so it is important to start the collection at a time such that 24 hours later the lab will be open to draw the blood. The normal results are:

Men: 85–125 ml/minute
Women: 75–115 ml/minute

In older people, the expected normal value decreases by 6 ml for each decade of age.

Specimens

The HUC accepts specimens at the desk from clinics, home care agencies, doctors' offices, and patients. Any time a specimen is brought to the lab desk, the HUC must check the label for the following information: patient name, registration or ID number, date and time of collection, and name of person who collected the specimen. The information on the requisition must match that on the label. All specimens should arrive and be handled using the standard universal precautions. The HUC makes sure there are orders in the computer for the requested test on every specimen. Each specimen is logged into the book with the date, time, and initials of person receiving the specimen. This begins the process that provides a method of tracking specimens if it becomes necessary.

Test Results

Sending test results out of the lab is as important as receiving specimens or patients. Test results must be sent out daily and the HUC is responsible to see that this is done in a timely manner. Results may be sent to a doctor's office, clinic, home health agency, nursing home, or other outside agencies. The ordering doctor may request that results also be sent to another doctor in situations when a patient has multiple care providers. The method of sending out results may vary depending on the type of test and urgency of reporting the results. The easiest and fastest method is to fax the test results to the proper destination. When faxing, keep in mind that this is confidential information and should be protected by using cover sheets and ensuring that the fax numbers are accurate and the equipment is in proper working order. Faxed results may be followed up by mailing the original result sheets. In some cases, it may be necessary to call results to the doctor, such as STAT orders or "panic" value results (too high or too low).

Test results are reported in many different formats. Since 1987, there has been an effort to standardize much of the way the results are presented internationally. The method is based on SI Units (International System Units). The International System is used in journal reports, but has not gained much favor among practitioners in the United States, where conventional units continue to be used (Table 20–1).

Telephone

Telephone triage is a big part of the lab desk duties. As any HUC knows, telephone management is always a test of patience and endurance. The phone will always ring when you are the busiest! The most common types of calls are to schedule patients for future appointments and to obtain results of completed tests. Patients call to change an existing appointment or to confirm a time. Patients may also call to review the preparation needed for an upcoming test. The HUC may be able to answer these questions, or it may require transferring the caller to another person.

The HUCs working in the clinics may call to obtain the proper procedure for ordering a certain test, or they may want to add tests to blood already drawn and in the lab. These calls may need to be transferred to the lab technicians who are running the test.

Health Unit Coordinator Knowledge and Skills Appropriate to Position

The experienced HUC who has spent any time working on a nursing unit may be qualified for this position. The skills needed on the nursing unit that carry over to the lab are good communication skills, the ability to work independently and to prioritize tasks, good time management and good decision-making skills, and the ability to work well with others, to name a few. The HUC interacts with all of the different departments in the hospital and many outside sources every day. This position requires a varied knowledge of hospital procedures, departments, computer systems,

Table 20-1 COMPARISON OF LAB VALUES

Name of Test	Results Expressed As	Standardized Result
Hematocrit	40–54 ml/dl	0.40–0.54
Hemoglobin	13.0–18.0 gm/dl	8.1–11.2 mmol/l
Serum albumin	3.3–5.2 gm/dl	33–52 gm/l
Cholesterol	<200 mg/dl	<5.20 mmol/l
Fasting glucose	70–115 mg/dl	3.9–6.4 mmol/l
Creatine kinase	55–170 U/l	55–170 U/l
Blood urea nitrogen	11–23 mg/dl	8.0–16.4 mmol/l
Potassium	3.5–5.0 mEq/l	3.5–5.0 mmol/l

and locations of services provided by the hospital to give the highest-quality customer service to the patient.

Additional Training

The hospital computer system may run on one brand of software with many functions, or several different brands of software that interface into the main system. It is important that the HUC in the diagnostic lab have a complete understanding of the software used in the department. This includes not only patient registration and billing procedures that might be part of the main system, but the laboratory information system (**LIS**). The LIS is a system that is used to print the specimen labels and keep a detailed record of each specimen. The information recorded on the label includes the patient's name, ID number, date, time, test to be run, the name of the person who drew the specimen, and the name of the person who performed the test. The LIS can track the date and time of all specimens done on a patient, whether or not the results are complete, and the reference ranges for that test. This can be vital information for many reasons, but one of the most common is for follow-up care. If the ordering doctor wants to know something about *how* the blood was obtained, it is easy to "see" who drew the blood. The doctor can go directly to that person and get the necessary information.

In addition to the computer, the HUC working in this area must be familiar with the information needed for billing purposes. The general information that is gathered for routine registration might also include ICD9 (diagnostic) codes or CPT (billing) codes. Some lab tests require specific forms to be completed and to accompany the specimen into the lab. Patients being crossmatched for possible blood transfusion during a surgical procedure routinely have that lab work done within 72 hours of surgery. If the patient is having the lab work done before that time, there is an "extended crossmatch" form that must be completed. These forms usually arrive with the patient from the doctor's office, but sometimes the HUC must call and request the form.

Anyone working in an area that might come in contact with body fluids must be familiar with the safety precautions for blood-borne pathogens and latex allergies. HUCs attend a training class and yearly update classes. Some of the safety precautions include *always* wearing gloves when handling specimens at the desk, and making sure all specimens are inside a plastic bag and sealed in case of spills.

Many chemicals are used in the lab testing area, and even though the HUC is mainly at the front desk, each lab employee is required to know what to do and who to contact in case of spills or contamination. The Occupational Safety and Health Administration (OSHA) is a federal government agency that mandates all employees be given training and other information on dangers posed by chemicals. It sets standards for worker exposure to hazardous substances and requires that such substances have warning labels. Some of the general precautions include:

1. Avoid accidents and spills
2. Avoid unnecessary exposure to chemicals
3. Do not remove or deface labels on chemicals
4. Wear protective apparel and equipment

Closing Thoughts

The diagnostic lab is an interesting place to work, especially for someone who does not like to do the same thing every day. Some days are busy and challenging, and others are calm and routine. In general it is a challenging and growing job. Understanding the computer system and all the different services provided in the hospital makes it easier to provide the customer service needed to please our customers.

Every week and every day is different. Before working in the diagnostic lab, I had worked on a medical-surgical unit and also in the internal medicine clinic. The experience from these areas helped to prepare me for the work in a busy area of service like the lab. It is rewarding getting to know and visiting with the regular lab patients and getting to meet new people each day. There is always something new to learn, so it is rarely boring. One never knows who is going to come to the desk or what they are going to need.

Review Questions

1. Explain the laboratory information system.
2. List five possible duties of the HUC in the diagnostic lab.
3. Describe the procedure for receiving specimens at the lab desk.
4. Name three laboratory tests that require fasting in preparation for them, and give their normal values.

Bibliography

Moore SB: Everything You Need to Know About Medical Tests. Springhouse, PA, Springhouse Corporation, 1996.

New England Clinical Laboratories Clinical Services Manual. 1994.

New Hampshire Medical Laboratories Procedures Directory. 1997.

Path Labs Laboratory Guide 1995.

Rakel RE: Saunders Manual of Medical Practice. Philadelphia, WB Saunders, 1996.

21 Educator in Hospital-Based Training Program

Patricia Noonan Rice

Common Abbreviations

ADA Americans with Disabilities Act

ASTD American Society for Training and Development

AVA-HOE American Vocational Association-Health Occupations Education

Objectives

Upon completion of this chapter, the reader should be able to:

1. Explain why hospital-based training programs were developed.
2. List the functions of the program coordinator in a hospital-based training program.
3. List the functions of the instructor in a hospital-based training program.
4. Identify the areas of additional knowledge that would be necessary for a position in a hospital-based training program and explain the reasons for needing them.

Vocabulary

Americans with Disabilities Act: Passed in 1990, the ADA requires employer accommodation of disabled individuals

Curriculum: A course of study in a school

Health unit coordinator (HUC) practitioner: One who is currently employed to perform the HUC duties in a health care facility

Objective: Something aimed at, a purpose or target

Practicum: A hands-on opportunity to apply classroom theory to practice

Preceptor: A HUC who provides coaching and mentoring to a HUC student during the practicum experience

Syllabus: A summary or outline of a course of study

History of Position

When the health unit coordinator (HUC) position was introduced to health care in the 1940s, most people were trained on the job. Employers would hire first, then train. As health care technology grew, so did the HUC responsibilities. It soon became apparent to hospital administrators that it was more cost effective to hire people who already had received formal training for the HUC position. It was also apparent that the delivery of high-quality health care depended on consistently trained employees. It was from these circumstances that HUC training programs in community colleges and vocational centers evolved.

However, HUC training programs are not available in all communities.

The lack of community college-based HUC training programs has led to the development of hospital-based training programs. Some hospital-based HUC training programs are offered to employees as part of their orientation. However, some hospitals have realized the benefits of providing a hospital-based training program first and then placing the successful students in open positions. A hospital-based training program of this type is cost effective because the student pays the hospital for the training instead of the hospital paying the new employee to learn. A hospital-based training program provides health care facilities with a pool of qualified applicants for their HUC positions.

Position Responsibilities and Duties

In the hospital setting, this position may consist of two components: program coordination and instructing. The dual responsibilities may be performed by one or more people.

Program Coordinator Responsibilities

Responsibilities for a HUC program director as defined in the National Association of Health Unit Coordinators' (NAHUC) *Essentials and Guidelines for Health Unit Coordinator Education Programs* (hereafter *Essentials and Guidelines*) are as follows: "The Program Director shall devote full-time to the sponsoring institution with primary responsibilities for the educational program to include organization, administration, periodic review, continued development, and general effectiveness."

Instructor

Responsibilities for a HUC instructor as defined in the NAHUC *Essentials and Guidelines* are, "The Instructional Staff shall be responsible for achieving the objectives for each course assigned by the Program Director, for evaluating students and reporting progress as required by the sponsoring institution, and for the periodic review and upgrading of course material."

Health Unit Coordinator Knowledge/Skills Appropriate to Position

Program Coordinator

The program coordinator should have knowledge of the basic management functions: planning, organizing, influencing, and controlling.

Planning

Planning focuses on achieving goals. The program coordinator might plan to achieve the goal of providing students with the basic knowledge about HUC duties and the environment in which they will work.

Organizing

Organizing is creating a mechanism to put plans into action. The program coordinator would develop the means to accomplish the goal.

Influencing

Influencing or directing is the process of guiding the activities of the organization's members toward goal attainment.

Controlling

Controlling is comparing actual performance to predetermined objectives and taking action to modify performance to meet goals. Controlling is an ongoing evaluation process.

In addition to possessing management skills,

the HUC program coordinator should be certified in health unit coordinating.

Instructor

The HUC program instructor should be a certified HUC and have had previous work experience as a HUC. First-hand knowledge of HUC responsibilities is good preparation for teaching. Students will respect an instructor with a working knowledge of subject matter. Being a HUC content expert is just the beginning. The HUC instructor must have the ability to organize and present material in a way the students can comprehend. A positive attitude toward teaching is necessary, as well as knowledge of continuous quality improvement.

The qualifications and job description for an instructor in a hospital-based training program will likely be as unique as the hospital itself. A hospital-based training program probably will not be governed by the same rules as an accredited learning facility. Therefore, a teaching degree may not be required for the instructor position. An instructor in a hospital-based training program will likely have HUC experience coupled with a training and development background.

A **HUC practitioner** can uncover numerous training opportunities in most hospitals. Training experience can be gained by facilitating continuing education sessions and in-services, teaching computer classes, precepting HUC students, assisting with new employee orientation, developing policies and procedures, and participating in committees.

Seminars as well as trade journals and books from professional associations can provide a wealth of learning opportunities for the HUC practitioner interested in instructing. NAHUC, the American Vocational Association-Health Occupations Education (**AVA-HOE**), and the American Society for Training and Development (**ASTD**) offer resources to instructors. All of these activities and more can lead to professional growth and a position as an instructor in a hospital-based training program.

Additional Training Required

Knowledge of Group Dynamics

The HUC instructor has to know how to direct and guide group learning and group activities. The HUC instructor needs to understand the roles people play. Group leadership skills are an essential for teaching. The HUC instructor must play the role of facilitator to guide the group process. An effective group leader provides proactive influences and receives feedback from group members. The HUC instructor must be able to encourage class participation. Allowing students to participate in discussion and search for answers themselves is more interesting than listening to a lecture.

Open-ended questions can be used to encourage participation. Open-ended questions cannot be answered with a simple "yes" or "no," so they stimulate thought and discussion. Deferring questions back to the students also encourages participation. Nonverbal reinforcement such as nods, smiles, and eye contact can encourage participation and create a positive atmosphere, too. The HUC instructor should give praise that is specific and sincere.

Knowledge of the Principles of Adult Learning

In most cases, HUC students are adults. The needs of the adult student are different than those of children. Adults have certain learning preferences and expectations. Adults want to know why a skill is important, they want an opportunity to practice the skill, and they want to be able to identify opportunities where they will use the skill. Adults bring their own unique experiences to the classroom and draw on their experiences in the learning process. Learning about individual learning styles and having adult students do a learning style inventory can be beneficial. Also, a refresher on effective study tips may be necessary.

Adult students have more responsibilities. Many HUC students have family and work obligations in addition to school obligations. An adult student's personal life affects his or her academic performance. An instructor can assist with this process by offering time management in the **curriculum.**

Knowledge of Instructional Methods/Tools

A HUC instructor needs to know how to develop instructional methods and tools. In addition to lecture, the instructor should present the subject material in a variety of ways. Each student may respond differently to the information presented. The HUC instructor needs to develop many ways to teach a topic to be certain that it is understood by all. Instructional tools should be developed for visual, auditory, and kinesthetic (hands-on) learners. Ideas for instructional methods and tools can be found in instructors' guides. The authors of HUC textbooks usually write instructors' guides to accompany their books. NAHUC's *Education Program Procedure Guide* lists resources such as textbooks, audiovisual aids, and classroom activities. Instructional tools are discussed later in this chapter.

Knowledge of Cultural Diversity

Our society is becoming more diverse. The ability to communicate with members of other cultures is a necessity. "Changing demographics means that more of us can expect to work with people who come from different backgrounds and thus have different customs and attitudes" (Adler and Elmhorst, *Communicating at Work*). Understanding how communication is affected by cultural conditioning can help an instructor adapt and develop appropriate teaching techniques. A HUC instructor should learn about different cultures and subcultures. Cultural differences bring an opportunity to strengthen the learning experiences with different perspectives. Cultural diversity can also be included in the curriculum to prepare HUC students to work with the public.

Knowledge of the Americans with Disabilities Act

The passage of the **Americans with Disabilities Act (ADA)** in 1990 expanded the scope of discrimination laws against people with disabilities. Specifically, this means discrimination is prohibited against a person if he or she can perform the essential job functions. Essential job functions are defined as the fundamental job duties of the employment position that a person with a disability holds or desires, but they do not include the marginal functions of the position. The essential job functions would be developed by the human resources department of the sponsoring institution (hospital). The human resources department would also be responsible for defining the physical and mental requirements for the position. Under the ADA, an employer must make reasonable accommodations for disabled people. The HUC instructor would need to work closely with the human resources department to ensure compliance with the ADA both in the classroom and the practicum sites.

Knowledge of Word Processing Skills

A HUC instructor in a hospital-based training program may be responsible for his or her own clerical support. Competence with a word processing program can ease the task of developing tests, instructional tools, and worksheets and maintaining records and correspondence.

Procedures and Functions Specific to Position

Program Coordinator

Planning Functions

Needs Assessment

The first step in planning a hospital-based HUC training program is a needs assessment. The program coordinator would assess the current job requirements, current training methods, recruitment and retention methods, turnover rates, and optional training methods. A job analysis can be performed to gather and analyze information about the HUC position. The HUC managers in the hospital can provide valuable input to the needs assessment and job analysis.

Program Objectives

Once the need for a hospital-based HUC training program is established, program **objectives** and requirements would be developed. Program objectives would state what the student will be able to do on successful completion of the program. The objectives include the knowledge that will be gained to perform the specific HUC job functions.

Program requirements would include the entry-level requirements for a HUC student. Entry-level requirements for a HUC student in a hospital-based training program will vary. The basic requirement would be a high school diploma or equivalent. The program coordinator should confer with the human resources department to check the legality and validity of any screening tests that would be administered.

Policies

Policy development is another responsibility of the HUC program coordinator. Policies can be defined as general guidelines that regulate organizational activities. Policies protect both the hospital-based training program and the student. Sound policy development can aid in making objective decisions. Policies regarding fees, refunds, and withdrawals have to be decided. The health policies of the sponsoring hospital have to be adapted to the HUC program. Student policies include rules regarding attendance, participation, dress code, confidentiality, liability insurance, examinations, and grades.

Curriculum

The HUC program curriculum would be based on the needs assessment and program objectives. The program coordinator or instructor may be responsible for developing the curriculum. Tools for developing curriculum include HUC textbooks and instructor guides and the NAHUC *Essentials and Guidelines*. Course descriptions, including course title, length, and content, should be written. In a hospital-based training program, course content is based on what is necessary for the students to learn to prepare them for the job.

Preparation/Organization Functions

Budget Development

Budget development is a function of the HUC program coordinator. The sponsoring hospital will have its own guidelines for developing and implementing the program budget.

Practicum

The program coordinator will secure **practicum** sites for the HUC students. Affiliation agreements set forth the responsibilities of the training department or site and the practicum department or site for providing instruction and experience. Hospitals usually have affiliation agreements with schools of medicine, nursing, and other allied health professions. Samples of affiliation agreements between the hospital and other schools should be readily available to the hospital-based instructor.

Other Responsibilities

Ordering supplies and textbooks and scheduling rooms and instructors are all part of the preparation process. The program coordinator may also be responsible for organizing special events such as the graduation ceremony or job fair.

Recruitment/Registration Functions

Recruitment

Recruitment functions may include the development of brochures and advertisements. It might also include giving presentations about the program to various groups such as high school students, and being present at job fairs.

Registration

Registration functions include interviewing prospective students and collecting fees.

Evaluation/Review Functions

Evaluation is an ongoing process. The program coordinator evaluates instructors (Fig. 21–1) and preceptors and performs student/employer follow-up. Evaluation criteria should be based on the program objectives. Evaluations may be in the form of questionnaires or may include site visits. An advisory committee is a valuable resource for the hospital-based HUC training program. Advisory committee members should include HUCs, HUC supervisors, HUC faculty, and a current and a former program student. It is important to note that even the best designed evaluation tool is worthless if the information obtained is not analyzed and used.

Academic and guidance counseling must be made available to the students under the guidelines of the sponsoring institution (hospital).

STUDENT EVALUATION–PROGRAM INSTRUCTOR

	Poor			Excellent		
1. Knowledge of subject material (adequate background, preparation)	0	1	2	3	4	5
2. Organization	0	1	2	3	4	5
3. Ability to present material in an interesting manner	0	1	2	3	4	5
4. Subject content relevant to practice	0	1	2	3	4	5
5. Allowed adequate time for content covered	0	1	2	3	4	5
6. Encouragement of class participation	0	1	2	3	4	5
7. Openness to student response, questions, and comments	0	1	2	3	4	5
8. Demonstrated professionalism, acted as a role model	0	1	2	3	4	5
9. Availability	0	1	2	3	4	5

Suggestions:

Strong Points:

Weak Points:

Figure 21–1
Instructor evaluation.

Instructor

Teaching Functions

Lesson Plans

The HUC instructor should develop class plans and objectives based on the curriculum. A daily lesson plan with specific objectives should be created and shared with the students. An objective is a target or a purpose. Class objectives should define what the students are to learn. Objectives should be written to measure what students have learned. Knowledge is reflected by the ability to remember or recall previously learned material. Words that can be used in knowledge objectives include *define, describe, identify*, and *state*—for example, "state the five components of a medication order." Comprehension is defined as the ability to grasp the meaning of material. Words that can be used in comprehension objectives include *conclude, explain, illustrate*, and *interpret*—for example, "explain the reason for patient preparation before an x-ray of the large intestine." Application is being able to select and use learned information. Words that can be used in application objectives include *demonstrate, operate*, and *prepare*—for instance, "demonstrate communication skills."

Health unit coordinator students should be provided with a **syllabus**. A syllabus is a schedule or guide for students to prepare for class (Fig. 21–2). The syllabus should include the course title, class dates, times, and location, and the instructor. The syllabus should briefly describe the lesson for each class meeting so that students can prepare in advance.

Classroom Preparation

The HUC instructor is responsible for classroom preparation. This includes everything from lighting and seating arrangements to properly functioning equipment (Fig. 21–3). It is important to create a comfortable learning environment because discomfort can be a distraction. Tables with ample working space and a well lit room are essential. Supplementary references should be readily available to the student. A simulated work area is necessary for skills practice (Fig. 21–4). The HUC instructor can elicit help from students to personalize the classroom. Giving students responsibility for their environment can increase their comfort level, thereby enhancing the learning experience.

Instructional Methods and Tools

The HUC instructor is responsible for developing instructional tools and audiovisual aids. Transparencies, games, demonstrations, videos, and bulletin board displays are examples of instructional tools. The instructor should also develop worksheets, quizzes, and tests based on the written class objectives. A variety of types of questions should be used. HUC textbooks and the NAHUC *Education Program Procedure Guide* offer many suggestions for instructional tools. However, the hospital-based HUC instructor should learn to develop other tools as well.

The first step for instructional writing is to research and develop the topic. For HUC procedures, research may include observing the task being performed and cross-referencing with other hospital policies. It is important to cross-reference other sources such as NAHUC's *Essentials and Guidelines* and the NAHUC Entry Level Competencies. Research can be expanded with HUC textbooks.

The next step after researching and developing the topic is to organize thoughts and ideas. The HUC instructor should identify the key points that need to be explained, such as "determine what computer functions were most widely used by new HUC employees," and then write the key points as measurable objectives. Once objectives are written, an outline is developed to define the lesson further. With a clearly developed outline, an instructor is prepared to compose.

It is important for an instructor to express ideas clearly and effectively because he or she writes to explain or inform. Written instructions have to be complete and concise. Misunderstood instructions can undermine an entire lesson. Tests and

HEALTH UNIT COORDINATOR PROGRAM
SYLLABUS

1/16		
P. Teacher	Introduction, History of HUCs Chapter 1–HUCing: An Allied Health Career	8:00–11:00
B. Instructor	Medical Terminology, Anatomy & Physiology Units I & II: Word Elements & Skin	12:00–3:00
1/17		
P. T.	Chapter 2–The Nursing Department Chapter 3–The Hospital Environment Hospital Tour	8:00–11:00
B.I.	Medical Terminology: Unit III, Musculoskeletal	12:00–3:00
1/18		
P.T.	**TEST Chapter 1, 2, 3** Communication Skills & Cultural Diversity	8:00–11:00
B.I.	Medical Terminology: Unit IV & V, Nervous System, Eye & Ear	12:00–3:00
1/19		
P.T.	Telephone Workshop	8:00–11:00
B.I.	Medical Terminology: Units IX & X, Urinary & Reproductive	12:00–3:00
1/20		
P. T.	Chapter 4–Communication Devices	8:00–11:00
S. Speaker	Guest Lecturer: Customer Service	
B.I.	**MEDICAL TERMINOLOGY TEST**	12:00–3:00

Figure 21–2
HUC course syllabus.

worksheets should be challenging because of the subject matter, not because of the wording.

Once the content is satisfactory, the tool (test, worksheet, activity) can be formatted. A hospital-based HUC instructor benefits from having word processing and computer presentation skills. The best designed tools are worthless if they are sloppy or illegible.

Performance Feedback

The HUC instructor is also responsible for providing the student with performance feedback. Class time should be allowed to review all tests and assignments to reinforce lesson objectives. The student should regularly receive progress reviews or reports. Report cards and certificates are examples of progress reviews. Adhering to lesson objectives enables the instructor to give unbiased evaluations. When students fail to meet objectives, the instructor and student can develop a plan together to meet the goals.

Counseling

The HUC instructor may also provide academic counseling. Students should be made aware of the times that the instructor is available for academic

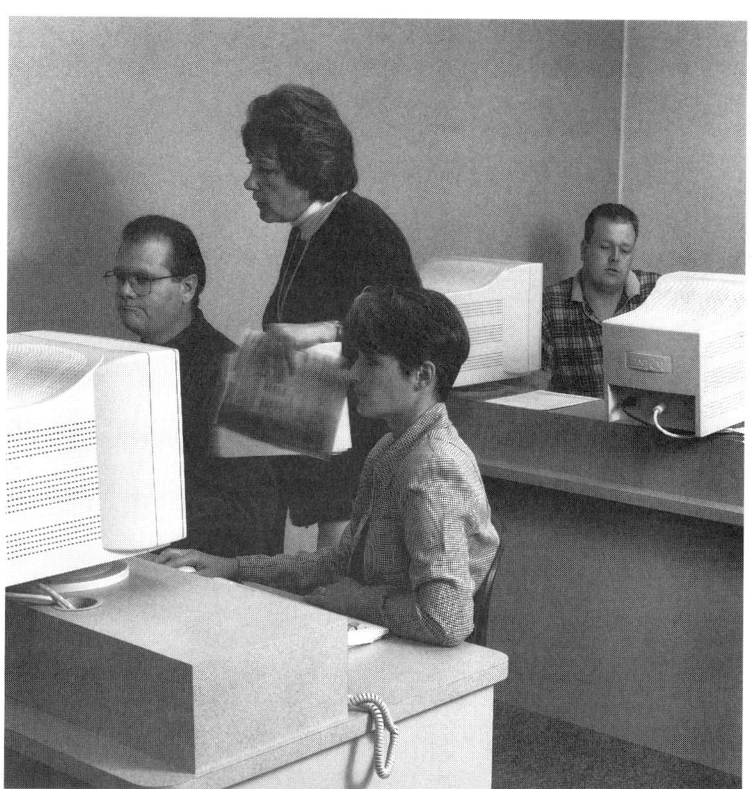

Figure 21–3
HUC classroom.

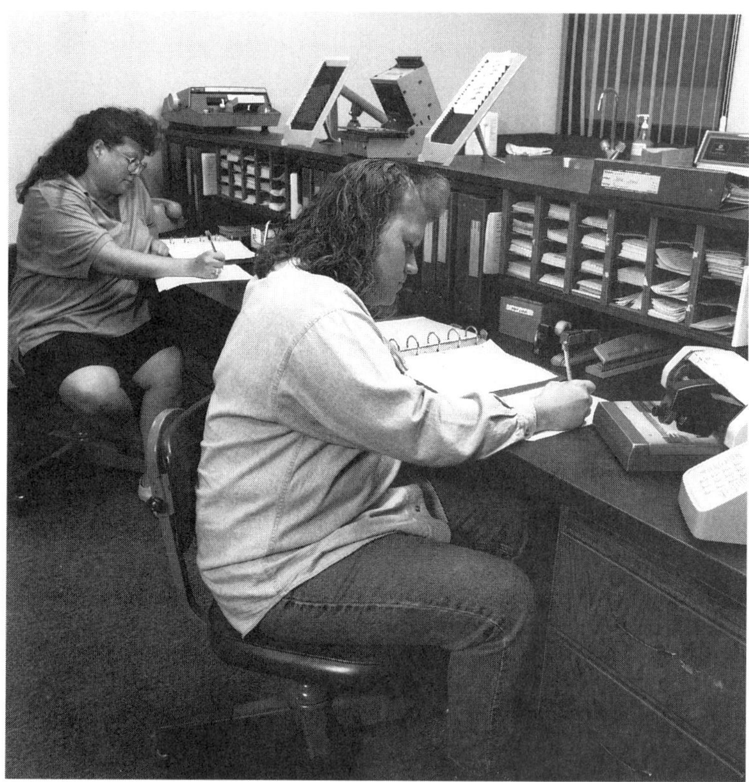

Figure 21–4
Simulated workstation in classroom.

counseling. The HUC instructor should have office hours set aside for counseling. Students need to know that counseling is private and confidential.

Practicum Functions

The hands-on portion of a hospital-based training program is the practicum. The practicum involves assigning HUC students to HUC **preceptors** to learn about the job duties firsthand (Fig. 21–5). The practicum provides the HUC students the opportunity to practice what they have learned in the classroom. The hospital-based training program provides the ideal practicum experience. The HUC instructor should be involved with preceptor selection and offer preceptor training. A preceptor is a role model and a coach.

A practicum skills list should be written, with measurable objectives and goals. Both the preceptor and student should know the performance expectations.

The HUC instructor should be available to the students and preceptors at all times during the practicum. In addition, the HUC instructor should make regular rounds of the practicum sites. The HUC instructor needs to be visible enough to ensure that the HUC student does not feel abandoned and yet distant enough to allow the student to learn and grow with the assistance of the preceptor. The HUC instructor in a hospital-based training program must support the HUC student and preceptor equally. Often this balancing act requires the instructor to practice his or her own diplomacy skills.

The practicum allows the HUC student to practice employability skills, and the student should be evaluated on those skills. This is also the ideal

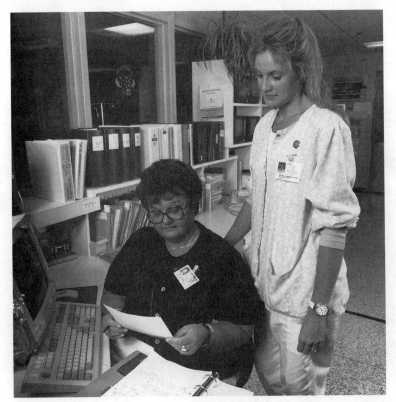

Figure 21–5
HUC student with preceptor.

time to discuss job search skills and employment opportunities (Fig. 21–6). The practicum is a crucial part of the learning process in a hospital-based training program.

Quality Improvement Functions

The HUC instructor should work closely with the program coordinator to ensure continuous improvement of the HUC program. Evaluations by students and an advisory committee can provide valuable input for self-evaluation.

Continuing Education Functions

The HUC instructor of a hospital-based training program may also be the provider of continuing education for HUC employees (Fig. 21–7). The HUC instructor will find that many of the responsibilities and functions of teaching the HUC program can be transferred to providing continuing education. Continuing education helps HUCs keep current in their field. NAHUC states that continuing education is essential and a life-long process. Continuing education is important because it serves as a means of maintaining or improving professional competence. Continuing education may be mandated by the employer or it may be used for HUC recertification. Continuing education for HUC recertification must meet NAHUC requirements.

Perhaps the HUC instructor of a hospital-based training program can best serve his or her former students by enlisting their help with continuing education. Once the HUC students graduate and

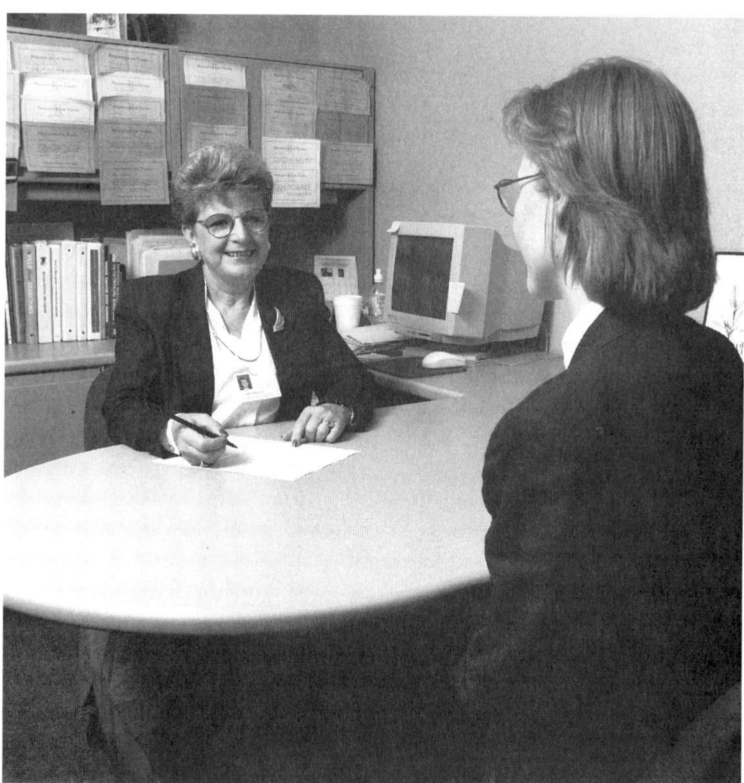

Figure 21–6
A job interview.

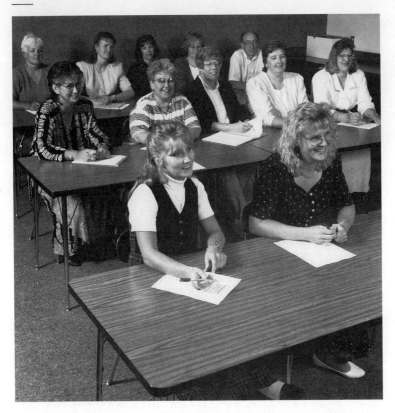

Figure 21–7
An in-service meeting.

are employed, the HUC instructor can continue to give them opportunities for professional growth by sharing the responsibilities for continuing education. HUC practitioners can assist with in-services and other continuing education offerings. Professional growth opportunities for HUCs ensure the continuation of the HUC education cycle.

Closing Thoughts

Reflection

In addition to having management skills, the importance of continuous evaluation and improvement cannot be overemphasized. Coordination of a hospital-based training program is a continuous cycle. It is important to pay attention to detail. The HUC Instructor needs creative skills to present information in as many ways as necessary for the student to understand. Change is inevitable, so flexibility, patience, and humor are necessary attributes for survival. I found out firsthand the many things that don't happen as planned. I learned to "think on my feet," and to be flexible and change directions if necessary. Scheduling conflicts, classrooms or speakers not being available, and faulty equipment are just a few of the unexpected events in the course of a program. I learned to stay focused on the main program objective: to provide the student with the best training possible.

Satisfaction

The most satisfying aspect of being involved in a hospital-based HUC training program is watching someone master a new skill or playing a part in someone's professional development. I have had the thrill of watching HUC students progress to HUC practitioners to HUC preceptors and beyond. I have the opportunity to convey my respect for the HUC position and see that respect grow in others. Most important, the instructor of a hospital-based training program has the opportunity to have fun and enjoy!

Review Questions

1. Explain why hospital-based training programs for HUCs were developed.
2. List the functions of the program coordinator in a hospital-based training program.
3. List the functions of the instructor in a hospital-based training program.
4. Identify the areas of additional knowledge that would be necessary for a position in a hospital-based training program, and explain the reasons for needing them.

Bibliography

Adler RB, Elmhorst JM: Communicating at Work: Principles and Practice for Business and the Professions, 5th ed. New York, McGraw-Hill, 1996.

Blanchard K, Hersey P: Management of Organizational Behavior: Utilizing Human Resources, 6th ed. Englewood Cliffs, NJ, Prentice Hall, 1993.

Certo S: Modern Management: Diversity, Quality, Ethics, and the Global Environment, 6th ed. Englewood Cliffs, NJ, Prentice Hall, 1994.

Mathis RL, Jackson JH: Human Resource Management, 7th ed. Minneapolis, MN, West Publishing Corporation, 1994.

National Association of Health Unit Coordinators (NAHUC) Education Program Procedure Guide. Philadelphia, NAHUC, 1996.

National Association of Health Unit Coordinators (NAHUC) Essentials and Guidelines for HUC Education Programs. Philadelphia, NAHUC, 1995.

National Association of Health Unit Coordinators (NAHUC) Informational Handbook. Philadelphia, NAHUC, 1995.

22 Hospital-Based Home Care

Jo-Ann Polis Wilkins

Abbreviations

AA	Administrative assistant
AAA	Area agency on aging
HCA	Home care aide (more recent term in use in some agencies)
HCC	Home care coordinator
HHA	Home health aide
HMO	Health maintenance organization
HV	Home visit
IDC	Interdisciplinary conference
LTG	Long-term goals
POC	Plan of care
SNV	Skilled nursing visit
SOC	Start of care
STG	Short-term goals

Objectives

Upon completion of this chapter, the reader will be able to:

1. Define and describe a hospital-based home care agency.
2. Name and describe clerical positions available in a hospital-based home care agency.
3. Describe a nonclinical management-level position in home care.
4. Follow the steps in a referral (intake) from initial call through staffing arrangements.

Vocabulary

Active client: A patient currently receiving services from a home care agency

Custodial care: Assistance with basic comfort and activities of daily living in the absence of the need for skilled care

Homebound: (Medicare definition) Unable to leave the home without a considerable and taxing effort and not on a regular basis

Evolution

Home Care in 1897

Home care has come full circle in the past 100 years. In the 19th and early 20th centuries, hospitals were places to be feared; only the hopeless and dying cases were taken to the hospital. Home care was a way of life for most people. Babies were born at home, injuries and illnesses were treated at home. People injured at work, from the cotton fields to the coal mines, were patched up and carried home to heal or die in their own bed. Doctors came to the patient's home to provide treatment, but the care was provided by family and neighbors. Many women became nurses by learning to care for loved ones at home.

Hospital-Based Home Care in 1997

For many years, hospitals have used outside home health care agencies for their patients needing home care, but in the past decade, more organizations have been developed from within the hospi-

The abbreviations listed for this chapter are those that a HUC working in this area would be expected to know. Only those in boldface type are used in the text and appear in boldface when they are used for the first time.

tal system. Hospital-based home care is a program coordinated within the hospital system that provides for multidisciplinary, high-quality care in the home (Fig. 22–1). The goal is to provide the patient the opportunity of returning to an independent function at the highest level possible. The physicians and staff team together with the family and patient to develop the necessary plan of care (**POC**) that meets the physical, emotional, and educational needs of the patient and family.

New Roles

Traditionally, many positions in this field were held by nurses. As the demands of home care have increased, the nonclinical positions have been turned over to nonclinical professionals, health unit coordinators (HUCs) and certified health unit coordinators (CHUCs) These positions may include handling referrals, processing insurance coverage, and working with the discharge planner and the many other agencies it takes to return the patient home. The HUC has the demonstrated ability to prioritize these multiple demands and duties.

Home Care Coordinator

The number of patients requiring posthospital care continues to grow as the recovery times are shortened by rising health care costs and insurance requirements. In many cases, the planning

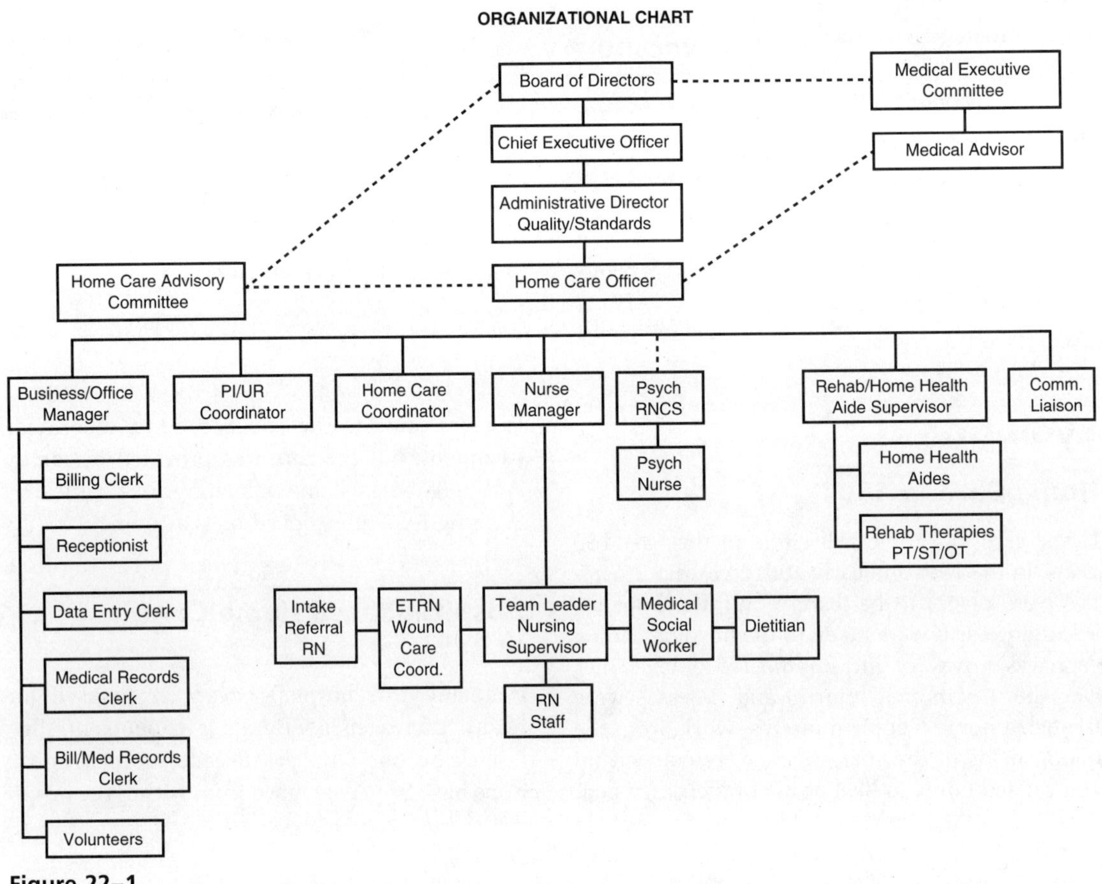

Figure 22–1
Organizational chart.

process for home care begins on admission. The home care coordinator (**HCC**) gathers all the necessary information and compiles a list of options for the team to review at the interdisciplinary conference (**IDC**).

The physician must write an order for home care in the patient's chart. The clinical team of doctors, nurses, and therapists do an assessment of the patient's needs at home. After the assessment of needs is determined, the HCC contacts the insurance carrier to determine the patient's eligibility for covered services. The HCC works closely with the discharge planner to ensure the patient has the right care for his or her needs. Patients may receive home visits (**HV**) from registered nurses, home health aides (**HHAs**), physical therapists, and many other professionals.

Becoming familiar with the regulations and guidelines of various regulatory agencies will be required for this position. Such agencies include but are not limited to the Joint Committee on Accreditation of Health Care Organizations (JCAHO), the Occupational Safety and Health Administration (OSHA), and Medicare. As an example, Medicare has strict admission criteria: the patient must be **home bound**, require skilled care (as opposed to **custodial care**), and the care must be intermittent (i.e., there is a finite end point to the service).

An HCC must learn about Medicare and other insurance carrier reimbursement guidelines. Like most things in health care today, the information is constantly revised and updated.

Frequently, other services (outside your department) are needed and may be available for the patient and family. Learning as much as possible during assessments and interviews may provide clues that will lead you to community resources that can be used to help provide the comprehensive care. Finding out what is "out there" locally or nation-wide is another area of learning. Some examples are support groups related to certain diseases; heart disease, cancer, Parkinson's and Alzheimer's disease, or veterans' organizations may have services geared toward specific age groups.

Intake and Referral

Referrals for home care usually come from the patient's doctor. The patient may be an in-patient or an outpatient. Referral calls can come from doctors with patients in other hospitals or facilities. Patient family members may be the first ones to initiate contact with the home care department. Regardless of how the referral is obtained, the procedure is the same. There must be a doctor's order, a completed needs assessment, and insurance verification and approval. A case manager is assigned, a plan of care is developed, all services are planned, and schedules are verified. In cases that go beyond the insurance coverage, financial planning becomes part of the routine. In some cases, it is possible to provide alternative sources of assistance, both public and private.

Active clients of the department are tracked if admitted to any in-patient facility such as acute care or rehabilitation. The appropriate discharge planner is contacted and made aware that the person is currently a patient of the hospital home care department, and is asked to notify that department when the patient is ready to return home and resume services. This is done to ensure continuity of care, especially if the patient is in another facility.

The person handling the intake and referral desk must be familiar with the different eligibility guidelines required by the governing agencies, insurance companies, Medicare, and Medicaid, in addition to the policies and procedures of the hospital and department. Ongoing education is required to stay current in this area.

The communication and problem-solving skills that HUCs have developed will be an asset in this position. Intakes and referrals demand attention to detail and prioritizing of time and duties. The person must be able to work with professional staff members, physicians, and outside agencies, as well as patients and family members.

Home Health Aide Scheduler

The primary responsibility in this position is to assign the aides (HHAs or HCAs) to meet both the needs of the patients and their caregivers or family members. This also requires scheduling adequate staff to meet fluctuating volume demands, including weekends and holidays. Time-off requests are reviewed and, if necessary, part-time and per diem staff are called to ensure that staffing is adequate to meet the needs of the department.

Field supervisory visits with the HHA supervisor are scheduled in compliance with department policy and existing regulatory requirements. The HUC arranges team meetings and continuing education in-services. Records are maintained for all field visits, meetings, inservices, and conferences. These records are used for personnel requirements and departmental statistics.

Medical Records Clerk

A medical record is initiated and maintained for all patients admitted for home care service. Protections are provided for the integrity of the medical record and patient confidentiality. Medical orders must be processed for a physician signature. Follow-up contact with the doctor's office is necessary if the signed orders are not returned within the required time frame. This may take a good deal of time, patience, and tact.

Inactive medical records must be prepared for storage or retrieval from archives on request. All HUCs are qualified and experienced in maintaining patient records as well as patient confidentiality. Medical terminology that is required for this position should have become a "second language" to the experienced HUC. This position requires good time management and interpersonal skills as well as the ability to work well with others. The HUC who chooses this position must have computer knowledge and be willing to expand into new areas of education.

Data Entry or Registration Clerk

All patients are registered using the information (computer) system of the hospital or department. This includes entering the diagnostic and insurance information. Data are entered for visit and supply charges for the billing department. Some coding may also be entered, using ICD-9 (diagnostic) or CPT (procedure) codes. This may require special training in coding records.

Any person operating in data entry must have excellent keyboard skills and computer knowledge, and the ability to work independently.

Receptionist

Many of the responsibilities of the receptionist are similar to those of the HUC. Incoming phone calls must be directed to the appropriate staff member. Calls must be assessed and prioritized as necessary. Visitors to the department are greeted and directed to the appropriate area or person. Departmental mail and other clerical duties may be performed by the receptionist.

Administrative Assistant

The hospital-based home care leadership team members have many demands on their time. Maintaining a calendar of appointments and meetings is a daily challenge for the administrative assistant (AA). The AA may be required to attend many of these meetings to take notes or minutes, then type and distribute them to the appropriate people. Mail and phone calls are a part of any AA's daily routine. The communications must be prioritized and channeled to the proper person. Whenever possible, the AA follows up on routine inquires and operational business.

Personnel files are maintained and kept current. These include home phone numbers, fax numbers, and pager and cell-phone numbers. It is necessary to understand the requirements of personnel certifications and licensing and to ensure the current copy is on file in the department. The department keeps operating certifications and licenses available for inspection by regulating agencies.

Department statistics are an important part of the duties of the AA. Tracking the number of patients and services being provided is critical to the operation of the department. Strategic planning, budget requests, and maintenance are based on statistics gathered, compiled, and tallied by the AA.

Computer skills are necessary in this position. The ability to understand software programs is valuable to anyone in this position. Basic training in word processing, database management, and spreadsheets are the minimum requirements. Advanced training will be an asset for the HUC and the department.

Scheduling the staff to accommodate the demands of the ever-increasing volume of patients is quite a challenge. An AA with a HUC background will use many of those skills while performing this task. Problem solving is essential when providing coverage 24 hours a day, 7 days a week, regardless of holidays, vacations, personal emergencies, or weather-related problems. The AA must juggle the staff so that people are working the days and hours they request and at the same time cover the department with the proper mix of services. On any given day/hour/minute, this can all change with a phone call; a staff member might be sick or have a sick child or relative. The nurse in the field may call and say he or she needs help with a difficult patient, or is unable to get to the last patient on the list because of car problems, or has a sick child. Any of these calls would require the AA to find a replacement to finish the daily visits.

Good organizational and time management skills are also used in this position. Scheduling periodic meetings for nurses, patient care conferences to update status and needs of patients, monthly staff meetings, and staff education may be part of the daily requirements.

As any HUC knows, whatever the job title, one of the duties always includes ordering supplies. In addition to routine office supplies, the AA may also order the necessary durable medical equipment. This includes such items as walkers, commodes, stool risers, and hospital beds. These items are loaned or rented to the patient for home use and are returned when the patient no longer needs them. Accurate records must be kept of this equipment. If the patient is renting equipment, the billing office needs to be informed. Maintenance of the inventory may also fall under the AA's duties.

Business/Office Manager

The HUC who accepts the role of business or office manager may perform all of the duties discussed so far in this chapter, with additional focus on supervision of others, financial responsibilities, and a greater level of independent decision making. In this position, management of the daily operations is the primary concern.

Management of personnel is a primary duty of any manager. This includes overseeing the duties and efficiency of all personnel. The payroll records and benefit hours are updated and maintained for all personnel. The business manager has the responsibility of interviewing and hiring new staff members. A more difficult aspect of the position is the discipline and dismissal of staff members. These duties require strong interpersonal skills and an understanding of how each employee fits into the operation and success of the whole department.

Billing and financial reports are a major concern of any organization or department. If the hospital-based home health department handles its own billing, the office manger is the person to oversee that process. This includes billing the patient or insurance company, dealing with billing problems, and making phone calls to patients or insurance companies. The manager must be familiar with and understand all federal and state regulations related to billing and collection activities. Many decisions must be made on a daily basis, and this requires good interpersonal and communication skills, in addition to leadership abilities.

Development and maintenance of the department budget, accounts receivable, and accounts payable are areas that can make the department a success or failure. The leadership team of the department develops the budget and determines how it will be managed. The manager is the person with the day-to-day accountability. This type of responsibility may require some additional education or a college degree.

Office equipment must be purchased and maintained. Computer hardware and software must be purchased and periodically upgraded. These are duties that the manager may see to personally or delegate to another staff member. In either instance, the manager must be knowledgeable and involved and have input on these decisions.

Community Liaison

This is an exciting and very challenging position. This person serves as a resource to internal and external customers on home health care and the variety of services offered by the home care department. Information on available services may be presented to other health care professionals, insurers, patients, and families, as well as to other institutions. Community groups provide opportunities for educational presentations on the home care department and the scope of services. Through these contacts, requests may come in for additional services that could benefit the community. The director may consider these ideas for future program development.

A HUC who is a "people person" should be right at home in this position. He or she will be able to take advantage of the relationships already established with physicians and staff members within the hospital to make this position a success. A public-speaking class is recommended to build confidence and learn how to use relaxation techniques in front of a large audience. Taking the course will also enhance one's resumé.

Closing Thoughts

The HUC can be a part of the home care team with a wide and varied scope of responsibility that depends on the size of the hospital or agency. The HUC's familiarity with the community, previously established relationships with physicians and staff, and general knowledge of medical terminology, diagnoses, treatments, and medications make the HUC a natural, and hitherto untapped, resource. Time management, interpersonal and communication skills, and the ability to work in an ever-changing environment are every bit as necessary in the home care department, as they are on any acute care unit.

A Final Thought:

Florence Nightingale: "My view you know is that the ultimate destination of all nursing is the nursing of the sick in their homes . . . I look to the abolition of all hospitals and workhouse infirmaries. But it is no use to talk about the year 2000."

Review Questions

1. Explain the chain of command in a hospital-based home care agency.
2. Name and describe in detail one clerical position found in a hospital-based home care agency.
3. List eight duties expected of the office manager.
4. The receptionist receives a call from Mrs. Chuc that her mother is forgetful, incontinent, and refusing hospitalization. She saw the doctor yesterday and is on medication for a urinary tract infection. She has Medicare Part A and John Hancock rather than Part B. Follow the course of action that should be taken with this referral and the hands it will pass through. Assume that the client is accepted for services.

Bibliography

Webster's II New Riverside Dictionary, revised edition. Boston, Houghton Mifflin Company, 1996.

23

Health Unit Coordinator Preceptor

Patty Sopko

Objectives

At the completion of this chapter, the reader should be able to:

1. Identify the four roles the title of health unit coordinator preceptor encompasses.
2. List six of the personal characteristics that the ideal preceptor should possess.
3. List five professional qualities that are necessary for the health unit coordinator preceptor.

Vocabulary

Advocate: Staff member responsible for the socialization process of the orientation program

Educator: Staff member responsible for the development of the educational plan for the orientation program

Mentor: Staff member who is recognized and well respected by both peers and managers for his or her leadership abilities and vision

Preceptor: Staff member who is responsible for an overall orientation program and whose position encompasses four roles: advocate, educator, role model, and mentor

Role model: Staff member who demonstrates desirable skills and qualities of a professional for trainees to model and incorporate into their own work habits

Overview

As a health unit coordinator (HUC) becomes proficient in technical, communication, and interpersonal skills over the years, the next step is to transmit this knowledge to future HUCs by serving in the role of preceptor. The role of a preceptor is a demanding one that, if done correctly, benefits not only the preceptor and trainee, but the institution as a whole. Statistics have shown over the years that a good orientation program, with an effective preceptor, has had a significant, positive effect on the issues of retention.

History

Little is written on how HUC precepting originated. It is believed that during World War II there was a shortage of nurses, and out of this grew a need to develop a nonclinical position that would allow the nurse to concentrate her efforts at the bedside. The term "ward clerk" was developed for the staff member who was responsible for all nonclinical-related tasks such as record keeping. The nurse initially oriented the "ward clerks" to the record-keeping responsibilities. Eventually, as more and more record keeping was required and more clerks hired, ward clerks took over the responsibility of orienting the new ward clerks, and nurses focused on orienting the new nurses.

As the role of the HUC expanded over the years, on-the-job training was replaced by educational programs, either through the hospital or in learning institutions. The first such programs were established in conjunction with vocational schools in the latter part of the 1960s. Now almost every state has at least one, and many states have several HUC educational programs in vocational and community colleges. These courses provide the foundation on which technical skills are built. They are then further developed on the nursing units with the assistance of HUC preceptors.

Definition

The title of *preceptor* encompasses four roles in one: **role model**, **educator**, **advocate**, and **mentor** (Fig. 23–1). A role model relationship is passive on both parts and requires one member of the relationship (the trainee) to be a novice and one member of the relationship to be an expert in a particular field. This role enables the trainee to observe an expert at work and model what is seen and adopt behaviors as his or her own. It is the initial relationship of the orientation period and continues until the trainee becomes confident in his or her ability to develop personal work habits.

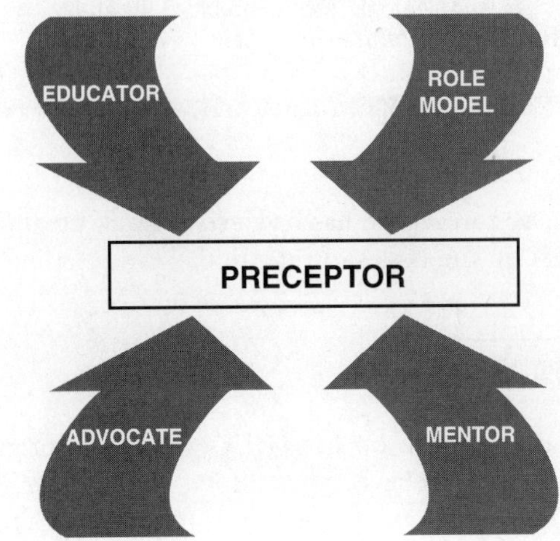

Figure 23–1
The roles of a preceptor.

The role of advocate is an ongoing relationship. This alliance should be initiated at first contact with the trainee and usually continues for years to come. In this role, the preceptor introduces the trainee to the workplace and is present to resolve any difficult situations that arise throughout the training period. After the orientation period, the advocate assists the novice to develop the skills necessary to resolve independently any difficult situations that might arise.

As an educator, a HUC preceptor has the responsibility of setting objectives, planning learning experiences, setting short- and long-term educational goals, providing continuous feedback and formal evaluations, and guiding the transition of a HUC trainee into a fully independent and functional member of the nursing unit team. As this role comes to an end when the trainee completes the orientation period, the preceptor and trainee move into the last type of relationship, if both desire it.

The mentor role is perhaps the most complex. It is a mutually chosen relationship between expert and novice. The mentor fosters and nurtures the growth, learning, and socialization processes that were initiated at the beginning of the orientation period. Mentors are respected for their expertise, personal traits, and promotion of the role of the HUC throughout the institution.

Hospital administrators must be made aware that to function effectively in all of these roles, the preceptor must be provided with the appropriate knowledge and tools. Most HUCs have received their training through hospital-based programs or on-the-job training that did not include concepts related to the development of educational programs. The ideal preparation for any type of preceptor would be a formal workshop that stresses key principles of adult education and assists the future preceptors in developing educational plans. This chapter outlines these key principles and elements of a sound educational plan.

Personal and Professional Qualities and Characteristics

Before setting up an effective orientation program, the most desirable applicants must be selected to fulfill the role of preceptor. It is not a role that every technically expert HUC can or will wish to fulfill. The desirable preceptor should be highly motivated to assume this additional role because HUCs who act as preceptors will be expected to maintain their current level of functioning in addition to providing a sound orientation and educational experience for a HUC trainee.

The ideal preceptor should possess some or all of the following personal qualities and characteristics: a high degree of professionalism, excellent communication and interpersonal skills, optimism, self-confidence, patience, and a nonjudgmental attitude.

Professional qualifications that are mandatory include technical expertise—at least 2 years' experience as a HUC in the specific institution; being based in a unit (HUCs who float on a daily basis do not provide the stability that is necessary during the initial orientation period); not being involved in any disciplinary issues; being well respected by the nursing staff and management; and being committed to being available for work during the initial weeks of the orientation period. It is also desirable to use HUCs who are full time or to use two part-time HUCs on the same unit who use the same approaches to fulfilling their job duties and responsibilities. Preceptor consistency is paramount to an effective orientation program that can be completed in a relatively short time, between 6 and 8 weeks, depending on the experience of the trainee.

When asked, trainees ranked the following characteristics as those of the most desirable preceptor: cooperativeness, kindness, patience, having wide interests, pleasantness, impartiality, a sense of humor, a good disposition, intervenes in difficult situations, provides recognition, flexibility, and technical proficiency. These characteristics seem to provide the secure environment that trainees are seeking as they acquire new skills.

Once preceptors have been selected, based on the aforementioned personal and professional qualities and characteristics, job duties and responsibilities should be discussed to ensure their ability to succeed in this role.

Job Duties and Responsibilities

Job duties and responsibilities can be divided into the four roles that were discussed at the beginning of the chapter. Role model responsibilities include adherence to the institution's policies and procedures; regular attendance at workshops and inservices to enhance knowledge base; excellent time management and organizational skills; being a team player; accuracy with the processing of physician orders and other HUC tasks; and effective communication and interpersonal skills. It is crucial that these behaviors are demonstrated at all times when functioning in the role of preceptor because the trainee is continually adopting personal work behaviors based on what is observed.

Responsibilities of the educator role include the design, implementation, and evaluation of educational and orientation programs to ensure that trainees are exposed to the optimal experiences and are becoming fully integrated members of the nursing unit. The educator guides the trainee to appropriate learning experiences and provides timely evaluations of progress. The educator must recognize individuality when planning these learning activities and provide direct supervision while moving the trainee from the role of observer to the role of HUC.

The advocate role responsibilities are more subjective and serve to assist with the socialization process. In this role, trainees need to be equipped with the necessary tools that will enable them to deal with inevitable confrontations and difficult situations. One of the most helpful and far-reaching responsibilities that the advocate can assume would be to assist the trainee to develop a peer support group that would give him or her the opportunity to share joint concerns, validate feelings, and resolve problems in the years to come. The advocate assists the trainee in the socialization process of the nursing unit as well, and the process is expedited when the preceptor displays a positive and impartial attitude toward staff members.

The mentor's primary responsibilities include encouragement of career advancement; promotion of the HUC role both at the nursing unit level and throughout the institution; encouragement of the growth and expansion of the HUC role; giving vision; and providing emotional support and encouragement.

Development of an Orientation Program

First and foremost, preceptors must be educated on the basic principles of adult learning (Table 23–1). By understanding these principles, the preceptor is better able to develop an orientation program that meets the needs of an adult learner.

A sound orientation program should be set up so that the trainee moves progressively through the development of the most simple of skills to the most complex in a manner that makes sense. A good starting point is always a classroom situation for the trainee who has no background in the HUC field. Classroom time should be focused on introducing the trainee to the topics (Table 23–2). This background information forms the foundation on which the technical skills should be built, so that the trainee understands the policies and procedures behind the task. In the absence of formal classroom time, the preceptor takes on this responsibility as well as guiding the trainee to develop the necessary technical skills. Medical terminology is vital as well, and if it is not available as a class in the hospital setting, the trainee should be referred to another source such as continuing adult education courses offered at area high schools or courses in a college setting. Attempting to cover medical terminology on the nursing unit is impossible in view of all of the technical procedures that must be covered during the orientation period, and a good foundation in medical terminology enables the trainee to acquire more quickly the skill of transcribing physician orders that is a large part of the HUC's role on a nursing unit.

Technical objectives should be outlined for trainees and given to them before their first day on the nursing unit. Technical objectives should list the skills that the trainee will have to be able to perform independently to complete successfully the technical part of the orientation program (Fig. 23–2). This type of outline allows the trainee to progress from the role of observer to an independently functioning member of the nursing unit and to see this progress clearly from week to week. Technical objectives should be set following the outline of the classroom topics and should encompass all skills expected of HUCs in the institution.

Once classroom and clinical expectations have been developed, evaluation tools should be created to match the objectives of both. Administering daily tests in the classroom setting is a good indicator of the trainee's understanding of written material presented. Tests should be administered based on material presented the previous day as well as medical terminology reviews that pertain to those particular subjects. Trainees should be informed that they are required to meet a certain average to complete the didactic portion of the training program. This ensures that the trainee reviews the material each night and continues to build the knowledge base that will make the transition to the nursing unit skills easier. Trainees who have no experience as HUCs should be expected to go through the classroom portion of the training program. Experienced HUCs, on the other hand, who are transferring to the institution from another should bypass the classroom portion of the orientation program and proceed directly to the technical portion.

The example document listing technical objectives in Figure 23–2 can also be used as an evalua-

Table 23-1 **PRINCIPLES OF ADULT LEARNING**

Principles of Adult Learning	Suggestions for Preceptors
Adults pursue accuracy rather than speed.	Proceed slowly from one duty to the next. Allow time to become proficient before demanding speed. Provide time for practice.
Adults have increasing self-reliance, autonomy, and inner directedness.	Keep them involved in all aspects of the learning activities. Meet daily to determine short- and long-term goals that will achieve the objectives of the orientation program. Allow self-paced learning.
Adults underestimate their ability to learn—they lack confidence.	Build on previously learned and mastered material each day before moving on to a new topic. Offer praise frequently.
Adults rely increasingly on prior knowledge and experience.	Tie learning to prior knowledge, current abilities, and skills. Teach through actual experience as much as possible.
Short-term memory declines while long-term memory improves.	Allow for frequent opportunities to practice newly acquired skills. Provide written material and instructions whenever possible.
Vision and hearing ability decline.	Take opportunities to instruct away from the nursing station whenever possible (e.g., review transcription of physician orders verbally in a remote spot). Make sure there is adequate lighting.
Energy level is lower and reaction speed becomes slower.	Arrange for breaks even if the preceptor cannot get away from the desk. Interactive training keeps energy levels up.
Adults are oriented toward solving immediate problems and making immediate applications.	When training, ensure that the trainee understands how to apply what is taught to everyday job duties and responsibilities. Do not give a lot of history or background information—give step-by-step instructions.
Adult individual differences are more pronounced than those of younger learners.	Use daily meetings to individualize teaching plans. Encourage individuals to select their own modes for learning and to set their own pace.
Adults need to feel comfortable taking risks and experimenting with what they have learned.	Rely less on significant risk-taking in planned learning activities. Offer praise and support often as well as constructive criticism aimed at the activity versus the trainee.

tion tool. Trainees should be given a listing of all technical objectives that must be completed by the end of the orientation period to consider the orientation period complete. Each week, the trainee and preceptor should go through the list of technical objectives together and update the trainee's progress. The length of time it takes the trainee to progress from observer to "doer" varies depending on the degree of difficulty of the skill. This list of technical skills can also be used to set goals for the next week on a new set of skills. Once the trainee has become adept at a skill and performs it independently, there is no need to continue to evaluate that skill (unless a problem

Table 23–2 CLASSROOM TOPICS

1. Health unit coordinating
   a. History of health unit coordination
   b. Job description
   c. General duties
   d. Dress code

2. Hospital environment
   a. Hospital philosophy
   b. Mission statement
   c. Hospital organization
      i. Administrative
      ii. Medical staff
      iii. Nursing service
   d. Hospital departments and services
      i. Business
      ii. Diagnostic/therapeutic services
      iii. Support services
      iv. Operational

3. Safety and infection control
   a. Disaster plans
   b. Safety codes
   c. Incident reports
   d. Isolation indicators/procedures

4. Communication/interpersonal skills
   a. Communication devices
   b. Taking messages
   c. Communicating skills
   d. Confidentiality
   e. Assertive vs. aggressive behavior

5. Patient's chart
   a. Documentation
   b. Imprinter card/holder
   c. Standard/supplemental chart forms
   d. Consents
   e. Maintaining patient chart
   f. Thinning the chart
   g. Chart copies

6. Transcription of physician orders
   a. Symbols
   b. Order sets
   c. Kardexing
   d. Signing-off

7. Orders
   a. Nursing observation orders
   b. Patient activity/positioning orders
   c. Nursing treatment orders
   d. Dietary orders
   e. Pharmacy orders
   f. Laboratory orders

Table 23–2 CLASSROOM TOPICS *(Continued)*

   g. Diagnostic/therapeutic orders
   h. Miscellaneous orders
      i. Consultations
      ii. Social service orders
      iii. Transfer/discharge orders

8. Health unit coordination procedures
   a. Admission procedures
   b. Discharge, transfer, postmortem procedures
   c. Diets
   d. Filing
   e. Maintaining forms/supplies
   f. Computer basics

arises), and attention should be focused on the remaining skills. It cannot be stressed enough how important the formal weekly evaluation meetings are to both the preceptor and the trainee. This weekly meeting helps keep the trainee focused and verifies where the trainee is in the orientation program. It also eliminates confusion on the trainee's part as to progress in the program, and allows estimation of when the training program should be completed.

Weekly evaluations should be enough for the trainee who seems to be progressing at a good rate. However, trainees who are having problems with specific technical skills need a more detailed daily evaluation (Fig. 23–3). This daily evaluation should be completed at the end of each day by the trainee and the preceptor. If problems persist despite these daily evaluations, the preceptor should direct the concerns to either the nursing unit manager or the director of the HUC training program.

Once the classroom, clinical, and evaluation aspects of a training program are developed, they can be used over and over from year to year. Only minor revisions, such as the addition of new tasks to the HUC job description or changes in policies and procedures of the institution, would need to be done. If the foundation is good, the program will serve the institution well for years to come.

Good measures of this foundation are program and preceptor evaluations that are completed by

Communication Technical Objectives

Communication Devices

Please mark each objective with the following:
1 = Trainee observed
2 = Trainee performed with assistance
3 = Trainee is able to perform without assistance

When a "3" is attained–the objective no longer need be evaluated.

Behavioral Objectives	Week One	Week Two	Week Three	Week Four	Week Five	Week Six	Week Seven	Week Eight	Comments by Preceptor
Answers the telephone properly identifying hospital, unit, name and title.									
Records and communicates phone messages accurately.									
Able to effectively communicate with the patient and RN via the unit intercom.									
Correctly uses the hospital paging system.									
Able to send documents accurately to various destinations via the fax machine.									

Figure 23–2
Technical objectives.

Daily HUC Trainee Evaluation Tool

Name________________________ Preceptor ________________________

Technical Skill: ____________________ Date: ________________________

Strengths	**Weaknesses**
____________________	____________________
____________________	____________________
____________________	____________________
____________________	____________________

Steps to Achieve Technical Skill:

____

____

____

Date for Completion: ________________________

Supervisor Comments:

Trainee Comments:

Figure 23–3
Daily evaluation.

the trainee at the end of the program. These evaluations can be quite eye-opening and alert the preceptor to aspects of the program that may need to be changed, including aspects of the preceptor as well as the program itself.

Effective Approaches to Precepting

The following concepts should be incorporated into the overall orientation program to enable the preceptor to conduct more thorough and effective one-on-one instruction. First and most important of all, the preceptor should contact the trainee before the first day on the nursing unit. This helps to initiate a rapport that will make the first day on the unit less threatening to the trainee. It gives the trainee a familiar face in the midst of an unfamiliar territory. It also allows the trainee the time to ask questions about the unit and to prepare for the first day.

While on the unit, the preceptor should present new skills to the trainee in a progressive demonstration method, as noted on the evaluation form. The preceptor should demonstrate the skill, then the trainee can perform the skill while the preceptor observes, and finally the trainee performs the skill alone. Each day should be planned so progression occurs from the easiest skill to the most complex. This type of planning reduces frustration and decreases training time. As the orientation program progresses, the preceptor should gradually reduce the amount of coaching provided so that the trainee becomes more independent. Too much coaching and constant supervision throughout the program will prove detrimental to the trainee when he or she finishes the program and is expected to function independently on a nursing unit.

Although too much coaching may cause problems in the future, this does not eliminate the need for daily feedback. Trainees need positive reinforcement to validate that there are skills they do well while they are learning the more difficult ones. Positive reinforcement should be given while the trainee is performing a new skill and again at the end of the day. This technique ends the day on a positive note, and the trainee leaves feeling good about what was accomplished that day and looking forward to another day.

Roadblocks to Success

Despite adequate preparation, throughout the course of the orientation program the preceptor may encounter certain roadblocks that are negatively affecting progress. The following tips may be helpful in dealing with the trainee and helping to overcome these obstacles. The biggest and easiest to overcome is trainee or preceptor fatigue. One-on-one training is intense and requires a vast amount of mental concentration and at times physical energy. Stop training at the first sign of fatigue, regardless if it is trainee or preceptor fatigue. It is a waste of time to continue training at this point. A quick break renews energy levels and allows for quicker processing of information than does a fatigued brain.

When working with experienced HUCs, the preceptor may also encounter a difficulty known as the "know-it-all" trainee. These trainees constantly resist learning new ways of doing skills they had perfected in other jobs. When you encounter trainees of this type, try to disarm them by purposely asking them to share their experiences and ideas. Use this technique sparingly and only at times when it appears that they are feeling uncomfortable with a procedural change involved in learning a new skill. This not only validates their experience and themselves as professionals, but may enlighten you with new ideas.

When matching up preceptors with trainees, it is most effective to use a specific learning style assessment tool to make the relationship more successful. Gregorc: Style Delineator, Myers-Briggs Type Indicator, or Witkin: Group Embedded Figures Test are examples of learning style assessment tools that can be used with both the preceptors and trainees to determine the most desirable pairings. Research shows that greater learning takes place, time needed for learning is reduced, and learners retain information longer when learning styles are matched.

Despite these tests, however, two people may still end up working together whose styles of learning vary greatly. If it appears that the preceptor and the trainee are having constant problems in communicating, it may be time to approach the trainee with a general question such as "Is there something I can do to make this program more meaningful to you and to help us communicate better?" The trainee may offer helpful suggestions that make the program run much smoother, or both parties may come to the conclusion that it is not in the best interests of either to continue the relationship, and perhaps a new preceptor should be arranged. This situation should not preclude someone being a preceptor again. It happens occasionally despite the best efforts put forth to match trainees with preceptors. Personality types vary between people all the time, and the best thing to do is recognize it and try to alter the situation to provide an optimal orientation program.

Closing Thoughts

Skilled preceptors are a valuable asset to an institution. Success as a preceptor is greatly dependent on adequate preparation by the institution. Although time and energy are needed up front to develop and implement a sound orientation program, the benefits are far reaching for the preceptor, trainee, and institution as a whole.

Review Questions

1. Identify the four roles the title of health unit coordinator preceptor encompasses.
2. List five of the personal characteristics that the ideal preceptor should possess.
3. List four professional qualities that are necessary for the health unit coordinator preceptor.

Bibliography

Buckley R, Caple J: One-to-One Training and Coaching Skills. San Diego, Pfeiffer and Company, 1991.

Cantwell ER, Kahn MH, Lacey MR, McLaughlin EF: Survey of current hospital preceptorship programs in greater Philadelphia area. J Nursing Staff Dev 1989;5:225.

Carroll P: Using personality styles to enhance preceptor programs. Dimensions of Critical Care Nursing 1992; 11(2):114.

Fox V, Rothrock J, Skelton M: The mentoring relationship. AORN J 1992;56:858.

Hill E, Lowenstein L: Preceptors, valuable members of the orientation process. AORN J 1992;55:1237.

Pryor F: Training the Trainer. Shawnee Mission, KS, Pryor Resources, 1996.

Schneller S, Hoeppner M: Preceptor development. J Nursing Staff Dev 1994;10:249.

24 The Health Unit Coordinator Supervisor

Nancy Fuerstenau Cutler

Objectives

Upon completion of this chapter, the reader should be able to:

1. List at least ten responsibilities of a health unit coordinator supervisor.
2. Identify the course base of clinical and business courses that a person should take in preparation for the position of health unit coordinator supervisor.
3. Name two Do and two Don't techniques of good management.

Vocabulary

Management: An organization's executives

Nonclinical/Clerical: Refers to the indirect tasks performed for a patient that support the direct or clinical patient care

Supervisor: A member of the administrative team who is accountable for managing a group and responsible for outcome

History

The health unit coordinator (HUC) **supervisor** position is a relatively new position in an institution's middle management structure. Formerly, a registered nurse (usually the nurse manager) supervised both the clinical and the clerical entities in a given department/unit. However, with many different reorganizations and paradigm shifts in health care **management** levels, in many hospitals it may become necessary to have a clinical and a clerical expert in designated supervisory roles. In parallel roles, the clinical manager and the clerical (HUC) supervisor are able to complement each other as their expertise dictates. A more harmonious department results as the manager and supervisor meld and balance their subordinates' clinical and clerical duties and responsibilities. Better support and better communication can be established with this type of supervisory composition.

Job Title

In today's health care world, the HUC supervisor may have a variety of job titles and may be responsible for subordinates in numerous units, areas, or buildings in the management structure of the health care system. Patient-focused care across the continuum is one of the optimum health care models being structured in organizations to take health care into the 21st century. Using this structure, a multidisciplinary team of caregivers is aligned under the management of a care coordinator. HUCs may also report to the more traditional nurse manager. In other instances, organizational hierarchy may direct that clinical professionals report to a registered nurse and that allied health care professionals report to an expert in his or her designated field. The HUC supervisor therefore can be found in several different positions under a system's organizational chart.

Overview of Position

Job Summary

The HUC supervisor is a health care professional responsible for providing competent and skilled HUCs to designated departments and nursing units in health care facilities. The HUC supervisor possesses expert knowledge in all facets of the HUC's duties and responsibilities. In carrying out the specific requirements for HUC supervision, this supervisor focuses on the institution's mission statement placing primary importance on the vision to assist in delivering the highest value to all internal and external customers.

Immediate Supervisor

The health system's organizational chart clearly depicts the line reporting structure of the HUC supervisor. The HUC supervisor most likely reports to a clinical service director, who usually reports to a clinical or patient care services vice president of the organization (Fig. 24–1). Modern health care systems comprise numerous entities. This composition can include any combination or all of the following: several hospitals, numerous clinics, a home health care division, and a variety of specialty services and centers such as physical medicine and rehabilitation, addiction treatment centers, and extended and long-term care facilities. Many systems are structuring "product lines and services" combining many of the traditional hospital departments under uniform management to address more appropriately patient flow and care needs. Numerous organizations have provided for career ladders for specific positions. The HUC position is one that fits well into selected career ladder models. There may be "lead"{C}-HUCs or "senior" {C}HUCs who assume specific managerial tasks and responsibilities. These lead or senior {C}HUCs are accountable to the unit or department manager or director.

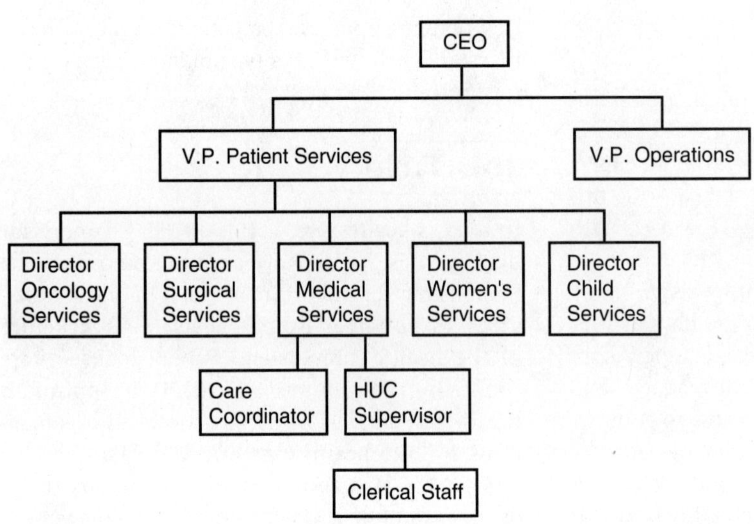

Figure 24–1
Skeletal organizational chart depicting HUC supervisor reporting hierarchy.

Position Responsibilities and Duties

The specific duties and responsibilities of the HUC supervisor include a myriad of tasks performed by all supervisors. This section highlights most of the jobs for which the supervisor is held accountable, and offers a brief description of each.

Hiring

The supervisor must possess expert knowledge of the duties and responsibilities of the HUC position. He or she needs to be skilled in the art of interviewing. With the correct job knowledge and interviewing skills, the supervisor is able to hire the correct person for the open HUC position. It is also extremely important to hire a HUC who is a graduate of a HUC program. These graduates most likely will enter the position with a higher level of qualifications.

Terminating

When terminating an employee, it is best to do so during the employee's probationary period (this is usually 90 days after the date of hire). If this is not an option, the supervisor must work closely with the human resources department (personnel) to follow the detailed protocol for terminating an employee. Clear, concise, and specific documentation is of utmost importance. There may be circumstances that require immediate termination of an employee (e.g., breach of confidentiality; theft), and supervisors need to be cognizant of these guidelines in the employee handbook and personnel policy and procedure manual.

Disciplining

Circumstances may arise (e.g., consistently reporting late for duty; repeated absences; continually working overtime without authorized approval) in which the supervisor will be required to confront and discipline the subordinate. The unacceptable behavior patterns may require additional support and counseling, and the supervisor should be aware of various options offered to the employee by the organization. The HUC supervisor will be expected to know the "steps of discipline" outlined in the personnel policies and procedure manual. Clear, concise, and specific documentation is a requirement the supervisor must fulfill.

Orientation

Every HUC supervisor should have a detailed orientation program when new employees are hired or transferred into a different department. The basic orientation usually begins with the overall organization orientation. This may cover the personnel policies and procedures, followed by a specific department/unit orientation. The unit orientation consists of individualized departmental policies and procedures and includes how they support the system's overall mission and vision statements. The orientation process usually concludes with the new HUC orienting to the daily routine side by side with a preceptor HUC. This preceptor may be the new HUC's mentor for a period of time after the actual orientation process is completed. The supervisor is responsible for scheduling and monitoring the employee's orientation process. Before completion of the employee's orientation, there should be a validation and evaluation process to ensure that the employee can function at the desired level of competence.

Training

It is paramount that the HUC possess the necessary knowledge, skills, and tools to perform the many aspects of the HUC position competently. Regardless of the HUC's education level at the time of hiring, the supervisor must be equipped with adequate training materials to evaluate the HUC's knowledge and skill level properly. The supervisor is responsible for all aspects of the HUC's training to ensure the desired competency level is attained and maintained. An excellent tool for the supervisor to use is a HUC performance-based development system. Training materials include medical terminology, anatomy and physiology, human relations, medical/legal aspects, transcription of physician orders, and telephone, computer, and other clerical duties requiring HUC management on a daily basis. HUC supervisors should encourage and promote National Association of Health Unit Coordinators (NAHUC) certification and recertification in conjunction with NAHUC membership. Continuing education is mandatory to keep employees aware and competent in current and changing practices and procedures. The HUC supervisor is responsible for scheduling and monitoring all training and continuing education classes for HUCs. The supervisor may also be the primary educator at these classes and in-services.

Health Unit Coordinator Coverage

The HUC supervisor is the most appropriate person to determine the amount of clerical support required for nursing units and departments. The supervisor possesses the knowledge needed to evaluate the quantity of work and the time needed to process all the clerical tasks. Therefore, using work volume and patient days, the HUC supervisor is able to establish first-, second-, and third-shift HUC coverage. Hours of service also dictate specific staffing parameters. One unit may require HUC coverage 24 hours a day; another unit's volume may be allocated only first-shift coverage and partial evening staffing. Weekends and holidays must be considered when establishing staffing patterns.

Health Unit Coordinator Staffing Schedules

Once HUC coverage has been determined for the nursing unit or department, the HUC supervisor's responsibility is to complete weekly, monthly, or quarterly staffing schedules. This is a meld of the required hours needing coverage and the full-time and part-time HUC positions allocated to the unit. All designated days and hours are filled in as blocks by the supervisor until the staffing pattern is completed. There are numerous staffing algorithms. These formulas consist of creating a pattern of days and hours requiring staffing. The supervisor's challenge is to complete the grid with the employees available. Requests and personal preferences are noted and taken into consideration as the schedule permits. Schedules are usually completed in 4- or 6-week intervals to allow employees to plan. Once schedules are completed and posted, it is normally the employee's responsibility to trade and arrange for a replacement if he or she cannot work a scheduled day. The supervisor is responsible to arrange for coverage in employee emergency situations and scheduled benefit time off (Fig. 24–2).

Health Unit Coordinator Staffing Budget

All supervisors are required to complete yearly budgets. An organization's budget process for the next fiscal/budget year usually begins months before the end of the current fiscal year. The finance department may offer budget workshops with an explanation of the next fiscal year's budget process and the forms to be completed. Two primary portions of the expense budget are the position control portion and the supply, equipment, and expense portion. The revenue budget comprises charges the unit or department generates for special care or procedures above and beyond the room rate charge. The staffing budget (Fig. 24–3) includes not only the hours for which the HUC was hired but also his or her benefit hours such as vacation and illness and holiday hours. Shift differential also must be taken into account, as well as merit increments. The other major components of a department's expense budget (Fig. 24–4) are supplies, maintenance, travel, and educational seminars. Considerations are needed for medical record forms, office supplies such as computer printer cartridges, and much more. Once the budget is prepared and accepted, the supervisor has the

Weekly Staffing Schedule							
NAME	09/20 Mon	09/21 Tue	09/22 Wed	09/23 Thu	09/24 Fri	09/25 Sat	09/26 Sun
C-4	**SURGICAL**						
J. Doe	---	7-3	7-3	7-3	7-3	---	---
M. Doe	7-3	3-11				7-3	7-3
S. Doe	3-11	---	3-11	3-11	3-11	---	---
V. Doe	3-11 (C3)					3-11	3-11
C-3	**MEDICAL**						
B. Jones	7-3	7-3	7-3	7-3	---	7-3	7-3
K. Jones	---	3-11	3-11	3-11	3-11	---	---
P. Jones	---				7-3	3-11	3-11

Figure 24–2
Weekly staffing schedule.

responsibility for remaining within those budgetary parameters. Review of revenue and expense reports must happen on a routine basis and variances must be documented, reported, and explained.

Evaluations

A new HUC's performance should be evaluated before the end of the probationary period. Performance appraisals are then usually performed annually. A performance appraisal may or may not

STAFFING BUDGET
Health Unit Coordinator Position Control

POS. #	HOURS	REG / JURY / ILL / VAC *PAY CODES* HOL/OT/											RATE	SHIFT
	FT/PT	99	98	97	96	95	94	93	92	91	90	89		
#1	FT	2080		40	80				48				10.00	
#2	PT	1040		24	40				24				10.00	2nd
#3	FT	2080		40	80				48				10.00	2nd
#4	PT	880		16	32				24				10.00	

Figure 24–3
Staffing budget.

EXPENSE BUDGET DETAIL

DEPARTMENT NAME: ______ DEPARTMENT COST CENTER: ______

PREPARED BY: ______ APPROVED BY: ______

FOR CALENDAR YEAR: ______ DATE PREPARED: ______

SUPPLIES/EXPENSES:

MONTH

	Jan.	Feb.	Mar.	April	May	June	July	Aug.	Sept.	Oct.	Nov.	Dec.
Printed Forms												
Office Supplies												
Repairs & Maint.												
Other Supplies												
Travel												
Emp. Dev. Seminar												

Figure 24–4
Expense budget.

be an indication for a merit increment. Performance appraisals should be scheduled well in advance, allowing both the HUC and the supervisor to be adequately prepared. If the employee and supervisor have been in the practice of open communication, a performance appraisal should contain no surprises. The most productive review sessions occur when both the supervisor and the HUC have come to the conference with forms completed for discussion (Figs. 24–5 and 24–6). The supervisor needs to remain open for negotiation and compromise. Do evaluations on time! When the performance appraisal is tied to a merit increment, the supervisor is required to complete forms for the human resources and payroll departments.

Supervision

A supervisor's schedule may call for meetings and conferences out of the departments, divisions, or units. Therefore, spending time with each HUC on a daily basis may be difficult. It is important that the supervisor interact with the HUCs as often as time permits. There may be peak periods during work hours when the supervisor needs to supply additional support to the HUC. The supervisor must also be aware of census and work load fluctuations to alter staffing for optimum productivity. HUC supervisors need to be knowledgeable of the HUCs' daily duties and responsibilities to ensure that all tasks are completed, orders transcribed in a timely manner, and customer needs are met. By daily interaction with HUCs, the supervisor can acquire a better understanding of how they perform their assigned daily duties. Communication becomes more frequent and praise and constructive criticism can be offered without defensiveness.

Resource and Liaison

The HUC supervisor should possess the expertise in the **nonclinical/clerical** functions required to

HEALTH UNIT COORDINATOR
Performance Appraisal Form

Employee Name: ______________________ Employee Number: ______________________
Job Title: ______________________ Department: ______________________
Supervisor: ______________________ Composite Performance Rank: ______________

PERFORMANCE ANCHORS

Rank 1: EXCEPTIONAL Rank 2: ABOVE EXPECTATIONS Rank 3: MEETS

Rank 4: IMPROVEMENT REQUIRED Rank 5: BELOW STANDARDS-PROBATION

PERFORMANCE DIMENSIONS

____ –Specific Duties/Responsibilities Related to Job Description/Competency List
____ –Professionalism
____ –Quality Improvement
____ –Communication Skills
____ –Support Processes

(Descriptions listed for all ANCHORS under each DIMENSION)

Supervisor Signature/Date: ______________________
Employee Signature/Date: ______________________

Figure 24–5
Supervisor's evaluation form.

run a nursing unit or department efficiently and effectively. When questions are asked or assistance needed by another department, the HUC supervisor has the opportunity to be an expert resource. This interaction and communication enhances the harmonious relationships between departments and units, fostering increased internal customer satisfaction. Quality improvement is a matter in which every supervisor takes an active role.

Payroll

Every supervisor is involved with the time and attendance functions payroll uses to issue employee paychecks. Most HUCs receive an hourly wage (vs. salaried employees). Therefore, records are kept when the HUC reports for duty and when the HUC is off duty. An employee's meal period is usually not included as work time, although normal break periods are considered as paid time. Many health systems pay their employees on a biweekly basis. Work hours are recorded for a 2-week period and totaled. This is the responsibility of the HUC. Record methodologies differ from institution to institution. Hours can be entered into a computer, punched into a time clock, or recorded on a time card. Time codes are entered with the number of hours to designate the appropriate type of hours to be paid (e.g., regular hours, sick time, vacation time). The supervisor's responsibility is to validate that the HUC has recorded the correct hours worked with the correct shift differential and the correct department/unit cost center. A supervisor may be required to sign individual time cards or a computer printout of the cost center and all employees' time. There is usually a deadline for supervisors to submit time and attendance records to payroll. Once this deadline has passed, the supervisor receives a printout of the time codes and hours to be paid each employee. The supervisor must check these sheets and make and report any necessary corrections. There is also a correction deadline. Super-

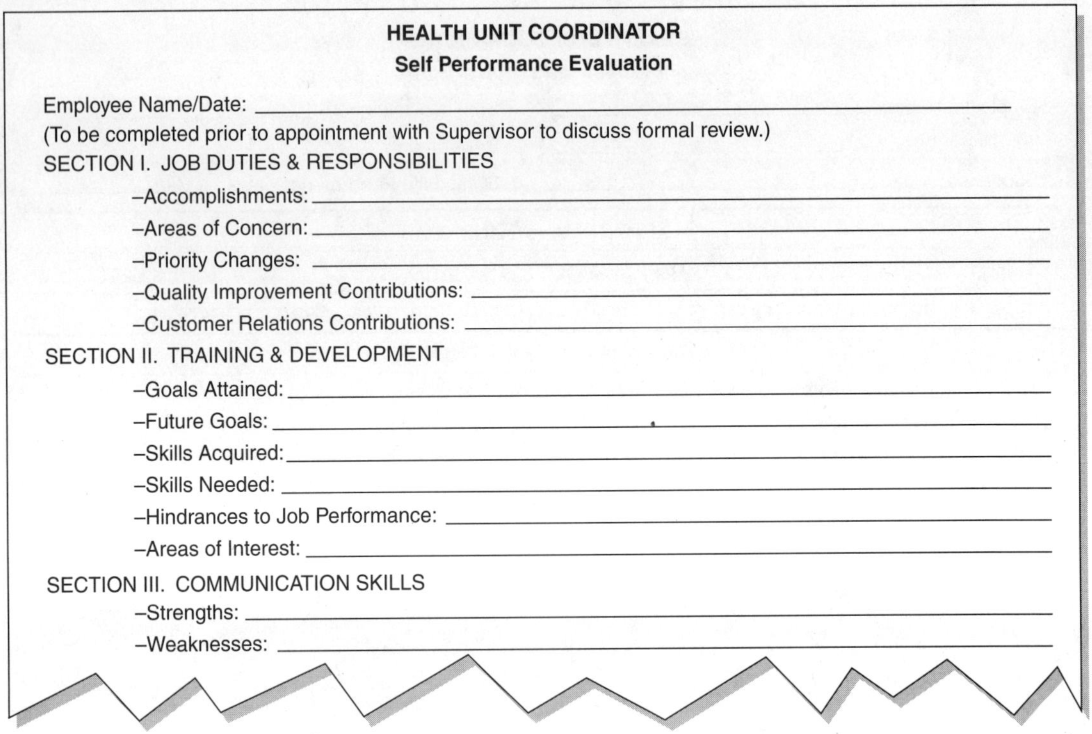

HEALTH UNIT COORDINATOR
Self Performance Evaluation

Employee Name/Date: ____________________

(To be completed prior to appointment with Supervisor to discuss formal review.)

SECTION I. JOB DUTIES & RESPONSIBILITIES

–Accomplishments: ____________________

–Areas of Concern: ____________________

–Priority Changes: ____________________

–Quality Improvement Contributions: ____________________

–Customer Relations Contributions: ____________________

SECTION II. TRAINING & DEVELOPMENT

–Goals Attained: ____________________

–Future Goals: ____________________

–Skills Acquired: ____________________

–Skills Needed: ____________________

–Hindrances to Job Performance: ____________________

–Areas of Interest: ____________________

SECTION III. COMMUNICATION SKILLS

–Strengths: ____________________

–Weaknesses: ____________________

Figure 24–6
Employee's self-evaluation form.

visors need to be extremely concise and accurate when validating employee time and attendance. No employee is happy when his or her paycheck is incorrect—even when the primary responsibility for time and attendance lies with the employee (Figs. 24–7 to 24–9).

Health Unit Coordinator Job Descriptions

The HUC supervisor is responsible for the department's or unit's HUC job descriptions. If there is no HUC job description, the supervisor is accountable for authoring the job description. The job description states the level of the position and salary grade or range. There will be a descriptive summary of the job and a detailed listing of duties and responsibilities. The job description must also state the education and experience requirements the HUC must possess. Along with educational stipulations, most job descriptions list applicant qualifications. There may be a general system-wide HUC job description with numerous addenda outlining specialty department/unit duty and responsibility differentiations. On an ongoing basis (at least yearly), the HUC supervisor must review and revise HUC job descriptions. There must be a process in place whereby all existing copies are updated and distributed to appropriate personnel.

Health Unit Coordinator Policy and Procedure Manual

Every position in a health care organization requires that its duties and responsibilities be outlined and explained in a policy and procedure

EMPLOYEE TIME CARD

Employee Name: Mary Doe

DATE	TIME IN	TIME OUT	TIME CODE	HOURS	SHIFT CODE	COST CENTER
M: 9/20	0700	1530	99	8.0	1	999.999
T: 9/21	1500	2330	99	8.0	2	999.999
W: 9/22						
T: 9/23						
F: 9/24						
S: 9/25	0700	1530	99	8.0	1	999.999
S: 9/26	0700	1530	99	8.0	1	999.999

CODES: 99=Reg Hrs 97=Ill 95=On Call 93=Orientation 91=Overtime
98=Jury Duty 96=Vac 94=Funeral Leave 92=Holiday Hrs

Figure 24–7
Employee time card.

(standards of practice) manual. These are the guidelines that can be used to assist in monitoring employee performance and subsequent productivity. The HUC supervisor is responsible for formulating these standards of HUC practice and reviewing and revising as necessary (at least annually). A mechanism should be in place to ensure that all holders of the manuals have the most current standards and that staff is made aware of all additions, deletions, and revisions. The primary content of the HUC policy and procedure manual pertains to the clerical (nonclinical) support functions the HUC performs in his or her intricate role as a member of the health care team. Detailed in the procedures are transcription, receptionist, and secretarial duties and responsibilities. Often the HUC policy and procedure manual cross-references other departmental policy and procedure manuals (e.g., lab, radiology, dietary) when featuring specific transcription protocols. The HUC policy and procedure manual is a critical element in an organization's documentation of transcription of physician's orders.

Health Unit Coordinator In-Services and Mandatory Meetings

Weekly, biweekly, or monthly meetings/in-services are important mechanisms for HUC interaction and communication. The supervisor is responsible for scheduling the in-service, preparing the agenda, obtaining a conference room, and securing guest speakers and materials. The content of the meeting may begin with informative updates and end with a period set aside for a continuing education offering approved for NAHUC contact hours. Every organization has state and federal mandates with which to comply. The JCAHO (Joint Commission for Accreditation of Healthcare Organizations) also has specific standards for adherence. These mandates and

TIME CARD SUMMARY

Employee Name: *Mary Doe* Employee #: *888444* Social Security #: *333-33-111*

Pay Period Begin Date: *09-20-96* Pay Period End Date: *10-03-96*

COMMENTS:	TIME CODE	HOURS	SHIFT CODE	COST CENTER
	99	*24.0*	*1*	*999.999*
	99	*8.0*	*2*	*999.999*
TOTAL ALL HOURS:		*32.0*		

Employee Signature: ______________________

Supervisor Signature: ______________________

Figure 24–8
Time card summary.

standards are reviewed and verified on a yearly basis with every employee (i.e., Occupational Safety and Health Administration fire and safety regulations, confidentiality statements, universal precautions, and annual tuberculosis skin tests). HUC supervisors are to schedule HUCs for the meetings and mandatory in-services. They must record attendance and rectify delinquent employees and records. The HUC supervisor records (or delegates the taking of) accurate and concise minutes for all in-services and meetings held. These minutes are permanently filed in manuals for records and reference.

Meetings, Task Forces, and Committees

As a part of the management team (usually termed "middle management"), the HUC supervisor is also required to fulfill specific leadership roles in the organization. This involves active participation in meetings and committees as appointed. Every member of management is expected vigorously to enhance the organization's mission and vision. Part of this obligation is fulfilled by diligent preparation for all meetings the supervisor attends. The supervisor must stay current and proactively respond to the goals and objectives of the committee. Many meetings require that the membership alternate in taking minutes. Participation in pilot studies, task forces, committees, and meetings is a responsibility and privilege. The HUC supervisor position demands a person who will grip the leadership role and participate dynamically to ensure his or her employer is the region's health care system of choice.

Equipment and Supplies

In the budget process, monies are set aside for minor and capital equipment. Before major equip-

TIME SHEET CO: 01				Department Name COST CENTER 999.999 Page 999		
EMPLOYEE NAME	TM-CD	HOURS	SFT	CST-CTR	BATCH	EMPL-NMB
Doe, Jane	99	32.00	1		100	111222
	Total	32.00				
Doe, Mary	99	24.00	1		100	888444
	99	8.00	2		100	888444
	Total	32.00				
Doe, Susan	99	32.00	2		100	333555
	Total	32.00				
Doe, Vickie	99	16.00	2		100	666777
	99	8.00	2	555.555	100	666777
	Total	24.00				

Figure 24–9
Time sheet summary.

ment is requested, authorized and approved substantial research and justification must be provided by the requester. The HUC supervisor completes the necessary process to procure equipment and supplies. This is an involved and precise process that requires initiative and follow-through. Budgets are scrutinized carefully and cuts are bound to occur. Strategic planning and alternative options must always be considered.

Quality Improvement

Change is the only constant. Everything can be done more effectively and more efficiently. As part of the system's middle management team, the HUC supervisor is involved in the on-going process of quality improvement. The HUC supervisor must be committed to satisfied customers. When areas of concern and problems arise, the supervisor must know and understand reorganization and reengineering principles that lend themselves to service quality. Process improvement, if implemented and executed properly, benefits everyone. Continual process evaluation is a major component of the HUC supervisor's duties.

Special Projects

This is the end-all, catch-all. What has not been accounted for and covered in any other description of the HUC supervisor's duties and responsibilities is captured here. Special projects can include such things as selecting new computer software applications and consequently training HUCs in the software functionality, or working with other members of management to promote awareness of and compliance with JCAHO standards.

Health Unit Coordinator Knowledge/Skills Appropriate to Position

The most desirable HUC supervisor is a person who has excellent interpersonal skills, a working knowledge of the HUC duties and responsibilities, and previous supervisory experience.

The HUC supervisor requires a base knowledge of management. Along with the management/business knowledge, corresponding skills in professional interaction are required. These skills include superlative communication skills. Any supervisor on a daily basis relies on verbal, nonverbal, and written communication. These skills are used in interviewing, performance appraisals, and day-to-day human relations, to cite just a few examples. The HUC supervisor is a self-starter who demonstrates initiative and follow-through. The budget process is one example of the business portion of the HUC supervisor's position. However, in today's ever-changing health care world, the HUC supervisor's knowledge of current and future health care trends is crucial. A dedication to and complete understanding of the organization's mission and vision are crucial.

The assumption that an excellent HUC will make a good HUC supervisor may or may not hold true. Many of the qualifications may appear to be the same, but the leadership capabilities and commitment to management cannot be overlooked. HUC supervisors should also be extremely sensitive to the organization's culture or climate. This cultural environment can work with or against a supervisor. Another positive management attribute is that the HUC supervisor is able to initiate change in harmony with the prevailing corporate culture, and not alienate staff by being "boss" and changing everything "STAT."

Additional Training Required

The HUC supervisor is a unique person. The value of the HUC supervisor lies in the fact that he or she is able perfectly to mesh the clinical and clerical worlds. Educationally, the HUC supervisor has an expert knowledge of the health care environment. To obtain this background, the HUC supervisor has preferably obtained a degree with a course base of clinical subjects (i.e., medical terminology and anatomy and physiology), business administration classes (e.g., human relations, management skills, communication skills), and transcription of physician orders.

Management Techniques

There are many management styles. Each supervisor is a unique person bringing his or her personality and experiences into the position. Nevertheless, there are several management techniques to "**do**" or "**don't**" do. Stephen Covey is a distinguished author in the field of self- and subordinate management principles. His writings served as guidelines and examples for the "do" and "don't" techniques that follow.

DO:

Always involve employees in the process of analyzing and solving problems. The more sincere and sustained this involvement becomes, the greater the innovation and commitment of the subordinates.

DO:

Express your individual needs, interpretations, and feelings with courage and conviction; nevertheless, always remember the needs, feelings, and convictions of others. This is mature supervision.

DO:

Have subordinates evaluate themselves using criteria they themselves helped to create up front.

In this type of win–win performance appraisal, when set up correctly, every employee can tell for himself or herself how "smoothly" the unit is running and how satisfied all his or her customers are.

DO:

An effective leader has the challenge to remain focused on the vision and values of his or her employer. This is an ongoing process where all involved continually "begin with the end in mind." When an effective supervisor and subordinates work together as a cohesive group sharing a core vision and values, there is deep commitment and tremendous unity. Everyone governs himself or herself. No one needs directing, controlling, or criticizing. No one will be backstabbing or finding fault. There will be no shift-to-shift squabbles or unit-to-unit defensiveness. Everyone understands why they are needed, who their customers are, and how valuable their unique contributions are to the success of their mission. All involved benefit mutually. Together, they have contributed to a unified victory, which none of the participants independently could have engineered. People worked together, communicated together, and produced a desired outcome. It takes a team: the physician writes the order, the {C}HUC transcribes the order, the caregiver initiates the order at the bedside, and the patient's response/outcome is noted. These are not random efforts, but the result of a well-developed and organized plan of care.

DO:

A supervisor holds his or her subordinates accountable for their duties and responsibilities, but does not neglect to affirm and convey confidence in their abilities. When a supervisor notices a problem, he or she is compassionate, not accusing. The real issue is not what the employee is or is not doing, but what the supervisor is doing in response to a given situation to build up the employee. Is there the need for further education or training? Never forget to treat employees exactly as the supervisor would want them to treat the organization's best customers. The only way for subordinates to give their manager their best is to know that they are appreciated and valued for their contributions to the system.

DON'T:

Don't lack confidence in the employee; in doing so, the supervisor cannot have confidence in the employee's work.

DON'T:

A supervisor is bound to be swept into difficult situations and confrontations. Be prepared! Don't get caught up in hook words and phrases. Don't let people see and take advantage of trigger points. Visualize the goal clearly in your mind. Rehearse responses carefully. Say and do and commit to only what you are comfortable with. Do homework and research. Use any and all available resources. Be clear in the outcome to be achieved.

DON'T:

Don't play "traditional" evaluation games. They are awkward and emotionally exhausting. Use win–win evaluation.

DON'T:

Don't run yourself ragged by constantly putting out fires in daily duties. You will exhaust both your physical and emotional banks and reservoirs. Rather, focus on the results to be accomplished on a daily, weekly, and monthly basis. Then prioritize activities to allow adequate time and resources to fulfill these commitments. There certainly will be emergencies, but if the supervisor is optimally organized and definitely in control, it will be easy to ensure the emergency does not grow in proportion from a ripple to a tidal wave. However, never lose sight of inner flexibility, and concentrate on the wisdom to know when to "shift gears" or take a "detour."

DON'T:

Remember "Transactional Analysis": don't be the supervisor "parent" addressing your "child" employee. *Do* communicate adult-to-adult. If you let fear replace cooperation, subordinates are constantly placed on the defensive.

DON'T:

Don't go into supervision with the unrealistic, starry-eyed belief that you can be all things to all people and that you now have the ability to right all the previous wrongs. It just isn't true, and it won't happen. That is an excellent way to set yourself up for failure.

Rather, concentrate on four "R's":

- *Regularly take time off* (60- to 70-hour weeks, week after week, can quickly lead to ineffectiveness and burnout).
- *Rest your mind and body* (learn to relax and get enough sleep).
- *Renew your spirit, mind, and body* (actively practice your religious beliefs, take time to enjoy your hobbies, take yourself on the vacation you're always promising yourself—see new sights, do new things).
- *Reflect* (look at where you've been—how you got there, learn from the past to plan your future).

Supervisors will never be successful in managing others if first they are not successful in managing all the aspects of "self." Nothing is free; everything has a price. Don't try to talk your way out of situations into which your behavior has led you. Actions always speak louder than words. A supervisor won't be convincing to others if he or she cannot practice what he or she preaches.

Be a manager with this philosophy:

Do be a manager who lights the way;
Don't be a condemning judge.
Do be a manager who is a model example;
Don't be a cynical critic.
Do be a manager who takes an active role in the solution;
Don't be a manager that employees see as part of the problem.

Always keep an open mind to be ready to explore new possibilities, entertain new alternatives, and try new options. By believing in employees, the supervisor positions himself or herself to be a positive force in their lives. When problems and differences arise, they do not have to become stumbling blocks; they can become building blocks to foster communication and advance progress. It is a win–win situation when there is cooperation instead of competition.

Closing Thoughts

Middle management members are hired to perform a job and quoted a salary for this job. Many times this will require a 200% effort. There will be 16-hour days and deadlines that had to be met yesterday. Nevertheless, the rewards are numerous. There is joy and satisfaction in witnessing objectives met and goals accomplished. As customer satisfaction rises, the HUC supervisor can realize that he or she had an integral part. Make no mistake; in the long run a manager will "reap what is sown." If, as a supervisor, you foster open communication and continual learning opportunities, and make a commitment to progress, your employees will grow and be an asset to you and your organization. Never forget, you are only as good as those who report to you. Subordinates can handle the simple, plain truth. It builds their confidence and tells them you value their trust and respect. Use your positive energy to focus your efforts on things that you can do something about. This increases your influence. Avoid reacting to situations, which creates negative energy. These are circumstances over which you have no control and your influence definitely decreases. Keep your promises. Meet your deadlines. Acknowledge and apologize for your mistakes. Learn and practice expert listening skills. We are always able to make a choice between being reactive and proactive. Be proactive. Don't take the easy way out by letting others influence you, control you, and limit your effectiveness. Be free to choose your own actions. Empower yourself and your employees. Don't empower problems to control your work environment. When you possess the important principles of HONESTY, CONSISTENCY, and FAIRNESS, your employees will be empowered to act and accomplish their duties and responsibilities without constant monitoring, evaluating, correcting, or controlling. Remember to walk the road of supervision with both feet planted firmly on the ground. Never run to the edge of the cliff and jump off expecting the right breeze at the right time to float your parachute gently to a nice, soft, grassy landing. Pack your own parachute. Make sure it's equipped with all the elements you'll need for good supervision and create your own climate of sunshine and good "work" weather.

Review Questions

1. List at least ten responsibilities of a HUC supervisor.
2. Identify the base of clinical and business courses that a person should take in preparation for the position of HUC supervisor.
3. Name two **do** and two **don't** techniques of good management.

Bibliography

Covey S: The 7 Habits of Highly Effective People. New York, Simon & Schuster, 1989.

25 Medical (Health Sciences) Library Assistant

Diane Faulkner

Common Abbreviations

MEDLARS	Medical Literature Analysis and Retrieval System
M.L.S.	Master's Degree in Library Science
NLM	National Library of Medicine

Objectives

Upon completion of this chapter, the reader should be able to:

1. Describe three aspects of library work.
2. Explain library procedure.
3. Prepare a catalog card.
4. Discuss use of journal information.

Vocabulary

Consortium: An association, fellowship, or coalition, collectively having vast resources

Library: A collection of books, pamphlets, magazines, journals, periodicals, and other materials arranged to facilitate reference.

Introduction

The minimum requirement for a hospital medical **library** is that it provide the books, journals, and other materials necessary to serve the immediate information needs of the professional staff and to support the programs undertaken by the hospital. The library remains just a collection of books unless a person is assigned at least on a part-time basis to assist requesters and provide library services such as reference and interlibrary loans.

This chapter is written to aid the inexperienced person (in librarianship) who finds himself or herself assigned to a hospital library with the responsibility of ordering the library materials, organizing the collection, borrowing from other libraries, or seeking out information. It is a varied, challenging, and rewarding responsibility for any health unit coordinator (HUC) to undertake. The hospital medical library personnel can provide a very dynamic and useful information service to the institution's community of health professionals.

Description of the Facilities

Ideally, the library should be in a room centrally located for the hospital staff and large enough to house the necessary books and journals. If possible, the room should function exclusively as a library to allow for maximum use of the materials. There should be adequate lighting, tables, and comfortable chairs. The library personnel should have a desk, typewriter, computer, and sufficient space in which to perform tasks. Convenient access to a photocopy machine is highly desirable.

Roles and Responsibilities

Librarians assist people to find information and to use it effectively in their personal and professional lives. They must have knowledge of a wide variety of medical and public information sources and trends related to publishing, computers, and the media effectively to oversee the selection and organization of library materials. Librarians manage staff and see to the development and direction of information programs for the public. They must be sure that the information is being organized to meet the needs of the users. Many of these same skills are used as a HUC. This makes for an easy transition from one position to the other (Fig. 25–1).

There are three general aspects of library work: user services, technical services, and administrative services. Increasingly, distinctions between these services are blurred and many library positions incorporate all three aspects of work. Even librarians who specialize in one of these areas may perform tasks from the others.

Librarians in user service, such as reference, work with the public to help them find the information they need. This may involve analyzing users' needs to determine what information is appropriate and searching for, acquiring, and providing the information.

Librarians in technical services, such as acquisitions and cataloguing, acquire and prepare material for use and may not deal directly with the public.

Librarians in administrative services oversee the management and planning of libraries. They negotiate contracts for services, materials, and equipment. They also supervise library employ-

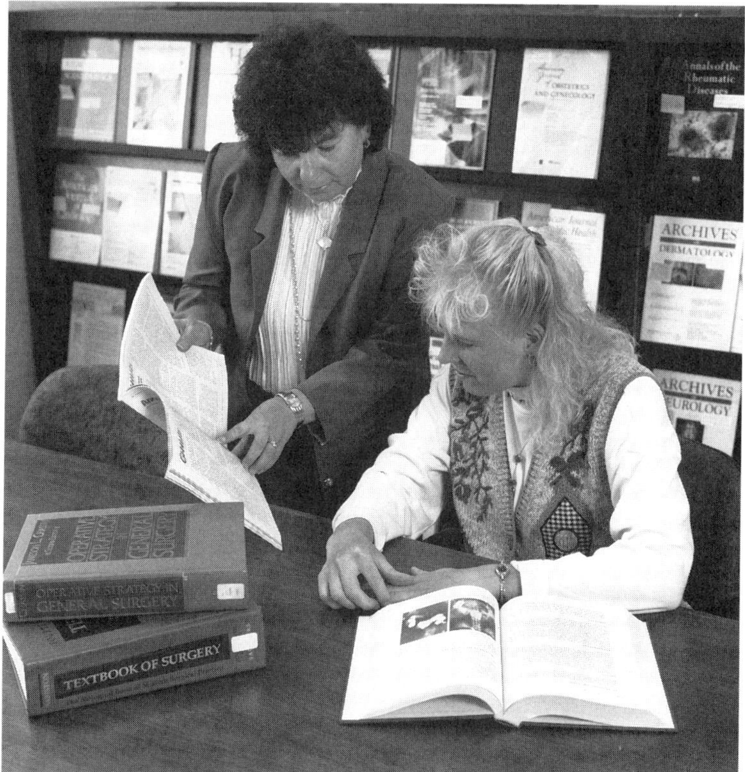

Figure 25–1
Helping to find information.

ees, perform public relations functions, prepare budgets, and direct activities to ensure that everything functions properly. There is ample opportunity for the experienced HUC to advance to any of these positions.

In small libraries of information centers, librarians usually handle all aspects of the work. They read book reviews, publisher's announcements, and catalogs to keep up with the current literature and other available resources. The chosen materials are purchased from publishers, wholesalers, and distributors. Librarians prepare new materials for use by classifying them by subject matter. Books and other library materials are described in such a way that users can find them easily. Assistants prepare cards, computer records, or other access tools that direct users to resources. In large libraries, librarians may specialize in a single area, such as acquisitions, cataloguing and bibliography, reference, special collections, or administration. Teamwork is increasingly important to ensure high-quality service to the public. This is something to which all HUCs are accustomed.

Librarians also compile lists of books, periodicals, articles, and audiovisual materials on particular subjects, analyze collections, and recommend materials to be acquired. They may collect and organize books, pamphlets, manuscripts, and other materials in a specific field such as rare books or genealogy. In addition, they coordinate programs such as public services; provide reference help; and help prepare budgets.

For the HUC who really enjoys working with computers, it is important to know that many libraries have access to remote databases as well as maintaining their own computerized databases. The widespread use of automation in libraries makes database searching skills important to librarians. Librarians develop and index databases and act as trainers to help others develop the searching skills to obtain the information they need.

Some libraries are forming **consortiums** with other libraries through electronic mail (e-mail). This allows patrons to submit information requests to several libraries at once. Use of the internet and other worldwide computer systems is also expanding the amount of reference information. Librarians must be increasingly aware of how to use these resources to locate information.

For the person working as a library assistant under the direction of a librarian, the duties might include registering patrons so they can borrow materials from the library. This is accomplished by recording the borrower's name and address from an application and issuing a library card. Most of this is now done using a computer.

Assistants collect and lend books, periodicals, video tapes. and other materials. When an item is borrowed, it is stamped with the due date on the material and recorded on the patron's identification card. Assistants inspect returned materials for damage, check the due dates, and compute any fines that may be owed. They review records to compile a list of overdue materials and send out notices. They also answer patrons' questions in person and on the telephone. A HUC's public relations skills are very useful in all aspects of work in the library.

The library assistants sort returned books, periodicals, and other items and return them to their designated shelves, files, or storage areas throughout the library. They locate materials to be loaned, either to a patron or to another library. Many card catalogs are computerized, so library assistants must be familiar with the computer system for their particular library. The services available on today's computers provide the capability of ordering cards by computer similar to e-mail.

Some library assistants operate and maintain audiovisual equipment, such as projectors, tape recorders, and videocassette recorders, and assist library users with microfilm or microfiche readers. They may also design posters, bulletin boards, or displays.

Assistants may have the added duty of being the site coordinator for satellite video and teleconferences for their hospital. These programs are usually continuing education conferences designed for educators, nurses, and other health practitioners. Most of these programs have to be subscribed to, and the coordinates need to match that of the satellite dish. Once a program has been selected, a room should be scheduled to accommodate the viewing. It may be necessary to tape the programs for those who are unable to attend. Flyers are sent to the appropriate departments to announce the offering. Registration sheets must be completed and returned to the company supplying the program for the participants to get credit for attending. Most of these programs last 1 to 2 hours and provide 1 to 2 contact hours of continuing education.

If the library is associated with the education department and they provide workshops for continuing education, the assistant might be asked to contribute some clerical support, such as phone registration or computer support for the upcoming workshops. When both departments are closely integrated, there are more phone duties than usual.

Organization

More than just a collection of books, journals, and videos, the hospital's health science library is an integral part of the hospital community. With dynamic library personnel and carefully selected materials, the library assumes an important role in supporting the patient care, research, professional education, and health facilities planning of the medical and nursing staff, the allied health personnel, and the hospital administration. The HUC strives to meet the needs of these same people, so the rapport that was developed should continue to command the same respect and trust in the library setting.

The Medical Library Personnel

Most hospital libraries are a one-person department. This person's duties should include selecting, ordering, organizing, circulating, and maintaining the collection. They obtain materials missing from the collection for the staff. They provide bibliographic and reference services. The hospital personnel should know who is responsible for the library, how to use the library, and of whom to make requests for information or additional books or journals. HUCs in the hospital have the advantage of the staff and physicians already being aware of them.

The Library Committee

A library committee is essential in a hospital setting. The committee established by the hospital may consist of the hospital administrator, two members of the medical staff, a member of the nursing staff, and the hospital library personnel. If the hospital has interns and residents, it is a good idea to ask them to select a person to serve as an honorary member. The library personnel may function as the secretary of the committee and prepare an agenda for each meeting's activities. In general, the library committee meets at regular intervals (monthly or every other month; some may meet quarterly). Its functions are:

1. To advise the library personnel regarding the selection of books and journals for purchasing.
2. To establish and to interpret the rules of the library to its users.
3. To serve as a link between the staff, the hospital administration, and the library.
4. To foster the development of the library.

Procedure Manual

Each library differs from another not only in physical ways but in the procedures used to do the necessary work. It is important to write down step-by-step descriptions of the procedures that are used routinely in the hospital, such as ordering books, getting journals ready to be bound, and disposing of old books and other obsolete materials.

Budget

Hospital libraries have various sources of revenue. Most are supported by the hospital budget, medical staff dues, or contributions. If there is an auxiliary department, they may be looked to for the funds to start a library or add to a library already established in the facility.

Another source of funds that can be used to establish a health science library or to expand an already existing library is a medical library resource improvement grant. Information about resource grants may be obtained from the National Library of Medicine, 8600 Rockville Pike, Bethesda, Maryland 20014.

It is useful for librarians to have a fixed sum of money each year that they can depend on. To have some idea of how much money is needed to manage the library, a budget should be prepared and reviewed each year. It should cover the expected:

1. Book purchases
2. Journal subscriptions
3. Library personnel salaries
4. Library equipment (e.g., telephone, typewriter, computer, shelving)
5. Library supplies (e.g., forms, mailing labels, packaging, postage)
6. Bindery costs (e.g., if journals are being bound)

Supplies

The use of specially developed library supplies can greatly assist in the organization and management of the library. These supplies are available from several companies, and the librarian may request catalogs to see what is available. Library supply companies can be found in the yellow pages of the telephone book, or the materiel management department could refer one.

Reports

A hospital medical library is a service unit in a hospital. Its effectiveness can be measured in part by how much service it provides. The hospital administration and the library committee should receive at least an annual report of library activities. The annual report should include:

1. Circulation statistics—the number of books and journals borrowed by the library patrons
2. Reference statistics
   a. Ready reference—the number of questions answered by a search by the library personnel of one or two books or journals
   b. Bibliographies—the number of bibliographies compiled
3. Interlibrary loan statistics
   a. The number of books or journal articles requested from other libraries
   b. The number of books or journal articles that one provided another library
4. Acquisition statistics
   a. The number of books purchased during the year
   b. The number of books discarded because of age
   c. The number of missing books
   d. The total number of books in the library
   e. The number of journal titles for which new subscriptions were entered during the year
   f. The total number of journal titles received by the library
5. Budget
   a. Amount expended for personnel
   b. Amount expended for books
   c. Amount expended for journals
   d. Amount expended for equipment
   e. Amount expended for supplies
   f. Amount expended for phone and postage
   g. Other expenditures
6. Special projects and exhibits
7. Library personnel attendance at workshops, meetings, or public relations events
8. Unusual events during the year, special visitors, or events that will complete the commentary on the library's activities for the previous year
9. Goals, objectives, and plans for the following year

Less detailed quarterly reports to the hospital administration may be required.

Book Selection

In the small working collection of a hospital library, it is important that the books be accurate, informative, up to date, and useful to the hospital staff. The library should contain basic texts covering the medical specialties. New books are acquired to update the basic collection or to keep the staff informed of the new developments in various areas of medicine.

Acquiring New Books

Each year, hundreds off new medical books are published. It is important to acquire for the library those that the staff should have immediately available.

How to Find Out What Is Being Published

1. Publishers' catalogs or announcements. Publishers are happy to put the library on their mailing list.

2. Book dealers' announcements. *A Select List of Medical Books in Print* is an annual free list of major medical books issued by American publishers. It is available through several dealers.

3. Advertisements or book sections in journals.

4. *Medical and Health Care Books and Serials in Print*. By R. R. Bowker.

5. National Library of Medicine (NLM) current catalog.

How to Select What to Buy

1. Order standard texts.

2. Order new or revised editions of books already owned. Check information on new or revised editions to see if the new edition differs substantially from the older editions.

3. Do a hospital-wide survey. Suggestions from the staff are always useful and should be encouraged.

4. Read reviews published in the book section of journals to become acquainted with books that are being published that would be suitable for the library.

5. Order items borrowed more than three or four times on interlibrary loan, within a reasonable period of time.

Gifts

1. Gifts are a wonderful way to receive additions to the library. They promote public relations with staff members and other members of the community.

2. Accept gifts with a "thank you" letter from the library to the donor.

3. Accept gifts with no strings attached, if possible. It is better not to accept gifts that cannot be disposed of when the material becomes dated. Receive all gifts graciously, and indicate that they may be placed on exchange or given to a library that needs them if they cannot be used in the donee institution.

4. Do not evaluate the gift for tax purposes. Accept the gift with a letter listing the items, giving identifying information such as the author, title, and date. The donor and his tax consultant should accept the responsibility for the tax claim.

Ordering Procedures for Books

After deciding to purchase a book, check the library's card catalog and files to be certain the book is not already in the library or on order.

Order Cards

Smaller libraries, without elaborate catalogs, may want to keep order cards. Include on the cards:

1. First author's last name and at least his or her first initial.

2. The exact and complete title.

3. The edition; make sure the latest edition is being ordered

4. Publisher's name, place of publication, and date of publication.

5. List price.

6. Date ordered and the purchase order number.

7. Name of person who recommended purchase (let them know when it is received).

8. Funds to be used if the library has several different accounts (e.g., memorial, budget).

Follow the hospital's purchase procedures, using the appropriate forms. Keep a copy of the purchase order if possible.

Where to Send the Order

The librarian may order directly from publishers or from dealers that specialize in medical and technical books. A dealer stocks books from many publishers, which should save time and effort on the part of the librarian. Select a dealer who:

1. Has a large stock so he or she will be able to fill the requests rapidly.
2. Has accurate and simple procedures.
3. Gives good service.
4. Is convenient to use. If the dealer is close, the librarian may call for rush orders or can make inquiries into orders that are taking a long time to fill.
5. Gives the standard library discount.

When the Book Arrives

Compare the book received with the order slip to see if you have received the right item. Check all the information you included on the order card. Check the book itself to make sure pages are in the right order, are all there, and so forth.

Fill in the date received and the actual price. Send the invoice that accompanied the book to the appropriate department for payment.

Suggestions

1. Order at regular intervals throughout the year.
2. Use as few dealers as possible, preferably only one or two.
3. Periodically check the order file to see that all the books have been received.

Dealers should notify the library within 30 days of the order about the status of each item. If this notification is not made, call the dealer to make sure the order was received.

Cataloging and Catalog Cards

A library card catalog is an index on 3 × 5-inch cards to the library's collection. Cataloging is transferring descriptive information taken from a book onto a card so that the user can tell if this is the book he or she wants and where in the library it may be found. Each catalog card contains the following information:

1. Author's full name if the book was written by one person. If the book was written by more than one person, use the first author mentioned. An editor is considered an author.
2. Complete title and subtitle.
3. Author statement, if there is more than one author. The names of the first two authors are contained on the catalog card. Additional authors are represented by the statement "and others."
4. Edition (if other than the first).
5. Imprint: place of publication, publisher, date of publication.
6. Pagination, number of volumes, note if volume is part of a series, and so forth.
7. Tracings: subject headings, second author's name (if there is one).
8. Call number (classification symbol and Cutter number) if the volume is classified. (This may be replaced by any designation of location that is used to locate the book.)

The basic catalog card is prepared by typing the information onto a 3 × 5 inch card (Fig. 25–2).

Call Number	Author's last name, first name Title. Edition. Place of Publication, Publisher, Date. Number of Pages. Illustrations. (Series) 1. Subject heading 2. Subject heading I. Second author II. Title III. Series

Figure 25–2
Catalog card.

A set of catalog cards includes the following:

1. Author or main entry card. This is the basic card. For each book, the set of catalog cards uses this basic card with the specific identifying information typed on the line above the author's name.
2. Title card: the basic card with the book's title typed on the line above the author's name.
3. Additional author cards: for the second author's name. A basic card is made with the second author's name typed on the line above the first author's name (last name first).
4. Subject card: for each subject heading used to describe the contents of the book, a basic card is made with the appropriate subject heading typed above the author's name. Usually not more than three per book.
5. Shelf list card: the basic card with business information such as price, date acquired, damage, date discarded, and the like, added. These cards are arranged by call number. This file is in the same order as the books on the shelves, and is usually kept in the librarian's office or staff area.

Catalog cards are printed by the Library of Congress. They may also be obtained from some book distributors and commercial firms. If you wish to purchase catalog cards with the description information printed on them, discuss it with a book jobber or write to the Library of Congress.

Filing Rules

1. Alphabetize word by word, and letter by letter within each word.

Example:
Hospital Management
Hospital Topics
Hospitals

2. Abbreviations and numbers are alphabetized as if they were spelled in full.
3. Ignore the *first* word of a title if it is an article (a, an, the).
4. Hyphenated words are treated as separate words.
5. "Mc" is always filed as "Mac."

Journals

A journal is a publication that comes out at regular intervals and is intended to be published indefinitely. Most journals contain several articles on different topics written by different authors. In most cases, journals have paper covers and are published with volume and issue numbers and date.

Why do we have journals? Journals started hundreds of years ago when scientists wrote letters to one another telling of their work and results. Later, letters were passed around among colleagues. Eventually, these were formally published as journals. Modern journals contain short communications of the results of experiments or clinical trials of drugs, descriptions of techniques or new diseases, and the like. It takes less time to publish a journal issue than it does to publish a book. Journals are published in countries all over the world and in many languages.

To keep up with the progress of medical knowledge, it is necessary to know what articles many journals contain. Because no library can subscribe to the many thousands of biomedical journals, indexes to the better journals are published. The major American medical index is *Index Medicus,* a monthly index of a few thousand English-language and foreign-language medical journals. By subscribing to *Index Medicus,* the librarian can see if an article has been written on any given medical subject in one of these journals.

The parts of a journal are:

Title
Volume
Dates (issue)
Pages
Contents
Advertising
Index

What kinds of information can be obtained from journals? In addition to the articles, journals contain:

1. Notices of meetings on clinical specialties
2. Book reviews

3. Advertisements for new books and journals
4. New items
5. Listings of society meetings and officers

What journals does the hospital need? As in the case of books, the selection of journals should reflect the needs and interests of the staff. Follow these principles in selection:

1. Select good-quality journals—ask the medical staff and consult core lists.
2. Select journals representing the medical specialties practiced in the hospital.
3. Select journals that are indexed in *Index Medicus, Abridged Index Medicus, Hospital Literature Index*, or a similar available index.

Ordering Procedures for Journals

A journal subscription is usually placed with the intention of continuing it indefinitely. After deciding to subscribe to a journal, complete an order form card with the journal title, publisher or issuing society, publisher's address, annual subscription rate, and the volume, issue, and date with which the order is to begin.

Order either through a subscription agent or directly through the journal's issuing body. Subscription agencies are service organizations that deal in handling subscriptions. They are helpful in ordering journals, claiming missing issues, renewing orders, obtaining sample copies, and so forth. In most cases, if you decide on a subscription agency, you would let them handle all the journal orders except those journals that come as a benefit of membership in a society, or that are government sponsored. You would receive an annual itemized invoice for all the orders. Subscription agencies may charge for their services, so be certain to check on costs and expenses before putting the subscriptions in an agent's hands. Agents act as liaison between you and the many publishers, so you would be able to establish good communication with one company instead of minimal contact with many. Subscription prices do change, so be certain to allow for this in the budget each year.

Binding Journals

Should you bind? Binding does protect the journals and it reduces the number of lost issues. However, binding is expensive, and it means that in order to circulate an issue, all the issues bound with it must circulate. Most libraries do not circulate their journal collections. It has been said that smaller hospitals should not bind their journals; medium-sized hospitals may or may not, and large hospitals should bind only those journals they will keep for 3 to 5 years.

Circulation

It is important that any book or journal in the medical library be available when it is needed. Except for a few important reference books, the books should be available so that users may borrow them for 1 or 2 weeks. The borrowing rules should be established by the library committee and all users should be told what the rules are. A simple circulation system for books would consist of:

1. A book pocket—this manila pocket is pasted on the inside of the back hard cover of the book. Usually, the pocket is marked with the classification number, the author's last name, the title of the book, and the date of publication. The name of the library is stamped on the pocket.
2. A book card—this must fit in the book pocket. The classification number, the author's last name, the title, and the date of publication are typed on the upper section of the book card.
3. To borrow a book, the user removes the book card from the book pocket, marks the date the book is being borrowed, and signs the book card.
4. The signed book cards are filed by author at the desk. The borrower of a particular book can easily be identified.
5. When the book is returned, it is initialed by the library personnel.
6. The book card is returned to the book pocket after verifying that it is the right book.
7. The book is returned to the shelf, ready to be borrowed again.

Weeding the Collection

What is weeding? The practice of discarding or storing superfluous copies, rarely used materials, and materials no longer of any use.

Why weed? To use the available space in the library in the best and most economical way. (Rely on interlibrary loan or borrowing arrangements with other libraries in the area for those little-used materials that would crowd the shelves.) To give the library a reputation of reliability, a collection that is up-to-date, and to make it functional.

When to weed? Continuously, by reviewing once a year.

Who should weed? Anyone who can select books can weed wisely. The final decision to discard or retain a book must be that of the librarian or the library committee.

What to weed? Books containing outdated information, duplicate copies of books, repetitious series, and old editions. Periodicals used very little. Items uncirculated for 5 years and not needed for reference may be suitable to discard. Relate this to who the user is, his or her future requirements, and the local situation.

The mechanics of weeding are as follows:

A. Disposition

1. *Discard:* Obsolete and outdated books of no historical value.

2. *Retain:* Good titles that cannot be replaced (out-of-print books and historical materials).

3. *Replace* regularly used items with a new edition or a revised edition if available.

4. *Replace* classics or notable volumes with better editions.

5. *Give away* or *exchange* duplicates of periodical titles that may be needed by other libraries.

6. *Recycle* or *sell* unneeded materials in accordance with library policy. Make sure that people or other libraries who purchase these materials are aware that they are old, possibly out of date, and perhaps of questionable reliability.

7. *Consult* subject specialists in your institution for advice on historical, rare, or specialized items.

Whichever weeding method is chosen, procedure must be followed. The book card is removed. It is verified that the book card is for that book. The shelf list card is dated and marked "withdrawn." If a book is the only copy of the title and is not being replaced, remove all catalog cards and the shelf list card. Shelf list cards are filed in the "withdrawn" file. Catalog cards are discarded. Each book is marked "discarded" over the ownership marks. The book pocket and date slip are removed. If possible, the library ownership marks are removed from books that are being sold or given away. Monthly and annual records are kept of withdrawn books. Replacement copies are ordered when needed. Each facility may have slightly different practices for disposing of weeded books.

Additional Services

Audiovisual Material

Common types of audiovisual materials are slides (projection and microscopic), tapes, motion pictures, records, and pictures. These materials need special shelving, environmental control, and a controlled circulation; they present special problems in terms of repair, and need special equipment to be used. The hospital library may only order, organize, store, and circulate these materials; or, the library may also provide the equipment.

The cataloging of audiovisual materials differs from that of books and journals. If the library has only one or two items, there is no problem remembering where they are, but a special area or shelf should be set aside for these materials.

MEDLARS

MEDLARS is an acronym for Medical Literature Analysis and Retrieval System, the computerized information system developed by and based at the NLM in Bethesda, Maryland. Several databases are mounted on the system. Of these databases, MEDLINE is the most heavily used and best known.

MEDLINE is a bibliographic database that, as the computerized counterpart of *Index Medicus,* is the primary source in the United States for information from the biomedical literature. As a bibliographic database, it contains references to articles that have appeared in thousands of journals. These journals have been carefully reviewed and selected for inclusion because of their importance to health professionals.

MEDLINE is international in scope, with approximately 75% of the citations published in the English language. It contains publications from 1966 to the present. The scope of MEDLINE includes such topics as microbiology, delivery of health care, nutrition, pharmacology, and environmental health. The categories covered by MEDLINE include anatomy; organisms; diseases, chemicals, and drugs; techniques and equipment; psychiatry and psychology; biologic sciences; physical sciences; social sciences and education; technology, agriculture, food, and industry; humanities; information science and communications; and health care.

Interlibrary Loans

Because no library can acquire and store all the materials available to users anywhere, libraries often agree to lend to other libraries that need a book or to borrow from a library that has the needed item. Usually there is an agreement between libraries or a contract with another library to locate needed materials.

Satellite Video Conferences

Satellite video conferences are another way of bringing up-to-date information right into your hospital for the medical staff. Coordinate the conference with the department that is in need of the information, set up the time and place, and send announcements by whatever media are available.

Book Sales

The department may offer the Heart Association Training Manuals for sale. They will be needed by all personnel taking the certification courses. Staff members and personnel may be interested in parts of the weeded collection. A fun book sale or trade can be done during library open house. The open house is also a good time to remind hospital staff what the library has to offer and what new books are available.

Another service the library provides is that of bringing health education information to the local schools. This may be done by speaking at career days, giving tours of the hospital and library, and inviting the schools to participate in library open house. A theme of the month might be developed to coincide with the various hospital departments or functions. During "Infection Control Week," a talk on hand washing could be given in the elementary school. Often, the subjects that seem most basic to health care workers are the ones for which education is needed most by the communities they serve.

Education Integration

If the library is integrated with the hospital's education department, the role of the assistant might expand even more than anticipated. The assistant may be required to assist with the department's clerical needs, such as registration for programs and workshops. Along with registration is record keeping from each program. These records may vary according to each hospital's policies, but should be maintained in accordance with Joint Committee on Accreditation of Healthcare Organizations (JCAHO) standards. Medical staff personnel are required to keep licenses current. If the hospital offers continuing education programs, the assistant may be required to supply the certificates of completion.

Training Beyond the Health Unit Coordinator

A master's degree in library science (M.L.S.) is necessary for librarian positions in most public, academic, and special libraries, and some school libraries. In the Federal Government, an M.L.S.

or the equivalent in education and experience is needed. Many colleges and universities offer M.L.S. programs, but many employers prefer graduates of the approximately 50 schools accredited by the American Library Association. Most M.L.S. programs require a bachelor's degree; any liberal arts major is appropriate.

Most programs take 1 year to complete; others take 2. A typical graduate program includes courses in the foundation of library and information science, including the history of books and printing, intellectual freedom and censorship, and the role of libraries and information in society. Other basic courses cover material selection and processing, the organization of information, reference tools and strategies, and user services. Courses are being adapted to educate librarians to use new resources brought about by advancing technology, such as on-line reference systems and automated circulation systems. Course options can include resources for children or young adults; classification, cataloging, indexing, and abstracting; library administration; and library automation. The M.L.S. provides general, all-around preparation for library work, but some people specialize in a particular area such as reference, technical services, or children's services. A Ph.D. degree in library and information science is useful when aspiring to a college teaching or top administrative position, particularly in a college or university library or in a large library system.

In special libraries, an M.L.S. is usually required. In addition, most special librarians supplement their education with knowledge of the subject specialization, or a master's, doctoral, or professional degree in the subject. Subject specializations include medicine, law, business, engineering, and the natural and social sciences. For example, a librarian working for a law firm may also be a licensed attorney, holding both library science and law degrees.

Closing Thoughts

My medical career began when I applied for my first position at a California district hospital. The challenges of working in the hospital atmosphere and seeing what I personally could do to make a difference kept me inspired to continue in this field. I became acutely aware of people's needs, not only patients', but also those of the health care professionals who needed information of every aspect to care for the patients. Speaking now from 14 years of experience as a certified health unit coordinator (CHUC) before transferring to our hospital's health science library 7 years ago, I thoroughly enjoyed being an HUC and have gained a wealth of knowledge since making the transition. Change creates the opportunity to expand our role in the health care community with great rewards and unlimited potential for success.

Review Questions

1. Describe the three aspects of library work.
2. Discuss the procedure for weeding the library collection.
3. Using this book for the information, prepare a catalog card for it.
4. List four types of information found in a journal.

26 Monitor Technician

Linda Sanford-Face

Common Abbreviations

Brady	Bradycardia
MASH	Mobile Army Surgical Hospital
MI	Myocardial infarction
NSR	Normal sinus rhythm
PVC	Premature ventricular contraction
V tach	Ventricular tachycardia

Objectives

Upon completion of the chapter, the reader should be able to:

1. Discuss the evolution of the monitor technician position.
2. List the responsibilities of the monitor technician when a patient is admitted to the monitor system.
3. Describe a typical day for a monitor technician.
4. Discuss additional training that might be necessary for the position of monitor technician.

Vocabulary

Arrhythmia: Irregularity in the rhythm of the heart

Dysrhythmia: Term used interchangeably with "arrhythmia"

Fibrillation: Rapid, random stimulation of heart muscle resulting in an ineffective quivering action

This chapter explores an "offspring" of the health unit coordinator (HUC), the cardiac monitor technician. The term "offspring" is used because the history of the HUC dates back to the period just after World War II, whereas the cardiac monitor technician position dates back to the 1960s, with the development of critical care areas in hospitals, and frequently it is certified HUCs who are trained into the position.

The current emphasis on coronary disease and care began in 1945. The demonstrated success of resuscitation stations on the front lines in World War II led to the emergence of special units for patient care. This translated to a broader concept, the intensive care unit, based on the success of the Mobile Army Surgical Hospital (MASH) units in the Korean War. Most American hospitals established intensive care units between 1950 and 1965. Coronary care units did not evolve until 1962. The HUC position was developed because of a shortage of nurses and a demand from the government for better record keeping in patient care. The position of cardiac monitor technician was also developed as the following trends in nursing began to emerge:

- The development of intensive care units
- The development of equipment specialized to cardiac care
- The demand for more "intense" nursing for the critically ill

The patient care process took more time; less time was allowed for proper record keeping—and hence the "birth" of the cardiac monitor technician.

The original training of the "monitor tech" was done by the nursing staff in the coronary care units. As the need increased, additional monitor technicians were brought in. Training was done by the experienced monitor technician. The success of the monitor technician program was acknowledged nationwide, and more advanced technology was introduced. In response, hospitals designed more formal programs of training to fit their needs and to reflect their protocols and equipment choices.

The addition of documentation responsibilities, the complexities of new equipment, and the quality of service provided led to the nationwide acceptance of the concept of the cardiac monitor technician, and the profession was established.

Physical Layout of the Work Environment

The physical layout of critical care areas differs from the general patient care areas in several ways. The "intensive care" areas, which include intensive care, cardiac or coronary care, and surgical intensive care, are usually housed behind double doors that stay closed to the general public. This helps to protect patient privacy and keeps traffic to a minimum in a fast-paced area.

The nurses' station is usually centralized so all patient rooms can be viewed from the desk. Some hospitals have the cardiac monitors at the nurses' station, but they are in an area away from the nurses' work area (Fig. 26–1*A*). Other hospitals house the monitoring equipment off to the side of the nurses' station in an "office"-like room with a door that can close off distractions from the nurses' station (Fig. 26–1*B*). Those that are housed in separate areas may have two monitor technicians on duty during a shift to assist one another during a crisis and to cover one another because the monitors cannot be left unattended. Another reason for having two monitor technicians on duty is that some areas have monitoring equipment set up to monitor more than one nursing unit, such as critical care and telemetry or intensive care and the monitors used in the emergency department.

The size and shape of the intensive care areas depend on the size of the hospital and the needs of the patients it serves. Smaller hospitals may have one combined unit, and larger hospitals may

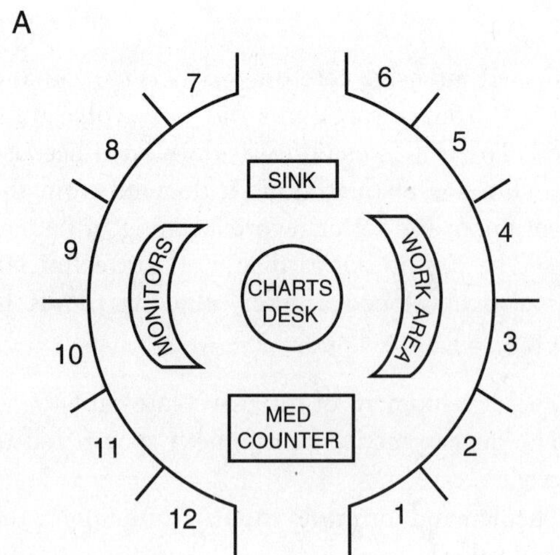

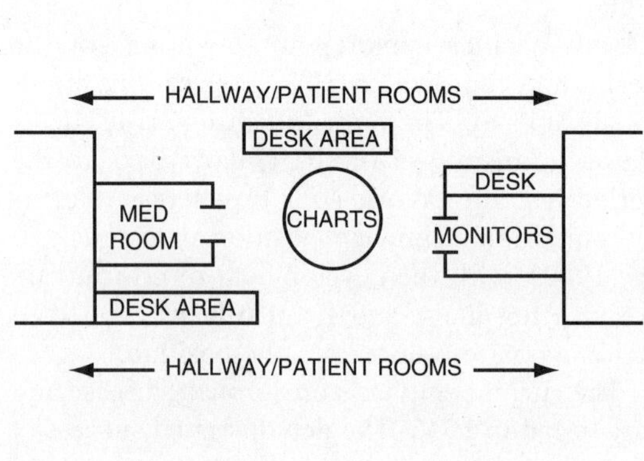

Figure 6–1
Physical layout.

have several units, each catering to the needs of a particular type of "critical" patient.

Educational Preparation

Proper identification of the rhythms as they appear on the monitor screen is crucial. The preparation for this responsibility is in the form of a basic electrocardiography (EKG) or **arrhythmia** course. The course typically includes:

- Basic cardiac anatomy
- Conduction system
- Correlation of waveforms with cardiac anatomy and physiology
- Correlation of the normal components of the EKG strip
- Recognition and significance of:
  - Normal rhythms
  - Blocks
  - Atrial arrhythmias
  - Ventricular arrhythmias
  - Asystole

The course of study ranges in length from 8 to 24 hours. An exam must be successfully completed for certification. The course is usually taught in the hospital setting, but in some areas it is available at local colleges.

Related Terminology

Terminology related to the position of a monitor technician is a combination of that taught during an HUC course and that taught in the basic EKG course. Terminology taught in the HUC course is general, covering an "A-to-Z" spectrum. The terminology taught in an EKG course is specific to the cardiovascular system. More in-depth general medical terminology courses may be offered through local colleges and may be helpful, if not required. Hospitals usually have a list of the terminology used in their particular facility with which it will be necessary to become familiar.

Position Responsibilities

Confidentiality

Confidentiality issues surrounding the monitor technician position are much the same as those confronting the HUC. Normally, any request for information about a patient is directed to the primary nurse and is handled by the HUC. Patient confidentiality is of the utmost importance and should not be breached for any reason.

Most states now have laws that govern and protect the rights of patients to decide who is allowed information about their illness, course of treatment, and prognosis. Breach of confidentiality is not only grounds for termination but could be grounds for a lawsuit should the wrong comment be overheard. Discussions concerning patient cases need to be held discreetly because passing visitors or family members may overhear information not meant for them. The main issue is the protection of patient privacy as well as rights. Monitor technicians should become familiar with the laws governing the "Patient Privacy Act" in the state where they work.

The log books, the report sheet, and the EKG strips are considered legal documents and contain personal information pertaining to the patient. This information needs to be guarded and given only to those involved in the case and who have permission to see it. Do not be afraid to ask someone for identification before releasing any information, written or verbal. Not only does this protect the patient, it protects the employee. Any paperwork that must be disposed of, such as the report sheets, should be torn several times or shredded.

Some hospitals allow EKG strips to be given to instructors or students for teaching and learning purposes, but the patient identification should be deleted.

Other Responsibilities

It is a responsibility of the monitor technician to obtain the required education to qualify to apply for and maintain this position. Once in the position, it is equally as important to continue to learn. Continued learning leads to self-improvement, inspires self-confidence, promotes efficiency, and contributes to better patient care.

Monitor Technician Duties

Patient Admission

When a patient is admitted, the monitor technician is required to run an initial EKG strip of that patient's rhythm and rate as a baseline and for documentation purposes. In some hospitals, the monitor technician is required to admit the patient to the monitoring system; in others, it is done by the nurse at the bedside monitor.

The process of admission to the monitoring system is as follows:

Pertinent patient information is entered onto a shift report sheet.
The same information is entered into a log book.
A file is established to maintain EKG strips for the length of stay in the unit.
Past medical history is noted, if available.
History of present illness is obtained, if possible.

This information will be helpful in alerting the monitor technician and other coronary care unit staff to possible complications that could arise during this illness.

The Monitors and Electrocardiogram Strips

Most hospital settings require that EKG strips be run on all patients at specific intervals for documentation purposes. These strips may be run every 2 hours, every 4 hours, or more frequently on unstable patients, critical patients, or during the time a procedure is being performed. The strips are properly identified with patient information and placed in the log. In some facilities they are also given to the primary nurse for placement into the permanent patient record.

Proper identification of the rhythms from the monitors and the strips is crucial. The monitor technician is the first to observe the information and to report it to other members of the team for immediate review and evaluation.

The following are examples of some common rhythms and brief explanations of what they are. The strip in Figure 26–2 shows a normal sinus rhythm (**NSR**) with a heart rate between 60 and 100 beats per minute. NSR is defined as that rhythm seen in a normally functioning heart. The electrical impulse is generated from the sinoatrial node, which is also known as the natural pacemaker of the heart. The electrical impulses are transmitted through the conduction system, depolarizing the muscle and initiating the contraction that pumps blood into the ventricles and then through the body.

The strip in Figure 26–3 shows a sinus bradycardia with a rate of less than 60. Sinus **brady** is

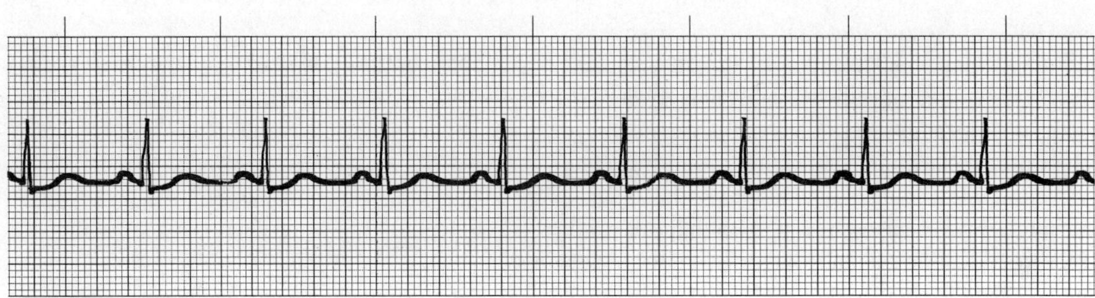

Figure 26–2
Normal sinus rhythm (strip). (From Cohn EG, Gilroy-Doohan M: Flip And See ECG. Philadelphia, WB Saunders, 1996.)

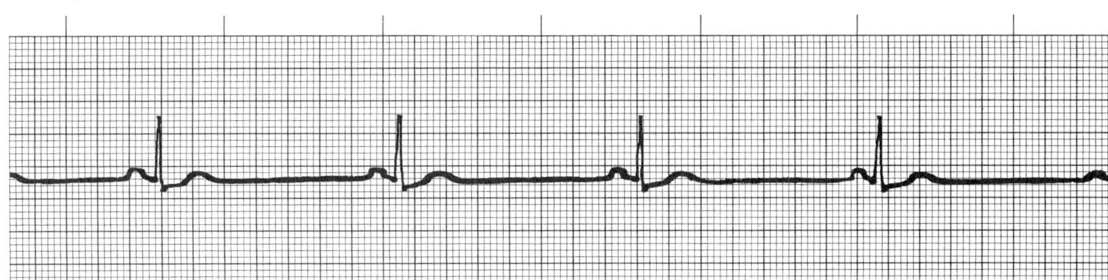

Figure 26–3
Sinus bradycardia (strip). (From Cohn EG, Gilroy-Doohan M: Flip And See ECG. Philadelphia, WB Saunders, 1996.)

defined as a rhythm producing a heart rate of less than 60 beats per minute. Sinus brady can be caused by drugs or severe damage to the heart muscle. It can be symptomatic of cellular degeneration in the sinoatrial node. If it is severe and persistent, life-threatening arrhythmias can result.

The strip in Figure 26–4 shows premature ventricular contractions (**PVCs**). PVCs are defined as uncoordinated firing of electrical impulses originating in the ventricles, usually indicating an irritable focus. PVCs can be caused by heart disease and electrolyte imbalances, particularly those in potassium levels. Frequent PVCs can lead to another abnormal rhythm known as ventricular tachycardia (**V tach**), which is a life-threatening arrhythmia.

The strip in Figure 26–5 shows an arrhythmia called asystole. Asystole is defined as a rhythm indicating the absence of electrical activity in the heart; it is also known as a "flat line." It may follow severe untreated sinus bradycardia, a high degree of heart block, or ventricular **fibrillation** (V fib).

The importance of having a knowledge of cardiac disease can be demonstrated here. What may otherwise be an abnormal rhythm might be the "expected" for a particular disease. For example, frequent PVCs would be abnormal for a person admitted with chronic obstructive pulmonary disease, but would not be unusual for a person with an acute myocardial infarction (**MI**).

Report

Reporting patient rate and rhythm is the responsibility of the monitor technician. It is yet another reason that proper interpretation of the strips is vital. The report is given to the oncoming monitor technician and the registered nurse in charge at shift change. The information is passed on to the physicians.

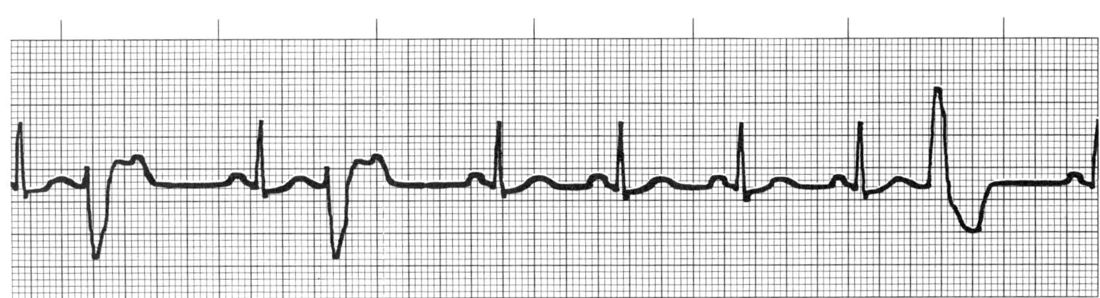

Figure 26–4
Premature ventricular contractions (strip). (From Cohn EG, Gilroy-Doohan M: Flip And See ECG. Philadelphia, WB Saunders, 1996.)

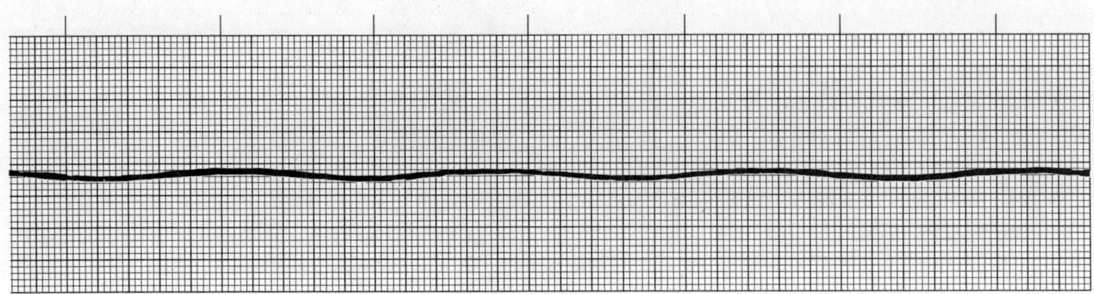

Figure 26–5
Asytole (strip). (From Cohn EG, Gilroy-Doohan M: Flip And See ECG. Philadelphia, WB Saunders, 1996.)

A report includes the patient name, age, date of admission, diagnosis, brief history of present illness, present rate and rhythm, and any abnormalities noted during the shift.

The information from the report sheet is verbally communicated in a similar format: "Room 101 is Mrs. Jones, a 50-year-old patient of Dr. Smith's with the diagnosis of possible MI. She was admitted this morning with severe chest pain which has improved. She has maintained a rate of 84 during my shift. She has a baseline of normal sinus rhythm. She has had occasional asymptomatic PVCs."

Documentation

The documentation involved in this position is usually limited to maintaining the logs and report sheets.

As EKG strips are run off at the specified intervals, the rate, rhythm and measurements of some of the waves are entered into the logs and or report sheets (Fig. 26–6). Other pertinent information such as patient identifying information, pulse, blood pressure, and date and time can be added to the full sheet.

Another type of observation record could be used for a 24-hour period (Fig. 26–7).

Information is recorded at intervals specified by policy. The comment area is used to record procedures done or to note what patient activity is occurring when a change is noted.

Log books contain the following information:

Date and time of admission
Patient name
Patient age

DATE	ROOM	NAME	AGE	DOCTOR	DIAGNOSIS	RATE	RHYTHM
6/1/97	201	Mary J. Doe	71	Jones	Chest pain	55	Sinus Brady

Figure 26–6
Log entry.

DATE	ROOM	NAME			MED RECORD #	DIAGNOSIS
6/1/97	201	Mary J. Doe			15554444	Chest pain
TIME	PULSE	B/P	RATE	RHYTHM	COMMENTS	
2400	58	100/57	60	Sinus Brady	Patient resting comfortably	
0200	55	90/50	57	Sinus Brady	Patient sleeping	
0400	50	85/50	55	Sinus Brady	Patient having pain	
0600						
0800						
1000						
1200						
1400						
1600						
1800						
2000						

Figure 26–7
24-hour record.

Medical record or admission number
Diagnosis
Physician of record
Date, time, and place of transfer
Date and time of death (if applicable)

These log books are often maintained by the HUC. They are kept for reference as well as utilization review and quality assurance projects.

Equipment

Continuous monitoring of cardiac rhythms and rates through visual contact with the screens and periodic running of the EKG strips is the basis of the monitor technician position. Knowledge of the monitoring equipment is essential to keep the monitors in working order at all times. Monitor technicians must know how to run EKG strips, how the alarms are set, and how to change the EKG paper. They are expected to deal with specific functions of the monitoring system during a patient arrest. Equipment varies from hospital to hospital and unit to unit. The monitoring information may consist of telemetry from one unit or several others. It may be part of a sophisticated computer system with links to ambulance systems and doctors' offices. Thorough knowledge of the equipment and the principles of its use makes the day-to-day operations somewhat easier (Fig. 26–8).

A Typical Day

A typical day for a monitor technician could consist of the following:

Receiving report on the patients from the previous shift monitor technician
Running strips on patients while receiving report

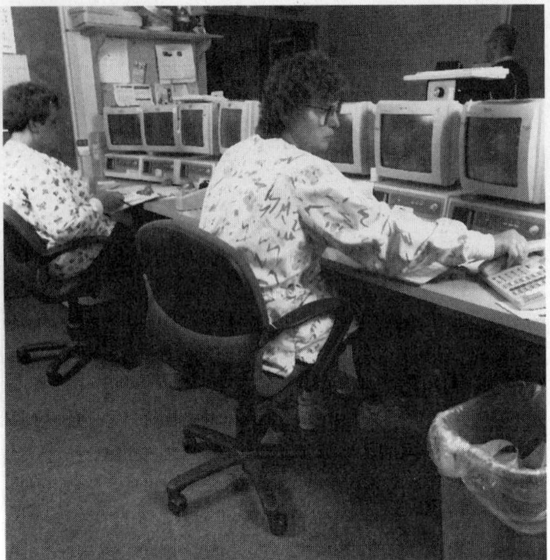

Figure 26–8
Monitor techs at bank of monitors.

Labeling the strips with the appropriate information
Initiating the shift report sheet from the unit census
Placing the information and strips on the report sheet
Reporting to the registered nurse in charge
Reporting to physicians as requested
Running strips at specified intervals per unit protocol
Logging strips
Checking paper supply in monitors
Replacing paper in monitors as needed
Watching monitors all the time while accomplishing other duties
Running strips on any unusual or changed rhythms and **dysrhythmias**
Reporting changes to the nurse
Being sure a replacement is available when leaving the monitors for breaks and lunch or any other reason
Completing logs and records for the shift
Reporting off to the oncoming shift

Health Unit Coordinator Knowledge and Skills

Health unit coordinator knowledge and skills are transferrable because cross-training between the two positions is common.

Organizational Skills

Organizational skills and thought processes learned as a HUC help the monitor technician with developing proper and efficient logging skills as well as in organizing an effective work area. HUC training involves charting of vital signs and their significance. This is helpful to the monitor technician in correlating vital signs with what is being displayed on the monitors.

Computer Knowledge and Skills

Computer knowledge and skills are quickly becoming requirements for both HUCs and monitor technicians. Some cardiac monitoring systems are controlled through a keyboard that connects with admissions and discharge systems. Computer entry is part of order transcription and interdepartmental communications in many facilities. Specific skill requirements vary among institutions, as do the systems and software.

Additional Training

Additional training required is set by institution policy and protocol. Some typical areas of additional training are described in the following sections.

Cardiopulmonary Resuscitation

As a member of the health care team, the monitor technician is required to be certified in cardiopulmonary resuscitation (CPR). In addition to teaching life-saving skills, this course offers information about coronary artery disease, touches on the operation of the cardiovascular and pulmonary systems, and focuses on prevention and intervention relative to MI.

The course is taught in the hospital, and typically is offered on a monthly or quarterly basis to employees. Annual certification is required. The program also offers advancement to instructor and instructor trainer levels.

Advanced Electrocardiograph Courses

Advanced EKG courses are often offered by the education department of the hospitals to meet further requirements of various positions or to fulfill the desire for further knowledge and skills.

The course consists of the breakdown and interpretation of the 12-lead EKG. The activities of the heart will become clearer and the location of an MI can be identified.

The 12-lead EKG provides more information than a monitor strip and is used as a diagnostic tool and for progress reports.

Refresher Courses

Refresher courses and yearly testing for EKG interpretation and CPR are offered through the hospital and are usually required to maintain employment in the position. Field-related workshops and in-services training assist in maintaining or upgrading job-related knowledge and skills.

Hospital-Specific Training

Each hospital requires an orientation program. This usually lasts 1 to 2 days and consists of general information about the facility and its philosophy, mission, benefits, and policies.

A unit-specific orientation lasts from 2 to 8 weeks and consists of on-the-job training in procedures and functions of a particular unit. The length of the orientation depends on the trainee's ability to learn procedures and function effectively.

Trainees work directly with a preceptor in the same unit in which they will work. The trainee's performance is evaluated at specified intervals for progress and compatibility with the environment.

Closing Thoughts

The position of a monitor technician can be exciting and challenging. It also carries with it a great deal of responsibility. This position challenges you to acquire further knowledge and skills, not only for personal reasons, but more to ensure efficient patient care. The monitor technician is depended on for the accurate interpretation of rhythms and the ability to recognize potentially life-threatening situations. Through early recognition and intervention in these situations, the monitor technician can be a part of the health care team that will allow a grandparent the opportunity to attend the graduation or wedding of a grandchild or to return parents home to watch their children grow.

The monitor technician is a vital part of a health care team, whose success depends on cooperative effort.

It is hoped that this chapter has offered an insight into the world of a monitor technician—what is expected on the job as well as areas to turn to that will help achieve success, higher knowledge, and skills.

Review Questions

1. Discuss the evolution of the monitor technician position.
2. List the responsibilities of the monitor technician when a patient is admitted to the monitor system.
3. Describe a typical day for a monitor technician.
4. Discuss additional training that might be necessary for the position of monitor technician.

Bibliography

Dorland's Illustrated Medical Dictionary, 28th ed. Philadelphia, WB Saunders, 1994.

Isselbacher K, et al: Harrison's Principles of Internal Medicine, 13th ed. New York, McGraw-Hill, 1994.

LaFleur-Brooks M: Health Unit Coordinating, 3rd ed. Philadelphia, WB Saunders, 1993.

O'Toole M (ed): Miller-Keane Encyclopedia and Dictionary of Medicine, Nursing and Allied Health, 6th ed. Philadelphia, WB Saunders, 1997.

27 The Pharmacy Assistant

Jessie Shelby/Virginia S. Mazza

Common Abbreviations

LAF Laminar air flow

PCA Patient-controlled analgesia

TPN Total parenteral nutrition

Objectives

Upon completion of this chapter, the reader should be able to:

1. Identify five positions in a hospital pharmacy to which a health unit coordinator could aspire.
2. Explain the primary responsibility of a medication technician.
3. Discuss the purpose of the laminar air flow hood.
4. Describe the responsibilities of a pharmacy technician II.
5. List three responsibilities of the stock technician.

Vocabulary

Laminar air flow: Air flow in which the entire body of air within a confined area moves with essentially unidirectional velocity along parallel flow lines (nonturbulent)

Patient-controlled analgesia: A method of controlling pain in which the patient is able to regulate, within limits, the amount and frequency of the medication and self-administer it by means of a pump

Total parenteral nutrition: The intravenous administration of the total nutritional requirements of a patient to supply all the nutrients necessary during critical illness

Unit dose system: A system of preparing and dispensing medications in individual doses.

History

"Pharmacy assistant" is a broad title that may cover many different types of job responsibilities in the hospital pharmacy. Most of these are positions to which a health unit coordinator (HUC) could aspire. With the changes that have occurred in health care, the pharmacist has taken on a much different role. No longer is the pharmacist primarily the dispenser of medication. More and more, he or she takes on a clinical role and works closely with physicians in planning the drug treatment of the patient, developing protocol management, and assisting with product selection and drug interaction concerns. There are now pharmacists with expertise in the areas of cardiology, oncology, gastroenterology, pediatrics, geriatrics, and so forth. Many of the tasks once performed by pharmacists are now being carried out by support personnel. These tasks range from the clerical aspects of the pharmacy to preparing the drugs for delivery to the nursing units. This chapter explores the various positions that might be found in a large or small hospital pharmacy and discusses the responsibilities of each. The titles used here for the positions described are not necessarily the only ones that might be used for jobs of a similar nature.

Position Responsibilities and Duties

Medication Technician

The role of the medication technician (or pharmacy technician I) as described here is carried out primarily in a central or satellite pharmacy area. Many hospitals may have a decentralized pharmacy situation in which the pharmacists are located directly in the patient care areas, and the dispensing of the medications is handled in a central pharmacy or satellite. Key duties in this position are to receive and process the physician orders as they are entered into the patients' records by the pharmacist or the HUC on the nursing unit. Medication orders might also be received directly in the pharmacy on the physician's order sheet from the patient's chart. Routing telephone calls for medication orders is an integral part of this position.

Most hospitals now dispense medications for administration in what is known as a **unit dose system**. In this system, each dose of medication for each patient is sent to the nursing unit from the pharmacy in an individually packaged and labeled form. Many medications are prepared by the manufacturer in single-dose packages, whereas other medications are shipped in bulk and must be packaged into individual doses in the hospital pharmacy. This packaging is another responsibility of the pharmacy technician I.

The medication technician is responsible for the daily preparation of medications for each patient in the hospital. This includes review of the patients' records for medications that have been discontinued since the previous day, changes that may have been made in dosage or frequency, changes in the patients' locations, and any new medications that have been ordered.

Once the review of the patients' medication records has been completed, the supply of medications for a specific period of time is selected and organized in a properly identified container. It is sent to the nursing unit for distribution to the patients at the appropriate times. The actual system for doing this varies from one hospital to another, but the basic information necessary to complete the task will generally be the same. This will probably be a very time-consuming task because it involves many patients and even more medications. Accuracy is, of course, extremely important. Once the process has been completed, the pharmacist in charge checks to make sure that the medications have been correctly selected. The medication technician always works under the direct supervision of a pharmacist.

Many hospitals use a medication cart exchange system (Fig. 27–1). In this system, one or more carts, each containing a series of drawers for a given number of patients, are delivered to the nursing unit by the medication technician after the carts have been stocked with the necessary medications for a given period of time (usually 24 hours). The empty cart is returned to the

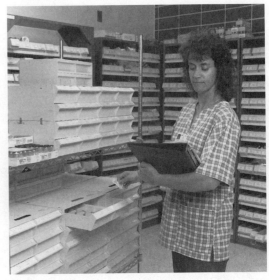

Figure 27–1
Medication cart.

pharmacy for restocking for the next time period.

The medication technician is also responsible for any new orders for medications that are received during the course of the day. These drugs are prepared and sent to the nursing unit as the orders are received in the pharmacy. The medication technician must be aware of the STAT orders that are received and make sure to process them and prepare the medications in a timely manner so that there is a minimum of delay in getting the drug to the patient for administration.

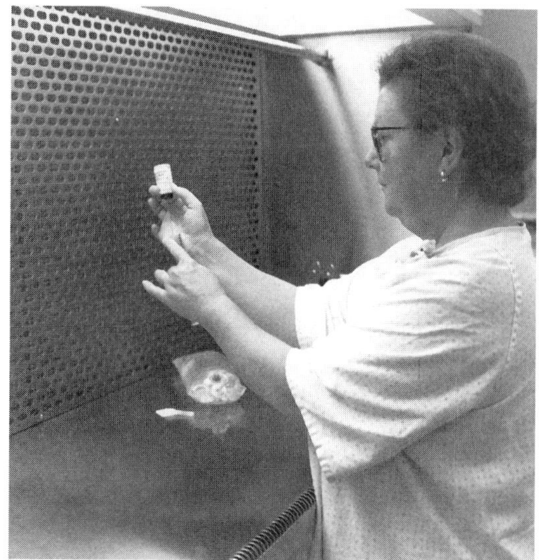

Figure 27–2
Laminar air flow hood.

Pharmacy Technician II

This position is also known as a sterile products technician. The responsibilities of a person in this position would include preparation of injections and infusion fluids (which could also include controlled substances) and the admixing of parenteral nutrition mixtures, cytotoxic drugs, and investigational drugs. Because all of these are substances that must be prepared and administered under sterile circumstances, the pharmacy technician II must have a thorough understanding of aseptic technique. The responsibilities of the pharmacy technician II include calculations and details of order entry beyond the scope of the medication technician.

To ensure the sterility of the products being prepared, the work of the pharmacy technician II is usually done in an environment of positive pressure. This prevents microorganisms in the air from entering the work area because air is always flowing out of the room. The preparation itself is done under a **laminar air flow (LAF)** hood that filters and controls the flow of air away from the work area and the worker (Fig. 27–2).

Injections prepared by the pharmacy technician II include antibiotics and controlled substances. Many times, narcotics are prepared so that the patients may administer the drug themselves in a system called **patient-controlled analgesia (PCA)**. There are other types of medications that may be prepared for intravenous (IV) use as well.

A primary responsibility of the pharmacy technician II is the preparation of **total parenteral nutrition (TPN)**. This mode of therapy provides all the vital nutrients that a patient requires for total nourishment when he or she is not able to take nourishment by mouth. The basic fluid is of very high concentration, and many other nutrients are added in the preparation of the mixture. This provides an ideal environment for the growth of microorganisms, and it is therefore extremely important that strict sterile technique is maintained in the process. Preparation of these products is done under an LAF hood (Fig. 27–3). Precise dosages of the components to be added to the mixture are also very important. Therefore, strict adherence to procedure is vital. Computerized equipment is often used in preparation of these products (Fig. 27–4). Accurate and complete documentation of the work is a prime responsibility of the pharmacy technician II.

Chemotherapy or cytotoxic drugs used for the treatment of patients with cancer are prepared by the pharmacy technician II. These hazardous substances are mixed under a specific type of LAF hood called a containment hood. It is important

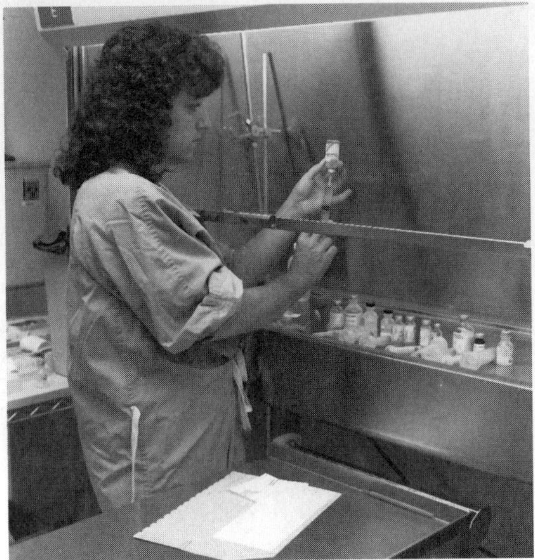

Figure 27–3
IV medications for TPN preparation.

that the technician and environment not become contaminated with hazardous drugs, so the special hood, gloves and gown, and other strict precautions are necessary. Attention to detail and proper dosage is vital. Accuracy in preparation is important, primarily because the life of the patient is at stake, but also because of the high cost of many of these drugs.

As with the medication technician, all the work of the pharmacy technician II is done under the direct supervision of a pharmacist and all medications are checked by that supervisor before being dispensed for administration to the patient. Documentation is critical. A system of checks and balances ensures that the patient is receiving the proper drugs in the correct dosages. These systems must always be adhered to in order to prevent serious errors.

Revenue Clerk

This is a position that may be known by many other names, but the general work it entails will be similar regardless of its designation.

Because of the high costs of medical care in general and medications in particular, it is important that treatments the patient receives while in the hospital are charged appropriately. This provides accurate records for insurance purposes. It also eliminates the need to increase base charges to all patients to offset losses due to expensive items that have not been charged to the patients who received them. The role of the revenue clerk in the pharmacy is to review the medication records on a daily basis and ensure that the drugs each patient received have been charged to the patient's account. A large number of medications are administered daily, so it is likely that only the most expensive drugs will be reviewed. This review acts as a system of checks and balances to the medical record because it is important that all medications the patient receives are documented on the medication administration record of the patient's chart. This is vital for insurance as well as legal reasons.

Each hospital has its own system for dealing with how the patient is charged for these medications. Figure 27–5 shows one manual or paper system that may be used. However, this often is done by means of a computer (Fig. 27–6).

There are other routine clerical duties that could be the responsibility of the revenue clerk, such as compiling statistics, reviewing billing information, completing reports, responding to requests for information, assembling and fil-

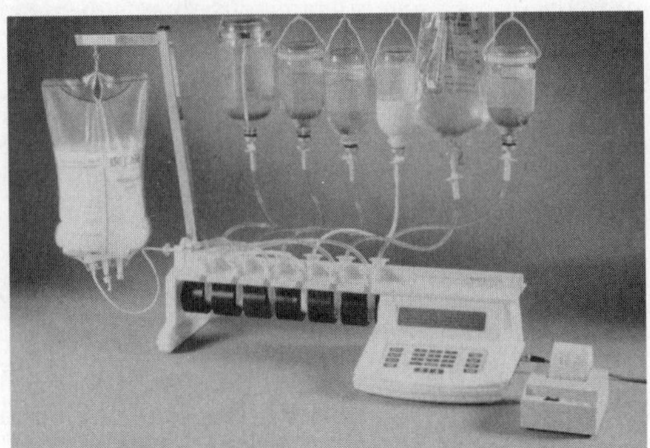

Figure 27–4
Automated compounder for TPN solutions. (Courtesy of Metrix Secure.)

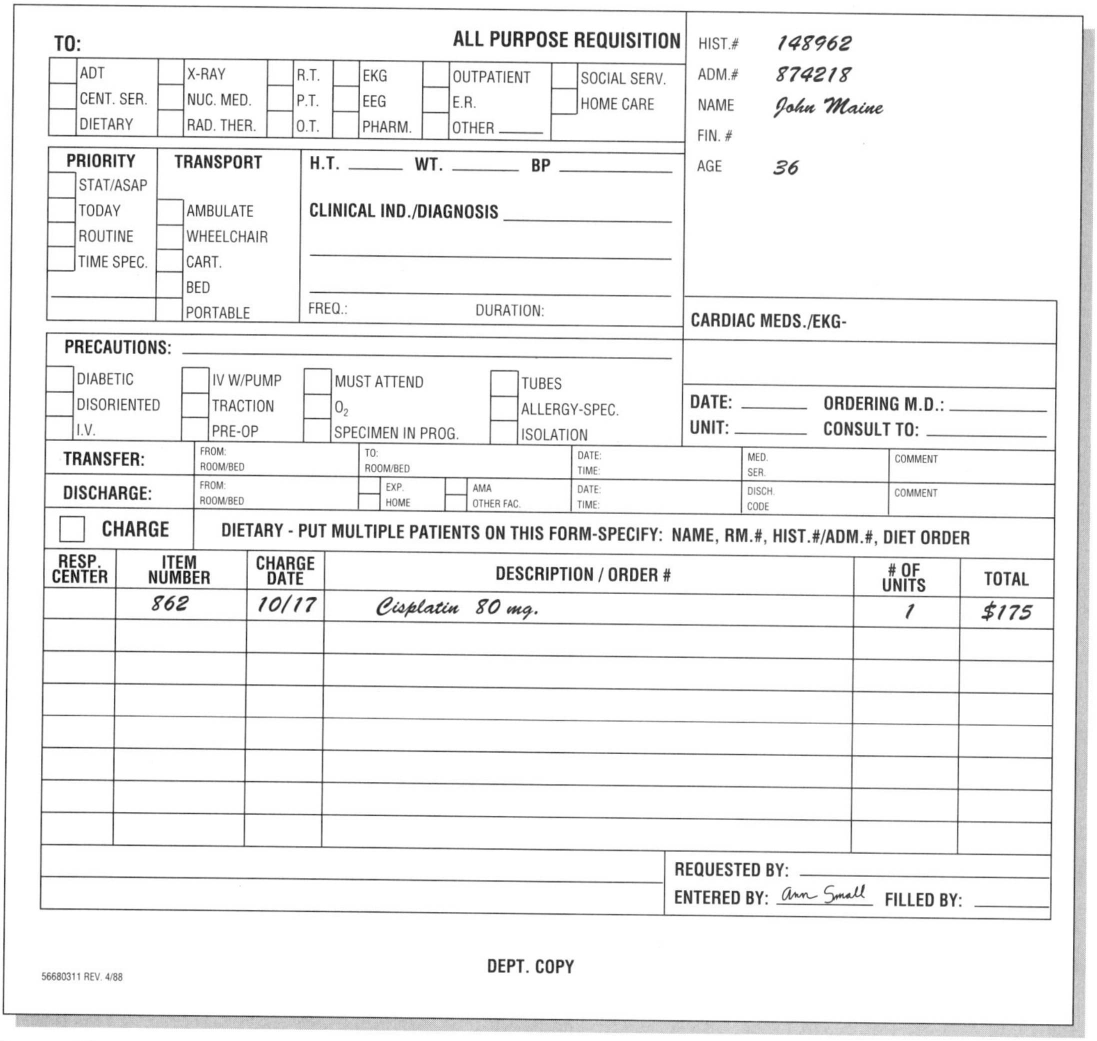

TO: ALL PURPOSE REQUISITION

HIST.# 148962
ADM.# 874218
NAME John Maine
FIN. #
AGE 36

☐ ADT ☐ CENT. SER. ☐ DIETARY ☐ X-RAY ☐ NUC. MED. ☐ RAD. THER. ☐ R.T. ☐ P.T. ☐ O.T. ☐ EKG ☐ EEG ☐ PHARM. ☐ OUTPATIENT ☐ E.R. ☐ OTHER ____ ☐ SOCIAL SERV. ☐ HOME CARE

PRIORITY: ☐ STAT/ASAP ☐ TODAY ☐ ROUTINE ☐ TIME SPEC.

TRANSPORT: ☐ AMBULATE ☐ WHEELCHAIR ☐ CART. ☐ BED ☐ PORTABLE

H.T. ____ WT. ____ BP ____

CLINICAL IND./DIAGNOSIS ____

FREQ.: DURATION:

CARDIAC MEDS./EKG-

PRECAUTIONS: ____

☐ DIABETIC ☐ DISORIENTED ☐ I.V. ☐ IV W/PUMP ☐ TRACTION ☐ PRE-OP ☐ MUST ATTEND ☐ O_2 ☐ SPECIMEN IN PROG. ☐ TUBES ☐ ALLERGY-SPEC. ☐ ISOLATION

DATE: ____ ORDERING M.D.: ____
UNIT: ____ CONSULT TO: ____

TRANSFER: FROM: ROOM/BED TO: ROOM/BED DATE: TIME: MED. SER. COMMENT

DISCHARGE: FROM: ROOM/BED ☐ EXP. HOME ☐ AMA OTHER FAC. DATE: TIME: DISCH. CODE COMMENT

☐ CHARGE DIETARY - PUT MULTIPLE PATIENTS ON THIS FORM-SPECIFY: NAME, RM.#, HIST.#/ADM.#, DIET ORDER

RESP. CENTER	ITEM NUMBER	CHARGE DATE	DESCRIPTION / ORDER #	# OF UNITS	TOTAL
	862	10/17	Cisplatin 80 mg.	1	$175

REQUESTED BY: ____
ENTERED BY: Ann Small FILLED BY: ____

56680311 REV. 4/88

DEPT. COPY

Figure 27–5
All-purpose requisition form.

ing patient information, and other duties related to the position. The revenue clerk might also assist hospital auditors in drug-charging explanations.

Stock Technician

In smaller hospitals, this position may be combined with the medication technician or pharmacy technician I role.

The pharmacy stock technician manages all controlled substances (narcotics) that are used throughout the hospital (Fig. 27–7). Every hospital has its own system for distributing and accounting for controlled substances. However, the need for accurate accounting of all controlled drugs is the same. Federal law governs the distribution and recording of all controlled drugs dispensed from the pharmacy. An example of a state-of-the-art dispensing system is shown in

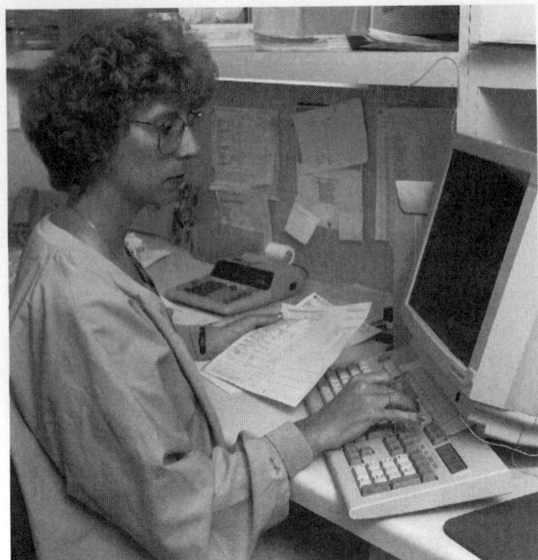

Figure 27–6
Revenue clerk.

Figure 27–8. In this system, the medications used are readily available and accounted for automatically on dispensing. This cuts down on manual record-keeping tasks and reduces the opportunity for diversion.

The person holding this position is responsible for managing and distributing all nonscheduled medications that are kept as floor stock on the nursing units. This would include such items as laxatives, simple pain relievers, lubricants, and nonmedicated IV solutions. In most cases, the HUC on the nursing unit submits an order to the pharmacy to replenish the floor stock, and the stock technician fills the order and delivers it to the nursing unit.

Another responsibility of the stock technician might be to review drugs used by anesthesia personnel and charge the patients appropriately. Those drugs that are used in surgery, as well as IV solutions used during surgery, might also be the responsibility of the person in this position. This would include ensuring adequate stock as well as documenting the charges.

The stock technician is responsible for the receipt, check-in, and storage of all drugs received in the pharmacy. The restocking of emergency carts is a task that is usually assigned to the stock technician.

These are the main tasks that a pharmacy stock technician might be expected to perform in any hospital; however, there are probably many other tasks specific to a particular hospital that have not been mentioned here.

Pharmacy Buyer

A buyer in a hospital pharmacy has far-reaching responsibilities. These include maintaining and monitoring pharmacy drug and IV fluid inventories as well as other supplies used and needed by the pharmacy department.

The person holding this position is responsible for the execution and maintenance of purchase orders for pharmaceutical stock (Fig. 27–9). This may be done electronically, by telephone, mail, or fax, or by other means. It is necessary to maintain a purchase order log and inventory control of pharmacy stock. This includes setting mini-

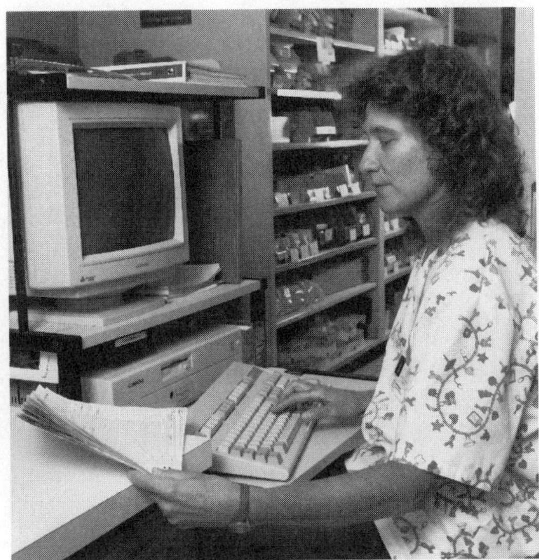

Figure 27–7
Stock technician.

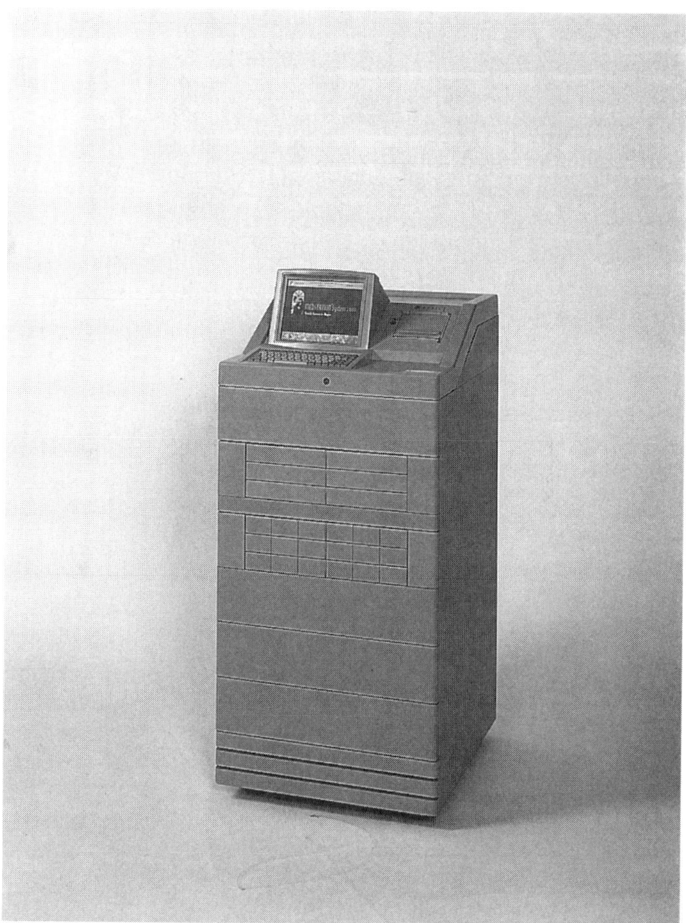

Figure 27–8
Automated drug dispensing system. (Courtesy of Pyxis Corporation.)

mum and maximum stock levels, minimizing stock outages, and overseeing rotation of the stock.

The person who functions as buyer for the pharmacy coordinates the return of outdated pharmaceutical items and handles the details of drug recalls. He or she is responsible for acquiring drugs that are needed on an emergency basis.

Keeping up with new pharmaceutical products on the market (e.g., by literature reviews) and meeting with pharmaceutical company representatives are additional responsibilities of the pharmacy buyer.

Health Unit Coordinator Knowledge and Skills Appropriate to Positions

All of the positions discussed in the previous sections can use the skills obtained through HUC education and experience. Having a working knowledge of the nursing unit is a tremendous asset when dealing with medications from the pharmacy perspective. Total familiarity with the medical record and an intimate knowledge of medical terminology also enhance the qualifica-

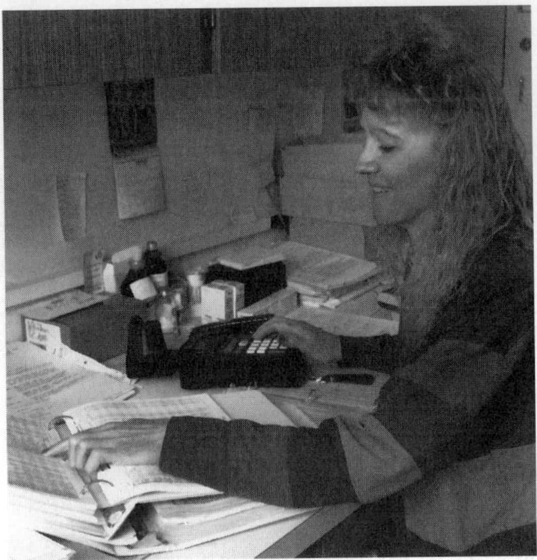

Figure 27–9
Pharmacy buyer.

tions of a HUC to function in any of the pharmacy assistant positions. And, of course, the HUC has a complete understanding of how hospital computer systems function. The HUC has the additional advantage of having interfaced with all the other hospital departments, which makes him or her aware of the intricacies of coordinating whatever is necessary to make the process flow more smoothly.

All of these positions require very good telephone skills and the ability to function as a team member. Problem solving and issues of confidentiality are also skills the HUC would bring to this position. In addition, the ability to prioritize and work independently are skills the HUC has achieved through educational and work experiences.

Attention to detail, a high degree of self-discipline, ability to work under stressful conditions, and good communications skills are essential for the positions in the pharmacy, and the HUC has had experience in all of these areas.

In addition, the HUC has a working knowledge of medication orders. This can prove invaluable when moving into a position in the pharmacy.

Additional Training Required

Although many of the positions that have been discussed here may not require any additional formal training, obtaining further education in courses such as basic chemistry, algebra, microbiology, and related health sciences is certainly desirable. Continually updating computer skills is necessary in most of these roles.

A thorough understanding of sterile technique and microbiology is necessary to qualify for the position of pharmacy technician II.

Certification as a pharmacy technician is an option available to pharmacy assistants and is encouraged. This may be a requirement in some hospitals.

The position of pharmacy buyer requires a 2-year associate degree in many institutions. This course work should include courses in math, accounting, basic statistics, chemistry, microcomputers, and other health care or purchasing-related courses.

Closing Thoughts

The pharmacy is an area of natural progression for a HUC. Because the pharmacy works so closely with the nursing units, it is very helpful to have workers there who are familiar with the day-to-day activities in the patient care areas. Being familiar with medication orders, understanding the importance of STAT, and knowing what receiving those drugs in a timely manner means to the nursing personnel can make the HUC the patient's best ally in the pharmacy.

Because so much of what the pharmacy assistant does occurs without direct supervision, the HUC, with that background as a given, becomes an instant performer in the role.

Pharmacy assistant is a position that allows a HUC to use the skills he or she already possesses and to learn new ones in an environment that can be very rewarding. There is probably no other area of the hospital that deals with greater numbers of patients than the pharmacy, and thus the pharmacy assistant can have a real impact on the care a patient receives.

Review Questions

1. Identify five positions in a hospital pharmacy to which a HUC could aspire.
2. Explain the primary responsibility of a medication technician.
3. Discuss the purpose of the laminar air flow hood.
4. Describe the responsibilities of a pharmacy technician II.
5. List three responsibilities of the stock technician.

SECTION THREE

THE HEALTH UNIT COORDINATOR IN THE HEALTH CARE INDUSTRY

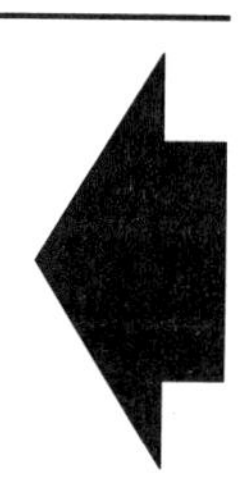

28 Agency Staffing Services

Karen DiFrancesco

Common Abbreviations

CNA	Certified nursing assistant
DHHS	Department of Health and Human Services
DON	Director of nursing
LPN	Licensed practical nurse
RN	Registered nurse

Objectives

Upon completion of this chapter, the reader should be able to:

1. Define supplemental staffing and the people it provides to health care facilities.
2. Identify the role of the scheduling coordinator.
3. Identify the technical and communication skills necessary in the role of the scheduling coordinator.
4. Explain the duties and responsibilities to both the agency and the clients contracting for services.

Vocabulary

Agency: A business whose primary function is to provide temporary nursing staff to health care facilities such as hospitals, clinics, and long-term care centers

Client: A health care facility that has contracted with the agency for services

Incident: An occurrence that is unusual in the normal course of events.

History

Agency staffing services evolved because health care facilities were experiencing shortages and were not able to employ sufficient staff to meet the needs of the patients requiring care. Much of this was due to increased patient admissions or turnover in staff. This caused in-house shortages of registered nurses (**RNs**), licensed practical nurses (**LPNs**), and certified nursing assistants (**CNAs**). Another need for agency staffing was created with the increase of psychiatric and mental health hospital discharges. Patients were sent out into the community unprepared to care for themselves. Fortunately, halfway homes and some residential facilities provided shelter for these individuals. However, professional medical personnel (e.g., RNs, LPNs, and CNAs) were needed to follow up on the patients' needs for care, counseling, and medication. Agency staffing popularity increased as people who provided the shelters now had a resource to provide high-quality clinical care. In time, the Department of Health and Human Services (**DHHS**) required residential (group) homes to meet specified regulations to offer services for the residents requiring attention.

Agency staffing is a desirable employment alternative for many health care professionals. RNs, LPNs, and CNAs are allowed to take responsibility for scheduling their own work time. This allows for versatility and flexibility in the employee's career. These people are quick to adapt to any health care environment and are skilled enough to adapt to the changes in health care settings. Often nurses have many years of experience when they decide to join an agency staffing service. Agency employees develop loyalty to the staffing agency because they understand the importance of their professional contributions to its success. They are effective team members dispatched into the community's health care facilities. Agency personnel perform their duties in a manner that provides positive feedback and ensures further requests from the health care facilities for their services in the future. Recently, health unit coordinators (**HUCs**) have joined the ranks of those employed by agencies.

This chapter explores the role of a scheduling coordinator in one agency staffing office. It must be realized that the information contained in this chapter is specific to the facility being described. Every nursing staffing agency is unique, and some of the situations described here may not occur in other agencies.

Education/Employment Experience

The scheduling coordinator should have the following educational and employment qualifications:

1. High school diploma or equivalent.
2. Completion of a recognized HUC program. National certification is desirable.
3. One or more years in a health care facility or medical office setting.

Position

The scheduling coordinator is directly accountable to the director of nursing (**DON**) and the administrator. He or she is also accountable to the **clients** and staff who depend on the services of the agency.

The scheduling coordinator is responsible for the supplemental staffing of health care facilities. These include specialty hospitals, general hospitals, and long-term care facilities (e.g., residential, skilled nursing homes, hospices).

Supplemental staffing also reaches out to those patients who have chosen to receive home health care nursing services. This includes staffing RNs with specialties in intravenous therapy, catheter care, wound care, and diabetes, to mention the more common areas of nurse clinician expertise. LPNs and CNAs are also staffed to the home care patient. Agency staffing has also helped to meet the needs of physician practices and ambulatory care clinics.

Required Skills

Communication

The most important skill one can possess is the ability to communicate effectively. The scheduling coordinator is fulfilling needs continually. It is important to have excellent communication skills because all transactions originate and are completed by telephone, fax machine, computer, or some combination of these methods.

The scheduling coordinator is at the hub of coordination of requests for service (Fig. 28–1). availability of staff (Fig. 28–2), and, ultimately, for the filling of requests (Fig. 28–3).

Medical Terminology

Medical terminology is the common language used by the facilities that agencies staff, as well as by the professionals who are contracted to those facilities. An effective scheduler is one who has a clear understanding of medical terms, particularly as they relate to the nursing specialties and the needs of the areas to be staffed. These areas of specialty include:

1. Medical/surgical (med/surg)
2. Telemetry
3. Intensive care unit/coronary care unit (ICU/CCU)
4. Neurointensive care unit, surgical intensive care unit (NICU, SICU)

FACILITY NEEDS

Log 2/9/97

1701	Hilltop Hospital needs RN- 3rd - ICU	2/9
1710	St. Jo's " " RN - 1st Med/Surg.	2/10
1711	St. Marks " " RN - 1st Med/ "	2/10
1712	Riverview Psyche needs RN 2nd Adol.	2/10
1720	St. Marks - cancelled Paula Smeak Ø needs for 3rd	2/9
1721	Hilltop Hospital needs RN 1st OB/GYN	2/10
1730	Rv - Psyche needs Psyche Tech 1st shift	2/10
1800	St. Jo's needs RN 1st shift OB/GYN	
1804	Wilmore Hosp. needs RN 1st .	2/10. 2/11. 2/12 - ICU.
1815	Mercy Hosp. needs RN 1st - onocology.	2/12
1819	Grace Rehab Hosp. needs RN 2nd SICU	2/11
1[illegible]	Holy Name Ho[illegible] " " [illegible] SICU	2/[illegible]

Figure 28–1
Facility requests form.

5. Pediatric intensive care unit, emergency room (Peds ICU, ER)
6. Obstetrics (LDRP)
7. Gynecology (GYN)
8. Psychiatry
9. Operating room, recovery room (OR, RR)
10. Supervisor (of hospital, home care, nursing home)
11. Home care
12. Office/clinic

Position Responsibilities

Clients

To obtain and maintain optimum rapport with agency clients, the scheduling coordinator will:

1. Contact clients to obtain their needs and meet those needs in a prompt manner.
2. Follow through with new client requests for information.
3. Maintain client information sheets in a current fashion, keeping all data updated.
4. Act as a customer service representative to clients regarding:
   a. Regular evaluations on agency employees
   b. Follow-through on any client complaints, **incident** reports, or concerns
5. Direct to the administrator any client concerns requiring his or her attention, such as incident reports, lateness, or attitude problems.
6. Accompany administrator on client appointments to assist with recruiting new health agencies for contract staffing.

STAFF AVAILABILITY		
Mary Smith, ICU	3rd Shift	2/9, 2/10, 2/11, 2/12
Lynn Moss, Med/Surg	1st Shift	2/10, 2/12, 2/15
Kevin Jones, M/S	1st	2/10, 2/11. - (2/10 - 8a. start x)
Cathy Drake, Psyche	2nd "	2/10, 2/11, 2/12
Peg Fritz	~	try to contact re: avail.
D.J. Tonka, OB-GYN	1st	2/9, 2/10, 2/11
Dave Frankie - Y RN	1st	2/8, 2/9, 2/10, 2/11
Becky White OB-GYN	1st	2/9, 2/10, 2/11, 2/12
Nancy Slim ICU	1st	2/9, 2/10, 2/11, 2/12, 2/13
Diane Kotel - onc.	1st	2/11 & 2/12
M[illegible]lle Jones SICU		2/10, 2/[illegible]

Figure 28–2
Staff availability form.

Employees

To obtain and maintain optimum rapport with employees, the scheduling coordinator will:

1. Facilitate the application process in the absence of the personnel coordinator.
2. Concentrate on the scheduling needs of the new employee. They are vital members of the organization. Only through proper orientation can staffing personnel function effectively in numerous health care facilities. The more thorough the orientation, the fewer mistakes will be made, and the end result will be a reputable staffing agency, with quality employees, whose services are in demand. This leads to ongoing requests from the contracting organizations.
3. Obtain availability from all employees on a frequent, regular basis and make every effort to place them at the preferred facility on the date that was requested. This is recorded on an employee request form (Fig. 28–4).
4. Supply employees with current information and updates through word of mouth, general mailings, and paycheck inserts regarding:
   a. Recruitment/referral bonuses
   b. Sign-on bonus
   c. Pay rate changes
   d. Miscellaneous notices pertaining to the agency
5. Counsel employees regarding:
   a. Excessive cancellations
   b. Late arrivals for assignments

REQUESTS FORM

FACILITY NEEDS	date: 2/9	
Facility	Need	Filled
Hilltop Hospital	RN 3rd Shift ICU 2/9	Mary Smith
St. Joe's	RN 1st Shift Med/Surg 2/10	Lynn Mos
St. Mark's	RN 1st Med/Surg 2/10	Kevin Jones
Riverview Psyche	RN 2nd Adol 2/10	Cathy Drake
Hilltop	RN 1st OB 2/10	
Riverview	Psych Tech 1st Shift 2/10	
Wilmore Hosp.	RN 1st shift ICU 2/10, 11, 12	
Mercy	RN 1st Shift Oncology 2/10	
Grace Rehab	RN 2nd Shift ICU 2/10	

Figure 28–3
Filled requests form.

c. Proper scheduling procedure
d. Procedure for completing time slips

6. Request evaluations of employees from clients when indicated. There may be occasions when an employee has a personality conflict with a person at the contracting facility. Should a nonprofessional incident occur between two people, a report is filed by the client and by the agency. To ensure proper documentation and follow-through, the agency requests an evaluation on

Figure 28–4
Employee requests form.

EMPLOYEE REQUEST FORM

Name: Lynn Mos

Phone Number: 738-6211

Preferred Facilities: St. Joe's, Mercy, St. Mark's

Preferred Shifts: First, second

Dates Requested: Feb 2, 3, 7, 8, 10, 11, 12

behalf of the client. It serves as a system of checks and balances. The DON for the agency decides on proper action. This could result in the agency employee not returning to that particular client and being staffed elsewhere.

7. Follow through with incident reports. The incident report is a permanent record of a happening that is unusual in the normal course of events. Some examples would be a fall resulting in a broken bone, administration of the wrong dose of a medication, or a theft of either the patient's property or that of the staff. An incident report protects the patient, agency/health care facility, and the employee. This report may be used in court as evidence of the occurrence. The incident is reviewed by the DON of the agency, the DON of the hospital, and the employee. In review, a course of action is agreed on and implemented to avoid another such occurrence. If further training of staff is needed, it is arranged. When it is the failure of equipment causing problematic circumstances, the safety/maintenance committee may decide to purchase new equipment or develop protocols more suitable for operation. In any event, care is taken to ensure above-standard training for the agency employees. An agency with numerous incident reports would eventually be excluded from use.

8. Promote and maintain a positive relationship with employees through personal interaction. It is necessary in agency staffing to create a caring, responsive base for the employees. The employees—RNs, LPNs, CNAs, or psychiatric technicians—are employed by the agency to provide their expertise to the health care facility. Although they are working in various health care facilities, it is important for them to have an established identity as team members of the agency. Telephone contacts, letters, and meetings help to establish an environment for team building among the administration and the professionals who are employed. When agency employees have a sense of security as team members and are able to see how they provide expertise to the community, they can appreciate that they are vital to the agency's success. The more comfortable the employee is going to a number of area health care facilities, the more marketable that employee becomes.

Agency

To provide optimum work flow within the agency itself, the scheduling coordinator will:

1. Organize his or her own work flow, maintaining scheduling as the top priority. It is crucial to have intense scheduling efforts by all schedulers. Failure to do so can jeopardize the success of the company. It is important to expend all of one's efforts in filling the highest percentage of requests possible. Health care facilities depend on well educated, up-to-date employees. Consistent, successful staffing reflects attentiveness to facility needs. When health care facilities call on agencies, they need to fill positions that directly affect the quality of care the patients will receive. By staffing the position in a timely manner, the facility and the agency employee both have their needs met. The result is fulfilling for the scheduler, the facility, and the agency. Morale of the agency is reflected in the employees' happiness and willingness to work and accept new assignments.

2. Keep the employee Kardex up to date and relay any changes to the financial department. Because the agency provides 24-hour coverage to the health care facilities, it is vital to have accurate employee information. Employee statistics (address, telephone number, availability, and any additional training directly related to their career) have to be recorded so the agency can comply with state requirements, both as an employer and as a provider of competent, legally qualified professionals. The finance department needs information to mail paychecks to employees' homes as well as for a database of the number of people employed and their qualifications.

3. Prepare time slips for payroll.

4. Separate mail and distribute appropriately.

5. Maintain records of employee bonuses.

6. Keep an employee and client contact person telephone list current. This is necessary to meet the needs of specific employees and match them with the health care facilities they request.

7. Maintain an inactive employee list. This is

done as a precautionary measure and reference. On occasion, some agency employees file Unemployment Compensation claims. This list serves as a ready reference as to when they opted to become inactive.

8. Record responses to advertisements. These data show the effectiveness of the advertisement in reaching the professionals desired for employment with the agency. A successful agency is one that is able to provide the type and number of employees requested by the health care facilities with whom the agency contracts. Effective advertising helps to accomplish this goal.

9. Prepare reports and projects as requested by administration.

10. Direct calls to appropriate people, screen calls, and take messages.

Unemployment Compensation

To protect the agency from Unemployment Compensation claims, the scheduling coordinator will:

1. Document all employee refusals of work, citing reasons for refusal, and work offered (Fig. 28–5).

2. Document all employee cancellations, citing reasons and work canceled. There have been incidents in which an employee files for Unemployment Compensation. The agency attempts to meet the needs of the employee. However, in agency nursing it is the employee's prerogative to refuse work. Documentation is very important in these instances. The scheduling coordinator records each call made to employees for the purpose of offering work hours. When the unemployment office contacts the agency, they are provided with a list of dates, times, and places of work offered. This releases the agency from having to pay unnecessary compensation to employees who have refused to take hours offered to them.

Record Keeping

It is important to have organized records for each of the contracted facilities. Although the personnel department is responsible for the employee records, the scheduling coordinator is responsible for the maintenance of facility requirements, records, and compliance.

Training courses for agency staff are necessary to meet clinical competencies required by the health care institutions contracting with the staffing agency. Specific guidelines are developed by the facilities. They may require competency in specific clinical areas, equipment use, or procedures.

EMPLOYEE REFUSAL FORM

NAME	DATE OF OFFER	WORK OFFERED	REASON FOR REFUSAL
Mary Jayeson	2/10	1st shift St. Joe's	will be out of town
Horace Held	2/10	1st shift St. Mark's	no babysitter
Jane Grayson	2/11	2nd shift St. Joe's	ill
Annabelle George	2/11	3rd shift Mercy	has house guests
Bill Henry	2/11	3rd shift Mercy	has other plans

Figure 28–5
Employee refusal form.

Staffing agencies providing health care workers to other institutions are not required to be licensed by the DHHS because no care is administered on the premises. However, the staffing agency must ensure that the requirements imposed by the contracting facilities are met. Current professional licensure/certification, adequate health and immunization status, and certain clinical policy reviews, such as Universal Blood and Body Fluid Precautions, are among the requirements.

The scheduling coordinator must develop a compliance checklist for each employee. He or she must then arrange for and ensure completion of these lists by each employee. The contracting facility has the right to do spot checks of the staffing agency files to ensure that the agency employees have met the requirements for competency. In addition to credentials, additional training may be implemented by the health care facility to ensure competence of specialties. For example, an acute care hospital may implement this requirement: "Please note that it will be mandatory that the agency be responsible for having all RNs credentialed in glucose testing. This will be done on a quarterly basis for quality control purposes. 'Facility' will not be responsible for keeping any paperwork regarding this. It will be the agency's responsibility to do this and keep appropriate records."

The DON for the agency advises the scheduling coordinator of how, when, and where the inservice for this will occur. It is the responsibility of the scheduler to contact all the appropriate personnel who work at that particular facility.

Other Responsibilities

In addition, the head scheduler is responsible and accountable for:

1. Overseeing daily operations of the scheduling table.
2. Developing new procedures when indicated.
3. Setting up monthly schedulers' meetings and preparing the agenda.
4. Problem solving when necessary. When dealing with staffing, there are times when a scheduled employee may have to cancel a particular shift. It is of utmost importance to restaff the position for the facility. There are times when the facility's census drops, and thus the coverage that had been arranged is not required. When this happens, it is important to call the agency's employee and let him or her know of the cancellation. It is the employee's option to remain unscheduled or be rescheduled at another facility.
5. Performing miscellaneous projects as assigned by the administrator, such as writing advertisements and recruitment efforts.
6. Being available to the on-call scheduler when problems or concerns arise on weekends or in the evening.
7. Directing to administration any concerns requiring attention.

Night and Weekend Schedulers

The agency is open 24 hours to take and fill requests. Coverage is supplied by the in-house scheduler and the on-call scheduler. The on-call scheduler is an extension of the office, and all information that occurred during the first shift is reported to the on-call scheduler. This is done verbally and by fax. The scheduling coordinator is a resource person available to all staff members who are working in the health care facilities. The position entails being a liaison to approve and confirm additional hours for agency staff once they are already at the facility. For example, an RN is working ICU and has 40 hours in for the week. The facility wants the nurse to stay and work another shift. The supervisor from the facility calls to verify if he or she can stay. The scheduler checks with the RN to confirm that a double shift is acceptable. The scheduler also confirms that this will be overtime. Then the scheduler is transferred back to the supervisor to approve the RN's acceptance of the shift and establish that it will be at another rate of pay, because it is overtime, at the beginning of the next shift.

To provide optimum work flow for the on-call

scheduler, the in-house scheduling coordinator will:

1. Keep the on-call scheduler informed of any changes in agency policy or procedure.
2. Give or fax night report to the on-call scheduler to include employee availability and client need, and any other information necessary.
3. Obtain a morning report from the on-call scheduler, documenting all activity. The night and weekend schedulers are extensions of the main office. As such, they need to have all the information that is available during business hours to fulfill their responsibilities.

This information includes but is not limited to:

1. New employee information.
2. New client information.
3. Marketing, expansion, and recruitment information (including times, dates, and locations of interview sites).
4. Inactive employees.
5. Clients no longer served.
6. Unemployment claims filed and documentation of work offered and refused.
7. Workers' Compensation claims pending.
8. Change in employee availability or requests not to send an employee to a particular facility.

The on-call schedulers maintain an ongoing log that documents attempts made to meet client needs and other information as it transpired during nonbusiness hours (Fig. 28–6).

Mental Health Services

Patients who may require the services of RNs from mental health services are given a designated emergency telephone number that will put them in contact with the scheduling coordinator. The scheduling coordinator collects information and evaluates the need to contact the RN. The scheduling coordinator is trained to triage as the patient cases emerge, following established guidelines. The scheduler has access to the records of every patient who would be given the designated emergency telephone number. The use of agency nurses specializing in psychiatric home care services has proven that the cycle of admission, discharge, and readmission can be reduced or stopped. Agency nursing staff work with people suffering from mental or emotional problems, often eliminating the need for hospitalization.

The scheduling coordinator needs to be an attentive listener and recorder to relay messages from patients to the appropriate RNs. The following information needs to be documented and relayed:

1. Date, time, and person calling.
2. Who the patient's nurse is (this also establishes if the patient is coherent. If unable to name, look up on master list of information provided). Reassure the patient that the nurse will be called immediately. The patient should be instructed to call back if the nurse has not called within a short time.
3. Any peculiar behavior regarding threat to self or to others, pill overdose, referring to self as another person, or any symptoms the patient specifically states.

The scheduler should then call the appropriate RN. If he or she is unable to reach the nurse, the DON should be contacted for intervention. Do not attempt to do clinical rehabilitation by phone; this is not the responsibility of the scheduling coordinator. The assessments are clinical in nature. This would be considered practicing or attempting to practice medicine, and one could be held legally responsible in the event a patient followed the advice and had a life-threatening event because of that advice or suggestion. When receiving patient calls, proper follow-through requires that a call always be placed to the nurse directly responsible for the clinical and counseling needs of the patient. It is important that the patient have a sense of trust in the system, and therefore a rapid return of the phone call by the patient's nurse is imperative. Triage is a critical responsibility and requires a scheduling coordinator to be an excellent listener and a stickler for details.

CALL OUT SHEET DATE February 9th, 1997

	NAME	PHONE	MESSAGE LEFT	NO ANSWER	OTHER
1705	Mary Smith	282-9090	Hill top Hosp. 3rd shift ICU 2/9	–	accepted 3rd shift @ HH.
1710	Lynn Mos	738-6211	St. Jo's 1st shift 2/10/97 Med/Surg	–	accepted 1st St. Jo's
1712	Kevin Jones	421-5155	St. Marks Hosp. 1st-med/Surg. 2/10/97	–	will work-OK. late start
	called St. Marks spoke w/Supervisor Jane Brown – Ok'd late start 2/10–Med/Surg.				
1715	Cathy Drake	829-6123	Riverview Psyche 2nd shift-Adol. 2/10		accepted 2nd shift @ RVP.
1722	Peg Fritz	832-9183	Please call and leave availablity for week of Feb. 20th '97		week of Feb. 20th '97
1725	Paula Smeak	383-2514	St. Marks cancelled your 3rd shift today @ 1500. *Please (Call back to CB)		
	confirm that you received this message and leave your availability.				
1730	D.J. Tonka	767-5400	Hill top Hosp. 1st 2/10 OB/GYN	✔	will call back
1800	Dave Frankie	427-8900	Riverview Psyche 1st shift 2/10	✔	
1805	Becky White	248-7612	St. Jo s 1st shift 2/10-OB/GYN	✔	
1807	Nancy Slim	487-2101	Wilmore Hosptial 1st 2/10, 2/11, 2/12-ICU		accepted 1st-2/10, 2/11, 2/12
18…	Di… Kot…	87…237	Mercy Hospital …/12-oncolo…		accepted …/12

Figure 28–6
On-call scheduler's log.

Professional Responsibility

Continuing Education

We are all members of a team in the health care field. The scheduling coordinator has a responsibility to pursue continuing education on a regular basis. By attending relevant in-services that relate to the community, health maintenance organizations, and health care providers, the scheduling coordinator can keep current in the ever-changing environment of the health care field.

Confidentiality

A staffing agency can contract with many different facilities. Many agencies have hundreds of nurses, all with many different areas of expertise. The quality of the people who work for an agency has a big impact on the success of that agency. The scheduling coordinator's professionalism is of utmost importance. He or she must demonstrate the ability and competence to deal with the requests of many different people in a timely manner. Voice, attitude, and willingness to pleasantly follow through with numerous requests and tasks will set the first impression of the agency. This is a reflection of the agency's professionalism and its ability to provide services to the public and its community.

There is extensive contact with the public and numerous health care facilities and the professionals who work at those facilities. In changing times, the scheduling coordinator will have the professional edge by respecting all he or she hears and holding all matters affecting facilities in confidence. Many agency nurses take positions because of downsizing or hospital mergers. Agencies also find employees from the ranks of health care workers who have been laid off because of chronic low census situations in their facilities. Should the staffing agency be privy to this information, these matters are strictly confidential in nature and not to be a topic for discussion outside of agency, employee, and administrative meetings. The scheduling coordinator must act with tact and skill when inquiries are received.

Health Unit Coordinator Skills

The technical skills used by the HUC can easily be transferred to the position of scheduler for staffing agencies. All HUCs have obtained skills in using the following systems:

1. Computer/printer/word processor/database
2. Fax machine and telephone communication
3. Pagers and paging systems
4. Filing systems (manual and computerized) for retrieval of client and employee information
5. Photocopying

When dealing with professionals, it is important to recognize and respect their areas of expertise. When contacting employees, have appropriate positions for them to consider. Consider timing when placing calls and have consideration for staff. For example, if a scheduled night nurse has worked four nights in a row, refrain from calling at 11:00 A.M. to ask a question regarding a shift. Courtesy and respect are just as important as knowing one's position description.

Marketing Health Unit Coordinator Skills

When seeking employment, a person needs to do an honest self-assessment regarding his or her strengths and weaknesses. Ask this question: "What do I have that would make a potential employer hire me, instead of another individual?" With regard to the position of a scheduling coordinator, experience in the medical field is of utmost desirability. Less time will be required to train a person who possesses working knowledge of how health care facilities function.

Health care facilities are service oriented. This is an important point to remember when having contact with anyone on the telephone. The scheduling coordinator is the first person to receive the calls. The way the telephone is answered is a reflection of the level of professionalism of the entire company. For those few seconds, the scheduling coordinator is the person who establishes the working relationship with staff, health care facilities, and the community. The "people" skills of empathy, understanding, care, and concern are revealed in the tone and inflection of the scheduling coordinator's voice and his or her promptness in dealing with the requests of the calling party.

Another acquired skill is that of familiarity with the community the agency is staffing. An agency can contract with as many as 300 different types of facilities. That same agency may staff as many as 600 employees. It is important to know location. When staffing health care professionals, one needs to take into consideration travel time, traffic conditions, and the possibility that the facility might want to staff them for a double shift (e.g., because of weather conditions or staff shortages).

A creative problem-solving ability is the scheduling coordinator's best asset. For example, an agency employee, when contacted, can work a specific shift, but public transportation is not available because of the hour. It is a reflection of resourcefulness to provide transportation for that employee to get to the health care facility with the staffing need. Thus, by providing transportation by office staff or another employee who is also dispatched to that particular facility, the needs of the facility are met. More important, it shows the employee the importance of his or her position.

Closing Thoughts

Experience is the HUC's best friend. Our position is versatile and demanding. A strong technical background, attention to detail, and a desire to learn and educate oneself are traits that can be carried with a HUC to create a career ladder of his of her making. The best way to prepare oneself for other positions is to work in as many different specialty areas as possible. When confident and comfortable, move onto another area. Transcription of as many different kinds of orders as there are patients ensures a thorough understanding of different aspects of the position. Flexibility, problem-solving ability, and respect for peers and coworkers are desired traits in a HUC. This background allows one to move into other areas of employment, thus preventing burnout. A caring attitude brought to the solution of problems is an asset to any person and creates a valued employee. Everything we do can add value to our personal career goals. We have skills that provide service to the health care system. It is up to us to evaluate and do our own needs assessment to fulfill our professional career ladder. The transition from HUC to scheduling coordinator is an inviting one. When a person makes this change, it can be done with ease. Proper orientation, focused priorities, flexibility, education, and a desire to learn with a friendly voice and smile make for a successful career move.

Review Questions

1. Define supplemental staffing and the people it provides to health care facilities.
2. Identify the role of the scheduling coordinator.
3. Identify the technical and communication skills necessary in the role of the scheduling coordinator.
4. Explain the duties and responsibilities to both the agency and the clients contracting for your services.

Community Mental Health Services

Audrey Langhorne

Objectives

Upon completion of this chapter, the reader should be able to:

1. Explain the purpose of community mental health services.
2. List and describe seven outpatient services that might be provided by a community mental health agency.
3. Explain the purpose of emergency crisis intervention service.

Vocabulary

Adjunct: An accessory or auxiliary agent or measure

Anxiety disorder: An excessive or unrealistic feeling of apprehension, worry, uneasiness, or dread, especially of the future

Attention deficit-hyperactivity disorder: Persistent pattern of inattention or hyperactivity—impulsivity that is more severe than is typically observed in people at a comparable level of development

Bipolar disorder (manic-depressive illness): A form of mood disorder in which the person experiences extreme and disabling mood swings that consist of either depression, sadness, decreased energy, sleep and appetite changes, and suicidal ideas; or a feeling of euphoria, grandiose ideas, or hyperactivity

Depression: A feeling of persistent sadness and helplessness with little drive for socialization and communication. The person does not enjoy anything in life, and may have suicidal ideas

Dyskinesia: Impairment of the power of voluntary movement, resulting in fragmentary or incomplete movements

Extrapyramidal: Refers to a functional unit involved in motor activities

Mental retardation: Deficient intellectual development. Levels of mental retardation determine the intelligence quotient: borderline, mild, moderate, severe, and profound.

Obsessive-compulsive disorder: Recurrent and persistent ideas, thoughts, impulses, or images (obsessions) or repetitive, purposeful, and intentional behaviors (compulsions) that are recognized (by self) as excessive or unreasonable

Continued

Vocabulary *Continued*

Parkinsonism: A group of neurologic disorders characterized by hypokinesia, tremor, and muscular rigidity

Schizophrenia and other psychotic disorders: A group of mental disorders characterized by disturbances of thinking, mood, and behavior. An altered concept of reality can result in delusions and hallucinations. Mood changes include inappropriate emotional responses and loss of empathy. Withdrawn, regressive, and bizarre behavior may be noted.

Tardive dyskinesia: A defect marked by involuntary repetitive movements of the facial area, found primarily in the elderly

Tic: An involuntary, compulsive, repetitive movement usually involving the face and shoulders

Tourette's syndrome: A syndrome of facial and vocal tics with onset in childhood, progressing to generalized jerking movements in any part of the body

Common Abbreviations

ADHD	Attention deficit-hyperactivity disorder
Admin Case Mgmt Sup	Administrative case management supervisor
Admin Services	Administrative services
Adult ICM Sup	Adult intensive case management supervisor
Adult OP Sup	Adult outpatient supervisor
BSU	Base service unit
Child Adoles & Family Services	Child adolescent and family services coordinator
Child/Adol OP Sup	Child/adolescent outpatient supervisor
CHIPS/CRR Super	Community hospital integration projects service/community residential rehabilitation supervisor
CMHS Contract Supervisor	Community mental health services contract supervisor
CRR	Community residential rehabilitation
EPDST	Early and periodic screening, diagnosis, and treatment
Evaluation & Case Mgmt Coordinator	Evaluation and case management coordinator
Fam Base Sup	Family base supervisor
Fiscal & MIS Sup	Fiscal and management information systems supervisor
FY	Fiscal year
HSI	Human services incorporated
MAX/CRR Sup	Maximum/community residential rehabilitation supervisor
MH Crisis Sup	Mental health crisis supervisor
MH/MR	Mental health/mental retardation
MH/SAP Sup	Mental health/student assistance program supervisor
MR	Mental retardation
OCD	Obsessive-compulsive disorder
PH/SOC Super	Partial hospital/social supervisor
Res Coord Sup/Child ICM	Residential coordinator supervisor/child intensive case management
Res Services Super	Residential services supervisor
SLA Super	Supported living arrangement supervisor
Support Serv. Sup	Support service supervisor

The abbreviations listed for this chapter are those that a HUC working in this area would be expected to know. Only those in boldface type are used in the text and appear in boldface when they are used for the first time.

Related Terminology

The terms listed below are common diagnoses for adults and children that a person working in a community mental health service would be expected to know. They do not appear anywhere in the text of the chapter.

Impulse-control disorder: The failure to resist an impulse, drive, or temptation to perform an act that is harmful to the person or to others, such as aggressive impulses, gambling, fire setting, and kleptomania.

Learning disorder: The inability to learn; occurs in children and is manifested by difficulty to learn basic skills such as reading, mathematics, writing, and other forms of language skills or motor skills.

History

Community-based mental health care came into existence in 1961 when the Joint Commission on Mental Health recommended that no more mental hospitals with a capacity of more than 1000 beds be built. Therefore, acute cases would be handled through agencies within the patient's home community. It was also recommended that large state institutions be closed or converted for the care of patients with chronic physical and mental illnesses. As a result, the Community Mental Health Centers Act encouraged the commencement of comprehensive community centers such as the one that is described in this chapter.

Community mental health service is a diagnostic, evaluative, and outpatient mental health program that offers a comprehensive array of services and activities to provide for the prevention, evaluation, diagnosis, treatment, and rehabilitation of mentally ill or emotionally troubled adults and children. Community mental health service is committed to the expansion of community-based mental health services and providing quality care that is responsive to the needs of the individual in the most appropriate, least intrusive manner.

Community mental health centers use professional staffs that include psychiatrists, psychologists, social workers, and master's-prepared counselors and caseworkers. In these centers, the staff is ready to understand and help with child and family difficulties, marital problems, school adjustment difficulties, fear, anxiety, depression, suicidal feelings, and other mental health problems, as well as serious and persistent mental illness. Services are provided to people experiencing difficulties regardless of race, color, creed, national origin, political affiliation, sex, sexual preference, handicap, ancestry, age, or disability. Bilingual services and services to the deaf and hearing impaired are also available in many centers.

Referrals are accepted from physicians, clinicians, hospitals, schools, churches, social service agencies, attorneys, families, and individuals.

It is interesting to note that in the 15th century, the Gheel foster-family tradition came into existence in Gheel, Belgium. This was a very early version of a community-based mental health agency.

Today, most general hospitals house a psychiatric unit, decreasing the rate of long-term inpatient care. The average patient is committed to a hospital in close proximity to his or her home, which eliminates adjusting to a strange environment and facilitates returning to families and friends within a shorter period of time to resume a "normal" lifestyle. Community mental health centers have become an integral part of the care of patients in their homes.

The following paragraphs provide an example of how an agency began and grew over the years as the needs of the **mental health/mental retardation (MH/MR)** population continually expanded. This growth was also influenced by federal, state, and local legislative changes that took place through the ongoing influence of advocacy groups.

The agency (Fig. 29–1), founded in 1972, initially provided information and referral service as well as active mental health outpatient care to one small community. It was hospital based, but within 1 year relocated to a community setting because of expansion of staff needed to provide services.

Over the next several years, because of the addition of community support services (after

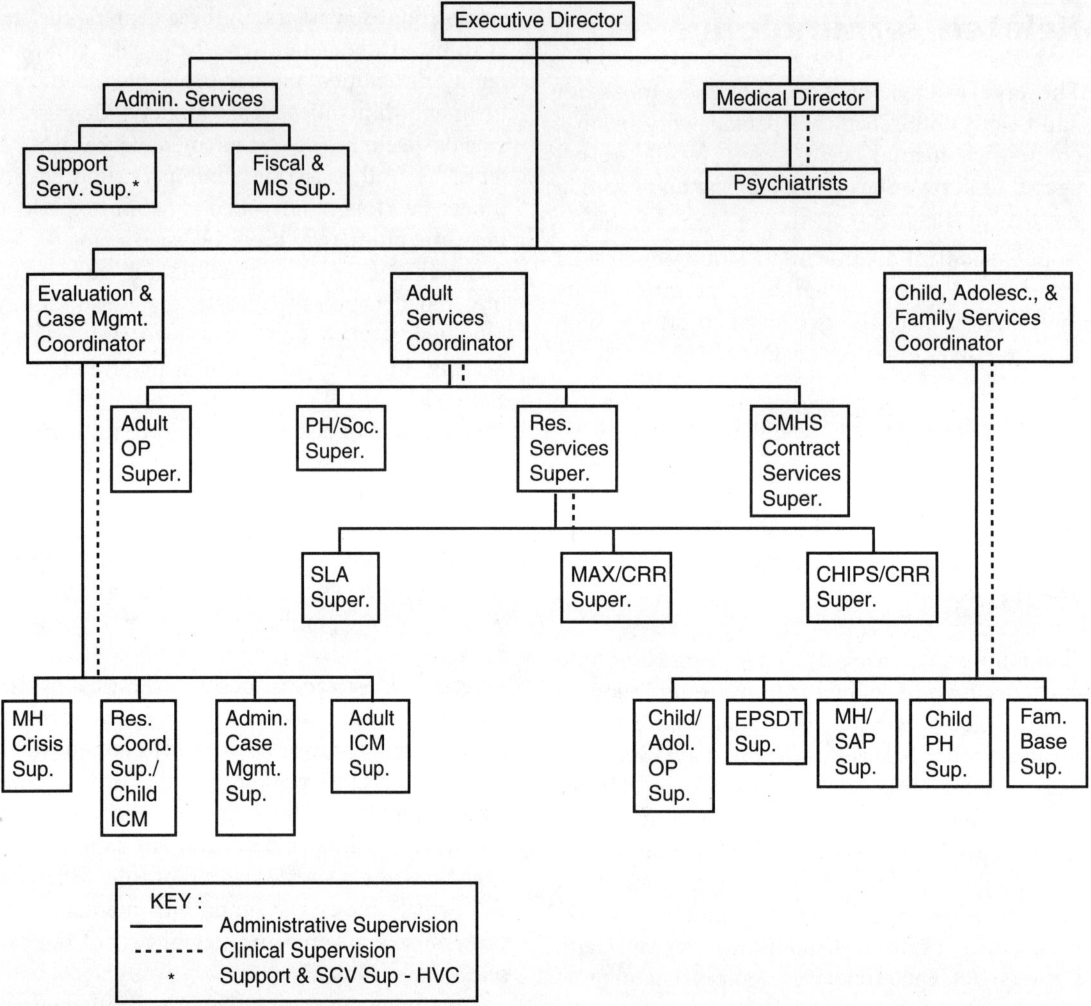

Figure 29–1
Organizational chart for a community-based mental health agency.

care), the crisis intervention services (24-hour/day program), partial hospital programs, and expansions into other localities and counties, the agency set up various satellite offices and moved administrative offices several times to accommodate the programs and staff.

Grants were applied for and received by the agency to initiate additional programs to meet the community's needs.

Collaboration with another county agency was begun to prevent duplication of services, provide specialized services, and implement prudent fiscal decisions.

In 1978, data collection and analysis were initiated. Through this, the agency was able to evaluate programs offered, create a strategic plan, and conduct research. One very important outcome of the analysis of data was the establishment of a transportation system enabling clients greater participation in the available services.

Quality assurance programs were initiated, residential programs for mentally impaired adults were constructed, and 12 work sites for mentally handicapped people were created in conjunction with the local county manpower program.

Through continued efforts to recognize and meet the needs of the community, the agency developed and implemented additional programs throughout the area. They became involved in major community fund-raising projects and expanded their programs so the deaf could be equally served.

In 1995, the agency became a member of a statewide network of community health centers formed to contract with managed care organizations and was granted a license by the office of mental health for a children's partial hospital program located in the local child development center.

Descriptions of the programs provided by this agency and many like it are found in the following sections.

Evaluation Case Management Services

Administrative Management Services

Administrative management services (base service unit) provides information concerning mental health services available in the community. The administrative management staff obtains initial information regarding a person's request for services through a phone contact with the person. The staff then schedules an appointment or provides referral information to the person for more appropriate services by other service providers. At the initial administrative management appointment, the staff works with the consumer to develop a preliminary service plan and then makes referrals to the most appropriate service and treatment resources. Administrative management also provides ongoing case management monitoring of special-needs cases and reviews all cases before closure from agency services.

Intensive Case Management

Intensive case management, available 24 hours a day, provides assistance to adults with serious and persistent mental illness and to children and adolescents with serious emotional disturbances, and their families. The program provides assistance in gaining access to needed medical, social, educational, and other resources. Activities are designed to provide an individualized approach to serving the daily needs of people and families to enable them to develop their strengths and improve the quality of their lives in the community. Staff in the program have limited caseloads and there are specific eligibility requirements for the recipients of the service.

Resource Coordination Services

Resource coordination services provides case management services to adults and children who have mental illnesses and require ongoing assistance in accessing and coordinating mental health and other social services, and assistance in monitoring the provision of those services. Activities are based on an initial assessment of the consumer's strengths and needs obtained from the consumer and, when appropriate, from family members. These activities include assessment, service access and monitoring, networking, coordination of services, problem solving, and advocacy. There are specific Department of Public Welfare eligibility requirements for the recipients of this service.

Outpatient Services

Outpatient services provides counseling to families and children who are experiencing difficulties because of family stress, school problems, emotional disturbances, or mental illness. The staff provides individual psychotherapy and group, family, and marital therapy. Specialized services include play therapy, behavior modification, school consultation, and medication management.

Partial Hospital Services (Child and Adolescent)

This program provides an intensive psychiatric day treatment program for socially or emotionally impaired children and adolescents who are experiencing difficulties in school and at home. The program also provides an outpatient alternative to in-patient hospitalization, or may serve as a transition program after in-patient hospitalization. Treatment services include individual, group, art, recreational, and family therapies. An educational component is provided in cooperation with an intermediate unit (specialized education). The program also provides a therapeutic/recreational summer program for socially or emotionally impaired children and adolescents.

Family-Based Services

Family-based services is an intensive, short-term, in-home treatment program designed to help families in crisis who are at risk of having a child placed outside the home because of mental illness or emotional disturbance. The program provides case management, family therapy, parent education, and other services that are needed to help the family's ability to manage current and future problems.

Early and Periodic Screening, Diagnosis, and Treatment

Early and periodic screening, diagnosis, and treatment (EPSDT) is preventive medicine; the program is designed to provide comprehensive health care to people younger than age 21 years who are eligible for medical assistance. The client is thoroughly evaluated for any disease or abnormalities and the evaluation determines the proper mode of treatment/therapy. The program has proven to be cost effective by treating the client before the situation becomes disabling.

Mental Health Student Assistance Program

The mental health student assistance program works with schools' student assistance teams in identifying students whose educational and developmental progress is hindered by social and emotional stresses. The program provides student support groups focusing on topics such as peer relationships, student–teacher relationships, and family difficulties. The program also provides in-home evaluations to "at risk" students and their families who have been unable to connect with treatment services.

Adult Treatment and Rehabilitation Services

Adult treatment and rehabilitation services provide counseling to adults who are experiencing personal difficulties, emotional problems, or serious and persistent mental illness. The staff provides individual psychotherapy, group, family, and marital therapy, and medication treatment. Adult treatment and rehabilitation services treat a variety of difficult personal situations, including job stress, child and family problems, and adjustment to life crises.

Partial Hospital Service (Adult)

Partial hospital service provides services to adults with a diagnosis of serious mental illness who require more intensive treatment than outpatient, but who do not require full-time hospitalization. The multidisciplinary team provides intensive, group-oriented treatment, individual therapy, medication assessment and management, socialization, and art, music, and recreation therapies. The program provides an alternative to hospitalization, and also serves as a transitional program for people returning to the community from the hospital. The partial hospital program also provides intensive rehabilitation and psychotherapy for improved vocational, social, family, and community functioning.

Social Rehabilitation Service

This program provides social and recreational activities for adults with significant psychiatric disabilities to assist them in developing social skills and enhancing the quality of their community living. The service helps adults identify, learn, and practice social skills related to daily living, community living, and leisure activities through informal and formal socialization experiences and community resources.

Community Residential Rehabilitation

Community residential rehabilitation provides a community-based alternative to institutional or hospital care. The program enables serious and persistently mentally ill adults to reside in a supervised, supportive community residential setting, while receiving the training and assistance needed to acquire the daily living skills necessary for independent community living.

Long-Term Supportive Housing Services

This program provides the opportunity for people with mental illness to secure permanent housing in the community. Staff assist people in accessing community-based social, educational, and vocational opportunities, as well as medical and psychiatric services. These services are intended to empower people to manage their own affairs, while maintaining a permanent residence.

Student Practicum

Students from various universities are placed in the agency for a period of one semester or 1 year. As a rule, students are in master's-level programs and are assigned a limited caseload. On completion of their practicum, the students receive an evaluation from the agency, which results in university credits.

Emergency Mental Health Crisis Intervention Service

This service, which is available 24 hours a day, provides immediate help for persons experiencing a mental health emergency or emotional crisis. The service provides a quick response—either in person or by phone—for assistance, support, guidance, and counseling during a mental health emergency. The purpose of the emergency intervention is to stabilize a crisis situation and to refer to appropriate treatment services to begin to resolve the problems. The service also provides assistance to voluntary or involuntary psychiatric hospitalization referrals.

Medications

The medications listed here are some that are most frequently used for patients with mental health disorders. However, the list is far from complete.

Ativan—Used for **anxiety disorders** and alcohol withdrawal syndrome treatment.

BuSpar—Used in the treatment of persistent anxiety, fatigue, insomnia, anxious mood, tension, upset stomach, palpitations, and dyspnea.

Clozaril—An antipsychotic known to help **schizophrenics** who have not been able to tolerate other antipsychotics, and without the signs of **tardive dyskinesia**; every patient must have a simple blood test weekly.

Cogentin—Used as an **adjunct** in the therapy of **parkinsonism**. Also used in the control of **extrapyramidal** disorders, with the exception of tardive dyskinesia.

Depakote—Indicated for use as sole and adjunctive therapy in the treatment of simple and complex absence seizures, and adjunctively in patients with multiple seizure types and for **bipolar disorders.**

Doxepin—An antidepressant; also used to treat anxiety and nervousness related to alcoholism.

Effexor—Used as an antidepressant.

Haldol—Indicated for use in the management of manifestations of psychotic disorders, **tics**, and **Tourette's syndrome.**

Klonopin—Used for anxiety states and for treatment of panic disorder. Also used to treat manic episodes.

Librium—Used for alcohol withdrawal syndrome.

Lithium—Indicated in the treatment of bipolar

disorder, prolonged intense moods, impulsiveness, agitation from stimulants, and conduct disorder.

Luvox–Treatment targeted for **obsessive-compulsive disorder (OCD)**.

Mellaril—An antipsychotic. Also used for children with combativeness or explosive, hyperexcitable behavior.

Norpramine—An antidepressant. Also used to treat panic disorder.

Pamelor—Same as Norpramine.

Paxil—Indicated in the treatment of anxiety symptoms, minimal agitation, insomnia, **depression**, and panic disorder.

Prolixin—Used for treatment of psychotic symptoms or severe agitation.

Prozac—Primarily used for depression.

Risupardal—An antipsychotic; indicated in the management of manifestations of psychosis and known to improve negative and positive symptoms.

Ritalin—Used in the treatment of **attention deficit-hyperactivity disorder** (ADHD) and aggression.

Serzone—Used as an antidepressant.

Stelazine—Used for the treatment of psychotic symptoms or severe agitation.

Tofranil—An antidepressant; also used to treat panic disorders.

Valium—Used for anxiety disorders and alcohol withdrawal syndrome treatment.

Wellbutrin—Used as an antidepressant.

Xanax—Used in the treatment of general anxiety (everyday occurrences) and panic attacks.

Zoloft—Indicated in the treatment of depression and anxiety.

Zyprexa—Prescribed for the management of the manifestations of psychotic disorders.

Medications by Category

Antianxiety agents or tranquilizers

Ativan
BuSpar
Klonopin
Librium
Luvox
Valium
Xanax

Antipsychotics

Clorazil
Haldol
Mellaril
Prolixin
Risperidal
Stelazine
Zyprexa

Antidepressants

Doxepin
Effexor
Norpramine
Pamelor
Paxil
Prozac
Serzone
Tofranil
Wellbutrin
Zoloft

Mood stabilizers

Lithium
Depakote

Anti-ADHD

Ritalin

Antiparkinson

Cogentin

The Health Unit Coordinator

The health unit coordinator (HUC) would be responsible for answering the phones, which could result in an intake (new patient/client), assisting with medication clinics, transcribing and receiving orders from the psychiatrist, calling prescriptions to the pharmacist, and scheduling appointments. Clients are received and referred to their proper appointments: medication clinics, group or individual therapy, psychological evaluations, and psychiatric evaluations.

One other duty is the processing of the authorization of release of information to acquire or release pertinent information from or to other agencies with which the client has had previous contact: psychiatric hospitalization, psychological counseling, prison, children, youth and family agency, pediatrician, correctional institution, and family doctor.

The HUC position takes form based on the needs of the agency. Courses such as introductory psychology, anatomy and physiology, medical terminology, and transcription and typing at a junior college are helpful. The subjects as mentioned are not required to become a HUC but enhance one's ability to perform the job well. Computer knowledge is an asset. Continuing education is required to maintain certification. It is essential to know how to handle an emergency and have the ability to help the client/patient feel comfortable in the environment.

Should the HUC wish to advance in the field of mental health—for example, as a social worker, therapist, or psychologist—education is needed at the university level.

Closing Thoughts

Community mental health services is an agency for the betterment of people in need of mental health therapy. The client is thoroughly evaluated and the modality of treatment is decided. The agency consists of a staff of psychiatrists, psychologists, social workers, master's-level counselors, and caseworkers. And, of course, the agency just wouldn't function without the HUC.

I have always worked in a medical environment: first in orthopedics, on to respiratory, and then covering the entire hospital as needed in any given day. My current employment is in community mental health. Regardless of what aspect of the medical environment you work in, you must be a nurturing soul. Working in mental health services makes you totally aware of what the human being is all about and that each person is an individual. Each day is a challenge and a caring attitude plus a sense of humor provide fulfillment on the job. I cannot remember a day when I said "I can't tolerate another day of this job." Community mental health services is truly an environment where you assist people in feeling better about themselves.

Review Questions

1. Explain the purpose of community mental health services.
2. List and describe seven outpatient services that might be provided by a community mental health agency.
3. Explain the purpose of emergency crisis intervention service.

Bibliography

Dorland's Illustrated Medical Dictionary, 28th ed. Philadelphia, WB Saunders, 1994.

30

Community/Vocational/ Technical Colleges

Nadine Stratford

Common Abbreviations

DACUM Developing a curriculum

PAC Professional advisement committee

Objectives

Upon completion of this chapter, the reader should be able to:

1. Explain the difference between a community college and a technical or vocational college.
2. Identify three positions in the community or technical college that would be appropriate for a health unit coordinator who aspires to a teaching career.
3. Explain the role of a professional advisement committee in health unit coordinator programs at the community or technical college.
4. List some of the health unit coordinator skills that are applicable to the classroom situation in a health unit coordinator program.

Vocabulary

Competency: Having sufficient skill, knowledge, or experience for some purpose

Curriculum: The aggregate of courses of study given in a school or college

Preceptor: An instructor, teacher, or tutor

Syllabus: An outline of the subjects of a course of study

Teaching: The purposeful imparting of information or skills to another person or group

Overview

Over the past few decades, the number of health unit coordinator (HUC) training programs in community, vocational, and technical college settings has risen dramatically. From the time of the inception of the HUC position in health care in the 1940s, on-the-job training was the standard for acquiring the necessary knowledge and skills. Because of the need to keep up with the rapidly changing health care industry, along with increasing time and budgetary constraints for individual facilities, formal HUC educational programs began to take shape in the 1960s. Over time, more and more health care institutions and other related settings have found that employing those who have completed a specific course of instruction in health unit coordinating is a practical and economical choice.

History

Community College

The community or junior college offers 2-year programs of study leading to associate degrees and certificates. These colleges do not offer bachelor's (baccalaureate), graduate, or professional degrees. Most community colleges are public institutions, receiving funds from the state, local school districts, or other public sources. Private 2-year colleges receive most of their funding from student tuition. Two-year colleges in general have six distinguishing characteristics: open admission, a local service region, low cost, a comprehensive educational program, diversified learners, and ties with community organizations. Community colleges offer education geared to the needs of the learners and their communities. These institutions also provide a more direct connection between preparatory education and the workplace than is customary with 4-year institutions.

The idea for a junior college was originally conceived as an extension of secondary education, and as a way to enable universities to focus on advanced work. Private junior colleges trace their beginnings back to the mid-1800s, but the public 2-year institution did not begin to gain momentum until after the turn of the century. In 1917, there were 5 accredited U.S. junior colleges, and by 1920 there were over 200 whose primary focus was on general and college-transferrable education. The evolution of other types of institutions, such as business schools and vocational education, into 2-year colleges, and the addition of junior colleges as part of universities spurred further growth. In 1947, the U.S. Commission on Higher Education advocated increased access to college and called for more tuition-free, public, 2-year community colleges. This encouraged extensive growth during the following decades, and by the late 1980s more than 40 percent of all undergraduate students were enrolled in community colleges.

The **curriculum** of the community college can be divided into five basic functions: collegiate, career, general, compensatory or remedial, and community education. Although these may vary in emphasis from institution to institution, most offer some form of all of them.

Collegiate

The collegiate function, also known as the college parallel or transfer program, offers the same type of courses as 4-year colleges and allows students to complete the first 2 years at a lower cost or closer to home.

Career

Career education is intended to develop skills and related knowledge to prepare for employment or to improve job skills. Also known as vocational, technical, or occupational education, these programs attract two of three students attending community colleges. Many institutions develop "customized" career education to prepare workers for jobs as requested by local companies.

General

General education emphasizes critical thinking, developing values, understanding traditions, respecting diverse cultures and opinions, and putting knowledge to use.

Compensatory or Remedial

Compensatory or remedial education consists of courses designed to teach students who are underprepared to take beginning college courses. This can be the starting point for many students who have come back into the educational system after many years of absence.

Community

Community education embraces adult basic education, continuing education, and community-based education. Offerings may include classes for credit or noncredit, and may vary in length from one evening to an entire term.

Vocational or Technical College/Education

Vocational or technical education prepares students for industrial and commercial occupations that do not require a university degree. It can include training in such fields as manufacturing, building, business, agriculture, and health services. Before the 19th century, vocational training was typically provided by a person's parents or through an apprenticeship. The Industrial Revolution of the early 19th century created a need for skilled workers that was greater than apprenticeship training could fulfill. As a result, the first vocational/technical training programs in the United States were offered in the 1820s. In the early 1960s, a government panel was formed to conduct a comprehensive study of vocational/ technical education, which led to the allocation of federal money for these educational programs in public secondary schools, resulting in the rapid growth of these programs during the 1960s. Later amendments broadened federal aid to include postsecondary and adult programs, programs for handicapped and disadvantaged students, sanctions against discrimination, and support services such as counseling and job placement.

Today, vocational and technical education programs are found in public and private secondary schools, industry, labor unions, penal institutions, adult education, the military, and community and junior colleges. Some 2-year institutions have based most or all of their curriculum around vocational and technical education. Although students concentrate their efforts on learning a job-related skill, there are additional academic requirements to ensure that they are competent in reading, writing, and math.

Health Unit Coordinator Programs

Traditionally, health unit coordinator (HUC) educational programs have been found in the community, vocational, or technical college setting, along with other programs geared toward a specific occupation. The length of the program varies, depending on how intensive and in-depth the course of study and clinical applications are. Programs may be short in duration with longer hours in the classroom, or single classes spread over several quarters or semesters. St. Philip's College in San Antonio, Texas offered the first college-credit HUC program in the United States in 1968. In 1987, New Hampshire Vocational Technical College in Manchester, New Hampshire organized the first associate degree program in Health Unit Coordinating, followed by Spokane Community College, Spokane, Washington, in 1990.

The course of study used in a HUC program is based on task-oriented skills and basic understanding of medical language and the field of health care. Several textbooks for the instruction of HUC students are available, and are the basis for planning curriculum. Common areas of study for most programs include (Fig. 30–1):

CURRICULUM

First Semester		Hours	Credits
510—324	HUC Procedures I	4	2
510—119	Medical Terminology	2	2
509—308	Anatomy & Physiology	3	2
801—355	Business Communications: Grammar & Punctuation	3	2
809—351	Applied Human Relations	3	2
509—301	Professional Ethics & Law	2	1
509—310	Emergency Care for Health Occupations	2	1
106—343	Medical Office Procedures I	3	2
510—312	Pharmacology for Health Occupations	2	1
103—303	Windows/Works	4	2
		28	17

Second Semester		Hours	Credits
801—356	Business Communication: Speaking & Writing	3	2
510—325	HUC Procedures II	7	4
510—326	HUC Practicum	12	6
102—130	Career Development	3	2
		25	14

Figure 30–1
HUC curriculum.

- The role and responsibilities of the HUC
- The health care industry and environment
- Communication and interpersonal skills
- Organizational, time management, and managerial skills
- Legal, ethical, and confidentiality issues
- Basic human body structure
- Medical terminology
- Transcription of doctor's orders
- Computer skills
- Use of other related equipment
- Job-seeking skills: resume writing, applications, interviewing

The ideal classroom circumstance provides a learning environment that includes ample space for study as well as a simulated work area that allows the students to develop application skills in a nonthreatening environment (Fig. 30–2). This might include a desk area that would be equipped in a way similar to a nursing unit desk, with all of the necessary supplies and equipment and a computer station to allow the students to practice those particular skills (Fig. 30–3).

In addition, most programs arrange for HUC students to have a clinical, "hands-on" experience with a **preceptor** at a local health care facility. This may also vary in length, but is necessary for the student to put practical knowledge to the test. A professional agreement between the college and the health care facilities may be put into place, whereby the facility agrees to provide the clinical experience and preceptors for the students, and the college assumes ultimate responsibility for the students and provides the necessary training needed to be successful as a HUC.

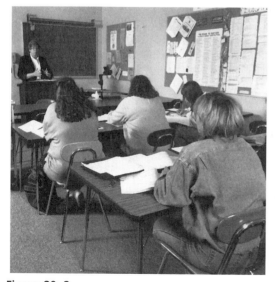

Figure 30–2
HUC classroom.

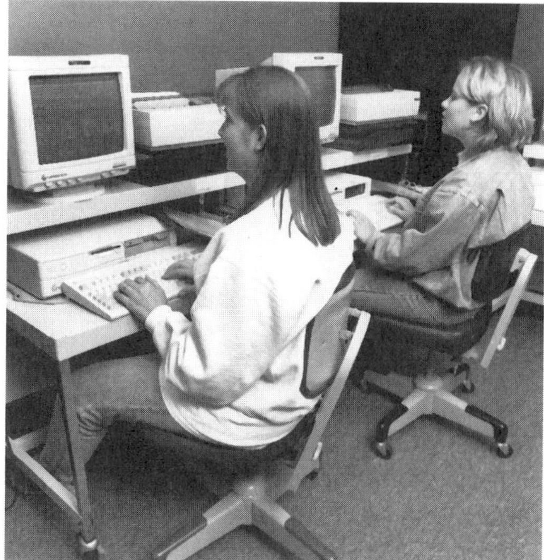

Figure 30–3
Classroom computer station.

The HUC program in a college setting affords students the many services available to other college students. Academic advisors/counselors are available to work with students on their educational goals and assist them with any other challenges and decisions. Many types of financial aid are available for students who need assistance in paying for schooling. Career guidance/job placement counselors assist in preparing students to enter into the workforce, and keep them aware of job opportunities.

Positions Available

Size and length of a program, along with whether the program is credit or noncredit, are key factors in determining faculty needs for a HUC program, and whether to use full-time or part-time adjunct instructors. Policies governing the faculty/student ratio are usually developed and approved by appropriate educational and academic administration in the individual colleges, following accreditation guidelines. In smaller programs, one faculty member is all that is needed to oversee all the aspects of a HUC course, whereas several instructors may be needed to guide the in-class academic activities and supervise clinical preceptorships in health care facilities for a larger group of students. Larger programs may also use the services of a program director who is responsible for the overall program.

The Program Director

In a program with several instructors, one may be designated as the program director. This position has the responsibility of supervising the instructors, assisting in the hiring of new instructors, reporting program progress to the division chair and professional advisement committee (PAC), representing the program at division, faculty, and PAC meetings, and assisting the division chair with budgeting for the program.

The Academic Instructor

The academic instructor is responsible for determining the pertinent curriculum for classroom instruction, along with preparing syllabi, assignments, tests, learning activities, evaluation tools, and competencies. In addition, the instructor assesses and maintains student grades and records, and keeps students advised regarding the program and their individual progress. Marketing the program by doing presentations for high school and college career fairs and for health care facilities may be an additional responsibility.

The Clinical Instructor

Arranging for and supervising student preceptorships in health care facilities, along with preparing the necessary skill checklists and evaluations, is the main responsibility of the clinical instructor. Orienting working HUCs as preceptors and maintaining a collaborative relationship with the health care facilities that train students is another area of focus for the clinical instructor. Precepting a student's clinical experience can be challenging for even the most seasoned HUC. Preceptor orientation may include an overview of the HUC course of study, basic adult learning styles, and skill level evaluation.

Qualifications

Qualifications for HUC instructors vary in the many educational programs around the country as a result of differing state, local, and college specific guidelines and regulations. A 1989 survey with responses from 45 states and 63 percent of technical teacher educational programs showed that some confusion does exist over the definition of postsecondary technical education, but that 17 states have technical teacher credentialing systems, and that work experience is deemed important in those states requiring teacher certification and in teacher education programs. For a HUC to be considered a candidate for an instructional position, the qualifications may include:

- A minimum of 5 to 6 years of recent, full-time, paid clinical experience in a health care facility
- Recent HUC or related educator experience
- National HUC certification

Some educational programs require a minimum 2-year or associate degree, or a teaching certificate if required in that particular state. In many instances, 2 or more years of work experience is considered equal to 1 year of education, or up to 3 years of academic training may be substituted for part of the required work experience.

The program director position usually has a minimum qualification requirement of a bachelor's degree, along with administrative or managerial experience.

Professional Advisement Committee

Health unit coordinator courses that have a PAC as part of the program provide an opportunity for local health unit coordinators to act as "advisors" for the course. Members of the committee include HUCs who are willing and have the time to serve, exhibit leadership ability, and have the technical expertise in the profession of health unit coordinating, along with representatives from admissions, student advising, and administration at the college. The committee should be a balanced representation of the geographic area the program serves and should include representatives for large and small health care facilities, professional associations, and recent program graduates. Some of the key activities of the PAC include:

- Assisting in the establishment of instructor qualifications
- Advising about skills and technical and general information to be taught
- Reviewing instructional needs for the program
- Assisting in surveys of local labor market needs
- Suggesting criteria for recruiting and selecting students
- Providing information concerning education and experience necessary for job entry and success
- Informing instructors of new methods, technologies, and industry trends

A lay member serves as chair of the committee. The chair works closely with college representatives, schedules meetings, gives assignments to members of the PAC, plans meeting agendas, leads the voting on issues, and represents the PAC on college advisory councils and in meetings that involve PACs from all programs.

Health Unit Coordinator Knowledge and Skills Appropriate for an Instructional Position

Basic Health Unit Coordinator Skills

The ability to teach the knowledge and skills used every day on the job as a HUC requires both practical experience and learning. An instructor who has actively functioned in the HUC role is well acquainted with the basic knowledge and skills of the job and, with additional formal or nonformal training in more technical aspects, can give a well-rounded learning experience.

Medical Terminology

As with many professions, the world of medicine and health care has its own language, abbreviations, and symbols. The HUC instructor needs to be well versed in both written and spoken medical terminology, along with having a working knowledge of basic human body structure, systems, disorders, and disease processes.

Health Care Environments

Also important is a thorough knowledge of the different health care environments, such as hospitals, clinics, care centers, offices, and the departments, staff, and specialties within that provide care, testing, treatment, and other services for patients.

Communication and Organizational Skills

Good communication and organizational skills are essential in any setting, and the HUC instructor draws on these skills continually to keep the learning experience understandable and meaningful for the student. In this era of rapidly changing technology, the instructor also needs to keep abreast of modern communication devices and their use in the health care industry, and have the ability to teach practical usage. Use of many of these devices is also essential in organizing classroom work and activities.

Legal and Ethical Considerations

The role of the HUC has expanded over the years, and the HUC has become recognized as an essential member of the health care team. With expanded responsibilities and accountability the opportunity for liability has also grown. Understanding the legal and ethical considerations that may be encountered in working in health care is necessary to instruct students in legally fulfilling their professional obligations as a HUCs.

Supervisory and Managerial Skills

In the health care setting, there are many opportunities for experienced HUCs to orient, precept, and train new HUCs and other personnel. The instructor who has had this experience can use many of the same orientation and precepting methods with a larger group of learners. Supervisory experience and managerial training is also helpful in overseeing the learning experiences and progress of students. Quality improvement training, which has been available in many health care settings, can be useful for evaluating and improving HUC educational programs.

Additional Training

Teaching is the purposeful imparting of information or skills to another person or group. There are several essential requirements for any instructor, whatever they are teaching: they must know the material they are to teach; they must be able to articulate the material in a manner understandable to the student; and they must manage the students to maintain focus on what is to be learned. Courses in teaching methods, public speaking, preparing and presenting workshops, and implications of adult learning styles can be useful for a HUC who is interested in teaching, in order to meet these essential requirements.

A new HUC instructor may not have experience in the development of curricula, creating a **syllabus**, or establishing competencies for a program that is being developed. Curriculum development involves evaluating and deciding on teaching materials and textbooks for use in a course of study, and organizing lectures, learning activities, and testing materials. A syllabus, or outline of the course and subjects to be covered, is created so that students have an overview and time line of what is to be studied. Competencies are established as the evaluation tool used to determine whether the student has met the skill level deemed necessary to complete a course of study successfully. Most colleges have specialists available to help guide new instructors and those involved in program development in these essential tasks.

Developing a curriculum for any course of study is accomplished by using a **DACUM (Developing A CurriculUM)** or a job analysis for the profession. A DACUM is created by bringing together a carefully chosen group of experts from the profession who, with the help of a facilitator, identify general areas of job responsibility, pinpoint specific tasks performed with each duty, and identify entry-level tasks. A job analysis is done on a broader scale, with the same type of expert group creating a questionnaire that asks about knowledge and tasks required, and other questions about the profession. The questionnaire is then sent out to as many in the profession as possible, with the same expert group compiling and analyzing the results. From this, "knowledge statements" are determined that reflect what knowledge one must have to function successfully in the profession. After the appropriate curriculum is determined, educational materials are chosen to coincide with outcomes of the DACUM or job analysis.

A syllabus gives a general overview of the course of study, rules and guidelines for the students enrolled, and a calendared sequence of what will be covered in the course. The purpose is to give the students clear expectations of what the course will cover, the time frame in which the content will be covered, and what is expected of the students themselves while enrolled in the course.

Competencies are evaluation tools that are done for each student at the completion of a course of study. Tasks and abilities based on the content of the program are listed, and students are measured and evaluated on their ability to demonstrate or perform those tasks and abilities

(Fig. 30–4). In **competency**-based programs, this evaluation takes the place of a letter grade as a reflection of successful course completion.

Marketing the Health Unit Coordinator as an Instructor

When the first HUC educational programs began appearing in colleges, the faculty of these courses were predominantly instructors with degrees in nursing. Although there are still nurses teaching in these courses today, many programs are now fully staffed with instructors whose background is exclusively in health unit coordinating. An instructor who has actively functioned as a HUC for a number of years, and who has taken the extra step of becoming a Certified HUC, brings essential knowledge and skills needed in the education of HUC students. The on-the-job experience, combined with practical learning, brings a well rounded perspective on the profession to the classroom setting, and gives students the opportu-

ORDER TRANSCRIPTION
Lab Collected

Student ____
Instructor/Preceptor ____
Date ____
Affiliate ____

Properly:		**Comme**
1. Recognizes type of order	x o	
2. Selects appropriate requisition or computer screen	x o	
3. Enters appropriate information	x o	
4. Notifies nursing staff if patient needs to fast	x o	
5. Notifies dietary if appropriate	x o	

____ Student needs more practice with this proc
____ Student's psychomotor skills are acceptab
____ Student's cognitive level is acceptable.
____ Student may advance to other procedures

Student's signature: ____
Instructor's signature: ____
Student's comments: ____

43

ORDER TRANSCRIPTION
Consultation

Student ____
Instructor/Preceptor ____
Date ____
Affiliate ____

Properly:		**Comments:**
1. Recognizes type of order	x o	
2. Gathers correct information	x o	
3. Selects correct form or computer screen	x o	
4. Determines correct physician to consult	x o	
5. Calls physician's office	x o	
6. Relays complete and accurate information to physician's office	x o	
7. Records date and time of phone call and name of person spoken to	x o	
8. Files information in proper place in chart	x o	

____ Student needs more practice with this procedure.
____ Student's psychomotor skills are acceptable.
____ Student's cognitive level is acceptable.
____ Student may advance to other procedures.

Student's signature: ____
Instructor's signature: ____
Student's comments: ____

53

Figure 30–4
Sample competency evaluation tool.

nity to have their instructor be a role model of health unit coordinating as well.

Closing Thoughts

Many years ago, the local community college in the area where I live offered a "ward clerk" course that was taught by nurses and grouped with other nursing courses and general education. The course was disbanded when the push came to hire master's degree–prepared instructors for all college courses, along with several local hospitals providing competition when they began to run their own courses. Some years later, the college's division that develops skill-based courses was approached by these same hospitals, who had found over time that it wasn't cost effective to run a HUC course, and wanted the community college to offer the course once again.

Because of my affiliation with the National Association of Health Unit Coordinators, I was contacted and asked what information I had with regard to availability of textbooks and access to a HUC job analysis. I was able to provide the college's program director with a current NAHUC Certification Board Job Analysis and give suggestions about what educational materials could be used. I was in turn asked to help develop the course outline and content, and to become one of the instructors. I was quite surprised to be asked because I did not have a postsecondary degree, but was assured that my years on the job as a HUC practitioner qualified me as an "expert in the industry," along with my supervisory and precepting experience, which gave me a good background. Courses I had taken previously in teacher development and adult learning styles added to my qualifications.

Being an instructor for a HUC course at a community college has greatly enhanced my already rewarding career as a HUC. I feel fortunate that I have a job that enables me to contribute to quality health care by working with physicians, nurses, and other hospital staff, and providing assistance to patients and their families. It is equally rewarding to help students to "catch the spark" of health unit coordinating themselves, and go on to use the knowledge and skills gained in health unit coordinating to begin a promising career in health care.

Review Questions

1. Explain the difference between a community college and a technical or vocational college.
2. Identify three positions in the community or technical college that would be appropriate for a HUC who aspires to a teaching career.
3. Explain the role of a professional advisement committee in HUC programs at the community or technical college.
4. List some of the HUC skills that are applicable to the classroom situation in an HUC program.

Bibliography

Kerschner VL: Health Unit Coordinating: Principles and Practices. Albany, NY, Delmar Publishing, 1992.

LaFleur-Brooks M: Health Unit Coordinating: 3rd ed. Philadelphia, WB Saunders, 1993.

Northwest Association of Schools and Colleges, Commission on Colleges: Accreditation Handbook, 1992 Edition. Seattle, Northwest Association of Schools and Colleges, 1992.

Olson SJ: Post secondary instructor programs and post secondary technical teacher certification: a national study. Journal of Studies in Technical Careers 1991;13(4).

Salt Lake Community College: Program Advisory Committee Handbook. Salt Lake City, UT, Salt Lake Community College, 1984.

The New Grolier Multimedia Encyclopedia. Danbury, CT, Grolier Interactive Publishing, 1993.

31 Criminal Justice Facilities

Charles S. Leyer

Common Abbreviations

CJF Criminal justice facility

CJIS Criminal Justice Information System

DME Durable medical equipment

ROI Release of information

Objectives

Upon completion of this chapter, the reader should be able to:

1. Identify the three levels of criminal justice facilities.
2. Describe the unique terminology used in the criminal justice facility.
3. Name three positions available to the health unit coordinator in a criminal justice facility.
4. Describe the duties expected of the health unit coordinator in the various areas of the criminal justice facility.

Vocabulary

Criminal justice facility: A general term used to describe a facility where those accused or convicted of a crime are detained

House of corrections: A criminal justice facility operated at the county level

Jail: A criminal justice facility operated at the local level

Prison: A criminal justice facility operated at the state or federal level

Pod: A unit in a criminal justice facility

History

Health unit coordinating in a **criminal justice facility (CJF)** can be an interesting, challenging, and enjoyable opportunity. The position is constantly evolving and provides a wide variety of work experiences. Before there were health unit coordinators (HUCs) in the medical departments, medical sections, and infirmaries of **jails**, **houses of corrections**, and **prisons**, the work was done by registered nurses and licensed practical nurses. When the workload became too much for the nursing staff to handle alone, they hired secretaries to do filing and assist with the scheduling of appointments.

The increased population of the facilities has seen a proportional increase in the number of inmates who have serious medical conditions and who are on more complex medication regimens. This has further increased the workload, and a number of facilities are now employing HUCs to transcribe physician orders and schedule appointments in and out of the facilities for consultation with specialists and for special testing. The HUCs are also usually responsible for ordering:

1. Paper supplies
2. Office supplies
3. Medical supplies
   a. Diabetic testing equipment
   b. Dressing supplies

c. Durable medical equipment (DME)
d. Oxygen and related equipment
e. Any other supplies necessary to care for ill or injured inmates

Description of Facilities

Jails are usually located in cities and towns and operated by the local authority, either the chief of police or the sheriff in the area. The primary use of a jail is to house people accused of a crime until their court appearance or trial. Depending on the outcome, one of the following may happen:

1. Released on bail pending trial
2. Housed in jail awaiting trial
3. Housed pending transfer to another facility (if found guilty)
4. Released if found not guilty

The jails are also used at times to house inmates who might otherwise be placed in a county facility.

A house of corrections (work house, county work farm) is a place of confinement that is used to house people who have been convicted of crimes against local ordinances, such as:

Driving under the influence of alcohol
Driving after revocation
Unpaid parking tickets
Repeated motor vehicle violations
Loitering
Prostitution

Usually the time spent in the house of corrections for these violations is 1 year or less.

People convicted of charges brought by the state often are housed in the local house of corrections if the sentence is less than 2 years. The house of corrections is the site where parole violators or probation violators are held pending evaluation by their probation agents for possible revocation.

Prisons are facilities operated by the state or federal government that usually house prisoners convicted of crimes and sentenced to terms of over 1 to 2 years.

Terminology

There are many abbreviations used by HUCs in their traditional role that take on an altogether different meaning in the CJF. Table 31–1 gives some examples.

Services Offered

In a jail setting, the scope of services provided depends in part on the licensed staff available. There must be the capability for emergency care and follow-up, as well as for dealing with preexisting health problems, acute or chronic, medical or mental health. The medications and treatments that an inmate required before his or her incarceration will be maintained. Medically necessary appointments are scheduled in larger facilities with the staff physician and in smaller facilities with outside contracted services.

In a house of corrections, the level of services is basically the same as in the jail setting, with most medical needs being met by the house of corrections physician and licensed staff.

In the state prisons, the level of care is governed by statute and the regulations of the state department of corrections. All the services covered in jails and houses of corrections are offered in prisons. Because of the length of sentences, longer-term and more intense treatment is often medically necessary. The medical services are directed by the code for the division of corrections for each state. In the federal prison system, there is generally a wider range of services offered. Eyeglasses and dentures are usually available at both the state and federal levels.

In general, facilities follow the practice of offering routine medications that the inmates were taking as ordered by their private physicians on the outside for medical or psychiatric conditions. The prison physician is the one who orders medications for newly diagnosed conditions. The medications are administered by registered or licensed practical nurses on the units or "**pods.**"

The facilities have a treatment room where the

Table 31–1 ABBREVIATIONS WITH DIFFERENT MEANINGS IN MEDICAL AND CRIMINAL JUSTICE SETTINGS

Abbreviation	Use in Medical Setting	Use in Criminal Justice Facility
NTG	Nitroglycerin	Not found guilty
PCN	Penicillin	Probabable cause not found
ROI	Release of information	Release/order in
FB	Foreign body	Felony bench warrant
OR	Operating room	Other order
OOB	Out of bed	Out on bail
O.T.	Overtime	Order to produce
REM	Rapid eye movement	Remanded into custody
TPR	Temp., pulse, resp.	Temporary release
MO	Mental observation	Motion
P.T.	Prothrombin time	Pretrial
VA	Veterans Affairs	Municipal video appearance
WT	Weight	Warrant return
DIS	Discharge	Charges dismissed

medical and nursing staffs can carry out assessments and minor outpatient procedures. In the facilities staffed by physicians, nurse practitioners, or physician assistants, minor suturing needed as a result of inmate altercations or accidental trauma can be accomplished on site.

It is interesting to note that many facilities across the nation are starting to charge inmates for services offered by the medical sections of CJFs, including community correctional centers (half-way houses). The fees can range from $0.50 for an aspirin to $2.50 for seeing the staff physician, nurse practitioner, physician assistant, or dentist. More is charged for visits outside the facility. In the past, the cost of medical services was covered entirely by the criminal justice system, but with the rising costs of medical and dental care in all types of units, the system must find ways to relieve the taxpayer burden. Many of the facilities are now charging the inmate accounts for over-the-counter medications that the prisoner may require or request. No inmate is ever denied services, even if they do not have funds.

This system has created the need for the use of a "charge slip" system, the application of which falls typically to the HUC. It is crucial to the success of the system that accurate information be entered by the HUC, particularly the inmate's

Criminal Justice Information System (**CJIS**) number and the medical record number (Fig. 31–1).

Positions Available

There are several positions available for the HUC in a CJF. The following sections address some of the more common ones.

Administrative Assistant

An HUC can be used as an administrative assistant, assisting the health services unit coordinator (usually the nursing supervisor) in coordinating the activities of the department. These duties may be varied, and usually include:

- Scheduling
- Maintaining records
- Compiling statistics
- Special projects
- Developing and using data collection sheets

The development and use of the data collection sheets is an assignment vital to the medical services system. The data would include collective numbers of inmates seen, by the units where they are assigned or by medical condition (Figs. 31–2 and 31–3). This information provides valuable tracking information to the medical professionals as well as to the personnel responsible for budgeting.

The administrative assistant also might be assigned to update and maintain the medical information worksheets, such as the daily fingerstick record, the daily diet sheets, and the blood pressure worksheets, which may be updated daily or weekly.

Medical Records #000098
COUNTY JAIL
REQUEST FOR WITHDRAWAL
SUPPLY ALL INFORMATION
PLEASE PRINT NEATLY 1132-1 R1

BOOKING NUMBER: 9999 9911

LAST NAME: Smith FIRST: John Jones

DATE OF BIRTH: 1 - 1 - 52

LEVEL AND POD: 6 B DATE: 4/17/97

CODE	CHECK HERE	MEDICAL	PRICE EACH
7880	1	First aid cream	0.50
7881		Hydrocortisone	0.50
7882	1	Acetaminophen (2 tablets)	0.50
7883		Aspirin (2 tablets)	0.50
7884		Ibuprofen (1 tablet)	0.50
7885		Decongestant (2 tablets)	0.50
7886		Antacid (2 tablets)	0.50
7887	4	Band-Aid (1 each)	0.50
		TOTAL	

I authorize the Sheriff's Department to charge my account for items I have received.

SIGN NAME: John Jones Smith

Figure 31–1
Request for withdrawal. (Courtesy of Milwaukee County Sheriff's Department, Milwaukee, WI.)

Health Unit Coordinator in the Health Services Unit

The HUC may be assigned to work in the record section of the health services unit. The duties there include:

- Filing
- Pulling charts
- Assembling charts
- Maintaining hard-copy records
- Updating computer records
- Maintaining card file records (if there is no computer system)

Health Unit Coordinator in the Booking Area

Being assigned to assist the medical department staff in the booking (intake) area involves processing charts and other records. This begins with ascertaining if the inmate has old medical records and obtaining them. If outside appointments are scheduled, release of information (**ROI**) forms are faxed to the hospitals, doctors, clinics, and other correctional facilities as indicated (Fig. 31–4). In-

	ANP	BLD WO RK	C X R	DEN TAL	DOC SICK CALL	EMER CALL FROM PODS	EME RM VISIT	ETOH PROT	HYPE RTEN SION	MED ORDER	OB-GYN	PHYS 1/2 WAY HOUSE	PHYS IN-MATE WORKR	RN TRIAGE	SCREEN REVIEW	STAT MEDS	TB	STD	VERIFI CATION
4/1/97	18	18	3	18	21	12	2	24	21	125	12	6	12	45	325	18	2	6	37
4/2/97	21	12	1	0	15	2	0	6	12	88	15	3	4	68	250	6	0	4	26
4/3	12	22	4	0	0	2	1	7	26	210	14	2	4	61	245	2	1	2	4
4/4	15	12	1	0	22	2	3	12	30	186	17	2	6	72	262	1	0	1	8

Figure 31–2
Data collection tool. (Courtesy of Milwaukee County Sheriff's Department, Milwaukee, WI.)

MONTH ______ HOC SICK CALL LOG **Page 3**

EAR/NOSE THROAT																															
EYE																															
GI																															
GU																															
STD																															
MUSCULAR																															
ORTHO																															
RASH/DERM																															
CARDIOVASCULAR																															
RESPIRATORY																															
WOUNDS																															
PHYSICALS																															
OTHER																															
COURT LIST																															
RN PHYSICALS																															

MONTH ______ HOC SICK CALL LOG **Page 2**

	1	2	3	4	5	6	7	8	9	10	11	12	13	14	15	16	17	18	19	20	21	22	23	24	25	26	27	28	29	30	31
INFIRMARY AND BLOCK																															
# I/M'S SEEN BY RN																															
# I/M'S REFERRED TO MD																															
# I/M'S REFERRED TO DENTIST																															
# OF PROTOCOLS ORDERED																															
# I/M'S REFERRED TO PSW																															
TOTAL MD VISITS																															
TOTAL PSYCHIATRIC VISITS																															
MD ASSESSMENT/COSIGNS																															

MONTH ______ HOC SICK CALL LOG **Page 1**

	1	2	3	4	5	6	7	8	9	10	11	12	13	14	15	16	17	18	19	20	21	22	23	24	25	26	27	28	29	30	31
ACC																															
# I/M'S SEEN BY RN																															
# I/M'S REFERRED TO MD																															
# I/M'S REFERRED TO DENTIST																															
# OF PROTOCOLS ORDERED																															
# I/M'S REFERRED TO PSW																															
TPC DORMS																															
# I/M'S SEEN BY RN																															
# I/M'S REFERRED TO MD																															
# I/M'S REFERRED TO DENTIST																															
# OF PROTOCOLS ORDERED																															
# I/M'S REFERRED TO PSW																															
FLM DORMS																															
# I/M'S SEEN BY RN																															
# I/M'S REFERRED TO MD																															
# I/M'S REFERRED TO DENTIST																															
# OF PROTOCOLS ORDERED																															
# I/M'S REFERRED TO PSW																															

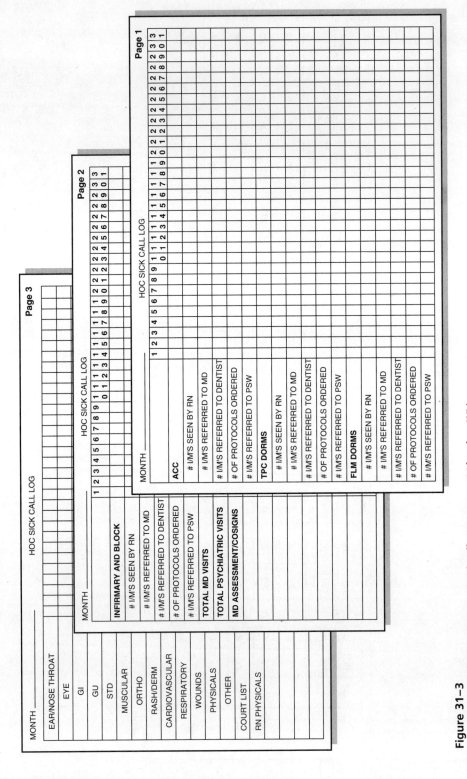

Figure 31–3
Logs. (Courtesy of Milwaukee County Sheriff's Department, Milwaukee, WI.)

COUNTY HOUSE OF CORRECTIONS

CONFIDENTIAL INFORMATION RELEASE OF INFORMATION	**INDIVIDUAL WHO IS SUBJECT OF RECORD**
CJIS NUMBER 999999111 **MEDICAL RECORD NUMBER** 000098	**NAME:** Smith John Jones **D. O. B.** 1 - 1 - 52
NAME AND ADDRESS OF AGENCY OR ORGANIZATION BEING AUTHORIZED TO RELEASE INFORMATION County Hospital	INFORMATION MAY BE RELEASED TO : MILWAUKEE COUNTY HOUSE OF CORRECTION HEALTH CENTER ATTN.: MEDICAL DIRECTOR 1004 NORTH 10TH STREET MILWAUKEE, WI 532323-1413

SPECIFIC RECORDS AUTHORIZED FOR RELEASE INCLUDES DIAGNOSIS, PROGNOSIS AND TREATMENT FOR PHYSICAL ILLNESS, MENTAL DISORDER, ALCOHOL, DRUG ABUSE, HIV TEST RESULTS OR ANY AIDS / AIDS RELATED DIAGNOSIS FOR THE FOLLOWING DATES:

Past history of Diabetes need current Med orders
" Seizures " " " "
Psych " " " "

PURPOSE OR NEED FOR RELEASE OF INFORMATION (BE SPECIFIC):

CONTINUITY OF CARE ✓

OTHER______ (SPECIFY)

I UNDERSTAND THAT I MAY REVOKE THIS AUTHORIZATION, IN WRITING AT ANY TIME EXCEPT WHERE INFORMATION HAS ALREADY BEEN RELEASED AS A RESULT OF THIS AUTHORIZATION. UNLESS REVOKED, THIS AUTHORIZATION WILL REMAIN IN EFFECT UNTIL THE DATE INDICATED. EXPIRATION DATE 9-1-97

AS EVIDENCED BY MY SIGNATURE BELOW, I HEREBY AUTHORIZE DISCLOSURE OF RECORDS TO THE MILWAUKEE COUNTY HOUSE OF CORRECTIONS AS SPECIFIED ABOVE.

SIGNATURE OF PATIENT: X John Jones Smith DATE: 4 - 17 - 97 WITNESS: Charles S Leyn CHRE	X______ SIGNATURE OF OTHER PERSON LEGALLY AUTHORIZED TO CONSENT TO DISCLOSURE(IF APPLICABLE) ______ TITLE OR RELATIONSHIP

Figure 31–4
Release of information. (Courtesy of Milwaukee County Sheriff's Department, Milwaukee, WI.)

formation received from these parties must be collated for the medical department staff in the booking area. It is also a requirement to assist in maintaining an adequate supple of forms and restocking them as needed from a central supply area. The rules of medical confidentiality subscribed to in a traditional health care setting apply to the medical and allied health personnel in a CJF.

Health Unit Coordinator in Main Clinic Area

An assignment to the main clinic area with a charge nurse involves transcribing physicians' orders, making appointments, and using the computer system to check on prisoner location and status. In CJFs, inmate locations and populations can change quite rapidly, even several times a day, as some inmates are released and others are moved to maximize space and staff. New inmates may be relocated as often as three or more times in several hours to:

Prebooking
Booking
Booking open waiting
Intake pod
Initial classification pod

The HUC may assist in "sick call visits." The inmate follows a triage process, beginning with submitting a request for medical attention (the request may also be generated by corrections officers/prison guards; Fig. 31–5). The nurse then sees the inmate and:

1. Writes orders as appropriate per standing protocol
2. Refers the inmate to the on staff nurse practitioner, physician assistant, medical doctor, or dentist, or
3. Sends the inmate to the emergency department of a local hospital if indicated

The HUC transcribes the orders and schedules appointments or consultations. If the inmate is sent to the local hospital, transfer arrangements must be made and applicable paperwork provided (Fig. 31–6). The visit information is recorded on the triage slip as well as on the flow sheet and in nursing notes (Fig. 31–7).

In the booking area, used for screening review, the HUC must oversee the completeness of the initial screening form (Fig. 31–8). The booking nurse needs someone to help process the paperwork, as well as to transcribe orders, whether they are new orders or restart orders, such as those used for inmates returning to the facility within 30 days. Psychiatric medication orders remain current for 90 days. Initiating the appropriate paper trail is important because some jails intake as many as 300 prisoners in a day.

Some inmates come in with medical orders from their private physicians. These orders must be verified by the nurse before being administered to the inmate. An ROI form is faxed to the ordering physician so the orders can be reviewed and validated. The nurse can then use standard protocols to initiate the order, and the orders are then transcribed by the HUC.

The CJF receives many inmates who are under the care of a psychiatrist. If the inmate has been in custody within the previous 90 days, the orders can be reinstated by protocol. The charts of these inmates must be pulled in the booking area so the orders can be restarted. Many of the CJFs contract for psychiatric services. The practitioner may spend 1 to 3 days assessing inmates and writing orders until a suitable treatment plan is developed. The HUC reviews the psychiatry notes and the doctor's order sheets and transcribes orders and schedules follow-up visits.

The federal and large state prisons offer dental services on site either by employing a dentist or contracting for the services. The local facilities usually offer only emergency dental care. It is not unusual for inmates to have poor oral hygiene, and many require dental visits.

The computer is widely used in any position a HUC might fill in a CJF. Because of the many location changes mentioned previously, it is imperative to enter data in a timely fashion. All departments within the institution are interdependent. The following are examples of shared information:

Text continued on page 527

Medical Record #000098

COUNTY HOUSE OF CORRECTIONS
Health Services Unit

Inmate Request for Medical/Dental Care

All information must be provided to receive care.

Inmate Name (*Please print.*) Smith – John Jones		Housing Unit 6 B
Date-of-Birth 1 - 1 - 52	Booking # 999999111	Provider's Initials
Please check the service requested. ☑ Medical **$2.50** ☑ Dental **$2.50**		*Circle appropriate title:* (RN) / LPN / NP / MD

This form is a request to be seen by a licensed staff member from the Health Services Unit. Completion of this form does not guarantee a visit with a health care professional. Response to this request will be based on a review of your Medical Records and is at the discretion of the Health Services Staff.

I understand that the necessary applicable funds will be deducted from my commissary account. I further understand that medical care will not be refused to any inmate based on his/her ability to pay. If no funds are currently available, a negative balance will be entered into my account. The negative balance will be deducted from any monies deposited.

Inmate's Signature	Date	Time
John Jones Smith	4-18-97	7:52 am

Distribution: White .... Inmate Yellow .... Fiscal Affairs Pink .... Health Services

Inmate request or description of problem. Please print clearly.

(1) High Blood Pressure need Meds (2) Bad teeth–Pull them
(3) Diabetic need meds

Do not write below this line.

Care provided:

(1) Monitor BP BID ×3 day –if ↑ Refer to NP/MD 200/120
(2) Motrin for Dental Problems –Refer to DDS
(3) Monitor FS if ↑ Refer to MD/NP
(4) Obtain & send ROI for HTN & Diabetic meds from PMD

Professional Providing Care	Date
Betty Jean Alexander RNC	4-18-97

Figure 31–5
Request for care. (Courtesy of Milwaukee County Sheriff's Department, Milwaukee, WI.)

COUNTY HOUSE OF CORRECTIONS
MEDICAL CONSULTATION AUTHORIZATION

CJIS: NUMBER: 999999111	MEDICAL RECORD NUMBER: 000098	RELEASE DATE: 7-29-98
NAME OF INMATE: Smith – John Jones		D. O. B. 1-1-52

REASON FOR REFERRAL: on cardiac medication and lithium

Please do EKG

(+) PPD in Past Plz Do CXR

CLINIC N.W.G.H. -out Patient	ADDRESS 5310 Capital Drive
DATE: 4-21-97 900 a.m.	PHONE: 447-8595 / 8550

FOR SECURITY REASONS, PLEASE <u>DO NOT</u> INFORM INMATE OF NEXT APPOINTMENT. THIS INCLUDES VERBALLY, VIA CARDS, LETTERS OR BY PHONE CALLS. THANK YOU

Primo R. Tamayo M.D. M. D.
PRIMO R. TAMAYO, M.D.
Betty Jean Alexander RNC R. N.
HOUSE OF CORRECTION R. N.

TO BE COMPLETED BY CLINIC / CONSULTANT

FINDINGS: (1) EKG – WNL NSR Report to follow
(2) C+R LLL infiltrate/noute Report to follow

RECOMMENDATIONS:

TREATMENT: Repeat C+R in 2 wks

RETURN VISIT DATE /TIME: call for appt

DOCTORS NAME: Doctor C Jones SIGNED: C. Jones M.D.

ONLY THE TREATMENT OR EXAMINATION REQUESTED ON THIS FORM IS AUTHORIZED. THE HOUSE OF CORRECTION WILL NOT PAY, FOR ANY CARE, EXAMINATION OR MEDICATION UNLESS IT IS AUTHORIZED IN ADVANCE BY THE HOUSE OF CORRECTION MEDICAL DEPARTMENT . CALL 427-4706 FOR DETAILS OR APPROVAL. THIS DOES NOT APPLY TO LIFE THREATENING SITUATIONS.

Figure 31–6
Consult authorization. (Courtesy of Milwaukee County Sheriff's Department, Milwaukee, WI.)

COUNTY HOUSE OF CORRECTIONS
HEALTH SERVICES UNITS

☑ Criminal Justice Facility ☑ House of Correction

BOOKING # 999999 111

INMATE REQUEST FOR TREATMENT DOCUMENTATION

INMATE NAME: Smith – John Jones	F	(M)	D.O.B. (MM/DD/YY) 1 - 1 - 52	MED RECORD # 000098

DATE	HSG UNIT	COMPLAINT #	ACTION	BY: INITIALS
4/17/97	BK	↑ BP ↑ FS Psych Hx	Monitor BP– FS Refer MD	
			if necessary–obtain Medical Record	BJA
4/18/97	3C	↑ FS 412	Call MD for orders	
			Call for Diabetes Info	BJA
4/19/97	HOC J2		Recd at House of Corrections	
			F/u on BP FS	
4/20/97	HOC H28	↑ BP FS Psych Hx	Recd FAXED info was on	
			Diabeta 5 mg BID & HCTZ 50 mg. 2D	
			Lithium 300 mg 2ID	
			Dilantin 200 mg	
			Cardiozem 120 mg. BID	
			Write order as above pu	
			Doctor Jones from County Hospital	BJA

MKS:mf
REVISED: December 16, 1996

FILE: TREATDOC.FRM

Figure 31–7
Documentation of treatment. (Courtesy of Milwaukee County Sheriff's Department, Milwaukee, WI.)

COUNTY HOUSE OF CORRECTIONS
Initial Screening Form

1139-1 R1
000098

Name: *Smith – John Jones*
(Last) (First) (Middle)

Form Completed
Date: *4-17-97*
Time: *12:50 PM*

D.O.B.: *01-01-52* Race: *W* Sex: *M*

PREV ADMIT *Yes*
TB TEST *(+) in Past*

01. MEDICAL HEALTH

01. Are you ill or injured NOW? (Yes) No
Describe: *Sore head, GSW (L) Leg*

Have you been diagnosed with:

02. Asthma Yes (No)
03. Diabetes (Yes) No
04. Seizure Disorder (Yes) No
05. Heart Problems (Yes) No
06. High Blood Pressure (Yes) No
07. Ulcers (Yes) No
08. Tuberculosis Yes (No)
09. Hepatitis Yes (No)
10. Sexually transmitted disease Crabs or lice (Yes) No
11. Other medical conditions that require attention (Yes) No
12. Are you taking medications ? (Yes) No

Name/Type	Amount	Frequency	Last Taken	Present
Diabeta	*5mg*	*BID*	*this AM*	*yes*
Dilantin	*200mg*	*BID*	*"*	*yes*
Cardiozem	*120*	*BID*	*"*	*yes*
ASA	*5 gr*	*2D*		*no*
Lithium	*300mg*	*2ID*	*this AM*	*yes*
HCTZ	*50mg*	*2D*		*yes*

Do you NOW have:

13. Prosthesis/Brace Yes (No)
14. Cane/Crutches/(Wheelchair) (Yes) No
Other:
15. **Allergies** **(Yes)** **No**
Medicine/Food/Other
Kind: *PCN Tylenol*

WOMEN:
16. Current Pregnancy Yes No
If Yes, LMP *NA*
17. In the last 6 weeks, have you had a baby, miscarriage, or abortion Yes No

Do you NOW have:

18. Urgent Dental Problems Yes (No)
19. Eye Glasses/Contacts (Yes) No
20. On Person (Yes) No

02. SUBSTANCE ABUSE

01. Do You use (drugs) or alcohol? *never* (Yes) No
Drug(s) of Choice: *Coke*
Last time Used: *4-17-97 AM*
Amount Used: *2 hits*
How Used: Drank (Snorted) IV Smoked

02. Current signs of influence: Alcohol (Drugs) (Yes) No
Describe: *eyes dilated*

03. History of Drug/Alcohol w/Drawal Yes No
Describe

03. SUICIDE RISK

01. Have you ever attempted suicide? (Yes) No
02. Do you feel suicidal now? (Yes) No
03. Have you been hospitalized for a suicide attempt? (Yes) No

Does the inmate exhibit:
04. Suicidal Threats (Yes) No
05. Extreme Shame/Embarrassment (Yes) No
06. Extreme Depression Yes No
07. Withdrawn/Non-communicative Yes (No)

04. MENTAL HEALTH

01. Do you NOW have any Mental Health problems: (Yes) No
Where have you been treated for these problems?
County Mental Health Hospital
02. Have you ever been in special classes in school? (Yes) No
(ie, (LD) ED. Speech, etc.)

I have answered all questions correctly to the best of my knowledge.
I am aware that health care services are available to me while in custody.

WIS Number
Bar Code

Inmate Signature *John Jones Smith* Date *4/17/97*

Nurse Signature *Betty Jean Alexander* RNC Date *4/17/97*

Figure 31–8
Initial screening form. (Courtesy of Milwaukee County Sheriff's Department, Milwaukee, WI.)

Daily booking register
Release list
Inmate location
Inmate housing history
Inmate release date
Inmate Social Security number

The HUC will always be working in a fast-paced environment because most CJFs are full or have more inmates than they were designed and built to hold.

Skills and Requirements

To secure employment in the criminal justice system, it is necessary to take and pass a civil service examination and pass a security clearance, which is based on a background check. Once these processes have been completed, the applicant must sit for an oral review, which, if successfully completed, results in eligibility for employment by the facility.

There is a need for flexibility. The HUC may be asked to work in two or more areas on a shift, each having different computer systems. The HUC must master all these systems and possess excellent work habits to succeed.

The log entries and order transcriptions must be accomplished with 100% accuracy. The computer systems and applications differ from those in traditional health care settings, requiring the HUC to learn new material in this area. Above all, the ability to prioritize is critical to being proficient in this setting. Armed with these abilities, a HUC will be an asset in the CJF.

Marketing Your Skills

In marketing yourself for a position in the criminal justice system, you must demonstrate a commitment to using your skills toward the provision of the best care possible. The HUC is a valuable asset to the health care team in the provision of this care. Because of the increase in corrections costs, the effective and efficient use of a HUC and his or her skills allows the institution to use other members of the health care team more cost effectively and in their areas of expertise. A HUC has the basic knowledge and skills necessary to work within this system. Exhibiting energy and the drive to build on that knowledge base is important.

Closing Thoughts

Our job in criminal justice facilities is still evolving. It is up to us to find further opportunities to grow in our profession. The areas of expectation are unclear for our job classification in criminal justice facilities. We are on the ground floor of a new area requiring our expertise. The population of jails, houses of corrections, and prisons is expected to explode as more correctional facilities are built. Along with this, the population will grow older and have a greater need for acute medical care. What can a HUC do in a system that is not oriented toward medical concerns, but rather toward security? We can grow and help it move into the 21st century.

Review Questions

1. Differentiate between the three levels of criminal justice facilities.
2. Name five terms that have a different meaning in the criminal justice facility and medical settings. Give the meaning for each.
3. Name three areas where a HUC might be used in the criminal justice facility setting.
4. List four duties a HUC might be expected to carry out in each of the areas mentioned in question 3.

Early Intervention Program

32

Monica L. Lowe

Common Abbreviations

EIP Early Intervention Program

ICC Interagency Coordination Council

IDEA Individuals with Disabilities Education Act

IEP Individualized Education Program

IFSP Individualized Family Service Plan

OT Occupational therapy

OTR Registered occupational therapist

P.L. Public Law

PT Physical therapy

RPT Registered physical therapist

SLP Speech and language pathologist

SLT Speech and language therapy

Objectives

Upon completion of this chapter, the reader should be able to:

1. Identify the law and act that the Early Intervention Program is funded under.
2. Explain the eligibility requirements for the Early Intervention Program.
3. Describe the roles of the members of the clinical team.
4. List the ways that the office manager's role is much like that of a health unit coordinator.

Vocabulary

Disability: The incapacity to perform as expected.

Intervention: The assumption of a corrective role in a situation.

Multidisciplinary: The participation of people from many branches of knowledge.

Transdisciplinary: Sharing across the traditional lines of the specialties or branches of knowledge.

History

The Individuals with Disabilities Education Act (**IDEA**) was enacted by Congress in 1975. Before then, less than one third of children needing special education received it. Many thousands of children with severe or multiple disabilities received little or no education.

The general purpose of the act was to supplement the capability of the states to ensure that children with disabilities had equal access to a free and appropriate education.

Part H of Federal Public Law (**P.L.**) 99-457 is the specific section that oversees how and what kind of services and supports are provided in the Early Intervention Programs (**EIP**) throughout the country. Programs for preschool-age children became a priority in 1986.

The EIP programs are administered by the individual states. Each state can use the designated funds in a manner preapproved by the federal regulations. The states are required to use these funds to develop and implement a statewide, comprehensive, coordinated, **multidisciplinary**, interagency program of early **intervention** for infants and toddlers with disabilities or developmental delays and their families. Infants and toddlers are defined in age as from birth to 3 years.

Some states administer the programs within their own agencies; others subcontract to nonprofit corporations with the expertise to carry out the program.

Introduction

For the purposes of this chapter, the State of New Hampshire is used as the example. The State of New Hampshire has been divided into 12 regions. Region 9 encompasses several cities in a county in the eastern part of the state. The area agency for Region 9 is a nonprofit corporation that is designed to provide the services to this particular region. Each state, region, and area is responsible for how they chose to administer the program and approach the delivery of services. Region 9 is used to describe the program opportunities for a health unit coordinator (HUC).

Staffing

The concept used to accomplish the goals of the agency is that of teams. The team may consist of the following: registered occupational therapist (**OTR**), registered physical therapist (**RPT**), speech and language pathologist (**SLP**), special educator, child development specialist, social worker, program coordinator, service coordinator, and office manager.

Each member of the team contributes different areas of expertise and special talents to the team. Together, they provides services to the children and families in the region. The office manager offers a unique perspective, and that person is considered an equal and valuable member of the team. The office manager is relied on to maintain the records of the children enrolled in the program, keep the office and paperwork in order, and provide technical and clerical support to the entire team, including keeping minutes of meetings.

The Program

The EIP provides early identification, screening, evaluation, service coordination, and the provision of services either in the home, a center-based facility, or alternate site. Alternate sites might include nursery schools, child care centers, headstart programs, and approved private schools. The use of alternate sites is usually dictated by geography. In rural, sparsely populated areas, the alternate sites or the home are likely to be used.

The provision that the child receive services in a "typical setting" is a regulation that governs the program. "Typical setting" is defined as an environment that is natural to the child, or one that is comfortable and familiar to him or her.

The eligibility is limited to those 0 to 3 years of age who are suspected of having developmental delays, a diagnosed **disability**, or a condition affecting development, or are at risk of developing substantial delays if early intervention services are not provided.

The services typically available include the following.

Special education involves preparing a plan of education, taking into account the developmental and disability issues. The goal is for the plan as nearly as possible to approach the education that is age appropriate.

Psychological services are available for the child with behavioral problems alone or in combination with physical problems. The psychological services are designed directly for support of the child with the family members, contributing to the emotional and psychological well-being. Their ongoing assessments evaluate the psychological development of the child compared with the norms for his or her age.

The *occupational therapist* evaluates the stages of development with respect to the normal sequence of events. Plans of care are developed and carried out that deal with:

The parents' handling of the child relative to the disabilities or developmental delays
Feeding problems from the point of view of delivery of the food and oral motor function
Behavioral issues around constant crying
Stimuli and positioning with respect to normal development (e.g., in crawling) and fine motor development

Much of the occupational therapy (**OT**) planning is based not only on the OTR's evaluation, but also on those of the SLP and RPT.

Speech and language therapy involves the evaluation of the development with respect to speech sounds and swallowing. Detailed assessments are done of the mouth and tongue to determine what problems might exist as well as sound production, cognitive language delays, and expressive speech. There can then be an overlap with the OTR, who incorporates these issues into his or her care plan.

Physical therapy (**PT**) deals with issues of muscle strength and deformities. The RPT recommends exercises to stretch tight muscles and strengthen weak ones. He or she evaluates the child periodically to monitor progress. The overlap with OTR is the follow-through to maximize development of the skills that use these muscles.

Social services works with family dynamics and social and financial issues and provides support to the family members and caregivers.

Nutrition services are made available in cases that have a component attributable to malnourishment. They also advise when there is a second medical problem that requires attention to a therapeutic diet, such as diabetes.

Other approved services include consultations by physicians concerning special health needs of the eligible children. The mission of the EIP is to provide early help to children with developmental delays so they can reach their full potential. The goal of the program is to prevent or ameliorate the effect of the child's disability or delay when he or she later enters school. Care must be taken to ensure that the plan is developmentally appropriate for these young children. It is important that the services are sensitive to the cultural and language needs of the families.

The Referral Process

The initial contact may come from physicians' offices, parents, neonatal intensive care units, home health, and other agencies. The office manager gathers the information on a form (Fig. 32–1). Intake paper work and releases are prepared for the staff member who will do the initial interview. The office manager schedules an appointment for the interview.

The Intake Interview

The intake process begins with an interview with the family and child to gather more in-depth background information about the child's needs and strengths and to determine who will be the most appropriate team members to be assigned to the developmental evaluation (Fig. 32–2). At this time, releases are signed by the parents to exchange and request information from the child's pediatrician, the mother's prenatal physician, and the hospital where the child was born and any other facility in which he or she may have been treated. The Early Intervention Face Sheet is filled out at this time for use by the evaluation team (Fig. 32–3).

The Evaluation Process

The evaluation team is assigned to do the developmental evaluation based on the needs of the child and the family. An effective model for this process is the **transdisciplinary** model. This means that each team member, regardless of specialty training and expertise, is also trained to provide a variety of other services and information.

Typically, a play-based evaluation is done in the home or at the center. Toys and games are used and an initial evaluation of how the child has met developmental milestones, such as crawling,

EARLY INTERVENTION REFERRAL

Today's Date ____________________ 45 Day Date ____________________

Child's Name: ____________________ D.O.B. ____________________

Town of Residence ____________________ Phone ____________________

Street Address ____

Mailing Address (if different) ____

Mother ____________________ Father ____________________

Are the parents aware of this referral? ____

Referred by ____________________ Phone ____________________

Agency ____________________ Address ____________________

Reason for referral/primary concerns/diagnosis

____

____

____

____

____

____

Additional information

____

____

____

____

____

____

Person taking referral information

____

Figure 32–1
Early intervention referral form.

walking, and talking, is done. Each team member gathers information and prepares a report to be shared with other team members and the parents. This process involves the use of several developmental evaluation tools to measure the progress based on the baseline assessment databases (Fig. 32–4).

The team makes a decision about eligibility, and if the parents agree, the child is enrolled into the program. When the child is accepted into the

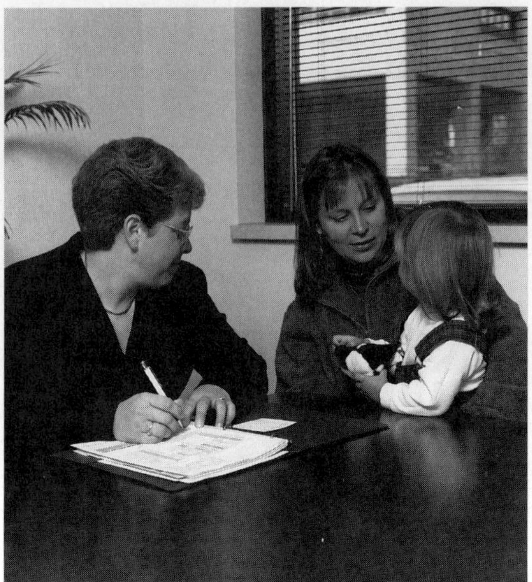

Figure 32–2
Early intervention intake interview.

program, a service coordinator is assigned to the case. The service coordinator is a therapist or special educator who oversees the services provided for each child. The service coordinator draws on the entire team's knowledge to provide well-rounded services for the family and child.

The interdisciplinary team and the family develop an Individualized Family Service Plan **(IFSP)**. The IFSP documents the child's outcomes, goals, and objectives. The document is reviewed quarterly by the interdisciplinary team and family to determine if goals have been met, in part or wholly. In this way, the goals are discontinued, renewed, or changed to reflect the progress or lack of it. At times, other services may be required. The service coordinator arranges these services and resources. They might include respite care, medical consults, financial assistance, and housing arrangements. This all can be accomplished only in the highly collaborative atmosphere that characterizes real teamwork.

Group programs are a major part of EIP. They are usually held in a parent/child setting like the center. The group meetings are usually under the direction of the service coordinator and include the participation of the therapists, educators, and the office manager.

Health Unit Coordinator Role

The HUC fits well into the office manager position of the EIP. The two roles have many of the same requirements and responsibilities.

The office manager is responsible for sending and following up on all correspondence and requests for medical records and information. This includes filling in the release forms completely, having them signed, and making sure they are up to date. Just as in a hospital setting, if a release has not been signed, vital information cannot be shared. If information has been properly requested from another source and it has not arrived in a timely fashion, a follow-up must be done. This is tracked by the office manager, who records the date the information is requested in the client chart and checks periodically to see if the request has been met.

The office manager is responsible for the client chart. This begins with "stuffing" a chart with the proper standard forms and releases. This chart is initiated with the intake interview and remains in use as long as the child is in the program. The chart is divided into sections, just as a hospital chart is. The reports are filed by the staff members. However, it is the primary responsibility of the office manager to maintain the charts in the correct order and to see that they are up to date and neat. Reminders may have to be given to staff members of deadlines for certain reports (Fig. 32–5).

It is also the duty of the office manager to control who has access to the chart and to be aware of its location at any given time. As in the hospital setting, the rules of confidentiality apply. If another agency, school district, or physician's office requests information, the parent or guar-

EARLY INTERVENTION FACE SHEET

Child's Name: ______________________ D.O.B.: ______________

Parents: ______________________ Phone: ______________

Address: ______________________ Alt Phone: ______________

SERVICE COORDINATOR: ______________________

TEAM MEMBERS: ______________ ______________

CONSULTANTS: ______________ ______________

______________ ______________

DAY CARE PROVIDER: ______________________

Phone Number: ______________________

Address: ______________________

____

PEDIATRICIAN: ______________________

Phone Number: ______________________

Address: ______________________

____

OTHER: ______________________

Phone Number: ______________________

Address: ______________________

____

DIRECTIONS TO HOME:

____

____

____

____

____

____

____

Figure 32–3
Early intervention face sheet.

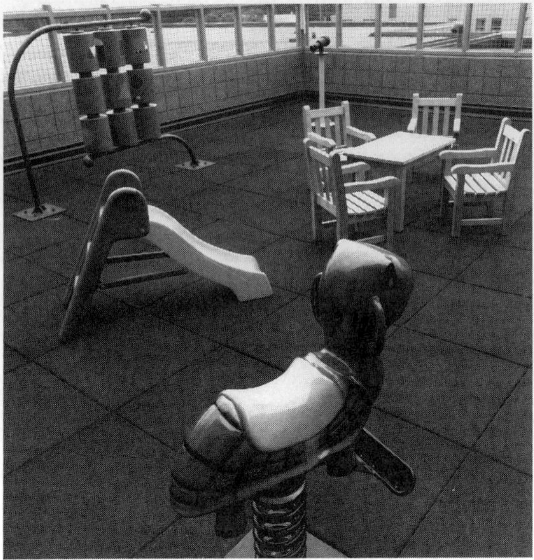

Figure 32–4
Play area.

ian would have to sign event-specific release forms giving permission for the release of information or to gain access to the record.

The various team members use different developmental evaluation tools to measure the child's progress. They are similar to the assessment tool used by a nurse in the hospital. It is important for the office manager to keep a well-stocked supply of these tools, evaluation kits, and toys for the team to use. It is important to be aware of the new developments in the field, so that new toys can be purchased as well as older standbys replaced before they wear out.

Often team members hand write individual sections of the evaluations and progress reports and present them to the office manager to compile a permanent record in the computer files. It is important for the office manager to become familiar with the computer programs in use. Competency in typing and word processing is a must.

The office manager is responsible for creating and compiling a database in the computer on each child enrolled in the program. This makes it easy for staff members to access any information they need, as well as produce reports on a monthly or bimonthly basis for each client and the activities of the agency as a whole. Information can be gathered from surveys to add to the completeness of reports presented at review and annual meetings.

An important daily responsibility is that of billing. EIPs have several funding sources, including Medicaid, grants, private insurance, and state and federal funds. It is of utmost importance that the office manager be detail oriented with the billing paperwork. Accuracy and attentiveness to detail is important because missing information in a submission for reimbursement could cause the entire request to be rejected (Fig. 32–6). When third-party payers, such as insurance companies, are involved, it is not unusual for the office manager to take on the role of liaison as the source and monitor of information flow between the agency and the payers. The billing paperwork is another source of information about services delivered for statistical information and tracking. In this part of the work, the office manager must be familiar with databases and spreadsheets. The office manager is in a position to formulate ways to track the information in the computer as well as create and generate forms that the team members use to provide the basic information. A creative person can develop forms that are user-friendly and support information for the program itself as well as billing information.

Quality Assurance

Each EIP is required to demonstrate quality assurance. In the State of New Hampshire, the quality of the individual program is reviewed by the Interagency Coordination Council (ICC). The tools used are not unlike an employee evaluation form. The strengths and weakness of the team are evaluated. The goals that have been set over a period of time are reviewed, and how well they are met is assessed. The whole team has an opportunity to reflect on the progress and paths the agency is taking. In this way, the service models are reassessed and improved on when needed. Similar types of quality assurance efforts are carried out in the other states.

Child's Name ______________________ DOB ______________

Referral Date ______________________ 45 Day Date ______________

Intake Date/Time ______________________________________

Assessment Date ______________________ Chart Set-Up ______________

Location ______________________________________

Team ______________________________________

Insurance Information

Primary Insurance ______________________ Policy Number ______________

Group Number ______________________________________

Secondary Insurance ______________________ Policy Number ______________

Group Number ______________________________________

I.C.D. 9 Code ______________________ Eligibility Verified ______________

Eligible Yes ☐ No ☐ Enrolled Yes ☐ No ☐ Date Letter Sent ______________

Service Coordinator Assigned ______________________________________

	Initial Paper Work		**Annual**		**Annual**	
	Date Due	Date Complete	Date Due	Date Complete	Date Due	Date Complete
Assessment Feedback						
Assessment Report						
IFSP Meeting						
IFSP Report						
6 Month Review						
Child Health Form						
Physician's Order						
Spedis						

	Date Due	Date Complete
School Referral School Referral		
School Transition Goal		
Discharge Discharge Form		
Discharge Summary		
Discharge Spedis		
Discharge Letter Sent		

Figure 32–5
Tracking sheet.

Early Intervention Services
Billing Sheet

Child's Name ____________ D.O.B. ____________ **Month/Year** ________

Primary Insurance ____________

Policy Number____________ Group Number ________ Discharge Date____________

Secondary Insurance ____________

Policy Number ____________ Group Number________

Estab. cat.________ Diagnostic Code________ Loc.of Serv.________ **Case Management/Service Coordination provided this month(circle one) Yes No**

Bundle Services		s	m	t	w	t	f	s	s	m	t	w	t	f	s	s	m	t	w	t	f	s	s	m	t	w	t	f	s
		1	2	3	4	5	6	7	8	9	10	11	12	13	14	15	16	17	18	19	20	21	22	23	24	25	26	27	28
Intake																													
I.F.S.P.																													
Evaluation	W4000																												
Re-Evaluation	W4000																												
Assistive Tech Services	W4001																												
Fam/Child Train.&Counsel.	W4001																												
Occupational Therapy	W4001																												
Physical Therapy	W4001																												
Speech Therapy	W4001																												
Social Work Services	W4001																												
Special Instruction	W4001																												
Special Instruction/Group	W4001																												

Therapy Codes *=eval.codes		s	m	t	w	t	f	s	s	m	t	w	t	f	s	s	m	t	w	t	f	s	s	m	t	w	t	f	s
		1	2	3	4	5	6	7	8	9	10	11	12	13	14	15	16	17	18	19	20	21	22	23	24	25	26	27	28
Note number of units and initials																													
SP/L or hearing eval	92506*																												
SP/L or hear.tharapy INDIVIDUAL	92507																												
SP/L or hear.therapy GROUP	92508																												
Swallowing/Feeding evaluation	92525*																												
Swallowing/Feeding treatment	92526																												
Theraputic procedure (ie ROM)	97110																												
Neuromuscular reeducation	97112																												
Gait training	97116																												
Therapeutic Proc.(group) 2 or more	97150																												
Myofascial release	97250																												
Manipulation(ie cervical,lumbosacral)	97260																												
Therapeutic function actictivities...	97530																												
Self Care/Home Management	97535																												
Phys. performance test-written report	97750*																												
Development of cognitive skills	97770																												
Other / Write in code																													

Service Coordinator Signature____________________

One Unit = 15 minutes
Two Units = 30 minutes

Therapists Signatures

Initials______ Signature____________________
Initials ______ Signature____________________
Initials ______ Signature____________________

Figure 32–6
Billing sheet.

Closing Thoughts

A way that my past hospital experience as a certified HUC has been beneficial to me has been to provide me with a strong knowledge of medical terminology. As the office manager, I review the child's medical record and the developmental evaluation reports to determine the most appropriate ICD-9 code to assign to the child (see Chapter 42). This code is used by the insurance company for reimbursement purposes, so it very important to assign the correct code. Having exposure to medical terminology has made this task easier and more accurate.

Individual team members each have a unique style of working, and with such a diverse team of professionals, this means constantly practicing and fine tuning your interpersonal and communication skills. Each team member's ideas are important, and we often brainstorm and share new ideas to develop new strategies and creative ways to deliver services, communicate with each other, and provide support for all team members. The office manager often sees the situation from a unique viewpoint, and can assist the team in keeping many issues in perspective.

The office manager is the one person who is consistently in the office. He or she becomes a grounding point for the rest of the team members. Team members are providing therapy to children in their homes, day care settings, and babysitters' homes during the day, and call into the office for important messages and information. It is the office manager who tracks down staff members to inform them of schedule changes and canceled visits. This allows the rest of the team to make changes in their schedules and use their time more efficiently.

Some of the routine daily tasks may seem dull or boring, but they are the foundation of a well-run office and team. I have had the opportunity to maintain a resource file of information to be shared with team members and families. It has been particularly rewarding to me to have been able to formulate the ways to track information and to develop forms that were accepted by my fellow team members. This has contributed to the quality of and ease with which the reporting is done in my office.

The office manager is someone who might not know all the answers, but knows where to find them. It is important to know that the HUC who is flexible and adaptable can bring the talents he or she has learned and mastered in the hospital setting to any EIP and become a valuable asset.

Review Questions

1. Under which Act and Public Law is the EIP funded?
2. List and explain the eligibility requirements to be entered into the EIP.
3. Name and describe the roles of two of the members of the clinical team.
4. Describe four ways in which the role of the office manager in an EIP resembles that of a HUC.

Bibliography

Internet
www.programs.gov
www.children with special needs.com

33

Home-Based Care

E. Anne Mason

Common Abbreviations

CHAP	Community Health Accreditation Program
CHPA	Council on Healthcare Provider Accreditation
DME	Durable medical equipment
DOH	Department of Health
DRG	Diagnosis-related group
HCFA	Health Care Financing Administration
HME	Home medical equipment
JCAHO	Joint Commission on Accreditation of Healthcare Organizations
NAHC	National Association of Home Care
NIV	Noninvasive ventilation
RCP	Respiratory care practitioner

Objectives

Upon completion of this chapter, the reader should be able to:

1. Explain the factors that have caused home health care to become a major part of the health care industry.
2. Identify the three main areas of home-based care.
3. List some of the services that may be provided by a home health agency.
4. Briefly describe the role of a health unit coordinator in home-based care.

Vocabulary

Competency: Capability of performing the requirements of a particular job at an acceptable level.

Enteral feeding: Delivering nutrition by way of the intestines.

Groshong catheter: A central venous catheter that differs from others in that it has a "biflow valve" that prevents blood from backing up into it between uses. This catheter is very safe for home care and does not have to be clamped or heparinized.

HCFA-485: Federally mandated form used to establish plan of care based on physician's orders

Homebound: Confined to the home because of a normal inability to leave home; consequently, leaving home requires considerable and taxing effort (Medicare definition)

Hyperalimentation: Providing all or part of the patient's caloric needs by the intravenous route

Intermittent care: Medically predictable, recurring need for service, usually at least every 60 days, with the skilled services being needed less than daily (Medicare definition)

Parenteral: Situated or occurring outside the intestines

Sleep apnea: Cessation of breathing during profound sleep, usually of a temporary nature

Wallaby: Phototherapy system developed to provide safe, effective home phototherapy

History

"Home-based health care" is an extremely broad-brush phrase encompassing a multitude of health services provided to the community outside the walls of traditional health care facilities such as hospitals, nursing homes, and clinics. The home was the primary site for health care long before anyone ever developed the idea of hospitals. The roots of home-based care actually date back to the 1880s, when community nurses brought health care services to those in need. Today, the home has again become a primary site for health care delivery.

State and federal health care funding throughout the years has been monitored and adjusted based primarily on those costs of health care provided through the hospitals. **DRGs** (diagnosis-related groups) were instituted in the mid-1980s. The cost of each diagnosis/procedure was bundled according to what was determined to be the "normal" course of events. The expectation was that a patient with a particular diagnosis would return home within a pre-established time frame. This predetermined amount of money was paid to the hospital. Hospital stays exceeding the "normal" course of events and fee schedule added a financial burden to the institution. Policymakers at this time embraced home care as the mechanism of choice to reduce hospital stays and physician office visits. They believed that wound dressings, routine blood work, and similar care could be done more cost effectively if the services were delivered at home.

Managed care came of age during the 1990s and rapidly changed the health care industry. The goal of managed care was to provide high-quality health services at reduced costs. In order to reach this goal, home-based care focused on expanding the utilization of skilled interventions and customer education. This, in turn, reduced the number of hospitalizations and the length of hospital stay.

With this in mind, and with reimbursement rates paid to hospitals by state, federal, and insurance sources being further reduced, patients are discharged earlier and usually require more intense levels of care at home. Their health status is much more fragile and unpredictable.

This reformed health care system has led to the very rapid increase in the number of home care agencies throughout the nation. According to the National Association of Home Care (**NAHC**), over 17,000 home care agencies deliver services to over 7 million people per year. Because of this rapid growth, during the 1980s state and federal regulations were implemented to protect the health and welfare of those in the community receiving home care. The Health Care Financing Administration (**HCFA**) and the Department of Health (**DOH**) are two of the predominant players in regulating services provided and in reimbursement.

Introduction

Today, soaring hospital costs, financial influences of managed care, and state and federal budgets demand cost-effective and high-quality services. In response to these demands, home care has become an effective alternative to institutional services. Home care agencies accept a greater share of the financial risk, which requires more efficient management of both resources and delivery. How the coordination of the two is performed has a direct effect on the organization's financial and clinical outcomes.

Another force that has become very powerful and influential is the consumer. The consumer's drive to live as normal a life as possible, maintaining his or her dignity and independence in the comfort of home, has prompted continued invention, evolution, and adaptation of home care services and equipment. The benefits of home care are:

- Shorter hospital stay
- Hospital, nursing home divergence
- Comforts of home along with enjoying the support of family and friends
- Increased morale from being at home
- Involvement of family and friends in treatment
- Faster recovery

- Higher level of personal independence
- Significantly less cost for care provided than in other settings
- Information, education, and support for caregivers

The growth of the aging population and the accompanying increase in chronic illnesses will continue to challenge the services provided by home care. Significant importance is placed on the choices available to the consumer who wishes to remain independent and at home during illness or convalescence. The Balanced Budget Act of August 1997 has parts that will influence many home care agencies in the future. As of January 1998, no specific guidelines have been published to support the changes in reimbursement that have been announced. The rapid growth of the home care industry has also led to the suspicion of fraudulent practices on the part of a small number of agencies, so that Medicare requirements will be much more stringent to protect the beneficiaries.

Change in the delivery of health care services is happening at an accelerated rate. Those participating in the provision of home care experience a challenging and rewarding opportunity in the much appreciated field of health care.

The goal of home care is to provide continuity of high-quality care outside the hospital or institutional setting through a fully integrated approach focusing on the consumer. This care, provided through various agencies in the community, requires specially educated personnel. They are people who are flexible and creative, possess common sense as well as a sense of humor, are independent as well as team players, and who see the client as a whole, part of a family and community, not just as a patient with an illness. The human factors involved in the provision of care affect the delivery of services.

Home care services are provided through proprietary agencies and not-for-profit agencies. These may be facility based (i.e., hospital or nursing home) or community based. Agencies may be publicly owned, funded by state, county, or local government, or privately owned.

This chapter focuses on three main areas of home-based care: the community-based home health agency, the home infusion therapy agency, and the durable medical equipment company.

Home Health Agency

Regulations in health care have created various types of agencies that fall under this category. Skilled professional services, paraprofessional services, and additional support services are provided or coordinated through these agencies. The coordination of these services is of primary importance in maintaining a person at home and in optimal health. The services are beneficial for people of all ages. From newborn infants and their mothers to the elderly, home health care provides much needed services in the comfort of home.

1. Skilled services provided may consist of one or all of the following: nursing, physical therapy, occupational therapy, speech therapy, nutrition services, rehabilitation services, respiratory therapy, pediatric care, or medical social work, depending on the individual needs of the client or as ordered by the physician.
2. Paraprofessional services are provided by a certified home health aide, certified occupational therapy assistant, or physical therapy assistant. The client receives assistance with personal care, activities of daily living, exercise program, light housekeeping, meal preparation, and running errands, as warranted.
3. Support services also coordinated or provided by the home care agencies are Meals on Wheels, social day care, and social work.

The physician plays an active role along with the registered nurse case manager in establishing each individualized plan of care, using the HCFA-485 form (Fig. 33–1).

The Service Coordinator

Various health care providers are involved in service delivery. One of these is the service coordinator. In this position, health unit coordinator

Department of Health and Human Services
Health Care Financing Administration

Form Approved
OMB No. 0938-0357

HOME HEALTH CERTIFICATION AND PLAN OF CARE

1. Patient's HI Claim No. | 2. Start Of Care Date | 3. Certification Period From: To: | 4. Medical Record No. | 5. Provider No.

6. Patient's Name and Address

7. Provider's Name, Address and Telephone Number

8. Date of Birth | 9. Sex ☐ M ☐ F

10. Medications: Dose/Frequency/Route (N)ew (C)hanged

11. ICD-9-CM | Principal Diagnosis | Date

12. ICD-9-CM | Surgical Procedure | Date

13. ICD-9-CM | Other Pertinent Diagnoses | Date

14. DME and Supplies

15. Safety Measures:

16. Nutritional Req.

17. Allergies:

18.A. Functional Limitations

1 ☐ Amputation
2 ☐ Bowel/Bladder (Incontinence)
3 ☐ Contracture
4 ☐ Hearing
5 ☐ Paralysis
6 ☐ Endurance
7 ☐ Ambulation
8 ☐ Speech
9 ☐ Legally Blind
A ☐ Dyspnea With Minimal Exertion
B ☐ Other (Specify)

18.B. Activities Permitted

1 ☐ Complete Bedrest
2 ☐ Bedrest BRP
3 ☐ Up As Tolerated
4 ☐ Transfer Bed/Chair
5 ☐ Exercises Prescribed
6 ☐ Partial Weight Bearing
7 ☐ Independent At Home
8 ☐ Crutches
9 ☐ Cane
A ☐ Wheelchair
B ☐ Walker
C ☐ No Restrictions
D ☐ Other (Specify)

19. Mental Status:

1 ☐ Oriented
2 ☐ Comatose
3 ☐ Forgetful
4 ☐ Depressed
5 ☐ Disoriented
6 ☐ Lethargic
7 ☐ Agitated
8 ☐ Other

20. Prognosis: 1 ☐ Poor 2 ☐ Guarded 3 ☐ Fair 4 ☐ Good 5 ☐ Excellent

21. Orders for Discipline and Treatments (Specify Amount/Frequency/Duration)

22. Goals/Rehabilitation Potential/Discharge Plans

23. Nurse's Signature and Date of Verbal SOC Where Applicable:

25. Date HHA Received Signed POT

24. Physician's Name and Address

26. I certify/recertify that this patient is confined to his/her home and needs intermittent skilled nursing care, physical therapy and/or speech therapy or continues to need occupational therapy. The patient is under my care, and I have authorized the services on this plan of care and will periodically review the plan.

27. Attending Physician's Signature and Date Signed

28. Anyone who misrepresents, falsifies, or conceals essential information required for payment of Federal funds may be subject to fine, imprisonment, or civil penalty under applicable Federal laws.

Form HCFA-485 (C-4) (02-94) (Print Aligned)

PROVIDER

Figure 33–1
HCFA 485 form. (Courtesy of the Health Care Financing Administration, Department of Health & Human Services, Baltimore, MD.)

(HUC) skills are very important. The ability to handle multiple tasks with ease is essential. The service coordinator interacts closely with the client, family, and allied health professionals. This position is extremely important in coordinating the delivery of services to the client. This is a diverse position requiring flexibility in a fast-paced setting.

The referral for home care services may be initiated by physicians, hospitals, clinics, community organizations, families, or the clients themselves. Once the referral is received, the nurse case manager assesses the client with regard to his or her clinical, environmental, and psychosocial status (Figs. 33–2 through 33–4).

At this point, in conjunction with the physician, a plan of care is developed and implemented. The care plan may in part be at the mercy of the third-party payor. Medicare, for example, requires that the services be **intermittent** and that the client be **homebound.** For this plan of care to be implemented successfully, arrangement and delivery of the various service components must be coordinated. The role of the service coordinator comes into play here.

Home health aide services, if required, can either be provided and scheduled by the agency itself or can be contracted out to an aide agency. If contracted out, the service coordinator must interact with the service coordinator of the aide agency. Efficient and accurate scheduling of aide services as well as nursing visits is essential to client health, welfare, and satisfaction. Coordinating staff and case assignments effectively and efficiently can significantly reduce mileage and travel time.

Medical terminology, acquired in the basic HUC course, facilitates understanding of the client's condition and many of his or her needs identified on the plan of care. This information is useful in scheduling the most appropriately skilled home health aide. By relaying pertinent information to the aide, the service coordinator contributes to an initial visit that is more therapeutic and satisfying to the client.

The service coordinator must also make referrals and coordinate other services/disciplines determined necessary for the client. Accurate documentation is necessary to ensure that the services are scheduled, provided, and reimbursable.

Effective communication and interpersonal skills are essential in this role. The service coordinator is often the only link many people have with the agency. He or she must possess "people skills" and have a genuine commitment to helping others. The person's perception of the agency is often determined by the impression given by the service coordinator.

One of the frequently used methods of communication is the telephone. Facial expression, a major component of verbal communication, is absent during this interaction. Special attention must therefore be given to tone of voice, the ability to listen, and the words used.

The service coordinator communicates regularly with clients, clients' families, and health care professionals. The health care professionals may be fellow employees or contracted services. It is important that the lines of communication remain open and effective, thus creating a dynamic interdisciplinary team. Teamwork is essential for the effective treatment of the client's medical needs and ensuring an optimal rate of recovery. The team's greatest desire is to optimize patient outcomes.

The service coordinator encounters various pieces of office equipment such as fax and photocopy machines, computers and printers, and pagers and paging systems. Proper management of office equipment and supplies is essential to the provision of client services.

The effectiveness of home care is based on client outcomes. The service coordinator may be required to enter and retrieve data to support the efficacy of the services provided by the agency. The information from these report will also be considered when reimbursement is discussed with current or new payor sources.

Confidentiality, another component taught in the HUC course, must be maintained at all times. A great deal of sensitive information is available in the health care record. It is the responsibility of all employees to follow the guidelines for maintaining confidentiality of client information. Con-

MERCY HOME CARE

OF WESTERN NEW YORK

Private Client Referral Form

Time________________ Date____________________

Source ____________________________ Discharge Planner/Social Worker____________________

Name ____________________________ Phone #______________________________

Address____

D.O.B. ________________ DX____

Equipment Involved____

Hospital__________________________ Room #______________ Phone___________________

Possible Discharge Date_______________ Type of Care__________ Hrs Per Week_______________

Responsible Party Name__________________________________ Phone #___________________

Relationship to Client____

Date and Document all interactions held prior to acceptance/nonacceptance of case.

Comments____

____

____

____

____

____

____

Date Accepted/ Not Accepted To Mercy Home Care Services_____________________________

If Not Accepted , Explain Why____

____

Survey Date________________________ Date Service to Start_____________________________

File Accepted Cases under Miscellaneous in Client Record, File Unaccepted Cases in separate binder.

MHC E-206/ 2/2/95

Figure 33–2
Private intake/referral form. (From Mercy Home Care of Western New York, Lockport, NY.)

Client ID: ______________ Referral Date: ______________ Revisions: ______________
SOC: ______________ Referral Time: ______________

MERCY LONG TERM HOME HEALTH CARE PROGRAM
Client Information Form

I. Demographic Data

Name: ______________ Sex: ______________
Address: ______________ Lives with: ______________
Phone Number: ______________ DOB: ______________

Directions to Home: ______________

Medicaid CIN#: ______________ Medicaid #: ______________
Medicaid #: ______________ Other Ins. #: ______________

Responsible party: ______________ Relationship: ______________
Address: ______________ Phone Number: ______________

II. Referral Source

Referred by: ______________ (Hosp/MD/Family/Other–please specify)
Admit Date: ______________
Potential Discharge: ______________
Phone Number: ______________

III. Medical Information

Primary Dx and ICD: 1) ______________ 3) ______________
2) ______________ 4) ______________

Allergies: ______________ Diet: ______________

Primary MD: ______________ UPIN #: ______________
Address: ______________ Medicaid Billing #: ______________
License #: ______________
Phone Number: ______________ Client's Hospital Preference: ______________

IV. Home Care Information

Services Provided

- ☐ RN
- ☐ ST
- ☐ PT
- ☐ OT
- ☐ HHA
- ☐ PCA
- ☐ Medical daycare
  Where:
  Phone:
  Days/week:
- ☐ Cab/WC Van carrier:

Waivered Services

- ☐ MOW #/week:
  Phone:
- ☐ MSW
- ☐ RT
- ☐ RD
- ☐ Social daycare
  Where:
  Phone:
  Days/week:
- ☐ Lifeline
  871-0176

DME Vendor
Phone:
Pharmacy:
Phone:
Aide Agency:
Phone:
CASA caseworker:
Phone:
RN Case manager:
Equipment used/needed:

Referral Code: **Discharge Code:**

Figure 33–3
L. T. intake/referral form. (From Mercy Long Term Home Health Care Program, West Seneca, NY.)

HOME CARE CONNECTION

INTAKE

Worker ______

PATIENT INFORMATION

Name ______

Address ______

______

Phone (H) ______ (W) ______

DOB __/__/__ Sex ______ Marital status ______

Social security # ______

Primary insurance ______

Secondary insurance ______

Physician ______

Office ______

Phone ______

PDX ______

SDX ______

CONTACT PERSON(S)

Name ______

Address ______

______

Phone (H) ______ (W) ______

Relationship ______

Name ______

Address ______

______

Phone (H) ______ (W) ______

Relationship ______

DATE: ______ **TIME:** ______

REASON FOR CALL ______

______

______

REFERRAL SOURCE ______

______

Medications ______

______

Secondary MD ______

SKILLED SERVICE

N PT OT ST MSS HHA OTHER

MERCY MEDICAL

Respiratory oxygen

A. Saturation % and date OR B. PO 2% and date

C. Liter flow ______

Type of equipment/supplies and length of time needed:

______

______

______

MHS LIFELINE

______

______

______

MERCY HOME CARE

______

______

______

MERCY LONG TERM

MEDICAID CIN# ______

MERCY HOME CARE

______

______

______

OUTCOME ______

______

______

HOME CARE CONNECTION **Client** ______

1. Request for Service ______

______

2. Is the client aware of call? ______

______

3. Mental Status ______

______

4. How are they living now? ______

______

5. What are the living arrangements? ______

______

6. What is the support system?

______ service request ______ non-skilled (custodial–help with ADL's or home chores)
______ general evaluation (non specific) ______ equipment
______ skilled need ______ long term sk/cus management (Medicaid)
______ PT, OT, ST, PSYCH, SN ______ Lifeline

7. What is the problem? ______

______

8. Does the patient need...

______ service request ______ non-skilled (custodial–help with ADL's or home chores)
______ general evaluation (non specific) ______ equipment
______ skilled need ______ long term sk/cus management (Medicaid)
______ PT, OT, ST, PSYCH, SN ______ Lifeline

9. Assess for

______ Safety ______ Transportation ______ Insurances ______ Advance directives
______ Meals ______ Meds ______ Entitlements

10. Ask if there is anything else we can do to help this person.

11. Outcome ______

______

______

______

______

Figure 33–4
Intake/referral form.

fidentiality of agency business should also be maintained.

Home Infusion Therapy Agency

The home infusion therapy agency provides cost-effective infusion therapies to be delivered outside of the hospital/clinic setting. Greater dignity and independence are maintained by the consumer. The consumer is afforded an alternative to being exiled to long stays in the cold sterility of the hospital or nursing home. Complex therapies can be delivered at home, work, or during recreational activities. Family members can be taught procedures previously thought of as only able to be delivered by trained health professionals. The following treatments are but a few of those available:

Intravenous antibiotics for infections
Chemotherapy for cancer
Parenteral pain control therapies
Hyperalimentation (TPN) in "failure to thrive"
Hydration for hyperemesis of pregnancy
Maintenance of central lines (e.g., **Groshong catheter**, Broviac catheter, Hickman line, ports)
Enteral feedings and supplies

Health Unit Coordinator Role

The physician contacts the home infusion therapy nurse with specific directions as to treatment modality. It is at this point that the HUC becomes very valuable in coordinating the individual facets of the treatment plan.

The pharmacist must be notified of the orders. The pharmacy itself may be agency, community, or hospital based. Other vendors must be contacted based on the individual client's needs. These needs may include supplies for wound care, a personal response system, or medical equipment. Referrals may be made to a nutritionist, physical therapist, or social worker. The HUC has the skills to organize the delivery of services. Laboratory tests need to be ordered and results relayed to the appropriate health professional. Ongoing contact with the client or his or her family is imperative.

The HUC is involved with the medical record from start of care to discharge; care plans are updated and physician orders completed and tracked. Discharge summaries must be sent and billing information generated. Data entry skills are essential.

A strong knowledge of medical terminology enables the HUC to understand the orders received, communicate with other health care professionals, and assist in demonstrating agency **competency** to the client. It is important for the HUC to recognize common medical equipment used in the therapies delivered by the agency. Two very common pieces of equipment are intravenous infusion pumps and enteral infusion pumps. The CADD-Plus infusion pump delivers a prescribed amount of intravenous medication (Fig. 33–5). The enteral infusion pump, Flexiflo Patrol, regulates the flow of a nutritional liquid into the digestive system (Fig. 33–6).

The HUC plays a pivotal role in the home infusion therapy agency.

Durable Medical Equipment Company

The durable medical equipment (**DME**) company provides the equipment necessary for a person who is ill or convalescing at home to maintain optimal function. Advances in home medical equipment (**HME**) technology have led to the development of portable equipment, which is very valuable in the home care arena. The client may require adaptive equipment such as a raised toilet seat, safety grab bars in the bathroom, or a bathtub bench. To maintain or assist mobility, it may be necessary for the client to use a cane, walker, or wheelchair. Products involved in wound care, ostomy care, incontinence care, and infection control are also available.

Many DME companies also provide home oxygen therapy services. This includes such items as:

Oxygen in tanks of various sizes
Oxygen delivery equipment

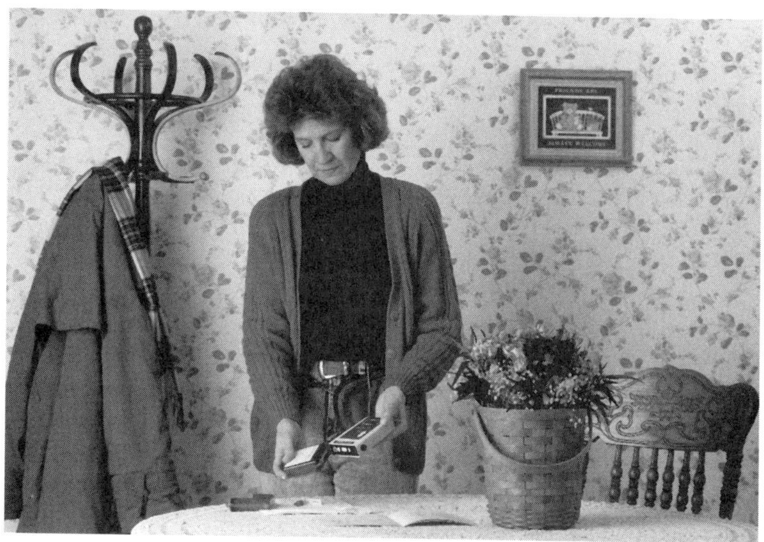

Figure 33–5
CADD pump. (Courtesy of Sims Deltec, Inc., St. Paul, MN.)

Ventilators
Noninvasive ventilation (**NIV**)
Pulse oximetry
Sleep apnea monitoring
Continuous positive airway pressure equipment

The third-party payors sometimes require that certain parameters be met before home therapy can be used. Arrangements are made with the respiratory care practitioner (**RCP**) to do home visits for evaluation and pretesting. The RCP is also scheduled to set up the equipment and do the follow-up teaching.

Advances in technology have made phototherapy for jaundice of the newborn appropriate for home use. The equipment comes in the form of a blanket, known as a **Wallaby.** It is very easy to use, has no side effects if used properly, and allows the baby to be held while receiving the therapy.

Nurses from an agency are usually needed to do daily heelsticks for blood draws.

Health Unit Coordinator Role

Many items require physician orders and are distributed according to regulations set forth by funding sources. The product orders must be received, filled, and distributed in a timely manner. The HUC's skills are very beneficial to this company, not only in the area of coordinating delivery but in the service representative arena dealing with customer inquiries. Much of the coordination must be done with outside agencies. Again, excellent communication skills are essential.

This type of agency requires the competencies, skills, and abilities of a HUC, as do those agencies previously mentioned.

Opportunities for Growth

Those participating in the provision of home care partake in a challenging and uniquely rewarding experience in the constant evolution of services. Effective delivery of services, whether equipment or personnel, is within the control of the HUC. The HUC must be able to work independently, problem solve, and make decisions within his or her scope of practice.

Many of these decisions must be made rapidly on notification of the situation at hand. These decisions may require referral to members of the health care professional team, rescheduling of aide services, notification of emergency personnel, rerouting of pharmacologic products, or reordering of durable medical equipment. Because of

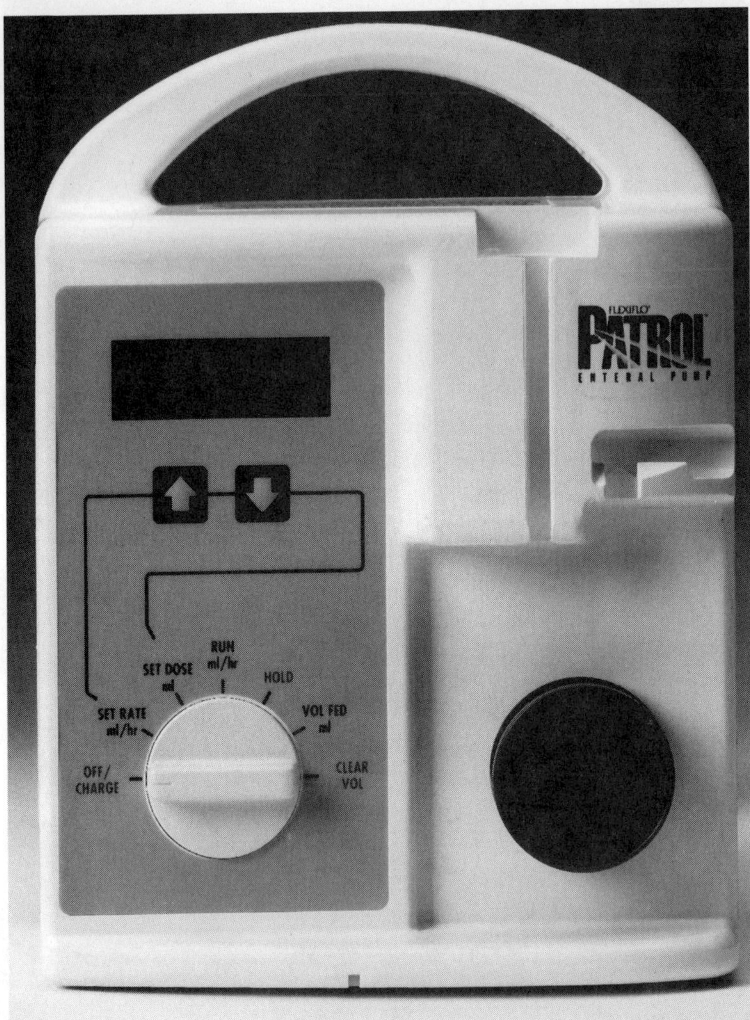

Figure 33–6
Enteral pump. (Photo used with permission of Ross Products Division, Abbott Laboratories, Columbus, OH.)

the nature of home care, the manager or supervisor is not always on site. Through effective listening, learning, and past experience, the HUC independently ensures the continued delivery of the most appropriate services.

Coordinating in any area of home care entails thinking "outside of the box"—being creative, expanding the norms. This ability enables the HUC to create opportunities for growth and betterment for the organization, employees, and customers (internal and external).

Knowledge of the community and the resources available in the community enhances the role of the HUC. This value is appreciated not only by fellow health team members but particularly by the clients, their families, and prospective clients. This often is the first step in the successful solution of a client's problem. The HUC is often called on to explain the role of the organization as well as direct calls appropriately.

A sense of humor and its uses are helpful in dealing with stress. The benefit of using humor in coping with stress is that it also helps conserve energy for dealing with larger issues. There are frequent demands imposed by the client, family, health professionals, or contract agencies.

The ability to embrace new technology is paramount. In all of the organizations previously mentioned, scheduling is a large part of the HUC role. Mapping is an example of augmenting effective and efficient scheduling. Through computer map software, the HUC can determine the location of an address, the distance between two points, and the most direct route to get there (Fig. 33–7). This is only one example of the many computer programs available.

Terminology specific to each of these areas of home care must be acquired. In the home care agency, new terminology arises from the language used by the various regulatory bodies. In the infusion therapy agency, familiarity and understanding of the intravenous lines and equipment enables the HUC effectively to order supplies, coordinate services, and communicate with the referral source, pharmacist, nurse, or family. HME has many abbreviations all its own.

The HUC in all home care agencies must become familiar with the regulations specific to the agency. It also helps to have a basic awareness of the regulations of other types of home health agencies in order to enhance the flow of services.

Quality Assurance

Accreditation bodies, such as Joint Commission on Accreditation of Healthcare Organizations **(JCAHO)**, Community Health Accreditation Program **(CHAP)**, and Council on Healthcare Provider Accreditation **(CHPA)**, have been rapidly embraced by the home care industry. It is not only important to believe that the agency provides high-quality care and services, but equally important for the agency to be measured against industry standards. Through this voluntary surveillance process, the organization ultimately knows that the services provided are of high quality and that improvements in organizational performance are continually being monitored. This accrediting process brings new terminology with which the HUC must become familiar.

The quality of service is important to all agencies. The HUC must be familiar with the quality improvement plan of the organization and must participate in quality measure activities (e.g., process teams, data collection, surveillance activities). The HUC may be involved in the distribution, collection, and data entry of the client satisfaction surveys.

Extra Training and Skills

The ability to create and understand spreadsheets and the use of databases adds value to a HUC on applying for a coordinator position in home care. Being well organized, detail oriented, and accurate are of unlimited value.

Some of the payment sources in home care are different from those encountered in a more traditional HUC role. It is important to know the regulations of each of those payment sources so that all services provided are reimbursable. The HUC involved in a DME company needs to become familiar with a new set of billing codes because these differ from the traditional billing codes (Fig. 33–8).

Scheduling of nurse and aide visits has become computerized, enabling direct linkage to payroll and billing (Fig. 33–9). Any additions, deletions, or adjustments must be made in a timely manner to ensure exact payroll and billing.

The HUC is one of the agency employees most often receiving or making telephone contact. Communicating as a caring, understanding, and knowledgeable individual enhances the interaction, whether it be requesting an extra shift from a home care aide, explaining the services of the agency to an inquirer, or discussing the most appropriate equipment for the client's needs. This expertise has a positive effect on the organization's business.

Providing high-quality customer service to both internal and external customers has become very important in a competitive industry. Although technology offers the potential for changes in service delivery, the need for personal interest and assistance remains a primary concern

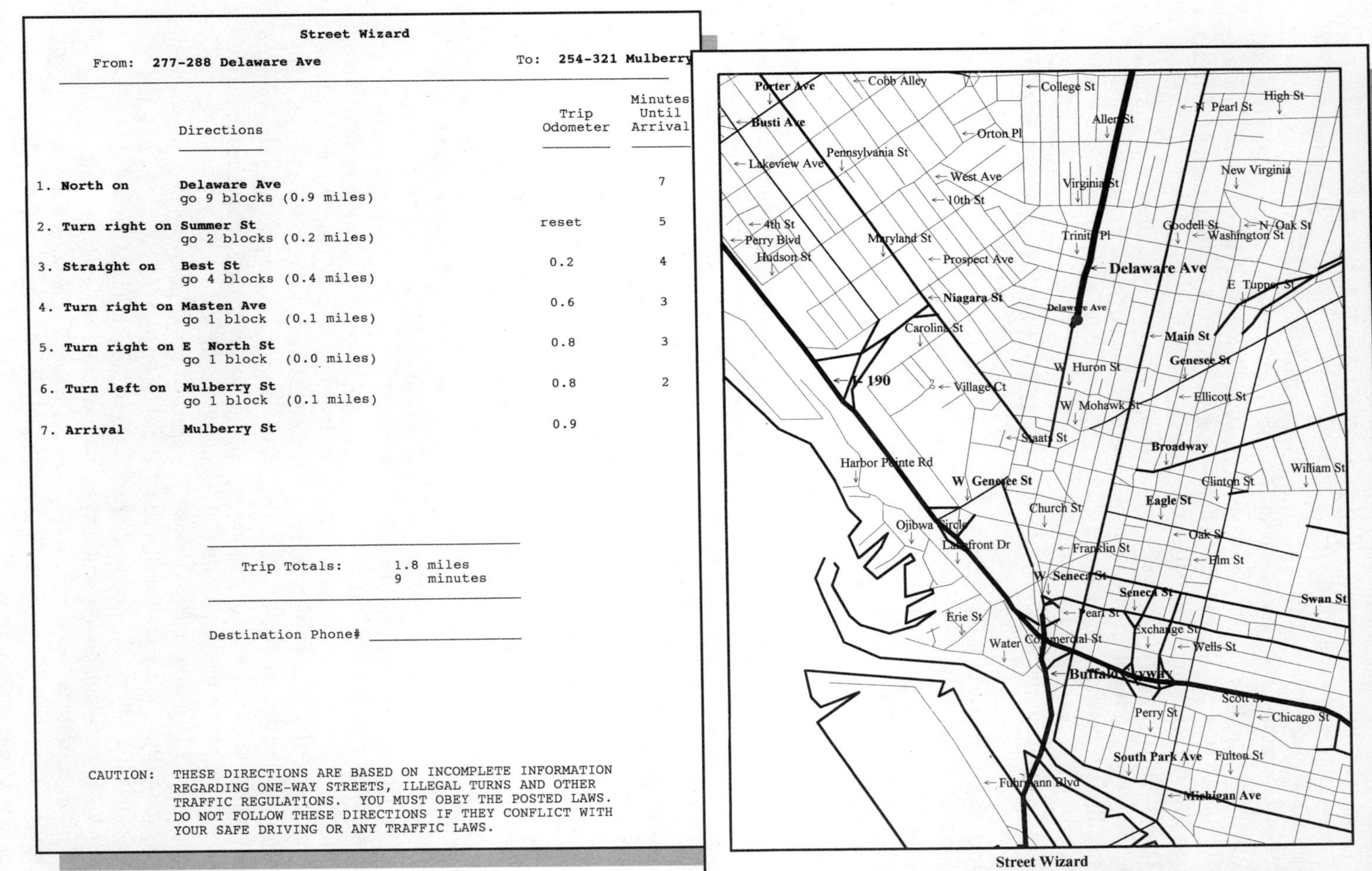

Street Wizard

From: **277-288 Delaware Ave** To: **254-321 Mulberry**

	Directions		Trip Odometer	Minutes Until Arrival
1.	**North on**	**Delaware Ave** go 9 blocks (0.9 miles)		7
2.	**Turn right on**	**Summer St** go 2 blocks (0.2 miles)	reset	5
3.	**Straight on**	**Best St** go 4 blocks (0.4 miles)	0.2	4
4.	**Turn right on**	**Masten Ave** go 1 block (0.1 miles)	0.6	3
5.	**Turn right on**	**E North St** go 1 block (0.0 miles)	0.8	3
6.	**Turn left on**	**Mulberry St** go 1 block (0.1 miles)	0.8	2
7.	**Arrival**	**Mulberry St**	0.9	

Trip Totals: 1.8 miles 9 minutes

Destination Phone# ____________

CAUTION: THESE DIRECTIONS ARE BASED ON INCOMPLETE INFORMATION REGARDING ONE-WAY STREETS, ILLEGAL TURNS AND OTHER TRAFFIC REGULATIONS. YOU MUST OBEY THE POSTED LAWS. DO NOT FOLLOW THESE DIRECTIONS IF THEY CONFLICT WITH YOUR SAFE DRIVING OR ANY TRAFFIC LAWS.

Figure 33–7
Mapping. (Courtesy of Adept Computer Solutions, Inc., San Diego, CA.)

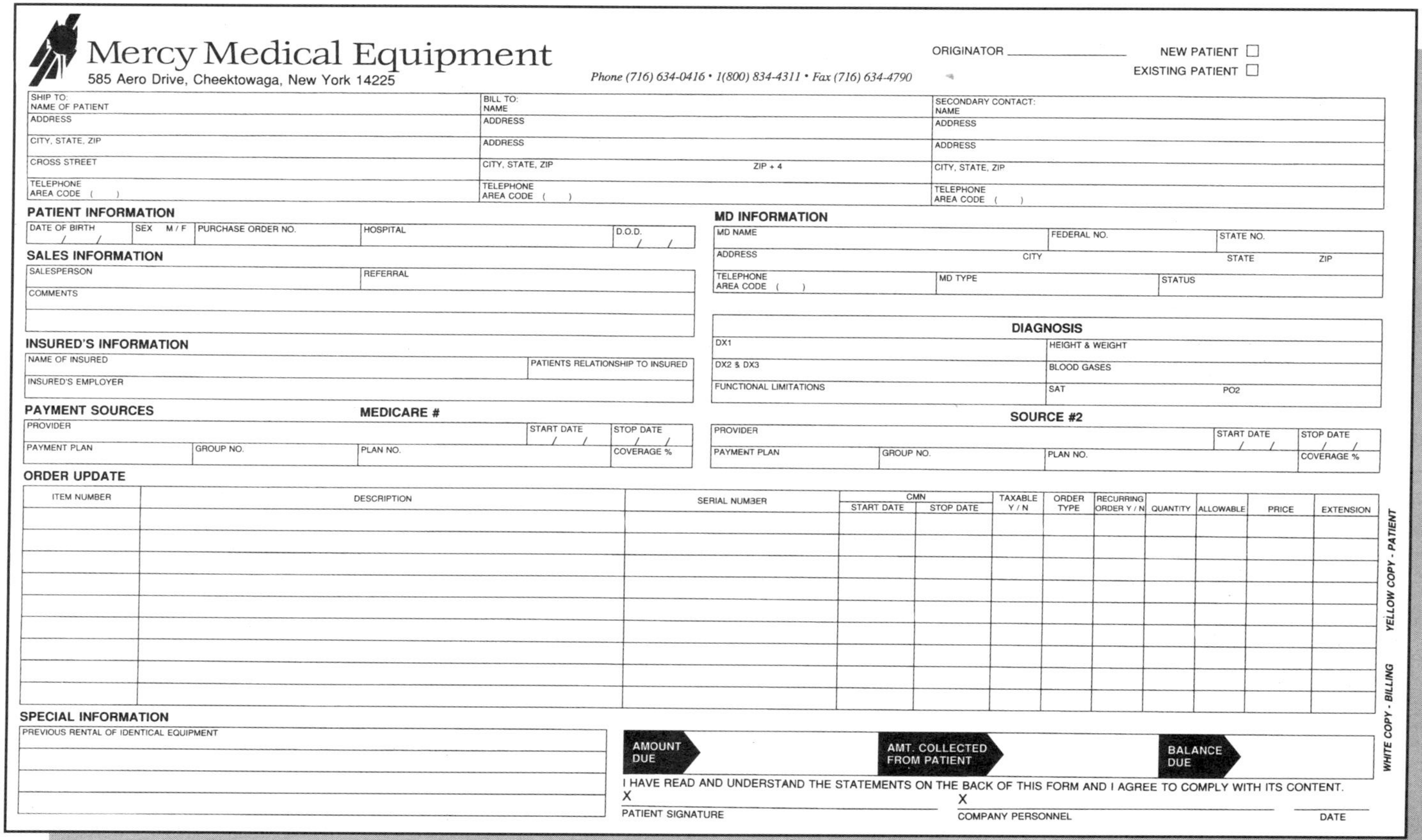

Mercy Medical Equipment
585 Aero Drive, Cheektowaga, New York 14225
Phone (716) 634-0416 • 1(800) 834-4311 • Fax (716) 634-4790

ORIGINATOR ______________ NEW PATIENT ☐ EXISTING PATIENT ☐

SHIP TO:	BILL TO:	SECONDARY CONTACT:
NAME OF PATIENT	NAME	NAME
ADDRESS	ADDRESS	ADDRESS
CITY, STATE, ZIP	ADDRESS	ADDRESS
CROSS STREET	CITY, STATE, ZIP ZIP + 4	CITY, STATE, ZIP
TELEPHONE AREA CODE ( )	TELEPHONE AREA CODE ( )	TELEPHONE AREA CODE ( )

PATIENT INFORMATION

DATE OF BIRTH / /	SEX M / F	PURCHASE ORDER NO.	HOSPITAL	D.O.D. / /

SALES INFORMATION

SALESPERSON	REFERRAL
COMMENTS	

INSURED'S INFORMATION

NAME OF INSURED	PATIENTS RELATIONSHIP TO INSURED
INSURED'S EMPLOYER	

PAYMENT SOURCES **MEDICARE #**

PROVIDER		START DATE / /	STOP DATE / /
PAYMENT PLAN	GROUP NO.	PLAN NO.	COVERAGE %

MD INFORMATION

MD NAME	FEDERAL NO.	STATE NO.
ADDRESS	CITY	STATE ZIP
TELEPHONE AREA CODE ( )	MD TYPE	STATUS

DIAGNOSIS

DX1	HEIGHT & WEIGHT
DX2 & DX3	BLOOD GASES
FUNCTIONAL LIMITATIONS	SAT PO2

SOURCE #2

PROVIDER		START DATE / /	STOP DATE / /
PAYMENT PLAN	GROUP NO.	PLAN NO.	COVERAGE %

ORDER UPDATE

ITEM NUMBER	DESCRIPTION	SERIAL NUMBER	CMN START DATE	CMN STOP DATE	TAXABLE Y / N	ORDER TYPE	RECURRING ORDER Y / N	QUANTITY	ALLOWABLE	PRICE	EXTENSION

SPECIAL INFORMATION

PREVIOUS RENTAL OF IDENTICAL EQUIPMENT

AMOUNT DUE | AMT. COLLECTED FROM PATIENT | BALANCE DUE

I HAVE READ AND UNDERSTAND THE STATEMENTS ON THE BACK OF THIS FORM AND I AGREE TO COMPLY WITH ITS CONTENT.

X ______________ PATIENT SIGNATURE X ______________ COMPANY PERSONNEL ______ DATE

WHITE COPY - BILLING YELLOW COPY - PATIENT

Figure 33–8
DME billing. (From Mercy Medical Equipment, West Seneca, NY.)

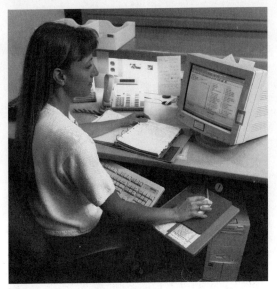

Figure 33–9
Entering visit list into computer.

for many people. Through demonstrating concern that the customer receives the best possible service to meet his or her needs, the organization will succeed. Each employee plays a determining role in the agency's degree of success.

Positioning for the Future

The formal education of a HUC is extremely valuable in many positions in the home care industry. It provides a broad base on which to build the array of skills mentioned in this chapter.

Before the interview, it is helpful to make inquiries regarding the organization to which you are applying. You may even be able to speak to someone who currently holds a similar position or has knowledge of the position requirements. Take previously used skills and relate them to the new position.

It is important to explore the organizational philosophy, vision, and mission. How do your skills, talents, and personal philosophy match?

Join a task force (temporary committee) or networking group as part of a professional or trade organization of students or workers in your related field (e.g., National Association of Health Unit Coordinators). This will help you handle the requirements of complex jobs. Learning task force skills allows you to be more flexible and open to problem-solving techniques that will be useful in any position you choose. These experiences make it easier to enter organizations at a more experienced level.

Become certified by your association. It could be the difference between two otherwise equally qualified candidates for a position.

Be open to applying current expertise to new situations. Flexibility in work habits and expectations is necessary. The health care scene is always evolving.

Closing Thoughts

If you choose to pursue a career in home care, job opportunities are nearly unlimited. In addition, home care creates opportunities for entrepreneurs. Those who possess vision and creativity and who feel empowered regarding their own destiny will be able to carve a future in home care. Job satisfaction results from performing vital services for people in your community who are striving to maintain their independence.

The HUC is part of the dynamic health care team. It takes the right temperament to work directly with people. If you feel the needs of the client are important to you, this is the first step. Those working in home care must continually strive to provide cost-effective, efficient services and not succumb to providing technical services only. The human connection must be maintained. Home care requires motivated people who are looking for a challenging job in a satisfying work environment.

Continuity of care is what the home care industry is all about. It requires many different types of specialists. The HUC plays a central role in the provision of continuity of care.

Roles and responsibilities vary with the type of position in the home care industry. What is universal is that people in home health care enjoy working with clients who trust them with their lives. Home care defines the term "caregiver."

Review Questions

1. Explain the factors that have caused home health care to become a major part of the health care industry.
2. Identify the three main areas of home-based care.
3. List some of the services that may be provided by a home health agency.
4. Briefly describe the role of a health unit coordinator in home-based care.

Bibliography

Briefings on JCAHO—Home Care. Marblehead, MA, Opus Communications, Inc., 1997.

de Sola Cardoza A: Opportunities in Home Care Services Careers. Lincolnwood, IL, GM Career Horizons, a division of NTC Publishing Group, 1993.

Health Care Financing Administration, Department of Health and Human Services, 6325 Security Blvd., Baltimore, MD 21207.

McAuley Seton Home Care: Groshong Catheter Policy. Cheektowaga, NY, McAuley Seton Home Care, 1997.

Mercy Home Care of WNY, 111 Main Street, Box 483, Lockport, NY 14095.

Mercy Long Term Home Health Care Program, WNY Medical Park, Building C, 550 Orchard Park Road, West Seneca, NY 14224.

Mercy Medical Equipment and Oxygen, 2170 Union Road, West Seneca, NY 14224.

Taber's Cyclopedic Medical Dictionary, 13th ed. Philadelphia, FA Davis Co, 1977.

Hospice Organization

34

Elizabeth A. Howe

Common Abbreviations

AIDS	Acquired immune deficiency syndrome
CHAP	Community health accreditation program
DPH	Department of Public Health
HHA	Home health aide
HMO	Health Maintenance Organization
JCAHO	Joint Commission on Accreditation of Healthcare Organizations

Objectives

Upon completion of this chapter, the reader will be able to:

1. Trace the history of hospice.
2. Describe the responsibilities of the health unit coordinator in the hospice setting.
3. Explain the communication unique to the hospice setting.
4. Describe a typical hospice house.

Vocabulary

Aerosolized: Made in a way that can be dispensed as gas

Hyperalimentation: Nutrition given by means other than into the GI tract (TPN)

Palliative: Producing comfort or alleviation of symptoms rather than curative

History

The term *hospice* goes back as far as the Middle Ages and originally meant a place of refuge that provided food and rest for travelers. Today, hospices provide an alternative form of care for the terminally ill. Hospice also provides emotional support for the patient's family.

The writings of Elizabeth Kübler-Ross in 1969 about death and dying heightened the awareness of the public. The modern hospice began in England, when Cicely Saunders founded the St. Christopher's Hospice near London in the late 1960s. In the mid-1970s she lectured about hospice at Yale University in Connecticut, and as a result the Connecticut Hospice Home Care was begun. Soon **palliative** care facilities and other hospices were established. The National Hospice Organization was founded in 1978. The main movement started in the United States in 1982, when Medicare enacted benefits for hospice. Medicaid followed in 1986. By 1988 there were 1200 hospice programs in the United States.

Description

Hospice Residences

Hospice is a philosophy of caring. It is seen as a compassionate approach to care, the goal of which is to help people live life fully, maintain their dignity, and keep personal control over their lives.

The provision of hospice services usually takes place in the home, but there are hospice residences for those who require extended care facilities or nursing home placement. The mission of such residences is to provide a wide range of services for individuals with advanced illness; meeting their needs while preserving their dignity. The goals are to improve or maintain the quality of life. They typically provide a full range of services to provide comfort and control of symptoms:

24-hour skilled nursing
Medical consultation
Dietary services
Nutritional programs
IV therapy
Palliative chemotherapy
Aerosolized medications
Hyperalimentation
Pharmaceuticals (usually charged separately)
Social services
Counseling
Occupational and physical therapy
Participation in clinical trials
Spiritual care
Age-oriented activities in a homelike atmosphere.

Hospice Care in the Home

Hospice enables people with terminal illnesses to decide where and how they wish to spend the remainder of their lives. It provides support, which helps patients minimize the time that they must spend in hospitals. With the increased cost of hospital confinement and aggressive life-prolonging measures, most patients wish to spend the rest of their lives at home surrounded by family and friends.

The criterion for admission to hospice care is a terminal illness with a physician certification of a life expectancy of 6 months or less. This prognosis is determined by the patient's physician. There must be agreement among all involved to focus on noncurative or palliative care. The patient must sign a statement indicating an understanding of the nature of the illness and of hospice care.

In addition to medical and nursing care, hospices provide spiritual care, physical therapy, dietary consultations, medical equipment (including walkers, commodes, electrical hospital beds, and oxygen equipment), medications needed (including morphine pumps [Fig. 34–1]) and trained volunteer services to fill the needs of the terminally ill and to support their families. More than 60 percent of hospice patients suffer from cancer; therefore the first priority is for the patient to be alert and as pain-free as possible. This is accomplished through monitoring and careful dispensing of pain medication. Hospices also care

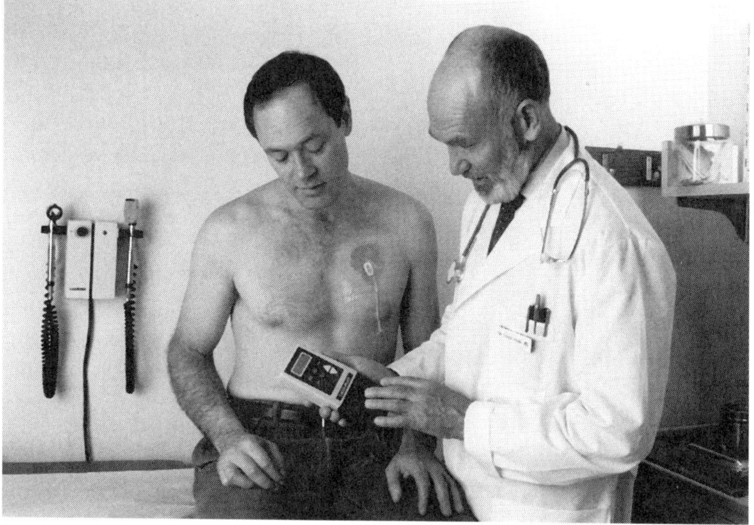

Figure 34–1
Patient with implanted port and ambulatory pump (#21). (Courtesy of Sims Deltec, Inc., St. Paul, MN.)

for patients with **AIDS**, which usually is a terminal condition; participate in specialized programs for children; and provide services to patients who are in extended care facilities.

Many patients worry about being a burden to family, but the team care concept that hospice provides alleviates most of that concern. Sometimes relationships are strengthened and families bond in such a way as to be described as a very meaningful experience.

Staffing

The team care concept is a major component of hospice care, whereby many people with different skills work together for the benefit of the patient and family. Team meetings are held to evaluate and coordinate care, which is individualized according to the needs of each patient. The medical director oversees the program from the medical aspect and attends the team meetings. Usually a hospice is a small organization with an affiliation with one or more local hospitals. It may employ its own nursing staff and home health aides or contract these services through local home health care service agencies.

Clinical Services

One of the questions that patients may ask is "Can I still have my own doctor?" The answer is "Yes." Once the patient and physician have discussed hospice, the patient's physician will continue to direct the plan of care and work closely with hospice. As long as treatments are palliative—for example, chemotherapy to reduce tumor size as a comfort measure—they can be provided in the care plan. Physicians may make home visits or call and leave medication, dietary, and treatment orders with the hospice nurse. Registered nurses, in addition to assessing the patient's needs, may teach family members to administer medications (injections) and to keep a record of those. The record would include time, amount given, site, and response. If the patient is receiving morphine by pump, the nurses monitor the pain control to assure that the patient is as pain-free as possible while still maintaining alertness. In order to maintain optimal pain control, the nurse is in contact with the family physician and makes adjustments as needed. Nurses are on call 24 hours a day and may visit patients at home one or two times a week. The nursing staff will inform the physician regularly as to the condition and any changes that are taking place.

Home health aides (**HHAs**) visit as needed to administer personal care, such as bathing, assisting with ambulating, and assisting the nurse with implementing the most effective plan of care. Home health aides may visit as many times a week as is necessary to maintain the patient's health, hygiene, and well-being.

Physical therapy and occupational therapy may be necessary to maintain strength and mobility as well as to help with circulation and to help improve the patient's quality of life. Therapists may instruct the family on proper techniques for exercises and the appropriate way to transfer the patient from bed to chair or commode, and back.

Volunteer Services

All activities (monthly educational meetings and support meetings) and fundraisers, such as bake sales, tag sales, and golf tournaments, are coordinated through the volunteer office. The volunteer coordinator also sets up the training program for new volunteers before they are assigned to cases. The volunteer training class can last up to 10 weeks. This program may be offered once or twice a year and includes guest speakers drawn from clergy, physicians, social workers, nurses, and funeral directors. Some hospices have separate training for bereavement, which involves different volunteers.

After a volunteer has successfully completed the training program, that individual is "buddied" with a seasoned volunteer for the few patient visits until a comfort level is established. The most important skills from the training class that the volunteer brings to the home are the following guides to good listening:

Do be attentive.
Do make eye contact.
Do focus on what is being said.
Do stay in the present.

Do not let your mind wander.

Do not sit with arms and/or legs crossed (gives message that what is being said is unimportant).

Most hospices use the same volunteer during the patient's illness and after the patient has died. This affords continuity to the family. Volunteers serve as companions and may assist by doing errands and providing respite for family members.

Support Services

Licensed social workers visit regularly to provide the patient and the family with emotional support and to assist the family in preparation for bereavement. Social workers also help the family obtain community services that are not provided by hospice. Pastoral counselors provide comfort and support whenever requested and will facilitate contact with community clergy. Bereavement support groups are usually attended a few months after the patient has died. There may be different and separate sessions for loss of spouse, loss of parent or sibling (particularly by youth or teenager), and loss of infant or young child.

Affiliations

Funding for hospices can be through Medicare (federal), Medicaid (state), **HMOs**, or private insurance plans, many of which have a co-pay policy. In the case in which insurance is insufficient, many hospices offer care on a sliding-fee scale or charitable basis whereby the necessary funds are provided through grants available through donations or fundraising activities. In 1983 the Medicare insurance program was expanded to include hospice care. A typical hospice is Medicare-certified and Medicaid-approved; in many states, because direct hands-on care is provided, a hospice license is needed. The license is generally issued by the state's Department of Public Health (**DPH**).

There is a National Hospice Organization, which encourages sharing of ideas and solutions at the national level. Some hospices have been accredited by the Joint Commission on the Accreditation of Healthcare Organizations (**JCAHO**) and others by the Community Health Accreditation Program (**CHAP**). The latter is similar to JCAHO—it is the accreditation arm of the National League for Nursing, which surveys home health and hospice. Through membership in national health care or accrediting organizations, quality of care is encouraged and monitored.

Role of the Health Unit Coordinator

When a patient is referred to and accepted into the hospice program, the information is sent to the local hospitals and ambulance services. Some hospitals have made special provisions with the local hospice enabling the family members to be with the patient throughout hospital stays. The HUC communicates the information to a liaison person in the event that a hospice patient is admitted to the hospital; that person notifies the hospice office, any home services (VNA, HHA), and any volunteers that the patient has been admitted.

In the hospice HUC role, excellent communication skills, computer skills, and a knowledge of medical terminology are necessary. Technology is constantly moving forward; visual phone systems are in the near future. Telephone etiquette is extremely important. Answering the phone promptly, with a pleasant, soft voice, and properly identifying yourself, while speaking clearly and courteously, will indicate to the caller that he or she has your undivided attention.

Computer skills are necessary for keeping patient census, equipment logs, schedules of nursing and home health aide visits, and keeping a record of the volunteer time log. Accurate patient census information is necessary for reports and data collection. This listing may include the patient's name, address, phone, physician, diagnosis, insurance information, and the date of admission to the program as well as the services that hospice is providing. Some of this information may be necessary for reports needed by the various agencies that license or provide benefits for hospice services.

1998 EQUIPMENT LOG

equipment/number	date	patient name	delivery date	pickup date
Bed-1640	4/21	EAH	4/24	7/18
Bed-1649	5/7	TML	5/7	

Figure 34–2
1998 equipment log.

1998 EQUIPMENT MAINTENANCE

item/number	date	cleaning	repairs
Bed-1640	7/18	7/20	replace headboard damaged in moving
Walker-1651	7/25	7/25	check wheel- rubs fixed
Bed-1652	8/15	8/16	OK

Figure 34–3
1998 equipment maintenance.

When a patient has been admitted to hospice, the HUC assembles a chart that may include the face sheet and financial record, referral form, physician progress notes and nursing notes, any ancillary department reports and consults, and the social services progress notes. Standing orders are faxed to the physician's office for signature, and any additions or deletions are then placed in the chart. The HUC will be highly involved in coordinating all the activities of the hospice team as well as relaying necessary information to patients and families.

The HUC will maintain the equipment log (Fig. 34–2) and the equipment maintenance log (Fig. 34–3). The HUC will also make the necessary arrangements to see that the equipment is delivered in a timely manner to the client. Arrangements will also be made for equipment repairs as needed.

Physicians' orders are transcribed much in the same way they are in the hospital. The HUC who is certified and has had advanced training may be asked to receive physician orders by phone.

Closing Thoughts

Hospice is a very important community service, as it meets the needs of the terminally ill for a quality of life that they deserve and gives emotional support to families and helps them through a difficult time in their lives. The philosophy of hospice is that every person deserves to live out life with respect and dignity.

The successful HUC will embrace this philosophy and become a supportive member of the team.

Review Questions

1. Mention five notable events in the history of hospice.
2. Name and describe three HUC responsibilities expected in the hospice setting.
3. Describe the relationship of hospice and the hospitals and the communication required.
4. List and describe six services that one might find in a hospice residence.

Bibliography

Highlights in Hospice History. Buffalo, NY, Hospice Buffalo, 1995.

Making the Most of Living. Cheektowaga, NY, The Hospice Association, 1997.

35

Long-Term Care/Skilled Nursing Facility

Madeline A. Clark

Common Abbreviations

ADL	Activities of daily living
IADL	Instrumental activities of daily living
NIPPV	Noninvasive positive-pressure ventilation
N/S	Normal saline
OBRA	Omnibus Budget Reconciliation Act
OT	Occupational therapy
PT	Physical therapy
RT	Respiratory therapy
SLT	Speech and language therapy
STAT	Immediately

Objectives

Upon completion of this chapter, the reader should be able to:

1. Explain design considerations that must be taken into account in a long-term care facility.
2. List areas in long-term care that were affected by the Omnibus Budget Reconciliation Act (OBRA).
3. Explain steps to take to improve communication with the hearing impaired.
4. Describe opportunities for a health unit coordinator in long-term care/skilled nursing facilities.

Vocabulary

Activities of daily living: Tasks that enable people to meet their basic needs

Custodial care: The care of a medically stable patient who needs assistance with activities of daily living, such as eating, bathing, dressing, and toileting

Debridement: Removal of foreign material or damaged and dead tissue

Hydrocolloid dressing: Flexible dressing made of adhering gumlike material that is covered with water-resistant film

Hypercapnia: Elevated carbon dioxide

Instrumental activities of daily living: Those tasks necessary for maintaining the home environment

Intermediate care: Prescribed care that can be provided on an intermittent, rather than on a continuous basis (e.g., physical therapy)

Continued

Vocabulary *Continued*

Skilled care: Twenty-four-hour-a-day prescribed care and oversight provided by licensed medical professionals who are working under a care plan directed by a physician. The care provided in the long-term care facility to marginally stable or severely deconditioned patients.

Subacute care: Care for those sufficiently stabilized to no longer require acute services, but still needing 3 hours or more of nursing or rehabilitation a day, having medically complex needs, or requiring physiologic monitoring.

History

Caring for sick and elderly loved ones in homes has been practiced since before the birth of Christ. As time went on, it became primarily associated with religious orders, who, as part of their mission, would care for the sick and needy in their monasteries and convents. In the United States, a family member would care for an elderly person in his or her home and would often open it up to others a well, feeling it was not much more difficult to care for two or three than one.

It is generally considered that in the "good old days" families took care of their elderly at home. In fact, it was not until recently that "elderly" took on a new meaning as the average life span increased. No more than 50 years ago, the caregivers in a family were in their late thirties and forties, taking care of "elderly" in their sixties and early seventies. Now the caregivers themselves are in their sixties and seventies. In the past, few people lived long enough to have to worry about burdening a family with dealing with a dementing illness. Now it is an all-too-common fact of life.

Many of the homes that were in existence at that time were old farms and mansions that had been passed down through generations. With interior decorating and some work to bring these houses into compliance with local and state fire codes, the owners provided a supervised communal living opportunity for the infirm and elderly whose families could not provide it. Most of what was provided is what we would now consider **custodial care**. In some states, the homes were licensed, but there was wide variation in the regulations that controlled their operations.

In 1987, the Omnibus Budget Reconciliation Act (**OBRA**) imposed many new standards and requirements on the industry. Nursing home/long-term care facility personnel are now mandated to have a certain educational background. Certification and continuing education are required for administrators and other key personnel.

There are now many nationally owned and operated facilities, some of which are actually campuses of **subacute care** facilities, **intermediate care** facilities, **skilled care** facilities, custodial facilities, rehabilitation, and congregate living or residential assisted living facilities. In some instances, a large building may have units devoted to each of these variables as well as specialty units for patients with Alzheimer's disease or stroke, or comatose patients.

Introduction

Long-term care includes a wide range of medical and nonmedical services needed when people are unable to care for themselves. This care may be temporary, needed while recovering from an accident or illness. It may be needed during an extended period of disability or as a result of the normal aging process. The nonmedical needs consist of the basic self-care tasks known as **activities**

of daily living (ADL) or support chores known as **instrumental activities of daily living** (IADL).

Long-term care needs can be met in the home, the community, or in facilities. It is estimated that 12.8 million Americans need some assistance in the long-term care continuum. Of these, 2.3 million require facility living. The 21st century will be marked by a dramatic increase in the size of the older population as the "Baby Boomers" age. An accepted fact is that the number of people needing long-term care will double in the next 25 years.

Nursing homes/long-term care facilities typically provide more medical services than are available at home and fewer than are available in the hospital. The care in long-term care facilities, although less costly than that in an acute care facility, is nonetheless expensive. It has to be considered that the term of care is in months and years rather than in days. The funds come from a variety of sources. About 13% is from Medicare, 60% from Medicaid, and the remainder from Veterans Administration benefits, private insurers, and patients' private funds.

Long-term care facilities can be classified by ownership in much the same way that hospitals are:

The *federal government* maintains extended care facilities, some of which are associated with Veterans' Administration hospitals. Others are veterans' homes or soldiers' and sailors' homes. Some states maintain Extended Care facilities, but not as many as in the past. It is not unusual for county governments to operate these facilities, many of which were extensions of the old county "poor farms."

Churches, religious groups, and fraternal organizations are very involved in providing this level of care. Examples of these are the facilities owned and operated by the Carmelite Sisters (Homes for the Aged and Infirm), the Masons, and Jewish facilities. Typically, these facilities have a nonprofit status.

Proprietary homes are those that have a for-profit status with the Internal Revenue Service. They are usually the facilities that are part of a national or regional chain owned and operated by a corporation set up for that purpose. They may also be part of a health care system, usually a subsidiary of a larger corporation, but with its own board of directors and some local or regional control.

The amount of time spent on tasks that are traditionally associated with health unit coordinating is far less in the long-term care facilities. The physician visits are less frequent and the patient population is more stable, influencing the time needed for order processing and chart preparation. In many places, the health unit coordinator (HUC) is asked to take additional training to be multifunctional.

Description of the Facility/Unit

In the past, too often the nursing homes/long-term care facilities were viewed as hospitals for the chronically ill. Although they are part of the continuum of care, they should be considered places where people live and where health care and many other services are provided.

Special consideration must be given to ensure an atmosphere that will reduce the likelihood of falls. Simple design techniques that can accomplish this are described in the following sections.

Bathrooms

Doors should be wide enough to allow easy access using a wheelchair or walker. Flooring of a material that does not get slippery when wet is preferred. Tubs, showers, and floor should have nonskid strips or mats. Grab bars must be securely attached to walls and low enough or within easy reach around tubs and shower stalls and toilets (Fig. 35–1). Portable elevated toilet seats should be available.

Beds

The best choices in beds are those that can be lowered to 18 inches to reduce injury if there is a fall.

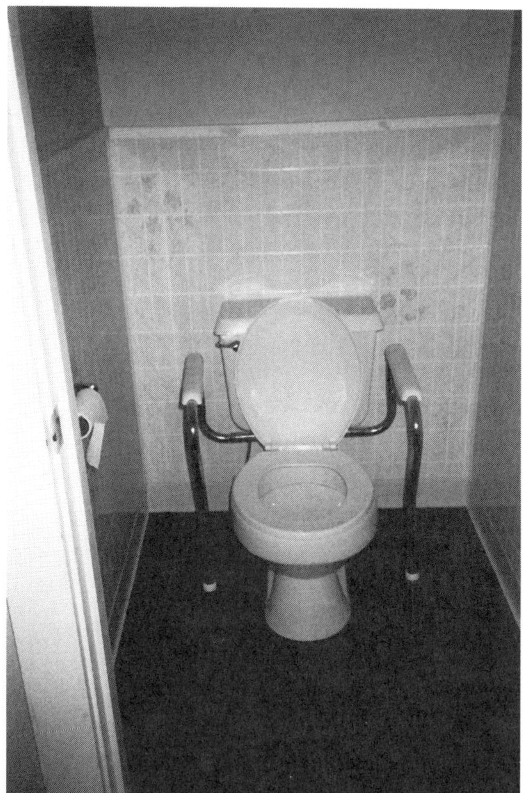

Figure 35–1
Toilet with supports. (Courtesy of The Inn at Deerfield, Inc., Deerfield, NH.)

The beds should be adjustable to allow for safe transfers and to a height comfortable for the caregivers. Mattresses should be firm on the sides to provide firm seating. The wheels, if any, should have a locking mechanism. Side rails should be appropriate to their intended use. Split side rails are best when transfers have to be assisted. Full side rails without gaps are best to ensure that a person will not slip out of bed, although some patients have been known to sustain injuries trying to climb over side rails. Some facilities have padding on the floor around the bed to break the fall if one should occur. An easily accessible call bell is provided.

Elevators

Elevator doors should be time delayed and outfitted with very sensitive pressure recoils. Buttons should be low enough to be used by someone in a wheelchair, easily visible, and marked in Braille. The floor should be slip free and should be level with the landings. The inside must be large to accommodate wheelchairs and other equipment. The emergency button and phone should be clearly marked and easily accessible.

Floors

Floors should be maintained with nonskid, nonglare wax. Throw rugs, if used at all, should have nonslip backing. Carpets and rugs should be of solid colors rather than a busy, distracting print, and the edges should be tacked or taped down. There should be no uneven surfaces such as thresholds and drops between different types of flooring surfaces. Spills and liquids must be wiped up STAT. Signs or other warnings are useful to alert patients of flooring changes and hallway turns.

Lighting

Light switches should be located and accessible outside the room as well as near the bed. The lights should be bright enough to compensate for people with limited vision and appropriate for the activities to be performed in the room. There should be night lights in the rooms, bathrooms, and lining the hallways. Special attention must be paid to the adequacy of lighting on stairs and in halls. Some facilities have successfully used floor-level lighting to reduce glare.

Rooms

There should be an unobstructed pathway from the bed to the bathroom. If furniture is in rooms, it must be remembered that low-level coffee tables and ottomans create tripping hazards. Floors must be clutter free (extension cords are particularly hazardous). Chairs, night tables, and over-bed tables should be secure and untippable because they might be used for support. In no case should these items be on wheels. Furniture should have rounded edges.

Seating

A wide variety of chairs should be available, and physical or occupational therapy should be consulted to choose the most appropriate for each patient. Chairs must be in good repair. If the chair is fitted with a safety belt, it should be positioned so that it will come low over the pelvis and be capable of being made snug enough so the patient cannot slide under it. The seat belts are provided in self-release and assisted-release models to fit various circumstances.

Overall Safety

The buildings are required to meet certain life safety codes with respect to evacuation and sprinkler systems, fire and smoke detectors, and other directions given by the Fire Marshall's office. Stairs should have secure handrails on both sides of staircases as well as hallways leading to them. Visibility can be improved with paint to outline each step. The steps should be covered with a nonskid material. In day-to-day fall prevention, the stairs should always be clutter free.

Staffing

A unit in a long-term care facility is typically staffed with a nurse manager who is a registered nurse (RN), other RNs, licensed practical nurses, and certified nurse's aides or assistants. In many facilities, the certified nurse's aides provide most of the hands-on care. There may be one HUC or, more likely, shared resources, with one HUC covering two or three units or two HUCs covering all the units. Only in the largest facilities will there be HUCs on the second or third shifts. If HUCs cover more than one unit, they wear a pager to be immediately available when needed in the other unit.

Onsite Ancillary Services

Depending on the size of the facility, the some or all of the following services will be available onsite:

Activities and recreation
Admissions
Business office
Dietary
Infection control
Laundry (may be done offsite)
Medical records
Rehabilitation
Physical therapy (**PT**)
Occupational therapy (**OT**)
Speech and language therapy (**SLT**)
Respiratory therapy (**RT**)
Social services

Offsite Ancillary Services

Offsite ancillary services include:

- Diagnostic imaging
- Electrocardiography, Holter monitoring, pacemaker checks
- Laboratory
- Pharmacy
- Physician appointments (usually with specialists such as the general surgeon, urologist, orthopedist, psychiatrist, and ophthalmologist)

Consultant Services

Consultant services include:

- Dentist
- Medical transcription (may be contracted)
- Pastoral counseling
- Podiatrist

Special Problems Encountered in the Long-Term Care Facility

Bowel Incontinence

Bowel incontinence may be seen in any of a number of diseases and disorders in the long-term care facility. Neurologic diseases are often accompanied by fecal incontinence, as is senility. In many cases this can be avoided by using a bowel program. A low-residue diet and reminders may be sufficient to avoid incontinence. In the neurologically impaired, a low-residue diet accompanied by enemas every 1 to 3 days is effective. There is a device that allows the retention of the irrigating fluid that has been reported to help establish continence. Anticholinergic drugs that reduce intestinal motility are introduced into the regime if other modalities are not effective on their own.

It is particularly important to try to establish continence in female patients because fecal contamination is often the cause of urinary tract infections.

Urinary Incontinence

Urinary incontinence is a silent epidemic, affecting approximately 13 million people, 85 percent of whom are women. It is an embarrassing condition that is often untreated because people are ashamed to discuss it with their doctors. Others do not seek help because they believe the condition is untreatable. Treatment in fact is effective, at least to some extent, in 80 percent of cases.

Incontinence can be based on a number of factors, and is of several types. Some women have a combinations of more than one of these types.

The most common form of incontinence is *stress incontinence*, which is characterized by leakage of small amounts of urine, often triggered by coughing, sneezing, laughing, or otherwise straining the abdominal muscles. It is not unusual for this type to develop during pregnancy and persist after childbirth. The incontinence may worsen with further pregnancies and definitely with age.

Urge incontinence occurs in women 65 years of age or older when the bladder goes into spasm. A pattern is established and may be made worse by caffeine ingestion, bladder infections, and certain medications.

Some women have *overflow incontinence*, which is characterized by the sensation of urine remaining in the bladder even when attempts have been made to empty it fully. Small amounts of urine may leak out continually.

Incontinence need not be an inevitable consequence of aging. There are several simple things that can be done in a long-term care facility to help deter incontinence:

- Perform Kegel exercises, which consist of tightening the muscles that are used to stop the flow of urine. The elderly can easily squeeze these muscles for 5 seconds, rest for 10 seconds, and repeat for a total of ten times. The sets of ten should be done three to five times a day. This is something anyone working in the area can remind the patients to do.
- Limit or eliminate the intake of alcohol and caffeine (in coffee, tea, cola, and chocolate).
- Encourage patients to lose weight to the optimum for their age and height. Extra weight puts extra pressure on the bladder outlet.
- Encourage the patients to cross their legs when sneezing or coughing. A university study found that this is an effective way to close off the urethra.
- Use a urination schedule if the person has urge incontinence. Cue him or her to go to the bathroom every 2 or 4 hours.

The physician might consider devices such as pessaries to hold up the bladder and urethra. Newer devices include a urinary control insert, which involves a small, balloon-like device being placed in the urethra and inflated. It remains in place until it is time to void, at which time it is removed with a string. There is also a soft patch made of a foam material that can be worn over the urethral opening until the wearer has to urinate. Both of these devices have permitted incontinent women to go out and socialize for limited periods of time without having to worry about incontinence.

Medications such as anticholinergics, antidepressants, decongestants, and estrogen replacement therapy may help, depending on the type of incontinence. Often, treating the symptoms of a bladder infection with antibiotics or sulfa drugs disposes of a contributing factor to incontinence.

If nothing can be done to improve the incontinence, disposable leakage barrier briefs and diapers are available in many sizes and configurations that are very useful for the bed-bound or chair-bound incontinent person. Ambulatory patients are sometime bothered by the effect these gives to their outer clothing, and may prefer pads.

Nutritional Status

Maintaining the nutritional status of a long-term care facility population is difficult. It is challenging to prepare a menu that meets all of the special dietary needs of the people with diseases that require special diets, and yet meets the wants of the other people as well. Appetites are influenced by eating habits of long standing. It is understood that a certain amount of scheduling must be done for meals, but a little flexibility must be built in as well. There are people with no special dietary requirements such as low-salt or American Diabetes Association diets, but who need ground food and additives to their liquids to make them thicker. The presence of ethnic diversity among the population adds further to the problem.

It does not take much to cause dehydration or weight loss in the elderly, so these parameters must be monitored closely and the dietary department made aware of any problems.

Pressure Sores

A pressure sore (bed sore) is an injury to the skin and the tissues under it. It is so named because the most common cause is unrelieved pressure on a particular area. When pressure is maintained in one place over a prolonged period of time, the small blood vessels feeding these superficial areas can be squeezed shut (the same principle that is used to stop superficial bleeding). These blood vessels no longer supply the nutrients and oxygen to the tissues. After a period of time, the tissues are starved and die, and a sore or ulcer forms.

Pressure sores are also known as pressure ulcers and decubitus ulcers. Their seriousness depends on the amount of damage there is to the skin and underlying tissue. The damage can range from discoloration of unbroken skin to deep wounds that reach muscle and bone. Healing open pressure sores can be complicated by infection and by pain that further limits mobility.

Treatment of a pressure sore depends on three principles, described in the following sections.

Pressure Relief

Pressure relief is accomplished by using special surfaces to support the body, such as air mattresses, overlay cushions, and sheepskin. These surfaces relieve and reduce pressure only if used properly. One way to check their adequacy is for the caregiver to place his or her hand, fingers extended and palm up, under the support surface at the location of the pressure point. If there is less than 1 inch of support material between the hand and the pressure point, there is not enough support. Care must be taken to do the hand check as gently as possible to prevent causing further pain.

Good Body Positioning

The following interventions help to relieve pressure:

Use foam pads or pillows to prevent pressure directly on the sore.
Maintain the body in good alignment.
Avoid sitting directly on the pressure sore.
Avoid using donut or ring-shaped cushions around the pressure sore (they tend to reduce the circulation).

The body position should be changed at least every hour while seated in a chair and every 2 hours while lying in bed. Until a routine is set, a timer can be used as a reminder.

Proper Care of the Sore

The first step in the care of a pressure ulcer is cleaning. This can be accomplished by rinsing or irrigating with normal saline (NS) or a medicated solution. Loose material can be wiped away with a sterile gauze pad. It is important to use the right pressure when rinsing or irrigating. Too much can cause further tissue damage, but too little can result in ineffective cleaning.

Debridement can be sometimes accomplished

by vigorous irrigation if the material is loose. If not, the use of normal saline wet-to-dry dressings or enzyme preparations is indicated. There are also dressings that are left in place that allow the body's enzymes slowly to dissolve the dead tissue. This method cannot be used with infected wounds.

Other considerations in choosing the dressings are the location and condition of the sore.

Hydrocolloid dressings have come onto favor because they retain moisture and oxygen. Transparent dressings permit the caregiver to see the adjacent tissue. Normal saline wet-to-dry dressings must be changed at least daily.

The final choice of dressing is made based on:

- The type of material that will best aid healing
- The presence or absence of infection
- The frequency with which the dressing will need to be changed

Nutrition can affect the speed with which any wound will heal. If the patient's condition will otherwise tolerate it, a diet higher in calories and protein is recommended.

Preventing pressure sores is a goal in all long-term care facilities. Positioning is the key to the prevention of the sores. Some principles that are followed include:

- A 30-degree side-lying position causes less pressure on the hips than straight up on a side.
- When a patient is lying supine, the heels should be kept off the bed by placing a thin foam pad or pillow from midcalf to ankle (do not place pillow under knees).
- Use pillows or foam pads to keep knees and ankles from touching each other.
- If the head of the bed must be raised, do so as little as possible to prevent pressure on the lower body (30 degrees maximum). The exception to this is during feeding time and for 1 hour thereafter, during which the head of the bed should be raised to maximum height to avoid choking.
- Remind the patients to use good posture in the wheelchair and to sit upright.
- Change positions frequently.

Medications Used in the Long-Term Care Facility

The actual medications ordered in the long-term care facility do not vary significantly from those seen in hospitals. The major difference is that in most facilities, the pharmacy service is contracted out. Medications are set up on a regular delivery schedule. Changes in medication orders and new orders must be relayed to the contracted pharmacy in an expeditious fashion to allow them time to prepare, package, and deliver the medication. Certain medications may be in stock bottles (e.g., Tylenol, milk of magnesia, or Kaopectate), but most of them (including prns) are packaged in unit doses for each individual patient.

Equipment Used in the Long-Term Care Facility

To some extent, the equipment seen in a facility depends on the type of facility and the type of patients it serves. The equipment listed here may not be seen on all units, but is seen in most facilities.

Canes are used by many of the patients in a long-term care facility to give them the stability they need in their gait. At times, a cane is used as a prop just to give the people who lack confidence the ability to lean on something if they think they are losing their balance (Fig. 35–2).

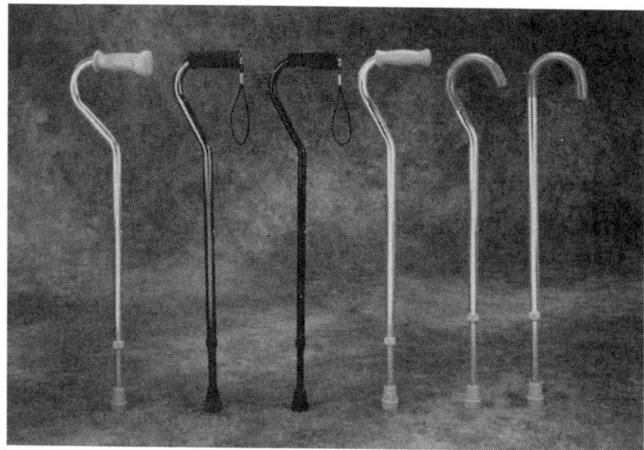

Figure 35–2
Single-point canes. (Photo used with permission of Guardian, a division of Sunrise Medical, Simi Valley, CA.)

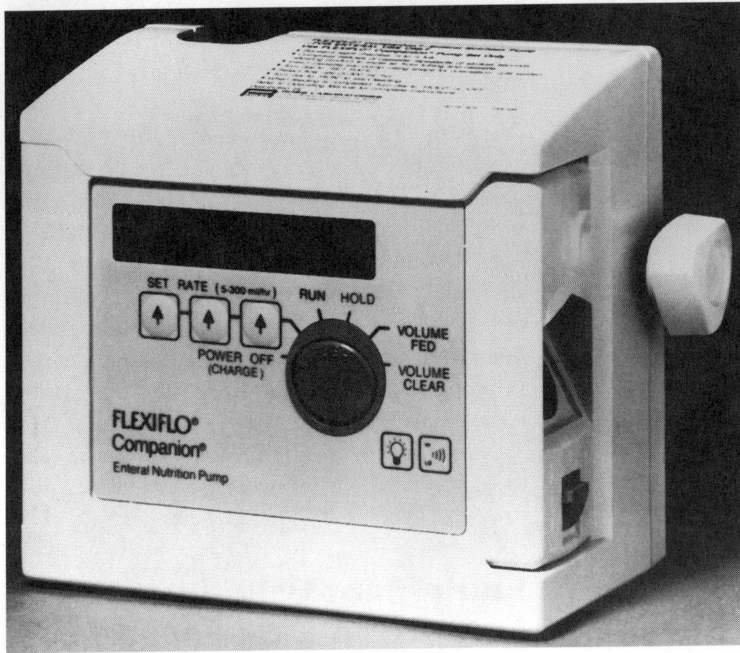

Figure 35–3
Enteral pump (portable). (Photo used with permission of Ross Products Division, Abbott Laboratories, Columbus, OH.)

Geri-chairs are made of padded, waterproof material. The typically have wheels and a seat belt. They are outfitted with a tray-type apparatus that can be placed in front of the patient.

Enteral pumps are used to regulate the flow of gastrostomy or jejunostomy feedings. They may be used continuously or intermittently. Some are fixed to an intravenous pole; others are portable (Fig. 35–3).

Infusion pumps are used for regulating the rate and volume of intravenous (IV) fluids and medications.

Noninvasive positive-pressure ventilation **(NIPPV)** devices consist of a small mask worn over the nose. It connects to a small therapy unit that is placed on a bedside table or nightstand. NIPPV is used during sleep to give a "breathing pressure boost" to people with sleep dysfunction from chronic obstructive pulmonary disease, emphysema, congestive heart failure, **hypercapnia**, neuromuscular disease, and hypoventilation of obesity.

Pneumatic lifts are used to assist in the transfer of paralyzed or otherwise immobile patients. They are designed in such a way that they can be used by one operator (Fig. 35–4).

Restraints as traditionally understood are no longer used in facilities. Posey belts and padded loose restraints may be used only when necessary to ensure patient safety. For example, if a patient is too weak to ambulate independently and is

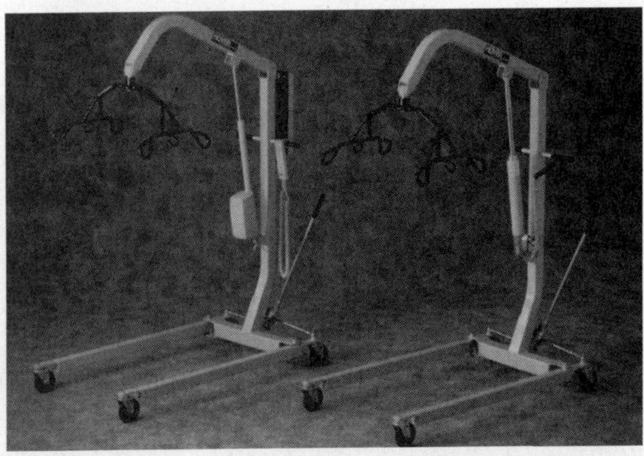

Figure 35–4
Pneumatic lifts. (Photo used with permission of Guardian, a division of Sunrise Medical, Simi Valley, CA.)

confused and tries to get out of bed at night, he or she may be restrained at night, but the restraints must be applied loosely and be removed every 2 hours. Restraint can be used to prevent a person from dislodging an IV device. These changes, as well as the abolition of the use of chemical restraints, came about with OBRA.

Tub lifts are usually water powered and are designed to be slid onto and then lower the patient into a tub (Fig. 35–5).

Ventilators are used for comatose patients and those with high cervical spine injuries, for whom there is no hope of recovery, as described in the special care unit chapters.

Walkers in a long-term care facility may be of various designs, from a simple folding walker to those with wheels and seats. The elderly need to be reminded that the walkers cannot be used on stairs or most uneven surfaces (Fig. 35–6).

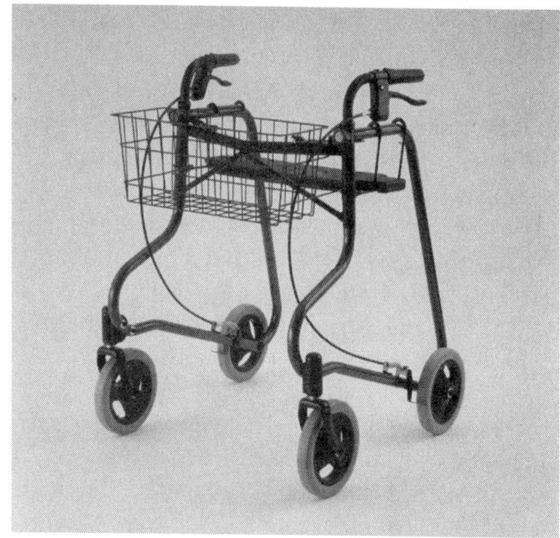

Figure 35–6
Walker. (Photo used with permission of Guardian, a division of Sunrise Medical, Simi Valley, CA.)

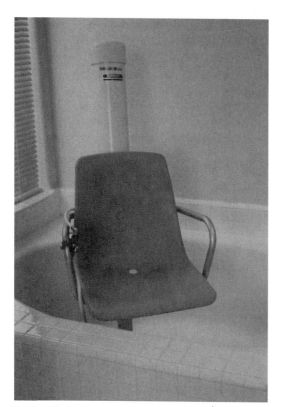

Figure 35–5
Tub lift. (Photo used with permission of Guardian, a division of Sunrise Medical, Simi Valley, CA.)

Communication

Communicating With the Patient

Many of the patients in a long-term facility are hearing impaired. There are certain steps that can be taken to communicate more effectively with them:

Attract their attention when you want to converse with them. Use their name, touch, or unimportant words until you have their attention.

Move closer to the listener to make your voice louder and clearer. Be sure to be in a direct line, so the sound won't fade. Face the person so they can see the word on your mouth.

Speak slowly and distinctly. The non–hearing-impaired person can hear and understand. The hearing impaired cannot. They often combine uncertain hearing, guesses, and body language into words and then into meaningful thoughts. This is a slow process, and the circuits can become overloaded by words that are too rapid, weak, or slurred. Listening then stops.

If it is noisy, move closer. If you see signs of uncertainty, stop; something may have been missed. It is interesting that most often the missed word is at the beginning of the phrase, so simply repeating it slowly and distinctly will clarify things.

Do not shout. Loudness alone usually does not help and the listener often gets the errant message that the speaker is angry. Save important conversations for times when near-ideal hearing conditions can be provided.

The HUC is often engaged in conversation by patients who are ambulatory and often lonely, just looking for attention. Occasionally having them help in some small way contributes to a feeling of self-worth. Speaking to them with respect adds to this as well.

Communicating About the Long-Term Care Facility Patient

The rules of confidentiality apply in this type of facility, as they do in any other. Information communicated about patients must be limited to that which is necessary for their care, and may be limited by the type of "release of information" permission granted by the family. If the patient needs to be transported by wheelchair van or ambulance to health care appointments, the lab, or x-ray, it is important to inform the transport personnel about special needs of the patient, both physical and emotional.

Legal and Ethical Considerations

Many people in the long-term facilities are cognitively impaired, so they may rarely be consulted about their plan of care. The planners at the facility must be aware of and look for the windows of opportunity. When a patient with some amount of cognitive impairment makes a decision, it is sometimes overridden by the medical community or the family.

Sensitive and empathetic discussions should be held about advanced directives and should include the patient. Many patients are openly hostile only because they are concerned that their wishes about resuscitation, hospitalization, and aggressive treatment will not be followed.

Patients' rights demand that medications, if refused, should not be given hidden away in food. If this is the only way patients can swallow the medication, it is fine to do so, but not surreptitiously.

The use of physical and chemical restraints is limited since OBRA. The only time restraints can be used is if the patient is endangering his or her own safety. Even then, the restraints must be removed at intervals.

Family members of severely impaired people are cast into the role of patient advocates and they must be fully informed of the patient's rights. If no one is available to serve in this capacity, there is a public advocacy system.

There must be system to record, communicate, and review the wish for Do Not Resuscitate (DNR) orders. The discussion must involve the patient and the family and be duly noted in the chart. No legal case has been reported in which a physician or facility has been found liable for respecting a DNR order so instituted.

There are occasionally problems arising over conflict among decision makers. Examples include:

- A competent patient can abandon treatment—but the physician cannot abandon the patient.
- If the physician believes the patient is making a poor choice because of lack of knowledge, it is incumbent on the physician to inform and educate the patient.
- A physician is not required to honor a patient's treatment choice.
- The physician may withdraw from the case with proper notification of the patient.

When a patient lacks the capacity to makes medical decisions, a surrogate decision maker is needed. The surrogate may be next of kin, someone to whom the patient has granted durable power of attorney, or a guardian appointed by the court.

The difficulty encountered in most facilities is in honestly determining the patient's "capacity" to make decisions, particularly if the decision is an unpopular one.

Health Unit Coordinator Roles in the Long-Term Care Facility Setting

Traditional Health Unit Coordinator Role

The role of the HUC on a unit of a long-term care facility is not different in many ways from that on a comparable hospital unit. It is essentially a question of volume in many of the units, because the physician's visits are typically less frequent and therefore there is a significant decrease in the numbers of orders.

The communication required in processing orders is necessarily different because many of the ordered services are contracted out. The outside agencies must be notified and services scheduled at times that do not conflict. If an outside appointment is needed, arrangements may have to be made with special transportation such as a wheelchair van or ambulance.

It is the responsibility of the HUC to see that the appropriate release forms are available to go with the patient.

Each facility has a procedure that is followed with the pharmacy service they use. The process may involve using the fax to communicate orders, or simply a phone call with card-copy follow-up. It is important to be aware of the status of orders to be sure the medication is available when it is needed.

Additional Health Unit Coordinator Roles

Most facilities that attempted to cross train HUC and nursing assistant roles have found that the duties of each require a different type of person. The long-term care industry has been particularly innovative in finding other roles for HUCs that use their skills and knowledge.

Assisting in the Business Office

There are several tasks accomplished in the business office that require computer skills possessed by HUCs. With very little training other than in facility procedures, the HUC can prepare bills, enter data into the computer, or use the word processor to prepare correspondence.

Training in insurance billing would be a plus for the HUC who aspires to transfer to this department. The billing for Medicare and Medicaid is done by strict regulations. Each private insurance company has different billing expectations, as does private billing.

Coordinating Admissions

The HUC can assist the assigned admission coordinator in tracking and gathering the information that is needed in preparation for admission. HUCs can schedule appointments for site visits by interested parties and those for the admissions nurse to do interviews with prospective patients offsite. One facility reports that the HUC became so proficient at coordinating the activities of the admissions office that she became the focal point of the department in a full-time position. The other admissions staff became multifunctional, better using their education and talents, at a considerable savings to the facility.

ICD coding can be done by the HUC who has received formal or in-service training in coding and its application. This task is accomplished by some HUCs on the unit as patients are admitted or as their diagnoses change. In other facilities, the HUC is assigned to the records room to do coding for the whole facility (see Chaps. 42 through 44). They are occasionally requested to assist with filing in the medical records department when there is a need.

Managing Central Supply/ Materiel Management

Many experienced HUCs have contributed savings to the long-term care facilities that employ them by demonstrating ways to establish a system for inventory and the ordering and tracking of supplies. In any health care facility, retrieving charges is a problem. The organizational skills possessed by a HUC make him or her a natural to find practical ways to deal with this problem. In many long-term care facilities, this a perfect match for multifunctioning. Each facility is unique, with its own built-in problems with respect to charges. This position often offers the right HUC an opportunity for independent decision making as well as a chance to be creative in problem solving.

Preparing for Surveys

Long-term care facilities must keep records to meet the standards of as many as four regulating bodies. Those that are accredited by the Joint Commission on Accreditation of Healthcare Agencies (JCAHO) must operate by those standards 365 days a year and be prepared to show compliance with standards. This is no less true with the licensing process of the state, Veterans Administration, and OBRA.

The HUC can participate in this preparation by maintaining the collection records that are needed and reminding the people responsible when certain schedules need to be met. In one facility, the HUC keeps the appropriate records and see that they are up to date in a very organized file of notebooks. She was complimented by the JCAHO surveyor for her efforts.

Quality Assurance

Meeting the standards of OBRA has helped to provide a quality of care that was not previously universally achieved. To be federally certified (to receive Medicare or Medicaid funds), the following are required:

Licensed charge nurse on site 24 hours a day
Registered nurses 8 hours a day, 7 days a week
Certified nurses aides
Full-time social worker in facilities of greater than 120 beds
Medical director
Licensed nursing home/long-term care facility administrator
Qualified therapeutic recreational therapist (several alternatives)
Licensed pharmacist (employ or obtain services of)
Rehabilitative therapists (employ or obtain services of)
Qualified dietitian (employed or scheduled consultations)
Dentist (employed or obtain services of)
Pastoral services (employ or obtain services of)
Physician services (employ or obtain services of)

In many of the long-term facilities that contract pharmacy services, quality assurance of the medication program is part of that contract. The pharmacy studies each patient profile and sends reminders when blood work should be done, recommends times to change to another drug, and collects data about responses to medication to present to the physicians.

The HUC can assist in this data-gathering process as well as in following through with the orders for blood work once the physician has been notified.

The quality assurance departments of long-term care facilities develop methods to accomplish outcomes monitoring for the patients in the facility. Peer review is carried out by the various departments.

Closing Thoughts

If a HUC enjoys being in a position where skill and knowledge are appreciated, the long-term care facility may well be the place to go. Many of the long-term care facilities still do not use HUCs, so when they decide to, the HUC has an opportunity to bring new ideas to them. The perception of long-term care facilities as a second-rate opportunity for HUCs no longer exists.

The staff members of these facilities are appreciative of the support a competent HUC can provide. The job is not boring because of the multiskilling aspects. I have known more than one person who started as a HUC in a long-term care facility whose ability to diversify led to a position of higher responsibility and authority. I would recommend that the HUC who ventures into the long-term care facility be experienced and certified.

The door continues to open for the expansion of our profession. The only thing that can limit our horizons is ourselves.

Review Questions

1. Explain three design considerations that must be taken into account in a long-term care facility and relate them to the safety issues they deal with.

2. List two areas in long-term care that were affected by OBRA and explain how they were affected.

3. Describe two specific measures that can be taken to improve communication with a hearing-impaired person.

4. Name and describe three opportunities for HUCs in long-term care/skilled nursing facilities.

Bibliography

Compton's Interactive Encyclopedia. Compton's NewMedia, 1995.
http://www.healthtouch.com
http://www.cmwf.org
http://www.meridianneuro.com
http://www.fni.com
Merck Research Laboratories: Merck Manual of Geriatrics, 2nd ed. Rahway, NJ, Merck Research Laboratories, 1995.
Stone RG, ed: Gerontology Manual. Puget Sound, WA, University of Puget Sound, 1996.
Taber's Cyclopedic Medical Dictionary, 18th ed. Philadelphia, FA Davis, 1997.

Multispecialty Clinics

36

Diane Helms

Common Abbreviations

DOB Date of birth

TDD Telecommunication device for the deaf

Objectives

Upon completion of this chapter, the reader should be able to:

1. Discuss the benefits of a multispecialty clinic.
2. List positions open to health unit coordinators in multispecialty clinics.
3. Describe the technical skills needed to work in a multispecialty clinic.
4. Explain the type of problem solving done by health unit coordinators in the multispecialty clinic setting.

Vocabulary

Demographics: The recording of certain characteristics of a particular segment of the population

History

Group practice or multispecialty clinics have been in existence since the late 1880s, when William Worrall Mayo and his two sons, William James and Charles Horace, started the Mayo Clinic, a group practice of surgical specialties, in Rochester, Minnesota. Within 25 years, both the Geisinger Medical Center (Danville, PA) and the Marshfield Clinic (Marshfield, WI) were established with a much broader range of specialties (e.g., surgery, pediatrics, obstetrics). Over the next 50 years, growth was slow, but the last 30 years have seen multispecialty clinics expand because of improving technology, insurance restrictions, and escalating health care costs.

Description of Facilities

Today, multispecialty clinics are facilities that provide a variety of health care services on an outpatient basis. Located in both large cities and small towns, these clinics vary in size from one building with as few as 6 physicians to multiple-building complexes with as many as 600 physicians. Their service areas vary from small sections of urban areas to geographically large rural areas. Multispecialty clinics frequently have access to at least one hospital to provide in-patient services for their patients. They may also be involved with medical research and medical education, providing residency programs for medical students and clinical rotations for laboratory, radiology, medical assistant, and health unit coordinator (HUC) programs. The services provided by multispecialty clinics may include a small number of specialties (e.g., obstetrics/gynecology and pediatrics), a specific area of specialty (e.g., orthopedics, orthopedic surgery, orthotics, physical medicine, and physical therapy), or a broad range of almost all major specialties. These clinics usually provide basic laboratory and radiology services, but may also provide more sophisticated diagnostic services (e.g., computed tomography, magnetic resonance imaging, ultrasonography, and nuclear medicine scanning), therapeutic services (e.g., physical and occupational therapy, radiation therapy, chemotherapy, and cardiac rehabilitation), urgent care services, and ambulatory surgery.

At multispecialty clinics, patients are able to see one or more physicians, have lab and diagnostic testing done, receive their results, and have treatment prescribed, often in 1 day. This is a major benefit for all patients, but especially for those who travel a distance for their health care.

Types of Positions Available for Health Unit Coordinators

Job Outlook

In general, the outlook for employment as a HUC in multispecialty clinics is good. The current trend in health care is toward an increase in outpatient services. In an attempt to control costs, many services that formerly required hospitalization (e.g., arteriograms and chemotherapy) are being performed in an outpatient setting. Because of advances in technology, many surgical procedures (e.g., arthroscopy and laparoscopic cholecystectomy) are now performed on an outpatient basis. In larger clinics, some departments have extended hours, creating several different shifts. If you are interested in a HUC career in a multispecialty clinic and there is none in the area, commuting or relocation to be closer to such a facility may be necessary.

Potential Health Unit Coordinator Employment

There are a number of employment opportunities available at multispecialty clinics for people who have graduated from an accredited technical college HUC program. They include:

1. Appointment coordinator—assesses patients' appointment needs and schedules their appointments and tests in a timely and appropriate manner by making decisions consistent with clinic policy and department protocol (Fig. 36–1).
2. Receptionist—greets and registers patients as they arrive for their appointments, verifies and updates patient **demographics** (date of birth [DOB], address, insurance, and so forth), answers phones, and oversees the patient waiting area.
3. Medical records secretary/clerk—pulls and dispatches charts for patients' appointments, files reports such as physician notes and test results in the correct area of the patient's chart, provides release of record information, and codes records for payment and research.
4. Medical complex messenger—delivers charts and interdepartmental mail to appropriate

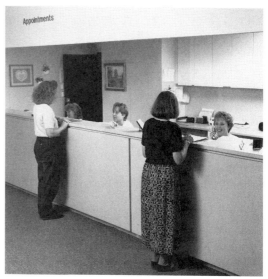

Figure 36–1
An appointment coordinator.

departments and escorts patients to diagnostic tests and appointments.

Positions Requiring Additional Experience or Education

There are other positions available to HUCs who have developed skills with additional work experience, who have sought additional education, or who have passed the National Association of Health Unit Coordinators, Inc., certification exam. Some of these positions include:

1. Department team leader—being responsible for time cards, scheduling workers for in-services or training programs, and overseeing the day-to-day operation of the department.
2. Medical assistant—screening patients on the telephone and in the office before their physician visit regarding their medical problems, taking and recording vital signs, and assisting the physician with procedures and examinations.
3. Medical transcriptionist—transcribing physicians' dictation regarding patients' medical history, problems, progress, and test results.
4. Pharmacy technician—assists the pharmacist by typing up labels, counting the number of pills needed for a prescription, and other tasks as directed.

Related Terminology

Medical Terminology

No matter what position is held in a multispecialty clinic, a HUC needs to understand and use the language of health care. This includes a complete understanding of basic medical terminology, anatomy and physiology, and medical abbreviations and symbols. For example, if a physician requests an ultrasound of the kidneys, a HUC without anatomy knowledge might order a lower abdominal ultrasound when an upper abdominal ultrasound would be required.

Interpreting Medical Abbreviations and Symbols

It is essential to interpret medical abbreviations and symbols correctly. If a HUC does not know that SOB means "shortness of breath," this abbreviation may be mistaken for slang and the patient may not be directed to the correct department. CAD can stand for "coronary artery disease" or "central appointment desk." Marshfield Clinic in Marshfield, Wisconsin, has such a desk, and it is referred to as CAD! HUCs must know all the abbreviations and symbols used in the facility so they can appoint or direct patients appropriately.

Diagnostic Tests

Knowledge of tests and their required preparation is necessary to accurately and appropriately appoint patients at a multispecialty clinic. A HUC must be familiar with the names of diagnostic tests, the proper sequence if multiple tests are ordered, the preparations required for tests, and the departments where tests are performed. Knowledge of how long procedures take is also very important. If the HUC allots insufficient time for a procedure, the patient will be late to other scheduled appointments, causing delays and the possible need to cancel and reschedule.

Lab Tests

Health unit coordinators must be able to recognize and order tests performed by the laboratory department. They must know which tests require the patient to fast (nothing by mouth for a certain period of time). If this information is not correctly relayed to the patient, test results will be incorrect, which would result in an error or delay in diagnosis or treatment.

Deciphering Written Orders from Physicians

One of the most difficult tasks facing HUCs is deciphering physicians' handwriting. It is essential that what a physician is ordering or requesting is understood. If a physician's order cannot be read, the HUC must not guess, but should ask the physician for clarification; the patient's well-being depends on it. There is no substitute for experience and becoming more familiar with the working area and the physicians in the department, to understand what the physicians are writing and what they are requesting.

Health Unit Coordinator Knowledge and Skills Appropriate to Position

Communication Skills

Health unit coordinators must possess excellent verbal and written communication skills and interpersonal skills, and enjoy working with the public. Their ability to communicate effectively with patients, physicians, support staff (e.g., lab, or x-ray), and coworkers is essential; HUCs can hinder the delivery of health care by communicating incorrect or incomplete information. Using correct grammar decreases the possibility of misinterpretation, enhances credibility, and creates a good impression of the HUC and his or her department and institution.

When speaking to patients, it is important that HUCs use terms that can be understood; patients can be overwhelmed or confused by technical language. Patients need to be at ease and feel free to speak to HUCs regarding their medical problems. Tone of voice and body language can convey willingness to be of help. HUCs should always explain procedures thoroughly; patients appreciate knowing exactly what will be taking place. They may have to reassure nervous patients and repeat their explanation, especially for difficult or lengthy procedures. It is necessary for HUCs to provide detailed appointment and procedure directions in writing for patients who have hearing difficulties or trouble comprehending.

Patients may be anxious or upset because of their medical problems; it is important that HUCs communicate their compassion and concern.

Telephone Etiquette

A high percentage of a HUC's duties are handled over the telephone. Proper telephone etiquette is essential in communicating with patients, physicians, and coworkers. The phone should always be answered promptly—*before* three rings. The HUC must identify himself or herself and department, speak clearly and distinctly, and let the caller hear a smile in his or her voice. If speaking with someone at the desk, HUCs should excuse themselves and answer the telephone. If it is necessary to put a caller on hold, the HUC should get the caller's permission to do so and then keep them appraised of the situation (e.g., looking for medical assistant).

It is essential to respond to messages in a timely manner. Nothing is more frustrating for a person than a lengthy wait for a return call to get an issue resolved. Each call is important, whether it is a patient needing to reschedule an appointment or a staff member needing information.

Health unit coordinators must be courteous (use "please" and "thank you") and maintain a professional manner. They are representing their facility and creating a lasting impression for prospective patients.

Technical Skills

Knowing the functions of the phone system is as important as telephone etiquette. It is important to know how to transfer a call, set up a conference call, or forward a phone. Each multispecialty clinic has a system that best fits its needs. HUCs must be sure to take the time to learn all the functions of their phone system.

Some clinics have a telecommunications device for the deaf, or **TDD**. If HUCs know how to type, they will be able to communicate on a TDD. HUCs and the person on the telephone take turns typing to each other. They carry on the same conversation (scheduling appointments or providing information) as if they were speaking (Fig. 36–2).

Basic computer skills and typing accuracy are required of a HUC. A working knowledge of computer functions is required appropriately to schedule, change, cancel, and confirm appointments. A number of multispecialty clinics schedule patients' appointments and diagnostic tests on the computer. Each clinic has a program that suits its needs, and HUCs will learn the specifics of its system after they become employed. A knowledge

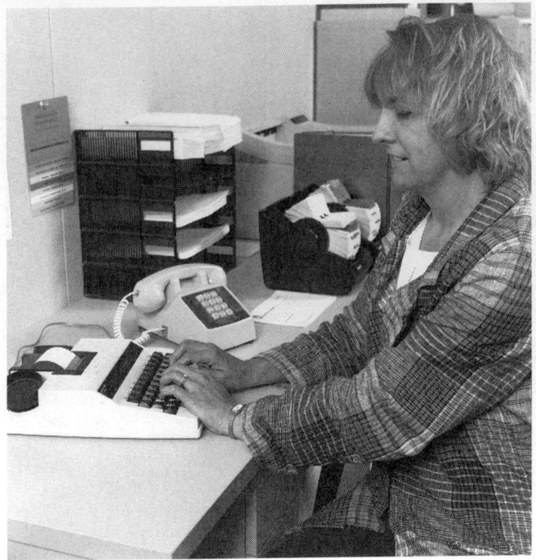

Figure 36–2
TDD equipment.

of personal computers, word processing, and spreadsheet programs is necessary to handle additional duties of typing meeting minutes or reports or collecting and compiling statistical data for research projects.

Knowledge regarding intercom and pager systems is necessary. Intercoms are convenient ways of communicating with the appointment desk, nurses' station, and physician's office. Pagers allow HUCs to contact personnel in other work areas or off site. Fax machines are one of the latest communicating devices in the medical field. They are used telephonically to transfer photocopies of medical records and information from one facility to another in a timely manner.

Health unit coordinators must be willing to learn new technical skills related to the position they hold to maintain satisfactory performance.

Problem-Solving Skills

Problem-solving skills are essential in working in multispecialty clinics. Many different situations will arise in which HUCs need good judgment and the ability to stay calm. The knowledge of the complete services of their clinic and the location of all departments ensures quick and effective problem solution. The ability to triage (assess the urgency of patients' medical problems) is important in assigning appropriate care for patients who walk in without an appointment or who call with a multitude of problems. HUCs must also know the limits of their expertise to be able, if necessary, to refer a problem to someone more qualified. Problem situations may cause patients or staff members to become impatient or angry. Listening for the facts and maintaining a professional demeanor help control the situation.

Stress Management Skills

Almost all health care jobs involve working under stress. HUCs experience stress while problem solving, when dealing with angry and impatient people, and when handling the numerous interruptions encountered during the day. HUCs may be on the phone with a patient when another line rings, or another patient comes to their desk complaining of a long wait, or a relative of a patient requests that they call a cab, or their physician informs them of an emergency with a patient at the hospital necessitating the cancellation of the remaining appointments of the day—all this in addition to the stack of return appointments on their desk needing to be scheduled. The ability to accept interruption as a normal part of the routine, manage time effectively, and meet deadlines helps in dealing with these everyday occurrences.

Additional Considerations

Confidentiality

Health unit coordinators have always had access to confidential information, and the use of computers has increased that access. It is their responsibility to maintain patient confidentiality at all times. Only access or discuss patient information within the scope of the position. Patients must not be discussed in areas where the conversation can be overheard by unauthorized personnel or the public (e.g., in hallways, elevators, cafeteria). Patient information should not be released to anyone but the patient or someone given written permission by the patient to receive it. Any breach of patient confidentiality could result in dismissal.

Requesting Medical Charts

Some multispecialty clinics keep their medical charts on-line in their computer system. Once a physician has dictated notes on the patient, they are typed on the computer and can be accessed at any time. If the records are not computerized, there will be occasions when HUCs need to request a patient's chart. The physician needs the chart to refer to when speaking to patients over the telephone. HUCs may need the chart to verify which tests the physician ordered to ensure proper scheduling of an appointment.

Abiding by Policies and Procedures of the Facility

Every employee should know the emergency procedures (e.g., fire, tornado) for their facility. The safety and well-being of patients and medical staff depend on HUCs knowing procedures during emergency situations. The facility also has policies on exposure to blood and body fluids, hepatitis B, and so forth. HUCs must know what precautions they are to take and what procedures they are to follow if exposed.

Each facility has its own dress standards. Clothing, whether uniform or conventional dress, should be neat and clean. HUCs should avoid current fashion fads. Little or no perfume or fragrance should be worn. Careful attention should be given to personal appearance and grooming habits. Appearance is important, and it makes an impression on patients, visitors, and medical staff.

Precepting New Employees and Student Unit Coordinators

Health unit coordinators have the opportunity to train new employees and student unit coordinators. HUCs can give them the chance to apply their knowledge to actual working situations. Precepting is very important because it is during this period of training that employees and students can demonstrate their ability to work with the public and staff and show they can deal with difficult situations and manage their time appropriately. By sharing knowledge with new and perspective employees, HUCs help ensure a competent work force for the facility.

Additional Training Required

Specific Training

It is extremely important that HUCs stay current in their profession. They will be required to have additional training as changes take place within their facility and in health care itself. This training may include such things as new computer skills, insurance information, and cardiopulmonary resuscitation.

Specific Area/ Department Training

Training specific to the area could include a session on verifying patient demographics such as current address, up-to-date phone numbers, and insurance information. Another session might involve learning time frames for specific appointment types. A physical exam may require a time frame of 1 hour, whereas an office visit may need only 15 minutes. Lab time frames are different from diagnostic time frames. Another session may present new forms and questionnaires that accurately correspond to the appointment type. These training sessions are necessary to maintain the HUC's skill in appointment coordinating.

The 1990s have seen a great change in health care, and multispecialty clinics have become a major part of that change. HUCs can empower themselves by learning about new technologies and taking responsibility for their professional growth.

Marketing Health Unit Coordinator Skills

Your Facility

Personal and professional development through continuing education is important. HUCs make daily contributions in the health care field. By attending workshops, seminars, and night classes, HUCs can stay abreast of changes that are taking place. As new technologies emerge, it will be necessary to attend on-the-job training sessions and share information learned with the other HUCs. Be willing to change and grow within the position.

As you assume responsibility and accountability for nonclinical tasks, you may find that you can advance in your career. Some facilities have a career ladder whereby you may acquire more responsibilities, which will lead to professional recognition, increased wages, and career advancement.

Market Yourself for a New Position

You may decide to apply for a different position. A cover letter and resume may be required. Updating your resume takes less time if you have kept a record of your additional education and experience. It is wise to keep a portfolio containing certification information, professional organization membership, diplomas, and proof of attendance at workshops and seminars.

Belong to a National Organization

The National Association of Health Unit Coordinators, Inc. is the professional organization for

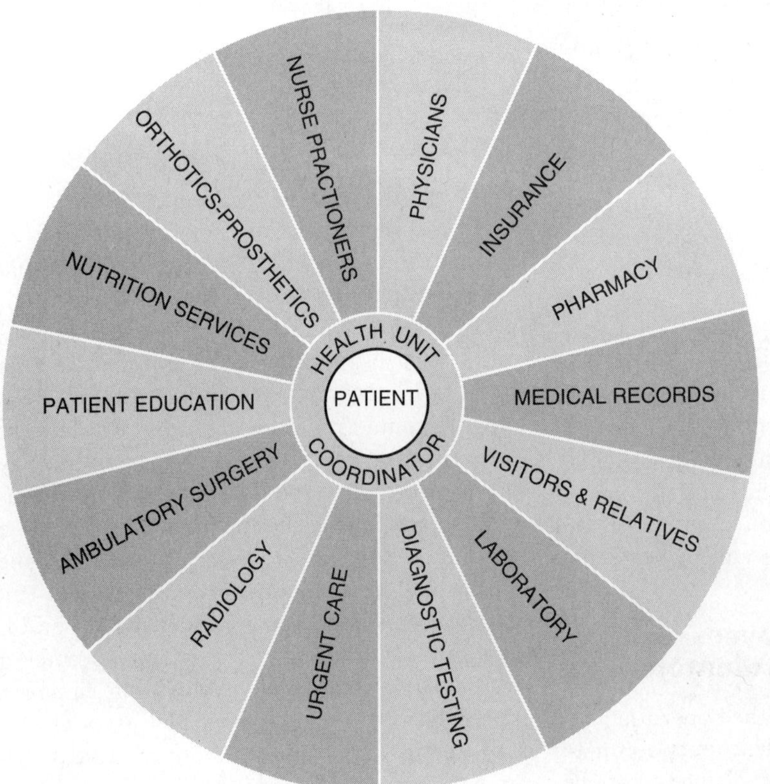

Figure 36–3
Coordination of a multispecialty clinic.

your position. It promotes health unit coordinating through continuing education, certification, recertification, and an annual national education conference. Membership in a local chapter provides the opportunity to participate by attending its educational meetings, networking with peers, serving on committees, planning workshops and seminars, and holding office. This may lead to involvement on the national level. You will find you can develop leadership skills that can in turn enhance your career.

Closing Thoughts

A HUC is a vital part of the appointment system. Only when patients have appointments will they receive the services of your facility (Fig. 36–3).

Health unit coordinators are essential members of the team that provides health care in multispecialty clinics. As a HUC, you provide patients with their first impression of your facility by your friendly and professional manner. You reinforce that impression through the competent way you schedule appointments and provide information. Your thorough understanding of the policies and services of your facility makes you as much a resource for other members of your health care team as it does for your patients. Your efficiency has a major effect on controlling costs for both your patients and your facility. Choosing to work as a multispecialty clinic HUC will provide you with an interesting, challenging, and rewarding career in the ever-changing field of outpatient health care.

Review Questions

1. Describe a major benefit for patients of a multispecialty clinic.
2. List and give a short description of five positions available to HUCs in a multispecialty clinic.
3. Describe the process for using the telecommunication device for the deaf.
4. Name two potential problem situations that might occur in a multispecialty clinic and tell how an HUC should deal with them.

Bibliography

Lipp MR: Medical Landmarks USA: A Travel Guide. New York, McGraw-Hill, 1991.

The World Book Encyclopedia, Volume 13 (M). World Book, Inc., 1997, pp 328–329 (Mayo Clinic).

37 Private Medical Office

Donna Knecht

Common Abbreviations

CPT Current Procedural Terminology

ICD International Classification of Diseases

Objectives

Upon completion of this chapter, the reader should be able to:

1. List the personnel who might be employed in a private medical office.
2. Name the positions in a private medical office that would be available to a health unit coordinator.
3. Identify the types of education courses that would be helpful when applying for a position in a private medical office.

Vocabulary

Computed tomography (CT): Recording a series of x-ray beams, then processing them by computer to display the scanned portion of the body in cross section

Diagnosis: The determination of a disease based on the signs and symptoms evidenced by a patient/client

Electrocardiogram (EKG): A graphic recording of the electrical potential variations of the heart muscle, received by electrodes placed on the body and recorded by an instrument called an electrocardiograph

Licensed practical nurse (LPN): A nurse who cares for patients/clients, licensed by a state authority, but without the educational training or experience required of a registered nurse

Medical assistant (MA): A multiskilled allied health practitioner who performs a wide range of roles in physicians' offices, clinics, and other health care settings

Medical terms/terminology: The language of medicine used to communicate with the medical community

Registered nurse (RN): A graduate, trained nurse who has been licensed by a state authority

Ultrasound (ultrasonography): Visualization of deep body structures using the reflected pulses of ultrasonic waves

X-rays (radiographs): The specially sensitized films recording the internal structures of the body when acted on by x-radiation (or gamma radiation) passing through the body.

Description of Facility

A private medical office can range from one physician practicing alone to several sharing office space and personnel, as well as small partnerships where a few doctors are all caring for the same patients. A private medical office can be dedicated to family practice or be a specialty practice.

This chapter describes a general surgeon's office in a small town in the Northwestern United States that does 45 percent surgery and 55 percent family practice and provides care not only to local townspeople but also to a large outlying rural area. The physician performs in-patient and outpatient hospital procedures with the usual office follow-up, does some surgical procedures in the office, and also practices family medicine. The office space consists of one surgical unit and another room for exams and treatments. There is a room for counseling patients with cancer and for family, birth control, preoperative, and diet counseling. There is a waiting room, reception area, billing area, nurse's station, the doctor's personal office, and room for the office manager. There is also one heat therapy room. Although the physical layout varies depending on the type of practice, many of the same rooms would be needed in any private office.

The organization consists of a doctor, nurse, office manager, receptionist, secretary, transcriptionist, insurance biller, cleaning person, and building maintenance person. Most private doctors' offices will be more similar than not. Although each medical specialty carries with it different requirements such as equipment and related knowledge (e.g., **electrocardiogram** [EKG] and treadmill for cardiology, or surgical table and instruments for general in-office surgery, or **ultrasound** for a large obstetrics clinic), in general each private office has the same needs in personnel.

In a small office, the duties of receptionist, secretary, transcriptionist, or billing clerk, for example, may actually be handled by one or two people, whereas the larger office or clinic, staffed with multiple physicians, may require a large number of people to handle these duties. The positions available, their job requirements, and how to gain these skills are all detailed in this chapter.

Related Terminology

All terminology learned as a health unit coordinator (HUC) can be carried into a doctor's office. Knowledge of medical terms related to specific areas of the doctor's practice will be helpful when dealing with the following situations.

Diagnoses

Knowledge of diagnoses helps with scheduling a patient for an office visit, knowing how soon a patient must be seen, and how lengthy a visit may be required. It is also helpful with scheduling tests or surgery in the hospital or those performed in the doctor's office. Proper **diagnosis** is required for billing and submission for payment to insurance companies.

Procedures

Knowledge of medical procedures aids in scheduling patients for lab tests, **x-rays**, ultrasounds, **computed tomography** (CT) scans, surgical procedures, and so forth. When billing patients, and especially for insurance purposes, knowledge of procedures is vital so that all payments requested have been included and are correct.

Medications

Knowledge of medications is vital, including brand name, generic, over-the-counter, and physician- or nurse-administered drugs. When a patient calls for a refill or with questions, the information must be transmitted to the nurse or doctor correctly so that they do not spend needless time researching a patient's chart or history and, most important, so that the patient receives correct information and proper care. This knowledge is also required for correct billing, to be able to answer questions about related lab work or diagnostic testing, and in relationships with pharmacies. Many pharmacies require a doctor's permission to change a prescription from a brand name to generic or vice versa, and will call to verify specific prescriptions and refills or to update a patient's chart when a patient has notified the pharmacist of a reaction to a specific drug. Again, it is imperative that information taken down and relayed be completely accurate.

X-ray and Laboratory Tests

Knowledge of diagnostic tests is important for scheduling tests not only in the office but also at the hospital and other facilities. Often patients need copies of results of tests to take with them for referrals or consultation visits. When results are called in, these must be correctly transmitted to the doctor or nurse and recorded in the patient's chart. Once again, this helps with giving a more accurate diagnosis for all billing and referral purposes, as well as for the patient.

General Medical Terminology

Because **medical terminology** is the language of medicine, anyone working in a private office environment needs this skill to communicate with the rest of the medical community. It is useful in scheduling the right procedures and tests and answering questions from insurance companies and patients. Being able to relate more fully to insurance companies and having the ability to deal easily with billing procedures, fill out claim forms, and deal with provider numbers, passport numbers, and names of companies, all lead to better job performance and better patient care. Any classes offered that relate to medical terminology will be very helpful to a potential employee in a doctor's office.

Types of Positions Available to Health Unit Coordinators

There are many positions in a private medical office to which a HUC could aspire. Many of the skills learned in the classroom or on the job can be readily applied to the private office situation. Several of these are described in the following sections.

Receptionist

The experience of a HUC in a hospital can lead directly to working as a receptionist in a doctor's office. The job description written for this doctor's office includes a lot of the same tasks performed by a HUC in a hospital. These tasks include greeting patients in person and by phone, scheduling appointments, scheduling tests and surgeries, compiling all results of tests on patients, scheduling follow-up appointments and referrals to other facilities, and filing all reports and notes in the patient's chart. Job requirements for this position include excellent communication skills and knowledge of general office equipment, including computers, because most offices keep appointments, records, and many other documents on computer. Experience with filing systems is helpful, and good language skills are a must.

Billing and Insurance Clerk

Because the HUC already has experience with and knowledge of diagnoses, procedures, diagnostic testing, and terminology, this is a position that could be handled with little additional training. This position requires filling out claim forms accurately and completely, the ability to talk with patients about their insurance claim, billing, and filing claims with insurance companies. Having good working relationships with others is very important. In most offices, computer skills are required, along with a willingness to take current procedural terminology (CPT) and International Classification of Diseases (ICD) coding training to keep abreast of constant changes in insurance company procedures.

The position of a billing clerk also requires basic accounting skills to be able to handle collections and payments as well as sending statements to patients each month. Good communication skills again are a must to act on delinquent accounts in a tactful but effective way.

Transcriptionist

Accurate typing and proofreading skills are necessary for this position, as well as a good working relationship with the doctor and staff. All the medical knowledge and familiarity with departments and procedures gained as a HUC can be used in this position. Learning the proper format used in each report and office is fairly basic, but the transcriptionist must pay particular attention to detail, making sure the reports are completely accurate in diagnosis, treatment, medication, and anything else that would be pertinent. Knowledge of proper formatting for letters and the like is helpful, and good language skills are necessary. Most offices require computer skills or the willingness to learn them, and filing of reports and charts may be required. Flexibility and a desire to learn new things are necessary because medical procedures and especially drug names change continually.

Medical Assistant

In some offices, a HUC can be trained to work as a **medical assistant** (MA) in a similar capacity as a **registered nurse** (RN) or **licensed practical nurse** (LPN). This requires assisting the doctor with patient procedures, physical treatments, calling in prescriptions to pharmacies, and calling other physicians and medical facilities to schedule consultations, diagnostic tests, and surgeries. Most insurance companies require preauthorization for surgery or procedures needed, and these phone calls also are usually made by the assistant. Often an MA gives instructions to patients for tests or lab work they are scheduled for and answers related questions, sets up annual physical exams, and recalls the patients annually for physicals. Depending on local or state requirements, in some areas MAs also give injections.

Office Manager

These duties vary with the size of the practice. In the smaller office, the office manager works in many different capacities. In smaller offices, the office manager may be expected to be cross trained to fill in for any other staff member who is unavailable for some reason. Experience as a HUC can make this much easier. In addition to all the aforementioned job requirements for the various positions, the office manager usually oversees the scheduling of office personnel, vacations, and leave, handles personnel management, payroll, and payment of all office bills, and often schedules the doctor's meetings, travel, and education.

Health Unit Coordinator Knowledge and Skills Appropriate to Positions

All knowledge and skills learned over the years in the hospital as a HUC can be carried into a doctor's office. Knowledge of transcribing orders, medications, lab work, diagnostic tests and x-rays, surgeries, and scheduling appointments with doctors and other institutions is used daily. Specific medical knowledge is used in all positions in a private medical office, as detailed previously, as well as general office practices, including filing, typing, and accounting. One of the important assets carried over from the HUC position is an effective working relationship with the hospital staff, associated private doctors' offices, pharmacies, and hospital patients. The importance of having good communication with all health care organizations cannot be emphasized enough to provide the very best health care for the patient. Phone manners, greeting patients pleasantly and efficiently, and good relationships with coworkers are also vital for the doctor's office to run smoothly. A private medical office works closely with other offices and their staff, pharmacies, nursing homes, home care agencies, and hospitals.

The professional knowledge gained from experience as a HUC is beneficial in working with all these facilities and institutions.

Additional Training Required

A person who is interested in working in this type of medical environment should take advantage of every opportunity for obtaining additional education and training. This may range from half-day seminars on various topics to courses in a vocational college or community college.

Computer skills, learning about insurance companies and their forms and billing claims, and mastering electronic billing all will be necessary to be successful in a doctor's office. Most offices use computers to schedule all appointments, update patient charts, and keep all medical records. Computers are also used for inventory and keeping track of medications. Some offices require courses on specific computer programs, billing programs, or any other subjects the office deems necessary.

As mentioned earlier, courses in CPT and ICD coding are very helpful. Courses in medical office practices can also be a great asset when seeking the positions that have been discussed here.

If the person is willing, there is much that he or she can learn from a private practice, and there are many opportunities to use the skills already learned as a HUC.

Marketing HUC Skills

Marketing oneself is sometimes the most difficult part of transition. Often, local job placement agencies and colleges offer classes or training sessions on personal marketing, such as resume writing, which can be very helpful.

In every situation, not only do you represent the doctor and the clinic, you also represent yourself to other institutions and practices. One can never know when an opportunity may arise.

When considering a change to any new position, it is important to do a thorough research of the facility being considered before applying. Knowing what services are provided and what the employer is seeking allows the applicant to tailor a resume to emphasize exactly those skills from the many that are acquired as a HUC. Each position places emphasis on different areas, and each application and resume should be prepared to fit the desired qualifications. The applicant should decide which skills are strongest and most enjoyable and then find a position that would best engage those skills. This provides for an interview with sincere enthusiasm about the position and a happy and effective employee once on the job.

A willingness to apply for a lower position in a particularly desirable facility can provide for future opportunities in that organization. In this case, marketing oneself more toward the facility itself as opposed to the position is desirable. Again, knowledge of the facility and its goals and services is essential.

Closing Thoughts

The basic knowledge gained as a HUC should enable you to go into any doctor's office and learn the requirements of running a private practice. The skills gained by HUCs are also required in private practice, and mainly you must be willing to learn different ways of performing the same skills. Although private practice is very similar in many ways to a hospital setting, the ability to adjust easily and apply the necessary skills appropriately is a valued trait. Working with many different departments in a hospital setting should have prepared you extremely well for this, and applying all these skills in a different setting can be a very rewarding experience. Many people enjoy the more personal aspect of a private office setting as opposed to the larger hospital setting. Long-standing personal relationships often are made with both the staff and pa-

tients. Whereas hospital patients tend to be transient, private doctors often see patients for years, sometimes a lifetime. Also the entire staff is usually close knit, with a sizable difference in number of personnel. Smaller offices rarely have night hours or shift work, although if these variable hours are appealing, a clinic with evening or weekend hours may be more enticing. A large hospital setting makes observing daily routines of different departments a bit overwhelming, but in a private office many duties may be performed in overlapping areas, even increasing the opportunities for learning and providing for a more varied work day. Whatever the desires or goals, the HUC should find a private medical office a place of many opportunities.

Review Questions

1. List the personnel who might be employed in a private medical office.
2. Name the positions in a private medical office that would be available to a HUC who wanted to work in that situation.
3. Identify the types of educational courses that would be helpful when applying for a position in a private medical office.

38 Private Medical Transcription Company

Joi Hieirling

Common Abbreviations

AT	Advanced technology
BMP	Windows bitmap
CD-ROM	Compact disk-read only memory
GB	Gigabyte
DOS	Disk operating system
MB	Megabyte
OJT	On-the-job training
PC	Personal computer
PCX	PC paintbrush
RAM	Random access memory
TIFF	Tagged image file format
VGA	Video graphics array

Objectives

Upon completion of this chapter, the reader should be able to:

1. Name the various educational options that could prepare a person to become a medical transcriptionist.
2. List the equipment that would be necessary to operate a private medical transcription company at home.
3. Identify the initial steps to take to start up a private small business.
4. List six opportunities for medical transcriptionists other than a private business.

Vocabulary

Dictaphone: A type of phonographic instrument that records and reproduces speech

Portfolio: A case in which important documents are carried from place to place

Transcribe: To produce in handwriting or typing a document that was originally created in another form

Transcriptionist: One who transcribes or performs the act of transcription

Overview of Medical Transcription

Medical transcription is the process by which a trained person produces a typed copy of a dictated report, using a standard format and proper medical terminology. In the past, medical transcription was done only in hospitals and physicians' offices. The volume of work and new technology forced a change in the field. Now, medical transcription continues to be done in hospitals and physicians' offices, as well as in offices of companies that specialize in medical transcription, and in private homes by people who have trained to be medical transcriptionists.

The abbreviations listed for this chapter are those that a HUC working in this area would be expected to know. Only those in boldface type are used in the text and appear in boldface when they are used for the first time.

Educational Preparation

In the past, medical **transcriptionists** were secretaries with knowledge of medical terminology, trained on the job **(OJT)** by hospitals to type the various reports. Some hospitals continue to train medical transcriptionists. OJT is now also available to medical transcriptionists from companies specializing in the transcription of medical reports.

In some states, educational options include attendance at a program or courses offered by junior colleges, universities, vocational/technical colleges, business schools, or trade schools.

Another choice is a certified home-based study program. Home study program information can be found in most newspapers and magazines. Not all courses are certified. The information will specify if the course is certified and whether a certificate is granted on successful completion. A certified home study program should be chosen to avoid any potential job difficulties.

Be aware that home study programs are not for everyone. A person needs to be self-disciplined, focused, committed, and able to manage under minimal supervision. It is important to have an area in the home where work can be done in total privacy and a designated time each day to work on assignments. Only a handful of people succeed in home-based studies and businesses.

On completion of the necessary course work in either option, a certificate of successful completion is awarded. This certificate should be placed in a **portfolio** containing the resume and other applicable educational records and certifications held by the person.

Applicable Health Unit Coordinator Knowledge

A medical transcriptionist is required to be skillful in interpreting and applying medical terminology in the following areas:

Anatomy and physiology
Laboratory
Radiology
Medications
Disease processes
Procedures and treatments

A grasp of basic grammar is needed as well as a mastery of keyboarding and a working knowledge of computers and dictation equipment. Possession of these skills enhances the ability to perform the tasks needed to **transcribe** medical documents.

Health unit coordinators (HUCs) already have several of the skills relating to the medical transcription field. Mastery of the medical language is essential because it is often difficult to hear a word over the **dictaphone** and discern its exact usage. Accuracy is required to be successful. HUCs use highly developed communication and organizational skills on a day-to-day basis. They are aware of the importance of confidentiality and possess the ability to prioritize tasks. This combination of knowledge and skills is easily transferable to successful performance as a medical transcriptionist (Fig. 38–1).

Certified HUCs (CHUCs) who expand into this role have new continuing education opportunities

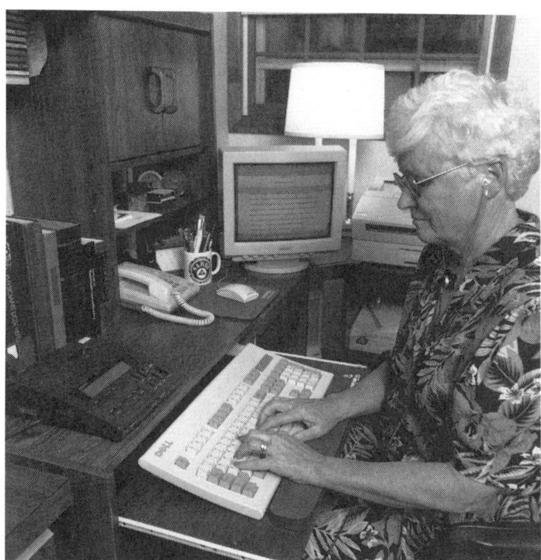

Figure 38–1
Home transcriptionist at work.

to help meet the requirements for recertification. Workshops and programs that will prove useful in either field include:

Computer languages and related terminology
- Disk operating systems (DOS)
- Windows
- Lotus
- WordPerfect
- Power Point
- Excel
- Accent

Advanced keyboarding
Advances in the medical fields
Communications

The private medical transcriptionist also can benefit from such program topics as small business, accounting basics, billing procedures, and marketing and advertising

Table 38–1 EQUIPMENT USED BY THE MEDICAL TRANSCRIPTIONIST

Equipment	Necessity	Nicety
Computer	X	
Printer	X	
Dedicated phone system	X	
Answering machine		X
e-Mail		X
Fax		X
Extra software		X
Dictaphone/transcriber	X	
Digital dictaphone		X
Copier		X
Scanner		X
Shredder	X	
Laptop computer		X
Pager	X	
Cellular phone	X	

Equipment Needed

Table 38–1 lists some of the equipment the medical transcriptionist might use.

Computer

The "best system" is an IBM-PC/AT-compatible computer with 486 processor or higher, 1 GB or higher hard disk, one 3.5″ floppy disk drive, one CD-ROM, at least one serial port and one parallel port, a 56 K modem, VGA color with video card, and an enhanced AT-style keyboard, with Microsoft Windows disk operating system software and the Corel WordPerfect word processing program installed.

Printer

The "best system" is a Hewlett-Packard DeskJet 694C color ink jet printer.

Phone System

A dedicated telephone line must be set up for the business. Call the local telephone company for a standard second line. They have many programs and will help set up the one best suited for the needs of the business. An answering machine can be set up on this line to record messages from clients when you are away. Any standard answering machine will do. There is a computer program (Pro Communicate by Ol Communique Laboratory, Inc.) that accomplishes this task when the computer is not in use.

Fax

A fax machine is convenient, but it is not a necessity. Preliminary reports can be faxed to customers and a hard copy can be delivered at a later date. This function also is available in various programs.

Special Software

Internet Access

Use e-mail to send and receive messages from clients. Advertisements can be placed on the internet/World Wide Web.

Programs

The computer system can be augmented with a spell-check medical dictionary, a billing and marketing program, and a speed-enhancing program.

Dictaphone/Transcriber

This is a tape player that has special features (Fig. 38–2):

An earphone to screen out background noises and enable dictation to be heard more clearly
A foot switch to keep hands free and allow the tape to be played, fast forwarded, and rewound
A variable-speed control to allow the tape to be played at any speed from very slow to very fast

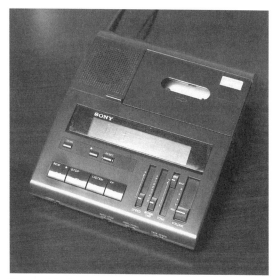

Figure 38–2
Dictaphone.

A back spacer to rewind a small amount to prevent accidental omission of a word or syllable
Tone adjustment to allow adjustment from high-pitched to low-pitched tones for better clarity
An erase key to clear tapes
A counter to measure the length of tape played for quick return to a specific location
A "cue," which is an electronic signal embedded into the tape when it is dictated. It serves to speed up a search to find a specific dictation quickly (useful for STAT reports).

Digital Dictation

Digital dictation equipment is state of the art and very expensive. Dictation is stored on a computer disk. The digital system equipment is similar to tape equipment. It is clearer than the tape, and it is easier and less time consuming to access reports on the digital system. Remote transcription units can be placed in the transcriber's home. The transcriber can access the reports, transcribe them, and then either send the hard copies over a modem to a printer at the client's facility, or print them out and deliver them the next day. This system is used mostly by hospitals and is known as an automated voice dictation system. The future will bring more digital dictation to this new and developing field.

Copier

This is a machine that duplicates an image or information that a client may require. It is often wise to have an additional copy of a receipt, form, or other document not accessible from the computer system.

Scanner

A scanner copies a picture or typed pages and places it into your computer as PC paintbrush (PCX), tagged image file format (TIFF), or bitmap (BMP), so you can insert it into a report or on a flyer or card. It can also be used as a copy machine.

Shredder

A paper shredder does not have to be expensive to be effective. A portable model that can be placed over the opening to an ordinary wastebasket is sufficient. It is needed to shred waste documents that may contain confidential information (Fig. 38–3).

Laptop Computer

A laptop can be used to make the job flexible. If a transcriber has to sit somewhere for hours, such as at a child's dance classes, and he or she has transcriptions to do, the laptop is an excellent vehicle with which to type and store work. On return home, the files from the laptop can be downloaded into the system and printed. This allows hours to be clocked in where there would have otherwise been wasted time.

Pager

Clients are happier when they have the security of reaching their transcriptionist when they need them. Pagers help to prioritize the workload and keep the transcriptionist accessible to the clients, family, and business in general. They are time savers. A pager with voice mail takes a verbal message. It can save the time ordinarily spent calling directly to a number to see what someone needs, and allows for prioritization.

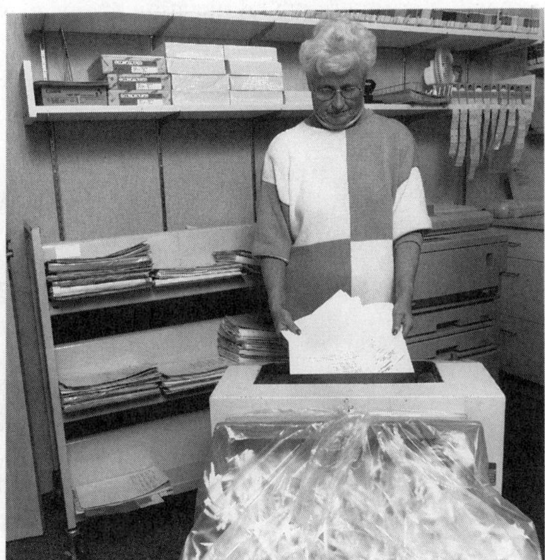

Figure 38–3
Shredding waste documents.

Cellular Phone

With a cellular ("cell") phone, urgent messages can be responded to immediately. Other calls can be left for later when the business line is available.

Starting the Business

When the required course work has been completed and a business plan has been conceived, it is time to take the steps to start the business. Contact the department of commerce and community affairs at the state level. They will have information about obtaining licenses and permits needed to start the business. They may also provide the individual with a "Start-Up Information Kit" and guidance about the department of the state from which to acquire a "Business Registration Kit." This kit typically contains necessary information and forms to register the business and the tax documents that have to be filed.

Check with local and county agencies to find out if there are any further regulations or restrictions. Contact the department of employment security to determine if the company is required to pay unemployment tax.

Junior and community colleges frequently offer assistance to start up small businesses. Assistance is also often available through groups of experienced retirees who offer their services at a nominal fee, as well as at the Small Business Administration offices.

A decision must be made about benefits if others are going to be employed by the business. The requirements depend on the rules of the particular state. They usually vary with the number of employees. If the individual owner works alone, it is wise to investigate all the insurance providers to get the coverage that is suitable. You may wish to maintain your own liability insurance in today's medical field, where everyone is named in various lawsuits, not just the individual doctor.

If you work alone and do not have benefits from a company, you may choose to purchase an insurance policy that would cover workers' compensation. This is recommended because you receive pay for only the work you complete. Insurance can be obtained at favorable rates through small business groups, some church organizations, and some social organizations.

There are several computer money management and billing systems that automate the billing process and record keeping. The availability of these programs does not preclude the need for bookkeeping skills by the person responsible for the business.

Marketing

In order to begin to sell the services to the potential buyers, the transcriptionist should organize all of the important documents into a portfolio. The portfolio should contain:

Up-to-date resume
All pertinent certificates
Business license
Letters of reference
Samples of work

Identify potential users of a medical transcription service in the locality the business will serve. Prepare and send a letter of introduction, describing the services offered, and request an appointment to meet with them. There are a number of potential users for this service (Table 38–2).

Other Opportunities

If HUCs with the required additional training prefer not to start their own business, there are other opportunities available to use their knowledge and skills.

Table 38–2 WORKING OPPORTUNITIES FOR THE MEDICAL TRANSCRIPTIONIST

Facility	Department	Type of Records
Hospitals	Medical records	History and physical exam Consultations Discharge summaries Progress notes Pathology reports X-ray reports Cardiology reports Operative reports Admission summaries Discharge summaries
Doctors' offices	Medical records	History and physical exam Admission summary Consultation reports Progress notes Test results
Independent labs	Medical records	Test results
Clinics	Medical records	Admissions Discharge summaries Progress notes Laboratory reports

Temporary Service Agencies

These services specialize in contracting temporary employment for a variety of positions. In some instances, the work may be done in the home; in others, it must be done on site in the workplace.

Transcription Service Companies

These companies often have workloads sufficient to hire additional transcriptionists or to subcontract some jobs to private transcriptionists in order to meet their deadlines.

Hospitals

Most hospitals have a transcription department. Inquiries should be made to the human resources department of the facility in which you are interested.

Outpatient Facilities

Some health clinics, laboratories, and physician's offices have a caseload large enough to warrant the hiring of part- or full-time personnel to do their transcribing.

Law Offices

Law offices that specialize in medical malpractice or personal injury cases are making use of the talents of transcriptionists. They are typically expected to transcribe and prepare medical briefs. They often can be of assistance in the interpretation of medical records and notes.

Miscellaneous Opportunities

In some areas, positions are also available in county health departments, coroners' offices, medical schools, and government medical facilities. Some transcriptionists offer clerical assistance to medical students.

A Day in the Life of a Private Transcriptionist

I have chosen to become a private medical transcriptionist for many reasons. The most compelling reason is flexibility. In my business, the following is an example of a typical day:

5:00 A.M. Wake up, shower, dress (on work days I wear scrubs; this helps keep me focused and reminds my family I am working), cook breakfast.
6:15 A.M. Wake up my daughter.
6:30 A.M. Finish breakfast.
7:00 A.M. Nebulize my daughter, make sure she has all the things she needs to bring to school. Pack up all tapes and transcribed reports for delivery.
7:30 A.M. Drive my daughter to school.
8:00–9:30 A.M. Drop off completed work and pick up new assignments from clients.
10:00 A.M.–1:30 P.M. Transcribe.
2:00 P.M. Pick up my daughter from school.
3:00–4:00 P.M. Transcribe.
4:00–5:00 P.M. Prepare dinner.
5:00–6:30 P.M. Eat dinner and clean up.
7:00–8:30 P.M. Help my daughter with her homework, or spend quality time with her.
8:30–10:00 P.M. Work on accounts and charges, and print bills for clients.

I type 4 1/2 hours per day, 5 days a week. When my daughter is out of school, I change my schedule to a 4-day, 10-hour-per-day week or a 3-day, 12-hour-per-day week depending on my personal need, so I can spend more time with my family. You are the boss! Work out your schedules to meet your needs and provide a great service for your clients with a quick turnaround time and an accurate product.

Closing Thoughts

I hope that this chapter has enlightened you in some of the other avenues of employment available to the HUC. Some personally prefer working in a home-based position because of the flexibility, *which enables them to adjust their* personal needs *to their* professional needs. *Some prefer to make their own hours and work status depending on their own needs, not those of a corporation. They can work full time or part time and any days they want. They could have every holiday and weekend off without any problem. Others prefer to work for someone or some company because it gives them a sense of job security. They are able to receive some form of benefits, which could include sick pay, vacation pay, limited pension plans, and possibly a health/life insurance program of some kind.*

In conclusion, we must always strive to maintain professionalism and continue to educate ourselves and to incorporate that education into our profession, which will keep us marketable and on the cutting edge of innovative ways to use our profession and talents. We are on a new frontier with the profession of certified HUC. Let's be creative and grow to new heights with this field. We are the base, only we can see how big we can grow, and we are the future.

Review Questions

1. Name the various educational options that could prepare a person to become a medical transcriptionist.
2. List the equipment that would be necessary to operate a private medical transcription company at home.
3. Identify the initial steps to take to start up a private small business.
4. List six other opportunites for medical transcriptionists other than a private business.

Bibliography

Harvey G: DOS for Dummies. Foster City, CA, IDG Books, 1993.

Owen B: Personal Computers for the Computer Illiterate. New York, Harper Perennial Publishers, 1990.

The Internet: A Guide for Health Professionals. Biomed General Corporation, Berkeley, CA, 1997.

39 Rehabilitation Facility

Donna Baker

Common Abbreviations

BVI	Bladder volume index
CMG/ EMG	Cystometrogram/ electromyogram
CVA	Cerebrovascular accident
EMG/ NCS	Electromyogram/Nerve conduction study
FEES	Fiberoptic endoscopic evaluation of swallowing
MPB	Motor point block

Objectives

Upon completion of this chapter, the reader should be able to:

1. List nine specialized programs that would be found in a rehabilitation hospital and briefly describe each.
2. Describe the members of the rehabilitation team.
3. Identify some of the special diagnostic procedures ordered for rehabilitation patients.
4. Describe the special equipment used to care for rehabilitation patients, and explain its uses.

Vocabulary

Aphasia: Loss of ability to speak

Autonomic dysreflexia: An exaggerated response of high blood pressure to a signal within the body

Bladder volume index: A noninvasive test to measure the volume of urine in a patient's bladder

Community skills practice: A planned outing into the community

Cystometrogram/electromyogram: A bladder function test to aid in the diagnosis and management of urinary incontinence

Dysphagia: Difficulty swallowing

Electromyogram/nerve conduction study: A test used to diagnose disease of nerves and muscles

Fiberoptic endoscopic evaluation of swallowing: A diagnostic procedure to evaluate a patient's ability to swallow

Hemiplegia: Paralysis of one side of the body

Modified barium swallow: An x-ray procedure done to evaluate the swallowing mechanism

Motor point block: A procedure used in managing situations where involuntary strong muscle contractions interfere with or prevent functional activities such as walking

Continued

Vocabulary *Continued*

Orthostatic hypotension: A lowering of the blood pressure after sitting upright

Paraplegia: Paralysis of the lower limbs

Physiatry: The medical specialty that deals with the diagnosis and treatment of patients with diseases and injuries that affect the neuromusculoskeletal systems

Quadriplegia: Paralysis affecting all four extremities of the body

History of Rehabilitative Medicine

Rehabilitation medicine is the branch of medicine that diagnoses and treats neuromusculoskeletal impairment, disability, and handicap and works to restore people with physical disabilities to their highest possible levels of physical, psychological, social, vocational, recreational, and economic functioning. Rehabilitation medicine tries to eliminate the disability or to moderate its impact by retraining the disabled person to live as normal and productive a life as possible.

Modern rehabilitation medicine developed during World War II, when Dr. Howard A. Rusk (1900–1989) demonstrated that physical and psychological rehabilitation was more effective than restful convalescence in restoring soldiers to the level of fitness sufficient for return to duty. He also found that people with physical disabilities best benefit from treatment by an interdisciplinary team addressing the multiple and complex problems created by the disability.

Rehabilitation medicine has since merged with physical medicine, a specialty that manages disease by means of physical agents such as light, heat, cold, water, electricity, and various mechanical agents including exercise, traction, manipulation, massage, and other devices. In 1947, rehabilitation medicine and physical medicine were formally recognized as one medical specialty, called physical medicine and rehabilitation, often referred to as **physiatry**. Physiatrists, physicians who specialize in physical medicine and rehabilitation, diagnose and set up treatment programs for the management of musculoskeletal pain syndromes and disabilities that result from injuries and diseases afflicting the neuromusculoskeletal systems. Most physiatrists perform electrodiagnostic studies, manage an interdisciplinary team of health care professionals, and plan long-term treatments for the disabled patient.

The practice of rehabilitation medicine ranges from short-term, outpatient management of various neuromusculoskeletal ailments and pain syndromes to long-term and comprehensive management of severe disabilities resulting from spinal cord injury, traumatic brain injury, stroke, injuries and disorders of bone, cancer, burns, various neuromuscular diseases, and congenital disorders, such as cerebral palsy and spina bifida. After onset of a major disability, the patient is admitted to an in-patient rehabilitation service if he or she is able to participate in the rehabilitation program and shows the potential significantly to improve functional performance.

Description of a Rehabilitation Facility

The rehabilitation facility specializes in the rehabilitation of each patient to his or her fullest potential of recovery from an acute, traumatic illness or accident or from a chronic, long-term illness or disability.

A rehabilitation facility as a free-standing facility specializes strictly in the rehabilitation of the patient. The free-standing rehabilitation facility does not have any of the acute care hospital services available such as an emergency room, operating room, cardiac services, and delivery room. The rehabilitation facility would need to contact, make arrangements with, and transport the patient to an acute care hospital for any services that would be needed. If a physician orders a computed tomography scan, for example, the health unit coordinator (HUC) makes arrangements with the acute care hospital for the test to be done, and arranges transportation for the patient to go to the acute care hospital for the test.

There may be several different specialized programs available to meet the specific needs of the patient. The specialized programs also provide a care plan for the patient's specific needs. Most programs include intense therapy for 3 hours per day with scheduled rest periods and meal times.

The following sections discuss some of the specialized programs that may be available in a rehabilitation facility.

Spinal Cord Injury Program

This may include patients with spinal cord injuries of varying degrees of severity. Both the severe and less severe injuries may involve paralysis. There are two general types of paralysis, **quadriplegia** and **paraplegia.** Quadriplegia is the result of a spinal cord injury in the cervical area (C1–C8). People with this injury may have poor ability to breathe as well as loss of movement and feeling in the arms, legs, and trunk areas. Paraplegia indicates a spinal cord injury at or below the thoracic area. People with this type of injury may have a loss of sensation in their legs and trunk, but do have sensation and movement in their arms. Patients with a spinal cord injury receive therapies and nursing care to bring them to the fullest level of function. Depending on the severity and location of the injury, this may be almost complete recovery, or may mean learning how to function using a wheelchair. Some patients may need to learn how to propel a wheelchair by using puffs of breath. They may need to learn to eat and perform other functions with the use of some special adaptive equipment. Nursing is responsible for teaching the patient how to become independent in self-care. Some of the other adaptive equipment is explained later in the chapter.

Some of the concerns involved with a spinal cord injury include loss of balance, muscle spasms, and pain that occurs with loss of sensation and movement. There is also a danger of development of pressure ulcers. **Autonomic dysreflexia** is an exaggerated response of high blood pressure to a signal within the body. It is an emergency situation and most commonly occurs in people with spinal cord injury at T6 and above. Other concerns may include **orthostatic hypotension** (a lowering of the blood pressure after sitting upright), loss of bowel and bladder control, breathing difficulties, and depression, frustration, and anger.

Cerebrovascular Accident or Stroke Program

The cerebrovascular accident (CVA) program includes patients who have had blood vessels in their brain damaged by a blood clot, weak vessels, or an aneurysm. A person's recovery depends on the area of the brain affected. The effects of some strokes may be barely noticeable, whereas some may involve a loss of vision, speech, coordination, emotions, or partial or complete loss of the use of the arm and leg on one side of the body (**hemiplegia**). Stroke patients may need to relearn how to do many tasks to return to their highest level of function. Some patients may lose the use of their dominant hand, for example; they would need to learn how to write or hold eating utensils with the less dominant hand. Some stroke patients may lose their ability to speak. This is called **aphasia.** Aphasia is a defect or loss of language function in which the comprehension or expression of words is impaired. They may need to learn other forms of communication, such as writing down their needs or using pictures.

Head Trauma Program

This program may involve patients with a closed head injury or one involving an open wound.

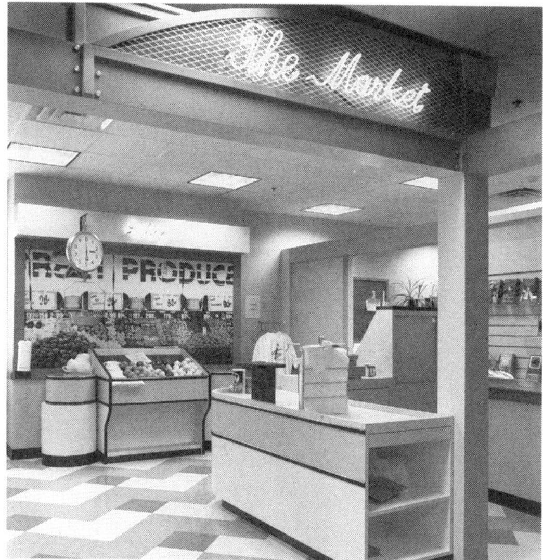

Figure 39–1
Independence Square grocery store.

Either way, there may be mild, moderate, or severe damage to the person's brain. The extent of recovery from a head injury is determined by the amount of brain damage that has occurred. Some of the common problems after a head trauma injury may be movement (motor) problems, speech problems, thinking (cognitive) problems, personality problems, perceptual changes, regulatory problems, or seizures. A patient's degree of injury is rated by the Rancho Los Amigos Head Trauma Scale of 1 to 8. As a patient's condition improves, he or she goes through certain identifiable stages of recovery. The eight stages can be broken into three general phases of rehabilitation. In the first phase of rehabilitation (level I, no response; level II, generalized response; and level III, localized response), the treatment emphasis is on sensory stimulation or "waking the person up." The goal of this phase is to increase the patient's awareness of self and his or her surroundings. In the challenging second phase of rehabilitation (level IV, confused-agitated; level V, confused-inappropriate-nonagitated; and level VI, confused-appropriate), the treatment emphasis is on structuring the environment. The goal of this phase is to control the person's agitation and confusion, and assist the person to direct his or her behavior in safe and productive ways. In the third phase of rehabilitation (level VII, automatic-appropriate; and level VIII, purposeful-appropriate), the treatment emphasis is on community reintegration. The goal of this phase is to assist the patient in participating successfully in the community.

To help reach the goal of successful participation in the community, the rehabilitation facility may have an Independence Square. The Independence Square may include a grocery store (Fig. 39–1), movie theater (Fig. 39–2), bank (Fig. 39–3), laundromat, or clothing store. It may also include a car and gasoline pump (Fig. 39–4, work area (Fig. 39–5), or a greenhouse (Fig. 39–6). The patient uses the Independence Square as part of the daily therapy routine. The patient may work on his or her specific needs, such as shopping in a grocery store or going to the bank. The patient is able to repeat tasks as needed without the fear of mistakes or the pressure involved in doing these tasks in the community. The Independence Square has become a very useful tool in commu-

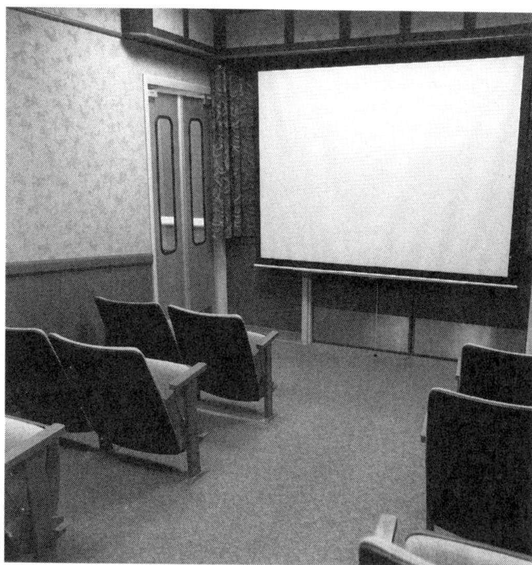

Figure 39–2
Independence Square movie theater.

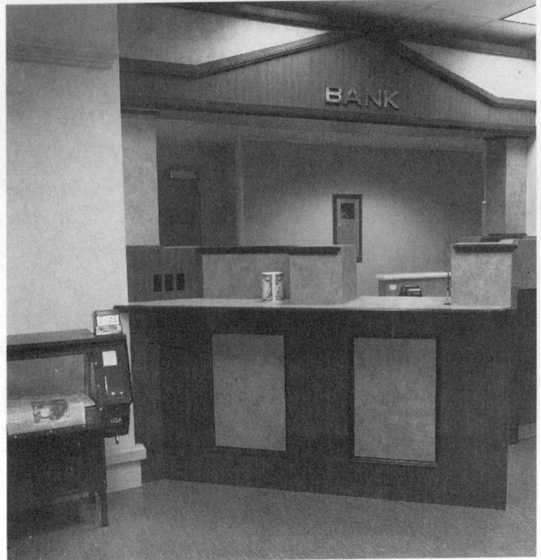

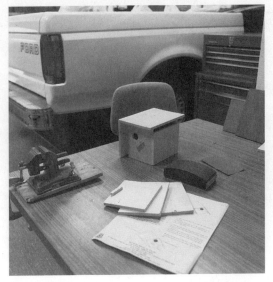

Figure 39–3
Independence Square bank.

nity reintegration without having the patient leave the grounds of the rehabilitation facility. Recovery from a severe brain injury usually takes months and years rather than days and weeks.

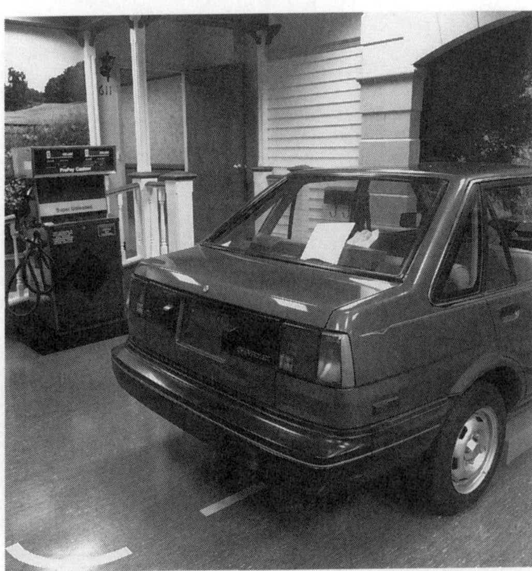

Figure 39–4
Independence Square car and gas pump.

Figure 39–5
Independence Square work area.

Arthritis Program

Rehabilitation for arthritis patients involves specialized therapy to improve their ability to per-

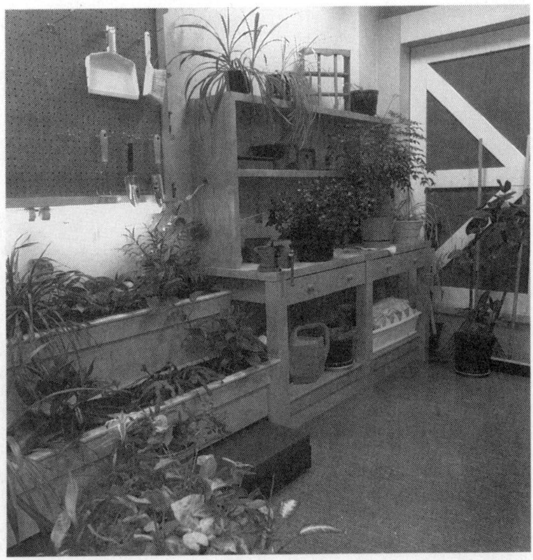

Figure 39–6
Independence Square greenhouse.

form the usual and ordinary tasks of daily living. Physical therapy and occupational therapy sessions are the most intense therapies used to work with arthritis patients. Pool therapy is commonly used to help the patients become more flexible and stronger by having them exercise in the warm pool several times a week. The warm water of the pool relaxes the muscles and the patients become more flexible as they exercise in the water. Also, the buoyancy of the water enables the patients to exercise with less strain on the muscles. Many times, the patients are able to do exercises in the water that they would not be able to do otherwise.

Burn Program

Recovery and rehabilitation from a burn can be quite extensive and involve a long period of time. Nursing may need to do a lot of wound care that may include very careful cleansing and treatments to the burned areas. Physical therapy involves painful stretching exercises to stretch the areas that have been burned to improve mobility. Burn therapy also includes neuropsychology sessions to help the patient cope with the disfigurement burns may cause.

Neurologic Rehabilitation Program

This program may include patients with neurologic conditions such as multiple sclerosis (MS) or Guillain-Barré syndrome. MS is a syndrome, not a disease, in which an acute spinal cord transection occurs. The cause remains unknown. MS may progress over several years, it can be severe, and it usually is recurring. Guillain-Barré syndrome is a rapidly progressive form of polyneuropathy characterized by muscular weakness and sensory loss. With these and other neurologic disorders, rehabilitation therapy helps the patient return to the highest level of function. These patients benefit from a rehabilitation program individually designed to help them live and cope with a neurologic condition. Along with the usual physical and occupational therapy, neuropsychology is very important in helping the patient and family learn coping skills for any neurologic disability.

Pediatric Program

This program is designed specifically with the pediatric patient in mind, and may include almost every illness or injury that may occur in a child. It is important for the therapy of a child to include the immediate family members as much as possible. Sometimes the child or his or her parents, or both, have expectations from the program of rehabilitation that are in excess of the child's potential. It is also necessary to have age-appropriate equipment, keeping the individual child in mind. The rehabilitation program is based on the philosophy that the child with a physical handicap is first a child, whose basic needs are those of a child. In addition to these basic needs, the child with a handicap requires services that will overcome or alleviate the handicap and help the child to attain the most satisfactory psychosocial and educational adjustments in the environment in which he or she must function for the remainder of his or her life. Periodic evaluations are necessary to assess the child's progress. The rehabilitation program is based on the motivation level of the child. Many parents think that by daily intensive work, a child will attain physical independence more rapidly. This pressure on the child often causes rebellion and retards progress.

Adult Day Care

This is a specialized program for the care of adults who need treatment or supervision during the day, but are able to return to their family in the evening. This program is very beneficial to caregivers who work during the day and are unable to leave their loved ones at home alone. Transportation, meals, baths, recreation, nursing, and a safe environment are some of the services provided by an adult day care service. Also, by providing social interaction, the program is able to combat the isolation that frequently occurs when an elderly or needy adult is otherwise alone.

Transitional Rehabilitation Programs

These programs provide for patients during a time of transition between being a full-time in-patient and returning to self-care or assisted care at home. At this step in the program, the patient may move into an apartment to begin the process of learning self-care. There is supervision and help available as the patient identifies his or her needs in moving toward the goal of self-care.

Work Injury Rehabilitation Center

This center has a group of specialists, including nurses and therapists, who work with patients on an outpatient basis who have been injured on or off the job. These patients do not need in-patient care, but need intense therapies to return to their current jobs. Occupational and physical therapy provides these patients with the strengthening and endurance exercises needed to help them return to their jobs as soon as possible. Pool therapy is also used for these patients.

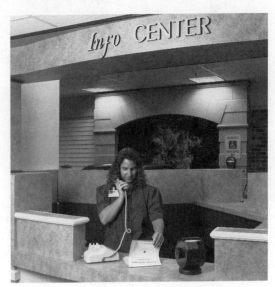

Figure 39–7
The health unit coordinator.

The Rehabilitation Team

The Health Unit Coordinator

The HUC is a very important part of the whole team approach of caring for the patients. The HUC is the one person with whom every other team member communicates. The HUC is usually the person depended on the most to know everything pertaining to the patient and his or her care (Fig. 39–7). The whole rehabilitation team shares the common goal of helping the patient recover and become as independent as possible.

Some of the other team members are described in the following sections.

Physiatrist

A physiatrist is a medical doctor who specializes in physical medicine and rehabilitation. The physiatrist is usually based at the facility and sees the patient daily. He or she manages the patient's medical care while the patient is at the facility.

Occupational Therapist

An occupational therapist is a specialist who teaches the patient how to gain independence in activities of daily living such as dressing, bathing, meal preparation, and others. Occupational therapy may also provide a driver retraining program to help a patient with a disability return to driving a motor vehicle safely.

Physical Therapist

A physical therapist is a specialist who helps the patient to gain strength, balance, coordination, and endurance. Also, the therapist works to improve bed movement, transfers, and walking or wheelchair skills.

Nurse Therapist

A registered nurse works closely with the doctors and the whole team to care for the medical, nursing, and therapy needs of the patient. The nurse therapist is usually one of the first contacts for the patient and family. He or she works closely with the patient and family, and provides nursing care for the patient. When primary care nursing is used, the same nurse and an alternate nurse care for the patient for the whole stay at the facility. This works well in providing continuity of care for the patient.

Speech-Language Pathologist

This person is a specialist who helps the patient with problems in communication, language skills, memory, thinking, and swallowing. There are many tools and equipment used to help improve a patient's ability to communicate. By using the special tools to detect swallowing difficulties, the speech-language pathologist can improve a patient's ability to swallow without choking or aspirating. By following the speech-language pathologist's recommendations, many patients are able to eat and enjoy proper nutrition without the use of a feeding tube. The speech-language pathologist also tests for any hearing problems the patient may have. Hearing aids or listening devices may help a patient return to a higher level of function sooner.

Recreation Therapist

This therapist is a specialist who helps the patient with leisure interests, social skills, and community re-entry. A recreation therapy session may include taking a bedridden patient outside on a warm day, or taking a spinal cord–injured patient fishing. These types of therapy sessions help improve a patient's outlook and possibly help reduce recovery time.

Respiratory Therapist

The respiratory therapist monitors the patient's breathing. This therapist would also teach the patient breathing exercises and give breathing treatments and education.

Nutrition Therapist

The nutrition therapist is a specialist who reviews the nutritional needs of the patient. The nutritionist closely monitors the patient's individual nutritional needs, including special diets and food allergies.

Case Manager

A case manager directs the whole rehabilitation team and is also a resource person for the patient and family. The case manager brings together many aspects of the patient's care, including education, team conferences, communication with insurance companies, and discharge planning. Discharge planning may include making arrangements for continued therapy on an outpatient basis at a facility close to the patient's home town, or making arrangements for a home health nurse to provide care for the patient at home.

Rehabilitation Associate

The rehabilitation associate is a specialist who works closely with the nurse to care for the patient's medical, nursing, and therapy needs. A rehabilitation associate is a certified nursing assistant with additional training in rehabilitation procedures.

Social Worker

The social worker addresses emotional and social concerns. He or she helps the patients understand the effects of their injuries and also helps them understand what resources are available in the community. If the patient is younger than 19 years of age, the social worker works with the school system to determine how the patient may be able to continue his or her education. The social worker also makes arrangements with a language interpreter when necessary. The social worker works closely with the patient, family, and case manager on the discharge process.

Orthotist

This is a person who specializes in a wide range of bracing systems and is able to determine the best options for the patient. The orthotist also provides artificial limbs for patients who have lost a limb because of injury or illness.

Neuropsychologist

A neuropsychologist works directly with the patient to find ways to make a more meaningful life. He or she also works with the rest of the treatment team to advise them on approaches that may work best for the patient. If needed, the neuropsychologist takes the lead role to explore chemical dependency issues that may be present.

Vocational Rehabilitationist

This is a specialist who helps the patient explore vocational options. These services are used when a patient is employable, but may not necessarily be able to continue in his or her previous line of work.

Pastoral Care Person

A member of the pastoral care department visits regularly to offer pastoral counseling, or can meet with the patient and family on an on-call basis. The pastoral care department coordinates with the patient's local pastor as well, when appropriate.

The most important members of the whole rehabilitation team are the patient and family members. All the aforementioned people must work together to provide the best care possible to the patient to help in returning each patient to his or her highest level of rehabilitation.

Knowledge/Skills Appropriate to Position

Transcription of Orders

The HUC is directly responsible for transcribing all the orders written by the physiatrist or the patient's physician. This may include entering the orders into the computer system and notifying the appropriate departments of the new order.

Chart Maintenance

The HUC is also responsible for maintaining the patients' charts. This may include the filing of any patient records, test results, and documentation into the patients' charts in a timely manner, so that the entire chart is available to the physician and nurse at all times.

The HUC is the central and most accessible person for everyone to contact. The HUC needs to possess excellent time management skills to keep up with the fast pace involved in working in a rehabilitation facility.

Communication

Communication skills are very important to ensure correct transcription of doctors' orders and ordering the many different treatments and tests that may be necessary during a patient's stay. Communicating directly with the patient and family also requires some skill to achieve the highest level of understanding for all involved parties. Many times a patient is not able to communicate his or her needs appropriately. It may be necessary to find out from the speech-language pathologist the most appropriate and affective way to communicate with the patient. Also, family members need to be informed of everything that is happening while their loved one is receiving rehabilitation therapy, or any tests that may be involved. The HUC must document in the patient's chart any communication with a family member or the patient so that the other team members will know what has occurred.

Confidentiality

Patient rights and confidentiality must be maintained at all times. Each facility should have the patients' rights posted and each patient should receive a copy of them. It is the responsibility of the HUC to know what the patients' rights are and to ensure that they are not compromised.

Medical Terminology

Medical terminology is a much needed skill for a HUC. The HUC needs to know exactly what the doctor or nurse is requesting and to be able to follow through with those requests or orders. Medical terminology is a tool needed to do the job effectively and efficiently. The local community college may have medical terminology classes available to the general public. Many of the common terms used in rehabilitation are explained throughout this chapter.

Pharmacology

Pharmacology knowledge is also very important to have when transcribing the many medication orders that may be ordered by the physiatrist or the patient's physician. A knowledge of medication, dosages, and frequencies can be a real time saver if there is a question regarding a medication order. Medication use in a particular setting is influenced by many factors, including physician prescribing habits and patient mix, as well as types and the technological advancement of programs offered by the hospital. The following medications may be anticipated to be frequently used in the rehabilitation setting:

Skeletal muscle relaxants—Lioresal (baclofen), Dantrium (dantrolene), Zanaflex (tizanidine)
Anticoagulants—Coumadin (warfarin)
Anticonvulsants—Dilantin (phenytoin), Tegretol (carbamazepine), Neurontin (gabapentin)
Genitourinary smooth muscle relaxants—Ditropan (oxybutynin)
Analgesics—Darvocet-N 100, Percocet, Vicodin
Antianxiety agents—Ativan (lorazepam), Xanax (alprazolam)

Diagnostic Tests

A general knowledge of laboratory and other test results is necessary to perform the job efficiently. Correct interpretation of the tests is necessary, and abnormal results need to be identified immediately so that the physician and nurse will have an opportunity to respond to the results promptly.

The physiatrist may order a variety of tests, activities, or procedures, and the HUC is responsible for communicating the order to the appropriate department to make arrangements.

There may be an order for a **cystometrogram/electromyogram (CMG/EMG)**. This procedure is done by the physiatrist, and is a bladder function test to aid in the diagnosis and management of incontinence.

Another test performed by the physiatrist is an **electromyogram/nerve conduction study (EMG/NCS)**. This is a test used to diagnose diseases of nerves and muscles.

It may be necessary for the physiatrist to perform a **motor point block (MPB)**. This is a procedure used in managing situations where involuntary strong muscle contractions (spasticity) interfere with or prevent functional activities such as walking, transfers, dressing, or other activities of daily living.

A **bladder volume index (BVI)** may be ordered. It is a noninvasive test to measure the volume of urine in a patient's bladder. A BVI is performed by the nurse.

There are two procedures for a speech-language pathologist to use to evaluate a patient for **dysphagia.** Dysphagia is a disorder of the swallowing mechanism. One test is a **fiberoptic endoscopic evaluation of swallowing (FEES)**. In this test, a flexible tube is inserted through the patient's nose by either a physician or speech-language pathologist. The patient is then given a liquid to drink and his or her ability to swallow can be followed by the light on the end of the tube. It is very useful when the patient cannot be moved because it can be performed at the bedside.

The other test that may be performed is a **modified barium swallow.** This is a radiographic evaluation performed in an acute care hospital with a speech-language pathologist in attendance to evaluate at the time of the procedure.

The physiatrist may also order a **community skills practice.** This is a scheduled, planned outing into the community. The purpose is to provide the patient with the opportunity to practice community skills before discharge. The physiatrist, nurse, and each therapist are involved in the decision as to what activities will be included in the community skills practice.

Equipment

Along with the aforementioned skills, it is necessary for a HUC to have knowledge in the operation of a fax machine and copy machine, and have excellent telephone skills. Telephone skills include knowledge of the functions and capabilities of the telephone system in the facility. If the facility has a telephone dictation system available, knowledge of the operation of this system will be necessary to assist the user.

Special Equipment

Environmental control units (ECU) are specialized equipment that allow people with limited movement to control appliances and equipment in their environment. These items are ordered at the recommendation of the specific therapists. This equipment assists the patient to select TV channels, to turn lights on and off, and to perform many other everyday activities that would otherwise be impossible.

An example of a specialized piece of equipment used to aid the spinal cord-injured patient in standing is a Power Lift Hi-Lo Stand in Table. This item is used by the Physical Therapy Department. Some examples of specialized equipment used by the occupational therapy department are a ball bearing feeder (Fig. 39–8), a friction feeder, a utensil holder (Fig. 39–9), and prism glasses (Fig. 39–10), which are used to allow a bedridden patient to read while remaining completely flat in bed. A net bed is a specialized bed used for an agitated head-injured patient (Fig. 39–11). This bed keeps the patient safe without the use of restraints and allows the patient an unobstructed view.

Marketing Health Unit Coordinator Skills

Because of the wide range of skills necessary, the HUC has become a very valuable asset to the health care and medical fields. Health unit coordinating has become a respected and valuable occupation.

Additional Training Required

A HUC can function in this position without additional training. However, just as in any other area of health unit coordinating, continuing education is very important. Workshops and seminars that deal with the rehabilitation patient are very useful,

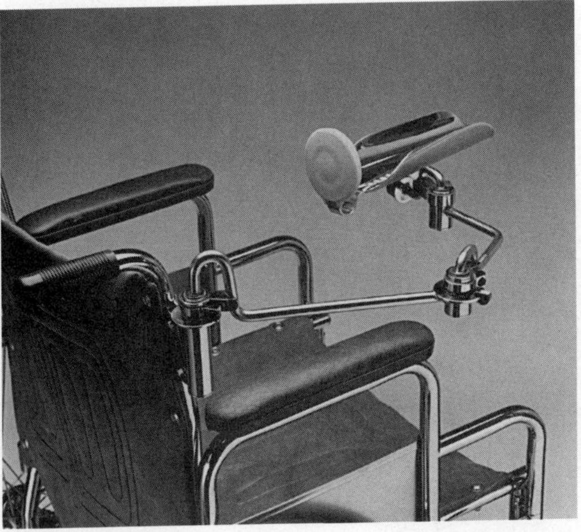

Figure 39–8
Ball-bearing feeder. (Courtesy of North Coast Medical, Inc., San Jose, CA.)

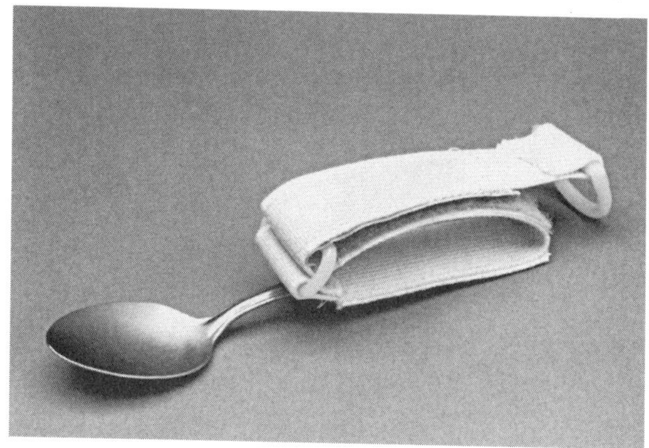

Figure 39–9
Utensil holder. (Courtesy of North Coast Medical, Inc., San Jose, CA.)

as are educational offerings that address communication skills and stress management.

Types of Positions Available

The types of positions available for a HUC in a rehabilitation facility may include staff HUC, HUC supervisor, and HUC educator. These positions vary from facility to facility.

Closing Thoughts

It is a very rewarding experience to be employed as a HUC in a rehabilitation facility. A HUC in a rehabilitation facility is able to

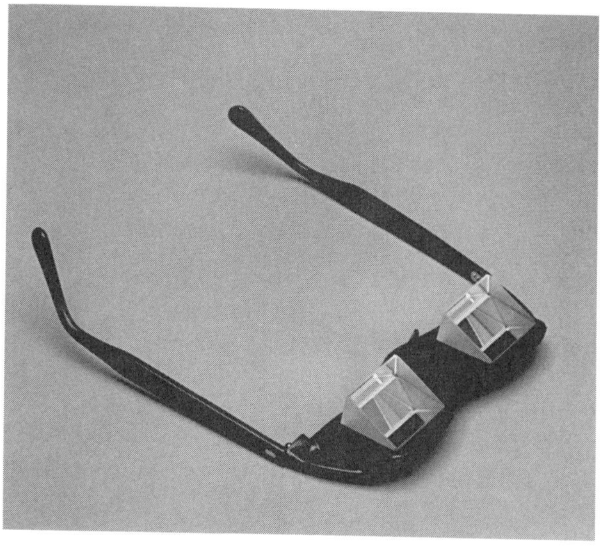

Figure 39–10
Prism glasses. (Courtesy of North Coast Medical, Inc., San Jose, CA.)

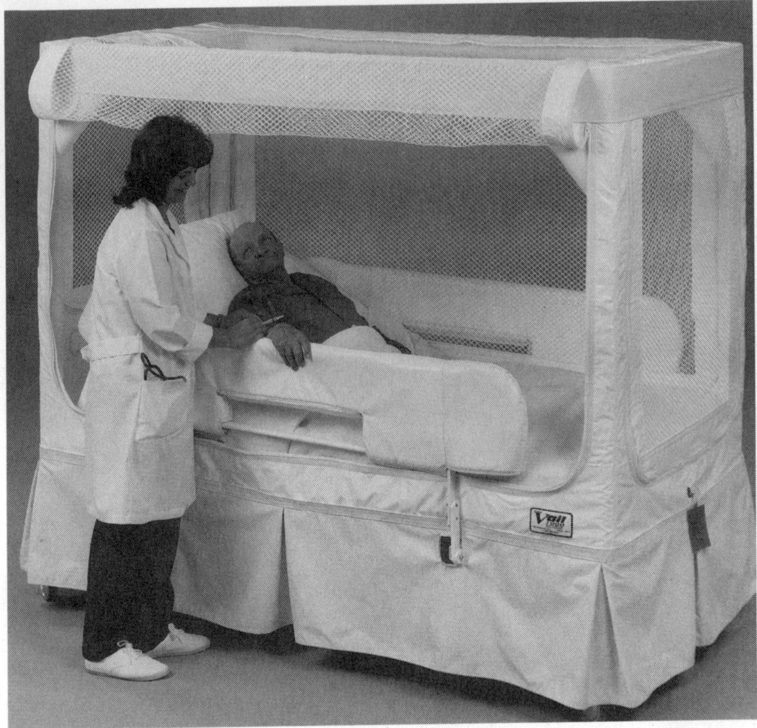

Figure 39–11
Net bed (Courtesy of Vail Products, Inc., Toledo, OH.)

witness the end results of each patient's hard work and determination: to be able to go home again and function at the highest attainable level, and to be as close to "normal" as possible. There is also a great sense of involvement when you are part of the "whole team" involved in helping the patients attain their goals. I have worked as a HUC in a rehabilitation facility for 25 years. I have found my work to be very rewarding, exciting, challenging, hectic, and chaotic at times. But, I think the reason I have stayed in this environment for so many years is the fact that every day is so different. You are never doing the same thing day after day. It has been very rewarding to work with such people as the nurses, doctors, pharmacists, therapists, and the patients and their families, among countless others. You can learn a lot from all of these people. I have always felt like a very important part of the team. As all HUCs know, you are expected to know "everything." This can be challenging, and also can keep you "on your toes." Health unit coordinating is a great career. I am very thankful and grateful to all of my coworkers for making it such a rewarding one.

Review Questions

1. List nine specialized programs that would be found in a rehabilitation hospital and describe each briefly.
2. Describe the members of the rehabilitation team.
3. Identify some of the special diagnostic procedures ordered for rehabilitation patients.

4. Describe the special equipment used to care for rehabilitation patients.

Bibliography

Gritzer G, Arlude A: The Making of Rehabilitation. Berkeley, CA, University of California Press, 1985.

Kottke FJ: Krusen's Handbook of Physical Medicine and Rehabilitation, 4th ed. Philadelphia, WB Saunders, 1990.

Madonna Rehabilitation Hospital: Spinal Cord Injury Patient/Family Information Booklet. Lincoln, NE, Madonna Rehabilitation Hospital, 1996.

Madonna Rehabilitation Hospital: Traumatic Brain Injury (TBI) Family Information Booklet. Lincoln, NE, Madonna Rehabilitation Hospital, February, 1995.

Rusk HA: Rehabilitation in Medicine, 4th ed. St. Louis, MO, CV Mosby, 1977.

40 Research Facility

Gloria Cornelius

Common Abbreviations

CRF	Case report form
DHHS	Department of Health and Human Services
FDA	Food and Drug Administration
IRB	Institutional review board
NIH	National Institutes of Health
PI	Principal investigator

Objectives

Upon completion of this chapter, the reader should be able to:

1. Explain what a protocol is and why protocols are used in research studies.
2. List the varied duties of a research coordinator.
3. Name five areas of interest that may be studied in a rural research center.
4. Identify the two government departments that enforce the regulations that apply to research.

Vocabulary

Adverse experience: Any undesirable experience occurring in a subject/patient during a clinical trial, regardless of whether considered causally related to the investigational product

Case report form: A form used to collect specific data for a research study

Clinical research associate: Same as a study monitor

Clinical trial: That phase of a research study that involves human subjects in the investigation

Inclusion/exclusion criteria: Those factors that determine whether a patient is eligible to participate in a research study

Informed consent form: A signed record of the subject's consent voluntarily to be part of a research study that outlines all the information the person would need to know in order to be informed about the study

Institutional review board: The group formally designated by an institution to review, approve the initiation of, and conduct periodic reviews of biomedical research involving human subjects, to protect their rights and welfare

Patient accrual: Obtaining eligible people to be part of a research study.

Continued

Vocabulary *Continued*

Principal investigator: The person under whose immediate direction a research investigation is conducted

Protocol: The plan of a scientific experiment or treatment that explains in detail exactly how the experiment is to be carried out

Randomization: Placing study participants (subjects) in a study in a manner that eliminates bias

Serious adverse experience: Any experience that is fatal, life threatening, permanently disabling, requires or prolongs hospitalization, causes a congenital anomaly or cancer, or overdose

Study monitor: A clinical research associate from the sponsoring pharmaceutical company who makes periodic site visits

Subject: A person who voluntarily participates in a research study.

Related Terminology

Protocol management: Ensuring that all aspects of the protocol's functions are being carried out.

Source document: The first place data are recorded, such as a hospital or clinic medical record, an original laboratory report form, or an original interpretive report for a diagnostic study.

Study design: A brief summary including classification and clarification of the protocol.

Description of Facility

Research facilities are established as an extension of medical education. Medical research focuses on human illness and disease. The research findings translate into improvements in patient care and health outcomes. Research can be conducted in all the areas of medicine. The research facility described here interfaces as one of the nation's largest links in national and international research chains. Studies of international import are done in molecular genetics, epidemiology (preventive medicine), and farm medicine.

The molecular genetics laboratory, which is headed by a PhD-level scientist assisted by research associates, studies human DNA to map the genes responsible for a variety of genetic diseases. In the cancer genetics section of this lab, many studies are being conducted to find the genes responsible for various types of cancer.

Epidemiology identifies the causes of illness by studying the disease distributions and determinants of human populations. Population-based studies are done in research areas. A defined population is taken, using the expertise of clinic physicians and information obtained from medical records. Clinical research is conducted in nearly every specialty area. The facility integrates research in the daily practice of medicine, thereby meeting patients' needs with the latest and most advanced treatments available.

Many research facilities have multiple regional centers in addition to the main facility. For example, this research center has 27 regional centers and includes an outreach network of more than 100 hospitals, clinics, and other sites. Off-site consultation is done in 47 specialties. These include cardiology, rheumatology, dermatology, child

---

The terms above are commonly used in the research environment but do not appear in the text of the chapter.

psychology, allergy, and oral surgery, to name a few. Approximately 400 clinical trials of medications and research projects are being conducted at any one time. Projects vary from genetics, epidemiology, and biostatistics, to fertility, health care, and numerous others.

A research facility interfaces with national organizations. The latest medical technology, research, and education are all blended together in the larger facilities. An annual budget may average over 12 million dollars. Prestigious medical publications are put out nationally every year to share the knowledge gained. Scientific lectures and symposia are designed to inform medical professionals and the public about new technology in research and health care, bringing experts from around the globe. A research foundation may collaborate frequently in multiinstitutional research studies with the National Institutes of Health (**NIH**), the U.S. Department of Health and Human Services (**DHHS**), and numerous other agencies. It may share scientific knowledge in the medical community locally, regionally, and nationally.

Funding for research is a vital consideration. Extramural funds are sought through grants and contracts. Resource development, patient endowments, and contributions are also used to aid in funding research.

Research facilities need not be part of a major university. Patterns of disease and health can be ascertained anywhere, and do not necessarily need to be found in an urban setting. Research facilities, such as the one described in this chapter, may be part of a clinic and closely connected with the practice of medicine. The facility can be considered a division of the clinic system—part of complete health care networking. A foundation may be established with a mission that engages in basic and clinical research. A research and education facility can also support the broad spectrum of medical education. It can be an active participant in public service initiatives whenever and wherever possible.

Areas of research interest vary depending on the location of the research center. Examples of specific areas of research interest for the facility we have been describing, which is located in a rural setting, include 1) agricultural medicine and health, 2) rural health services, 3) epidemiology of disease, injury, and premature death within rural populations, 4) genetic, immunologic, and environmental causes of disease, and 5) Department of Medical Education and hundreds of additional research projects.

The Role of the Research Coordinator

A clinical research coordinator deals with all members of a disciplinary team at the institution (Fig. 40–1). This team is made up of physicians and specialists who provide state-of-the-art diagnosis, treatment, care, and investigation of the disease process being studied. The researchers and participating staff members at each institution are generally referred to as the "member institution." The lead physician is known as the **principal investigator (PI)**. The mission for research involvement is to improve treatments and survival rates, and find cures for specific diseases. It also involves the discovery of new agents for treatment, obtaining new scientific information in the

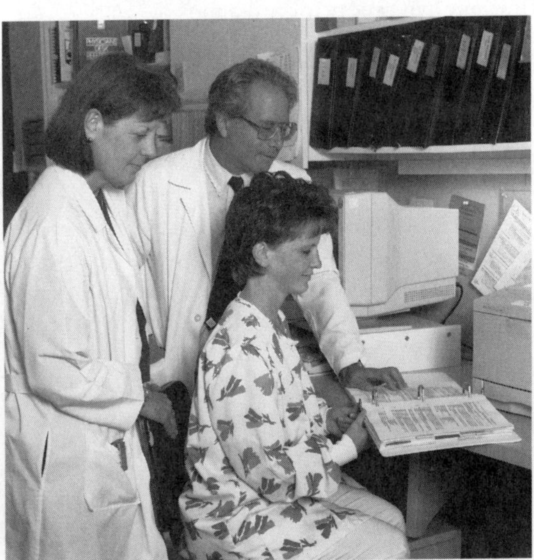

Figure 40–1
The research team—research coordinator, physician, and medical assistant.

biology, end results, causes, and potential prevention of the diseases being studied. It seeks to help obtain definitive answers to significant therapeutic questions about improved strategies for specific diseases.

Some **protocols** require review centers to provide central review of diagnostic pathology specimens and radiation films; provide a quality-control check in ascertaining patient diagnosis and eligibility for the protocols; and verify conformance to the guidelines set out in the appropriate protocol. Treatment protocols are step-by-step instructions for treating specific disease categories. All participants follow these protocols when treating eligible patients. All physicians at the participating sites or centers are expected to adhere to the protocol as closely as possible to increase the likelihood that the data gathered are usable and correct. Protocols can be therapeutic as well as nontherapeutic. They have specific aims to gather all data and answer the study question. The coordinator is an integral part of this.

There are many areas in clinical research trials open to a research coordinator. Job descriptions vary widely. Those working in a private clinic, for instance, may have duties that include administration, regulatory affairs, data entry, and patient care relating to studies that may involve totally different specialty areas. Others may have duties that concentrate on data quality control or eligibility concerns. Each type of employer, whether large or small, industry or academia, must develop individualized educational and experience requirements for its own needs.

Certain personality traits consistently lend themselves to this profession, including a tendency toward perfectionism, persistence, and a love of detail. Skills and knowledge are transferable from one specialty or job description to another, with a reasonable amount of additional education or training. Daily changes in health care and increases in the amount of necessary knowledge require constant learning and expansion of horizons to keep up with the new aspects of varied clinical trials. The types of positions, multiple disease sites, and protocol types vary from protocol to protocol. The main involvement for the coordinator lies in capturing data and coordinating the total protocol and its workings.

For any pharmaceutical protocols (**clinical trials** of new drugs), a study procedure manual is provided by the pharmaceutical company. The study procedure manual is a supplement to the protocol and **case report forms** (**CRF**) for a specific study. It provides guidelines and instructions to assist study personnel in implementing the protocol and must be used in concert with the protocol and with regulatory guidelines that govern good clinical research practices. The manual consists of a series of independent sections. This design allows revisions to relevant sections to be made in the event of amendments to the protocol or changes in management of the study. It also allows distribution only of relevant sections to individual members of the study team.

Whenever changes are made to the manual, revised sections are distributed to all study team members who hold copies of those sections. Copies of all versions of the procedures manual must be retained in the study file. There is constant contact between study personnel at the site and at the pharmaceutical company. Periodic site visits are scheduled at a frequency appropriate to the rate of **patient accrual.** These visits are estimated to be every 8 to 12 weeks for 2 to 3 days. During the site visits, the **study monitor** will:

1. Confirm the presence of signed **informed consent forms** for each patient
2. Review CRFs for logic, consistency, completeness, correctness, legibility, and compliance with the protocol
3. Verify CRF entries against the patients' medical records
4. Ensure the appropriate collection and reporting of **adverse experience** information
5. Inspect study files to confirm the presence of complete and appropriate study documentation
6. Review drug dispensing records to ensure proper management and documentation of the study drug
7. Check the adequacy of the study drug and other supplies
8. Check the status of study-specific lab serum samples, if appropriate

9. Meet with investigators and other study site personnel to discuss the progress of the study and any new or unresolved issues

Study site personnel contact the study monitor assigned to the site to obtain clarification about study conduct for case report form completion or to report clinically relevant information. Examples include the following:

- **Randomization**
- Entry of a new patient
- **Serious adverse experiences**
- Patient death
- Pending shipment of study drug or plasma samples

A research coordinator coordinates anywhere from four to six trials with pharmaceutical companies at any given time. The coordinator works directly with **clinical research associates** and managers nationwide.

On a local basis, the coordinator works directly with physicians, technicians, other research coordinators, research assistants, and all those involved directly or indirectly with the patient's care–including the patient. It is an excellent opportunity to participate actively in a team effort in every sense of the word. The coordinator is involved in patient education, and directly and indirectly involved with visits with trial participants. Numerous opportunities for professional as well as personal growth are afforded.

The coordinator works with the physician directly in screening a patient for research trial participation. All **inclusion/exclusion criteria** are gone through carefully and documented before a patient is even presented with the consent form and the feasibility of participation. The coordinator may present the consent form, with the physician answering study-related questions. Once a patient is entered on study, the coordinator follows a study flow sheet, interacting with all members of a medical team–informing them of assessments required by the protocol (e.g., physicians, lab personnel, medical assistants, radiology personnel, appointment secretaries, and others). Even if a patient on study is hospitalized, the follow-through and assessment required per protocol are carried out by the coordinator for the duration of the study, whether it be in a clinic setting, hospital setting, or outreach.

An example of professional growth would be the ongoing necessity to learn the basics about whatever disease a research protocol involves. When abstracting the data, the medical record is used and the research coordinator invariably "digs" for more information. Constants on a coordinator's desk are the drug handbooks, medical dictionary, the **Merck Manual**, and a lab reference handbook, as well as other resources.

In the area of personal growth, the opportunity to work independently yet interact on a one-on-one basis with patients, their families, and the medical team is afforded. The U.S. Food and Drug Administration (**FDA**) and the DHHS are the enforcing agencies that regulate the conduct of research. An **institutional review board** (**IRB**) in the institution practicing research is mandated by regulation of both the FDA and DHHS. Any research in an institution that deals with human **subjects**, whether patients or any other population group, must have the approval of the IRB. A research committee is also needed to serve as the reviewing body for all investigative or biomedical projects, grants, or contracts that use resources in a medical complex. Projects are reviewed for adequacy of scientific design, appropriateness of requested funding, and scientific merit of the proposal.

The coordinator is involved in a wide variety of activities. These include regulatory and administrative responsibilities. They also entail indirect and direct patient contact, indirect and direct protocol management, and multiple administrative activities, both internally and externally.

Health Unit Coordinator Knowledge and Skills

There are many areas of expertise in the research coordinator position that a health unit coordinator (HUC) would possess. These include a working knowledge of the medical record, a knowledge of medical terminology, and familiarity with drug names and abbreviations and their uses.

Computer skills are a requirement of the job in most instances. Much of the data and records is stored electronically. Patient records also are frequently stored in computers. The coordinator must be able to access these data.

In addition, the research coordinator must be able to organize, manage priorities, and have analytical skills. The ability to problem solve is essential. Flexibility and the ability to manage stress are skills the HUC has had many opportunities to practice. The handling of confidential information is equally important in the two positions.

Because the research coordinator deals with people from all areas of the medical environment, and especially patients, good interpersonal skills and good communication skills, including telephone skills, are vital. The HUC has had experience in all of these areas.

Additional Training Required

A post-high school education in science-related fields with a firm record of continuing education in science, health care, or research fields is desirable. A HUC or medical assistant certification is preferred. Work experience as a HUC for 3 to 5 years is a real asset, along with experience in multiple disciplines. Knowledge of two or more disease-specific areas is also helpful.

Ongoing education includes training sponsored by the pharmaceutical companies involved in the protocols. When a new protocol is initiated, the pharmaceutical company usually has an initiation meeting. At this meeting, a coordinator meets coordinators from all the sites that are participating in the study, both nationally and internationally. New techniques in computer data entry may be learned, along with specifics regarding a research protocol—for example, the study objectives, the overall investigational study design, treatment assignments, expected toxicities, and the collection of lab samples. On-site training is done for every protocol initiated by the clinical research associates from the participating pharmaceutical companies. Ongoing training through seminars and workshops is also provided. Advanced curriculum programs are offered for coordinators through Duke University. A certification program is encouraged strongly, but is not yet mandatory. Attendance at conferences and other continuing education offerings is encouraged.

Closing Thoughts

Research coordination enables you to be a part of a multidisciplinary team. It is very exciting and challenging to be able to participate in evaluating regimens for prevention and treatment of specific diseases. It offers the opportunity to help obtain definitive answers to significant therapeutic questions about improved strategies for specific diseases. Through research coordination, treatment and survival rates are improved and cures of specific diseases are discovered. Compiling data at participating institutions and readying the data for monitoring, evaluation, and analysis is a daily part of the job. The ability to interact and communicate effectively with physicians, researchers, medical complex staff, and pharmaceutical representatives is a must.

During my years as a clinical research coordinator, I have found the position to be a constant learning experience. Each day brings new challenges and opens up new opportunities. I find it a very rewarding and fulfilling position, in all respects.

Review Questions

1. Explain what a protocol is and why protocols are used in research studies.
2. List the varied duties of a research coordinator.
3. Name five areas of interest that may be studied in a rural research center.
4. Identify the two government departments that enforce the regulations that apply to research.

Residential Assisted Living Home

41

Winona Hardy

Common Abbreviations

AARP American Association of Retired People

ADL Activities of daily living

ALF Assisted living facility

CBRF Community-based residential facility

RALF Residential assisted living facility

RALH Residential assisted living home

RCF Residential care facility

Objectives

Upon completion of this chapter, the reader should be able to:

1. Discuss the purpose of residential assisted living homes.
2. List six other titles by which residential assisted living homes may be known.
3. Identify three positions available to health unit coordinators in residential assisted living homes.

Vocabulary

Hospitality: Cordial and generous reception of guests

Oversight: Supervision

Supportive: To keep from failing during stress

History

Many refer to residential assisted living homes as the "new kid on the block," whereas in reality they have been around for many years. Originally, they were a resource for poor homeless people in Europe. The care homes in the United States came into being years later. Before World War II in the United States, they served the widow well, as a source of income after a husband's death. Before nursing homes were introduced, a widow with empty bedrooms could care for two or three elderly in her home. The "homes" were family oriented, with no documentation needed. No special title was given to these care homes. Their function was based on a social model with personal care and housekeeping provided and **oversight** of the residents' medical needs. Women's organizations contributed time and money to these care homes for their social needs. It was a neighborhood or village project.

What is a residential assisted living home (**RALH**)? In the age of technology and communication, the home care of yesteryear has developed into a complete array of services. The controls imposed by licensing requirements, legal pitfalls, and the movement to an industry have made it a business first and a care home second. This change of focus has created the need for documentation, not only for reimbursement purposes but to prove the financial value of its very existence.

Introduction

In a normal life cycle, we come into this world dependent, develop to independence, then move to a stage of needing some assistance, and back to dependency.

It is in the stage between total independence and becoming totally dependent again that we move into a phase of needing more assistance managing our lives. It is at this time of life that we need to make a change in our environment. If 24-hour nursing service and constant medical care are not needed, residential assisted living is the appropriate bridge between independence and dependence.

Residential assisted living can provide that quality of life we all want to hold onto for as long as possible. It is an environment that allows for independence, within the scope of reality, and a maintenance of dignity, which is the true measure of quality of life for this stage in the life cycle.

The function of the RALH is to provide the help where help is needed and to allow the person to function without interference when help is not needed. It is also of prime importance that residents be encouraged to do as much for themselves as possible. When we take away people's independence unnecessarily, we have stolen a piece of their dignity. If a person needs help buttoning a button, then provide that help; however, if a zipper is easier to use, then make the effort to find the clothing articles that have zippers, thus restoring independence and dignity. All needs must be addressed, and where no solutions are possible it is our responsibility to be the residents' hands, ears, eyes, and "artificial brain."

People headed to dependency can often be maintained in an environment of **supportive** independence by just relieving the stress and anxiety of housekeeping and the pressure of taking their medications appropriately. A little help with bathing, eating, dressing, or some other activity of daily living (**ADL**) function can make the difference in how people live their everyday lives. Relieving a simple task that has become a burden can make the difference in whether someone lives a life defined by sickness or by wellness. In the RALH, helping someone with a need is normal, and allowing them to help themselves with minimal assistance is also normal. Keeping a person as independent as possible is the mission of an RALH.

The ever-present loneliness can be the breaking point for many people. Loneliness is a divisive existence that creates an environment of suspicion, fear, and divorce from reality, and often times brings about the separation of family and friends. The saying, "an idle mind is a devil's workshop," certainly bears truth in a lonely environment. An RALH offers a living environment that creates an extended family bond surrounded by daily reality. The residents miss their own families and friends. This loss is noted less as time is occupied by activities in the new environment. The RALH allows for independence, freedom, and privacy of space while giving the caring and knowledge that is needed so that the resident will not shrink from the daily rhythm of life. The RALH can provide the extended family environment that maintains the feeling of "I'm in charge," "I have a reason to wake up each morning," and the excitement of expectation. The social rhythm of a normal lifestyle becomes the reason for living.

In an RALH, it is important that the person's medical needs are met in a normal pattern of a family environment, not a medical environment. It is interesting to note that we are often asked what is meant by a family environment but seldom asked what is meant by a medical environment. Is it because we are unsure of what is meant by family, or are we afraid we are going to lose a piece of our past, question our present, and fear our future? A family environment should mean the equality of a lifestyle within the scope of love, kindness, politeness, and caring for each other, with the head of the family in charge of the structure of the functions within the family. Therefore, family means a group of people united in a cause, who do not need to be related. That is why this level of care can be a difficult environment to maintain. Medical needs can sometimes be overwhelming, especially when the medical discipline dictates precise procedure. The RALH can get caught between providing the necessary care in a manner consistent with good medical practice while at the same time trying to maintain the "extended family" environment. Functioning in a manner that meets regulation requirements and avoiding legal pitfalls can be demanding. In today's tort-crazy world, the RALH must always beware of the distortion of facts. Documentation is essential to the well-being of an RALH if it is called on to prove what was done or not done in a situation adverse or otherwise. Training in how to document facts is extremely important. Here is where a health unit coordinator (HUC) has experience that is transferable and valuable to the RALH work environment.

All of this is essential for the protection of the independence and dignity of the resident, while meeting medical and personal needs. The difference in the environments between the RALH, a social model, and a medical institution lies in the primary focus on daily living. In the medical environment, the primary focus is on the medical needs first and quality of life second. In a social environment, wellness and an active lifestyle are encouraged within the reality of each individual's capabilities. This means placing the emphasis on a wellness quality of life rather than a sick lifestyle. The medical needs are addressed in the daily activities in a more general way and are not the primary reason for the day's activities. The medical needs are met to ensure that the social needs can be enjoyed, thus promoting a good quality of life. In an RALH, independence and dignity are offered first and foremost, but provision of medical care must be a solid part of the home's caregiving philosophy, while remaining a largely invisible component (Fig. 41–1).

Description of Facility

In terms of size and space, many of the large residential assisted living facilities are difficult to differentiate from nursing homes. For the purposes of this chapter, smaller homes will be described.

Many of the smaller homes are large family

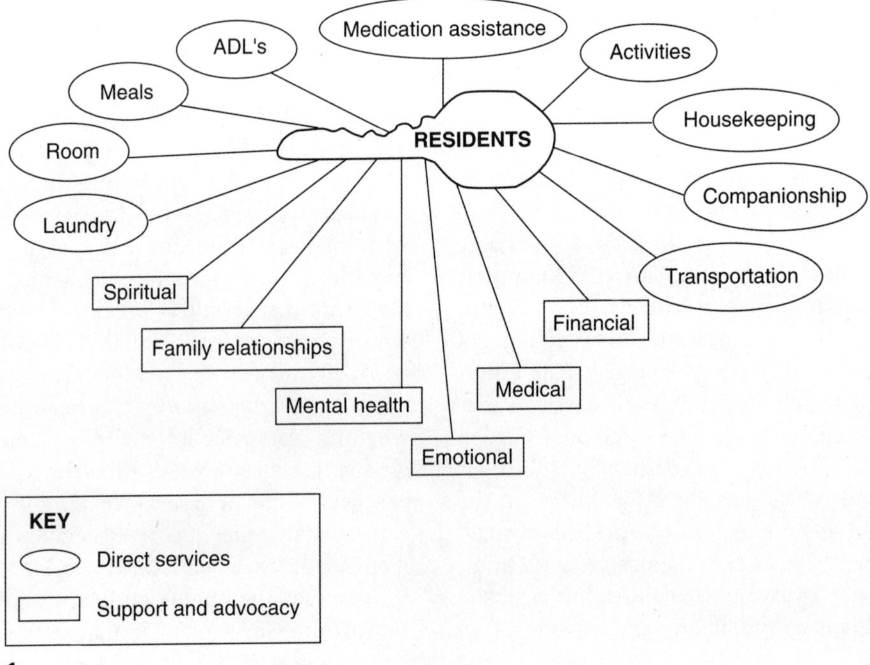

Figure 41–1
Chart showing services.

homes or farms that have been remodeled to meet the needs of the RALH. The renovations must also bring the homes into compliance with fire codes at the state and local levels.

Typically, there is an office area for the administrator and his or her assistant or manager. There is a kitchen, group dining area, and common living/family room (Fig. 41–2). The resident rooms may be private or shared companion rooms (Fig. 41–3). In some homes, each room has a bath, but in the homes occupying older houses, bathrooms are shared. A locked area is designated for the storage of medications and medical supplies needed by the residents. Residents who have physician orders to that effect may store and administer their own medications, but they must be stored in a locked box of some type.

In some homes, residents are given the choice of using the furniture provided by the home or bringing their own in from home. Every effort is made to decorate the rooms and the building as a whole in as "homey" a style as possible.

Some homes may be required to have a sprinkler system; all homes must have an electrical wired alarm system that alerts the residents and staff in case of heat or smoke. Reliable heating, plumbing, and electrical systems are musts for the comfort of the residents. The licensed homes are required to meet the federal life safety code and regulations of their respective states and cities or towns.

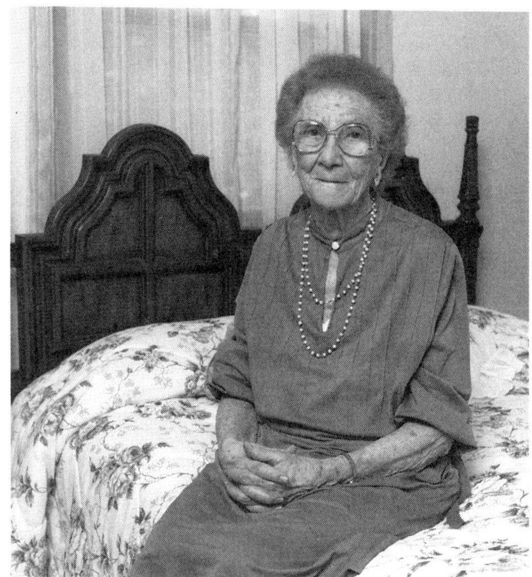

Figure 41–3
Bedroom.

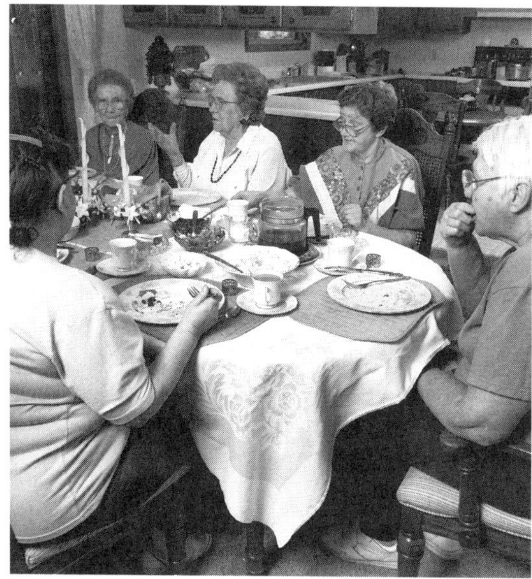

Figure 41–2
Community dining area.

Staffing

The staff of a small RALH is usually cross trained between core positions. The typical positions are:

Primary caregiver (residential care technician), a core staff member who is responsible for assisting the residents with their ADLs, reminding about and assisting with medications, assisting with snacks and meals, assisting with toileting when necessary, and doing exercises and other activities. It is not unusual in quiet periods to see the caregivers playing cards, reading, and doing crafts and other projects with the residents.

Cook, a core staff member who prepares the meals according to a meal plan. The cook also prepares snacks and is responsible for the cleanliness of the kitchen area and equipment.

Housekeeper, a core staff member who is responsible for the cleanliness of the home and small items of upkeep. Does resident laundry.

House manager, who is responsible for the day-to-day resident care. Often responsible for medication inventory and ordering. Schedules and arranges transportation for resident medical and other appointments. Plans structured activities.

Administrator, who is responsible for all aspects of the day-to-day running of the business. May be called on to fill in for others in an urgent situation.

Related Terminology

Names or labels used to identify RALHs can be numerous, confusing, and unhelpful in defining services offered. Therefore, we have to examine each home for its true purpose and services offered regardless of the title being used. Examples of titles used for facilities that provide similar services are:

Group home
Foster care home
Assisted living facility **(ALF)**
Community-based residential facility **(CBRF)**
Personal care home
Residential care facility **(RCF)**
Residential assisted living facility **(RALF)**
Residential assisted living home (RALH)

and approximately 27 similar titles. Within the past 10 years, the American Association of Retired People **(AARP)** conducted a survey and found that there were over 100 terms used nationwide to describe this level of care, so you can see that progress is being made toward standardization.

Use of Health Unit Coordinator Terminology

In an RALH, medical care is of prime importance to the resident's longevity and quality of life. Knowledge about a medical condition and restrictions of certain conditions are extremely important to the residents and their families. Understanding the individual's condition medically and mentally is important to the care of the resident. Knowing when residents are expressing themselves in the world of reality or their world of psychosis is necessary for the caregivers, family, and friends, in order to respond appropriately. An HUC has the experience, knowledge, and expertise to explain, in lay language, medical conditions to a resident and family. If not explained properly, to a resident's level of understanding, a simple medical condition could lead to a life of dependency. Knowing medical terms and being able to explain them to the residents in language they can understand can make the difference between crippling fear and the understanding and acceptance of one's condition. Fear can be more devastating to a person than a medical condition itself.

Health unit coordinators have medical knowledge and some observational experience of many medical conditions. They can realistically discuss a person's condition with other medical professionals, staff members, family members, and residents. As an employee of the home, and someone the resident trusts and sees daily, the HUC can answer questions on a continuing basis. When medical personnel are not available or the resident feels uncomfortable asking them questions, the HUC could be available to help relieve the stress and anxiety related to not knowing what is being said. Examples of this are the resident asking "what did so and so mean when they said such and such?", and "does that mean I am going to die?" Taking the time to explain something in understandable words not only relieves stress and anxiety but helps to maintain a healthy environment.

In the relationship between the RALH and the medical system, there is a need for someone who can communicate in language of medicine. For examples, see Table 41–1.

Table 41–1 TYPES OF COMMUNICATION IN A RESIDENTIAL ASSISTED LIVING HOME

Communication With	Types of Communication
Hospitals	Giving admission report Discussing discharge plan
Physician	Reporting illnesses and incidents Answering questions about symptoms
Home health agency	Reporting illnesses, incidents Communicating physician orders Reporting resident progress or lack of it
Dentists	Describing conditions
Podiatrists	Describing conditions Describing gaits
Pharmacist	Replenishing medications Checking inventory Describing side effects
Mental health professionals	Facilitating appointments Reporting behavior changes

Types of Positions Available for Health Unit Coordinators

Primary Caregiver

Knowledge, like a river, is a natural stream of information. HUCs have knowledge and experience in many overlapping areas. Some HUCs have been cross trained in the nurse's aide or assistant position. This cross training makes the HUC well qualified as the primary care giver in an RALH. Although regulations may not require a licensed certified nurse assistant, much of the training received in a certified nurse assistant course is needed and used in the personal care given in an RALH. Cross-trained HUCs would understand the individual care needs of those in their charge.

For many people employed in the assisted living field, the position of primary caregiver is the first step on the ladder to advancement. It is possible that HUC skills could be used in other aspects of the business at the same time, in a combined position.

House Manager

Many HUCs have management responsibilities on their units. They take care of scheduling, purchasing, networking, and other duties that make a hospital unit run smoothly. These same skills are important and necessary in an RALH.

Training new employees is of primary importance to teamwork, decreasing turnover, and delivering good services. An HUC has had the experience of training and precepting new employees and working as a team member. This knowledge and experience is of great importance in a managerial position such as assistant administrator or house manager in an RALH.

The ability to be creative is helpful in scheduling activities inside and outside the RALH. The person doing this type of planning must know the capabilities and interests of the various residents to ensure a well rounded program that meets everyone's needs (Fig. 41–4).

The transition from a medical environment that promotes dependency to a nonmedical environment promoting independence may be the most difficult task a HUC would face. A complete change in attitude can be difficult. However, HUCs should feel comfortable in bringing with them the technical knowledge and experience that allows them to be more relaxed while becoming oriented to the new environment.

Administrator

Many HUCs are well prepared to accept the position of administrator in a small home. A HUC has the experience of living within the constraints of regulations and the exact documentation of a Joint Commission on the Accreditation of

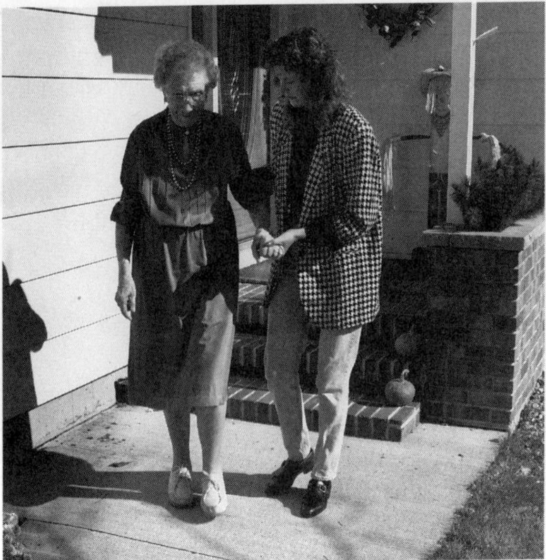

Figure 41–4
Going out to activities.

Healthcare Organizations (JCAHO) review. Some are aware of insurance, Medicaid, and Medicare reimbursement. All of the HUC skills and others are necessary to prepare a home to be in compliance on the unannounced annual inspections. A home may be inspected only once a year by a state agency, but it is important that the home be in compliance 365 days a year. Maintaining records and keeping operations of the home in daily compliance are important to the many informal inspections that occur daily. Family members are in the home often, as well as health care regulatory agencies who are reviewing every aspect of a home's operation. Homes are not in operation for annual inspection but to provide the best of care every day of the year.

Ongoing training of staff is the link that keeps the services flowing smoothly. One area of training that is extremely important and often forgotten is **hospitality**. If staff members are not trained in the aspects of hospitality, a financially rewarding client may be lost. This kind of lost revenue can never be retrieved. Staff needs to be made aware that lost revenue could be their raise or even their job. RALHs are in the hospitality business, even though it may not be advertised or thought of as such.

Being an administrator means taking charge of all aspects of the operation. A HUC is the "glue" that holds it all together on the unit; the administrator plays that role in the RALH. HUC background and training meet many of the requirements for the administrator position.

The educational requirement to be an administrator in a large home is usually a bachelor's degree or some college credits and several years of experience in health care. In the smaller homes, the educational requirements usually are somewhat less. High school diploma, GED, and years of experience in a health care field may satisfy the requirements for the small homes. HUCs meet these requirements, so they certainly may be ideal candidates for an administrator position.

Finally, HUCs have the temperament and experience to function through a crisis, an important trait for an administrator.

Health Unit Coordinator Knowledge and Skills Appropriate to Positions

Computer Skills

The documentation of all services offered and delivered in an RALH is crucial today and will be even more so in the future, as managed care exerts its influence at this level of care. Using computers to record information is becoming a must.

Organizational Skills

Health unit coordinators bring organizational skills necessary for the smooth operation of a home. A hospital unit depends on an organized operation to keep running smoothly; the HUC's skills define the operation and how it is maintained. All of these skills are necessary in an RALF. An HUC who wishes to become an employee of an RALF can be miles ahead of someone who needs extensive training in these skills.

Communication Skills

Verbal communication skills are essential. The person employed by the RALH will be communicating with:

Peers
State officials
Home health workers
Pharmacists
Physicians
Employer
Families
Residents

A different level of communication is required for each of these. It is paramount to be able to listen as well as speak clearly and to get feedback to be sure the communication loop is complete.

As the need for more accurate documentation overflows into the RALH industry, the use of electronic communication systems becomes mandatory. Today, if you do not have a fax machine to communicate with doctors and pharmacies, it can cause delays in the provision of timely medical treatment and the availability of medications.

The telephone is a major form of communication in the RALH. The same courtesy practiced in the hospital is required here.

Confidentiality

As previously mentioned, the assisted living industry has become regulated by state entities. The same rules of confidentiality of information apply here. Information must be given only to the appropriate people, and much of it only with the resident's permission.

Disposal of paper documents that contain resident information should be done by shredding. However, it is important to note that resident records must be maintained for a minimum of 7 years. Therefore, extreme care must be taken when disposing of any documentation. If in doubt, *do not* dispose.

Additional Training

Orientation

The orientation to an RALH includes the usual introduction to the facility, policies, philosophy, mission, benefits, job descriptions, work schedule, and more. Inasmuch as HUCs need to have a complete understanding of the services offered in their hospitals, so too must the employee of an RALH. For example, the staff of an RALH needs to understand the accommodations offered in the home:

Is it a shared bathroom arrangement?
If so, how many people per bathroom?
Are the rooms companion rooms or are they private rooms?
What activities are offered?
Is there an extra charge for transportation?
Are special diets offered?
What, if any medical care is offered?

These are questions that might be asked by families or potential residents interested in placement, state inspectors, home health agency workers, or other people involved in the industry. Each day is an opportunity for marketing the RALH.

Resident Assessment

It is vital to the successful operation of an RALH that an honest assessment of the potential resident to be admitted to the home be made before acceptance. If the home does not have the capability to care for a person for any reason, the home must not accept the person. Assessments are made before admission, shortly after admission, and periodically during the resident's stay. This ensures that the home can meet the resident's needs on an ongoing and often changing basis.

In many areas, there is training available to teach the employees of an RALH to use an assessment tool. HUCs are already aware of the importance of accurate assessments, and with this training are well qualified to maintain the resident' current assessment.

Continuing Education

Training for caregivers and administrators must be ongoing. Several states have regulations mandating certain amounts of required continuing education. Typical target areas for continuing education programs are:

Behavior management
Resident services plan of care
Business
Marketing
Licensing requirements
Electronic technology
Documentation
Hospitality
Social versus medical model

Continuing education courses are offered by several different sources. Some training may be offered by professional training agencies; some by trade associations; others by colleges. It is important that the employees of an RALH maintain a resource library to assist with accessing the training that is available to meet their needs and further their professional growth.

Closing Thoughts

Although a HUC has many areas of expertise and could specialize using any of their many skills, I know of nowhere where all of a HUC's skills can be better used than in an RALH. The tools and skills HUCs use in their daily routine are all used in an RALH.

An RALH can be more subdued and gentle in nature than a hospital, but at times can also be demanding and challenging. Understanding the doctors' routine and a hospital's routine is an advantage. This knowledge certainly could promote a better relationship between the RALH and the doctor or hospital in times of need. Given that HUCs have the experience of how to communicate with families during adverse times, they have the instincts and knowledge to work with families who feel guilt and uncertainty about their decision to leave the care of their loved one to a stranger in an RALH.

Health unit coordinators can pitch their numerous and diversified skills to the many job opportunities in an RALH. At this time, when managed care is becoming the centerpiece for health care, the need for the HUC's well rounded knowledge and experience becomes even more important. Although HUCs' extensive area of experience gives them the tools and skills to perform many jobs in an RALH, salary may be a concern. Most RALHs are small and cash flow may limit their ability to be highly competitive with salary and benefits. The rewards are many and varied when working with a particular group. It is up to you, the HUC, to know what group you would find to your liking. Whether it is adolescents, elderly, mental health, or developmentally disabled, it is your decision.

Review Questions

1. Discuss the purpose of residential assisted living homes.
2. List six other titles by which residential assisted living homes may be known.
3. Identify three positions available to HUCs in residential assisted living homes.

Bibliography

American Heritage Dictionary. New York, Dell Publishing Group, 1989.
Bridges B: Therapeutic Caregiving. Millcreek, WA, BJB Publishing, 1995.
Cox H: Aging, 5th ed. Guilford, CT, Dushkin Publishing Group, 1987.

SECTION FOUR

CLINICAL CODING

42 Overview of Clinical Coding

Lou Ann Schraffenberger

Common Abbreviations

APACHE Acute Physiology and Chronic Health Evaluation

CPT-4 Current Procedural Terminology, Fourth Edition

DRG Diagnosis-Related Groups

DSM-IV Diagnostic and Statistical Manual of Mental Disorders, Fourth Edition

HCFA Health Care Finance Administration

HCPCS HCFA Common Procedure Coding System

ICD-9-CM International Classification of Diseases, Ninth Revision, Clinical Modification

ICD-O International Classification of Diseases, Oncology

NCHS National Center for Health Statistics

SNOMED Systematized Nomenclature of Human and Veterinary Medicine International

SNOP Systematized Nomenclature of Pathology

Objectives

Upon completion of this chapter, the reader should be able to:

1. Explain the difference between a nomenclature system and a classification system.
2. List the major types of coding used in health care settings.
3. Identify the settings in which an ICD-9-CM coding system would be used.
4. State the purposes of coding.

Vocabulary

Classification: An arrangement of elements of a subject into groups according to pre-established criteria

Nomenclature: Systematic listing of proper names

Prospective payment: A system that pays the hospital in advance for a patient's treatment based on the DRG to which the patient has been assigned.

Introduction

Overview

Clinical coders have an important responsibility to assign codes that best describe the diagnosis and procedures performed by the physicians. This chapter describes the business of clinical coding and what a health care practitioner needs to know to become a competent, skilled clinical coder.

Clinical Coding Defined

Clinical coding can be described as transforming words into numbers. In health care, this means that long and complicated narrative descriptions of a patient's illness or procedures can be translated into a three- to five-digit numeric sequence. Codes simplify the descriptions and make them more manageable.

Types of Coding Systems

There are a variety of coding systems or organizations of code numbers. Basically, coding systems are of two types: **nomenclature** or **classification** systems (Table 42–1).

Nomenclature System

A nomenclature is a systematic listing of proper names. A disease or procedure nomenclature is a listing of the proper name or title of a disease or procedure. A disease or procedure nomenclature's purpose is to provide a uniform language that correctly describes the condition or treatment. Each disease or procedure is given its own unique number. Using the code number, instead of the medical words, allows for reliable communication between health care practitioners and external users of the information. Words can mean different things to different people. Using the codes from a nomenclature allows everyone to understand the same message. Examples of nomenclatures are the Systematized Nomenclature of Human and Veterinary Medicine International (SNOMED) and the Physicians' Current Procedural Terminology, Fourth Edition (CPT-4).

Table 42–1 NOMENCLATURE VERSUS CLASSIFICATION SYSTEM

Nomenclature	Classification
A systematic listing of proper names	An arrangement of elements of a subject into groups according to pre-established criteria

Classification System

A classification system is an arrangement of the elements of a subject into groups according to pre-established criteria. In a disease classification system, diseases and injuries are arranged into appropriate chapters, sections, categories, and subcategories. To facilitate analysis, a classification system must limit its size and maintain its ability to collapse or summarize to a small number of related groups or expand as needed. The system must provide a place within the classification for all diseases and injuries, even when each disease or injury cannot be identifiable by a separate code number. Specific disease entities are given separate titles and code numbers because of their importance or their frequent occurrence. Other conditions of less importance as causes of morbidity or mortality are grouped together in categories often labeled "other" or "not elsewhere classified."

Diagnoses not stated specifically enough to permit precise classification are often grouped together in categories labeled "unspecified." There is only one place to classify each disease or injury. Each category and subcategory in a classification system must be mutually exclusive.

A classification system is somewhat like a sorting system. Think of a disease classification system as a storage area with a large number of sorting bins. When preparing to store items, a person must remember "a place for everything and everything in its place." When a diagnosis comes in to be sorted (or coded), it is put in the appropriate bin depending on the type of disease. Cardiovascular diseases are sorted together. Obstetric conditions are sorted together. This sorting is very important when a person has to go back into the storage area and find something, such as all of the cardiovascular conditions or all the obstetric conditions. To determine how many of these conditions are stored, the sorter must be certain that all diagnoses are in their proper place or the sorting will be useless.

An example of a widely used classification system is the International Classification of Diseases, Ninth Revision, Clinical Modification (**ICD-9-CM**). Every diagnosis and procedure imaginable can be sorted, classified, or coded with ICD-9-CM. Every diagnosis or procedure has one unique code number that either describes that condition explicitly or that groups it together with similar vague or ill-defined conditions.

Major Types of Coding Schemes

There are a number of coding schemes available for use in health care, but the major systems are the ICD-9-CM, CPT-4, and Health Care Finance Administration (**HCFA**) Common Procedure Coding System (**HCPCS**).

ICD-9-CM

The ICD-9-CM contains approximately 10,000 codes describing diseases and procedures. ICD-9-CM codes consist of three, four, or five digits (Table 42–2). Diagnosis codes describe a patient's disease or condition. In the absence of a confirmed diagnosis, the patient's complaints or physical signs and symptoms may be coded. ICD-9-CM also contains procedure codes. These may include surgical operations, diagnostic and therapeutic invasive procedures, and noninvasive procedures, including radiology and other examinations. All hospitals and almost every other health care provider use ICD-9-CM to code patients' diagnoses and conditions. The procedure codes from ICD-9-CM, however, are almost exclusively used for in-patients in hospitals. Other health care providers are more likely to use CPT-4 to code procedures.

Table 42–2 SAMPLE ICD-9-CM DIAGNOSIS CODES

Code	Diagnosis
650	Normal delivery
540.0	Acute appendicitis with generalized peritonitis
414.01	Coronary atherosclerosis of native coronary artery

The responsibility for keeping ICD-9-CM current and up to date rests with two federal agencies. The National Center for Health Statistics (**NCHS**) is responsible for changes to the disease classification. The HCFA is responsible for updates to the procedure classification. ICD-9-CM is revised annually with new codes becoming effective each October 1. The ICD has been totally rewritten approximately every 10 years. ICD-9-CM was issued in 1979, so its revision is overdue. The Tenth Edition of ICD is expected between the years 2000 and 2002. It will likely be known as ICD-10-CM.

CPT-4

CPT-4 is a systematic listing of procedure descriptions and the code for procedures and services performed by physicians. Each procedure or service is identified by a five-digit numeric code (Table 42–3). CPT-4 contains the codes and a description or title for approximately 7000 services and procedures.

Hospitals are required for Medicare reporting purposes to code all outpatient procedures performed for Medicare beneficiaries with CPT-4. Hospitals may elect to use CPT-4 for other outpatient procedures and services. It is not likely that hospital in-patients will be coded with CPT. CPT-4 is required for most insurance companies, including Medicare, for the reporting of services. Physicians, ambulatory surgery centers, home health agencies, as well as many other health care providers use CPT-4 for billing of their services.

Table 42–3 SAMPLE CPT-4 PROCEDURE CODES

Section Numbers and Sequences	Procedure Codes
99201–99499	Evaluation and Management
00100–01999 and 99100–99140	Anesthesiology
10040–69979	Surgery
70010–79999	Radiology
80049–89399	Pathology and Laboratory
90700–99199	Medicine

CPT-4 is the property of the American Medical Association (AMA). A new revision of CPT-4 is published every year with the changes effective January 1. Each year, CPT-4 codes may be added, deleted, or have their descriptions modified. The AMA has a CPT Editorial Panel that oversees the ongoing development of the coding systems. The Editorial Panel is composed of 14 physician members representing major physician specialty groups. Two advisory groups provide input into the process. The CPT Advisory Committee comprises 60 physicians representing almost every medical and surgical specialty. The second group is the Health Care Professionals Advisory Committee, which consists of allied health professionals who use CPT for billing purposes. Members of this second group include podiatrists, occupational therapists, physical therapists, chiropractic physicians, and optometrists, as well as others.

HCPCS

The HCPCS is a coding system developed and managed by the HCFA, a federal agency in the Social Security Administration. HCPCS is a coding system based on CPT-4 but supplemented with additional codes for nonphysician services. Although the acronym refers to the coding system that includes CPT-4, HCPCS is most frequently used to refer to National Level II and Local Level III codes (Table 42–4). With the HCPCS coding system, the supplies, medications, services, and equipment provided to Medicare and Medicaid patients can be specifically and accurately reported.

The HCPCS is actually three different coding schemes or levels. HCPCS Level I is the CPT-4 nomenclature produced by the AMA. Level II and Level III codes were created by Medicare to supplement CPT-4, because CPT-4 contains a minimal number of codes to describe supplies, medications, equipment, and other services provided to Medicare and Medicaid beneficiaries. HCPCS Level II is also called national codes. National codes are alphanumeric codes beginning with A through V followed by four numbers. There are over 2500 National Level II codes covering supplies, medications, materials, injections, durable medical equipment, prostheses, and a variety of other services reimbursed under the Medicare and Medicaid programs in most states. The codes and descriptions listed in HCPCS, which are intended to be consistent on a national basis, are generally consistent with contemporary practice defined by HCFA. The national codes are updated yearly by the HCFA central office in Baltimore, Maryland, and are available from the U.S. Superintendent of Documents and various health care publishers.

The HCPCS Level III codes are also known as Local codes. Each individual state's Medicare carrier develops state-specific codes intended for use only in that carrier's region. Like the national codes, local codes are alphanumeric. The range of HCPCS Level III codes is from W0000 to

Table 42–4 HCFA COMMON PROCEDURE CODING SYSTEM

Level	HCPCS
Level 1	CPT-4 nomenclature
Level 2	National codes
Level 3	Local codes

Z9999. Local codes are often used to describe new procedures, services, or supplies that are not listed in CPT-4 or National Level II codes, or are used to describe procedures and services which have been deleted from CPT-4, but which the local carrier still recognizes and reimburses. Level III codes are obtained from the state's Medicare carrier and are updated as needed throughout the year.

Other Types of Coding Schemes

DSM-IV

The *Diagnostic and Statistical Manual of Mental Disorders,* fourth edition (**DSM-IV**), is used primarily in psychiatric hospitals, community mental health centers, developmental/mental retardation centers, mental health units in acute care hospitals, and by individual psychiatrists and other mental health practitioners. It includes definitions and diagnostic criteria for mental disorders in addition to the code numbers. This system is derived from ICD and the structure of its codes is similar; however, some of the codes are six digits long, as opposed to the maximum five digits in ICD. The American Psychiatric Association develops and maintains DSM-IV. DSM-IV is used by mental health professionals to assign a diagnosis as well as by coders to assign a code. DSM-IV codes usually are not used for reimbursement purposes but rather for internal databases and statistical purposes.

SNOMED

SNOMED is developed and maintained by the American College of Pathologists. It is not related to ICD. SNOMED provides preferred medical terms in 11 units or modules, including topography; morphology; function; living organisms; chemicals, drugs and biologic products; physical agents, activities, and forces; occupation; social context; disease/diagnosis; procedures; and a general linkage-modifier. Coding a diagnosis with SNOMED may involve codes from one or more of the modules. SNOMED was originally developed to aid in the computerization of diseases and operative information. SNOMED was developed from an earlier system, the Systematized Nomenclature of Pathology (**SNOP**), also developed by the American College of Pathologists. SNOP had only four axes—topography, morphology, etiology, and function—and was used almost exclusively in pathology departments.

ICD-O

Another classification system derived from ICD is the International Classification of Diseases for Oncology (**ICD-O**). This system is developed and maintained by the World Health Organization and is used almost exclusively in cancer registries. This system is used to classify neoplasms according to their site, behavior, and morphology. Although similar to ICD, this system is much more specific for the coding of malignant tumors and diseases.

Case-Mix Systems and Severity-of-Illness Systems

Case-mix systems classify patients according to some common characteristics. Severity-of-illness systems try to judge the severity or seriousness of a patient's condition.

Diagnosis-Related Groups (**DRGs**) is the major case-mix system in use today. Used by Medicare to reimburse acute care hospitals for care rendered to Medicare beneficiaries, DRGs divide patients into groups according to the type of medical condition they had or the type of surgical procedure performed. Instead of paying the hospital bill with the individual charges for services rendered for the patient, the hospital is paid a set price according to the DRG assigned. There are over 500 different groups, each with a unique payment determined for the particular hospital delivering the care. The DRGs are determined by the ICD-9-CM diagnosis and procedure codes assigned to the individual patient and, depending on the DRG, the age and discharge status (alive or dead) of the patient. DRGs are referred to as a **prospective payment** system because the hospital knows in advance what exact dollar amount they will receive for a patient's care if they have assigned that patient to a particular DRG. The completeness and accuracy of the ICD-9-CM diagnosis and procedure codes are extremely important because the hospital's reimbursement by Medicare will be determined by the DRGs the codes create.

A new system called Refined DRGs is being developed. DRGs do not always account for the severity of a patient's illness. Apparently, this new system will take into consideration more precisely the patient's complications and co-existing conditions to better predict and reimburse the cost of the care for the Medicare patients.

Other systems not necessarily related to reimbursement directly are severity-of-illness systems. Disease staging is a severity measurement system that uses ICD-9-CM codes and divides patients into one of four severity levels. Patient management categories are based on ICD-9-CM diagnosis and procedures and are combined with patient management paths to outline efficient care and determine cost weights.

In the Atlas System (formerly called MedisGroups), the diagnosis of the patient is not considered. Instead, patients are assigned to a severity level based on key clinical findings from the history and physical examination, laboratory, radiology, and other information contained in the patient's record. Some states, such as Pennsylvania, have mandated the use of Atlas for the reporting of all hospital admissions data to a central state data agency.

The Acute Physiology and Chronic Health Evaluation (**APACHE**) was developed for use in intensive care units (ICU) to predict the severity of their patients' illnesses. It uses 12 physiologic measures, including laboratory findings, to determine a score for each patient adjusted for age, previous health status, and reason for admission to the ICU. Like Atlas, APACHE does not consider the patient's particular diagnosis.

Severity-of-illness systems do not determine hospital reimbursement, but instead allow the hospital to measure the resources needed to care for the type of patients in their particular facility or patient care unit in the facility.

Purposes of Coding

For a variety of reasons, codes describing a patient's condition can be stored, retrieved, and examined as needed. Some of the major reasons coding is done relate to the creation of databases, health care statistics, reimbursement, and peer review.

Purposes of Coding
Statistical Databases Reimbursement Peer Review

Statistical Databases

Health care facilities use the codes to create disease and operation databases so that information about the patients and the types of services rendered can be readily available. These internal databases are used by quality management, utilization review, medical research, and medical education staffs to fulfill their missions. External databases such as those at the U.S. Public Health Service use diagnosis and procedure codes to determine the leading causes of morbidity and mortality in the United States. Medical and social science researchers often use external databases as a basis for their studies of disease management and health care policy.

Reimbursement

Medicare and other insurance companies require diagnosis and procedure codes for insurance claims processing. Codes describe the patient and the treatment rendered to the insurance company. Codes paint a picture of the patient to the insurance company and describe what was done for the patient. Medicare and some other insurance plans pay hospitals based on DRGs. DRGs are determined primarily based on what diagnosis and procedure codes were assigned to the patient.

The wide variety of uses for diagnosis and procedure codes requires accurate code assignments.

Even if reimbursement is not affected, reporting an incorrect code may result in subsequent conclusions, based on the code, that are inaccurate about a patient or about what the provider did for the patient.

Peer Review

Using the coded information about a provider's individual patients and the aggregate data it produces, health care professionals can perform peer reviews of the type and quality of care rendered to patients. Physicians' practices can be compared by the types of diseases, patient lengths of stay, and cost of care using ICD-9-CM and CPT-4 codes. Improving the quality of health care and outcomes measurement are major areas of interest today in the health care industry. These types of activities depend on good-quality coded information about the patients served.

Closing Thoughts

Clinical coding is the transformation of patients' diagnoses and procedures into numerical descriptions. The coded data are used for a variety of important functions. Reimbursement, peer review processes, and medical databases depend on the accuracy and completeness of the coding performed. The HUC's knowledge of medical science, ability to work with computers, and attention to detail make a coding career a realistic pursuit. The next two chapters describe in detail the coding process and the knowledge and skills required of the clinical coder.

Review Questions

1. Explain the difference between a nomenclature system and a classification system.
2. List the major types of coding used in health care settings.
3. Identify the settings in which an ICD-9-CM coding system would be used.
4. State the purposes of coding.

Bibliography

Abdelhak M, Grostick S, Hanken M, et al: Health Information Management: Management of a Strategic Resource. Philadelphia, WB Saunders, 1996.

American Medical Association: Physicians' Current Procedural Terminology, 4th ed. Chicago, American Medical Association, 1997.

American Psychiatric Association: Diagnostic and Statistical Manual of Mental Disorders, 4th ed. Washington, DC, American Psychiatric Association, 1994.

Brown F: ICD-9-CM Coding Handbook with Answers: 1997 Revised Edition. Chicago, American Hospital Publishing, 1997.

Bryant G, Prophet S: Growing demand for accurate coded data in new healthcare delivery era. J Am Health Info Mgmt Assoc 1997;69:42–47.

Buck C: Step-by-Step Medical Coding. Philadelphia, WB Saunders, 1996.

Frawley K, Asmonga D: Health Insurance Portability and Accessibility Act addresses healthcare fraud and abuse. Journal of American Health Information Management Association 1996;67:10–11.

Hirschl N: A closer look at ambulatory patient groups. Journal of American Health Information Management Association 1996;67:22–25.

Huffman E: Health Information Management, 10th ed. Berwyn, IL, Physicians Record Company, 1994.

Nicholas T: Basic ICD-9-CM Coding Handbook. Chicago, American Health Information Management Association, 1997.

Nicholas T: CPT/HCPS Basic Coding Handbook. Chicago, American Health Information Management Association, 1997.

Prophet S: Fraud and abuse implications for the HIM professional. Journal of the American Health Information Management Association 1997;68:52–55.

Prophet S: Classification systems: taking a broader look. Journal of the American Health Information Management Association 1997;68:46–50.

Rogers V: Ambulatory patient groups: an outpatient data management tool. Journal of American Health Information Management Association 1996;67:56–59.

Rogers V: Ambulatory Surgery Coding. Chicago, American Health Information Management Association, 1996.

Rogers V: Intermediate ICD-9-CM Coding Handbook for Hospitals. Chicago, American Health Information Management Association, 1996.

U.S. Department of Health and Human Services: International Classification of Disease, 9th ed., Clinical Modification. Washington, DC, USDHHS, 1997.

43

The Coding Process

Lou Ann Schraffenberger

Common Abbreviations

APG Ambulatory patient group

EDI Electronic data interchange

RBRVS Resource-based relative value system

UHDDS Uniform hospital discharge data set

Objectives

At the completion of this chapter, the reader should be able to:

1. Explain the coding process in the in-patient setting.
2. List the various types of ambulatory care settings where the ICD-9-CM classification system would be used.
3. Discuss the importance of coding for reimbursement for health care services.
4. List the four measures used to determine the quality of coded data.

Vocabulary

Abstracting: Locating key demographic and clinical information about a patient in addition to the disease and operation codes and entering it into a computer

Electronic data interchange: A type of hardware and software configuration that allows for the submission, edit, or payment of health care insurance claims

Encoders: Software programs to help in the encoding process

Grouper: Software program used to determine the diagnosis related group assigned to a Medicare or other patient paid according to a DRG system

Coding requirements vary depending upon the type of patient setting. In-patients are coded differently from those in the ambulatory care situation or a physician's office (Table 43–1).

Coding in the In-Patient/ Hospital Setting

Coders working in acute care hospitals will use the ICD-9-CM classification system for coding records of hospitalized patients. Most hospitals code records after the patient is discharged. Some institutions, however, perform "concurrent" coding or code the patient's diagnoses and procedures while the patient is still hospitalized.

The coding process begins with a thorough review of all the documentation contained in the patient's medical record. Ideally, the physician has documented on the face sheet or admission record all the patient's diagnoses and conditions. Careful comparison of these stated diagnoses with the information from the patient's history and physical examination, operative report, pathology report, discharge summary, and consultation reports will enable the coder to determine all the

Table 43–1 CODING REQUIREMENTS BY SETTING

	In-patient	Ambulatory	Physician Office
ICD-9-CM Diagnosis	X	X	X
ICD-9-CM Procedures	X		
CPT-4 Procedures		X	X
HCPCS Procedures		X	X

patient's disease entities. Often, the in-patient record is not complete at the time of the patient's discharge or at the time the coder is attempting to work with the record. This is when the coder's investigative skills, coupled with a knowledge of pathophysiology and pharmacology, are crucial. Often the in-patient coder is required to code incomplete records.

In addition to coding, the in-patient coder may locate key demographic and clinical information about each patient and enter this information into a computer. This process is referred to as **abstracting.** A common set of data elements is collected on all in-patient stays. This data set is known as the uniform hospital discharge data set, or **UHDDS.** These data elements, including the disease and operation codes, create a database for the hospital. Reports can be generated from this database for the hospital's internal purposes. The information necessary to complete an insurance claim for the hospital is transferred from this clinical database into the hospital's financial database.

Coding in the Ambulatory Care Setting

Ambulatory care settings may include hospital outpatient departments, ambulatory surgery centers, urgent care centers, community mental health clinics, rehabilitation centers, home health agencies, or just about anywhere that a patient comes for health care but does not stay overnight.

All these ambulatory care centers will use the ICD-9-CM classification system for coding the patient's diagnoses or conditions. In mental health centers, the psychiatrists and psychologists will also use DSM-IV to classify the patient's condition. Depending on the insurance company requirements, each patient procedure may be coded with CPT-4, HCPCS level II or level III (for Medicare or Medicaid patients), or ICD-9-CM.

The coding process begins with a thorough review of the entire ambulatory care record. Often these records are brief and may be limited to a history or physical examination, progress notes written by the health care provider, or test results. In the ambulatory surgery centers, the records are more extensive, often including operative reports and pathology reports. It is hoped that the physician has documented the patient's condition, but if not, the ambulatory care coder must be able to determine the conditions to code.

Often the coding of ambulatory care records is simpler than in-patient records because the patient has fewer and less complicated conditions and the purpose of the visit may be quite specific. This is not always the case, however. The work of the ambulatory care coder is often thwarted by a lack of documentation or very little information upon which to make a coding decision.

Coding for Physician Services

Coding for physician services often includes coding for patient visits in the physician's office as well as coding for the physician visits to patients in all other health care settings. It may also include coding for the professional component of a test or service, such as coding for a radiologist. Regardless of the type of physician services, all patients' diagnoses or conditions are coded with ICD-9-CM. All procedures performed by the physician as well as office visits are coded with CPT-4. Procedures are rarely, if ever, coded with ICD-9-CM for physician services. Other services ordered or directed by the physician may be coded with HCPCS for Medicare or Medicaid patients.

The physician-based coder is dependent on the documentation in the physician practice record or within test or procedure reports provided by the physician. Because of the wide range of services and types of patients seen, coding for these records can vary from simple to complex. Again, the coder may be stymied by the lack of documentation or the lack of specificity in the information supplied by the physician.

Relationship of Coding to Reimbursement

Coding is extremely important for the reimbursement of health care services. Regardless of the setting, the coder must be aware that the codes selected are communicated to the insurance company and are used to determine what benefits are covered and, often, how much money is paid. Therefore, to communicate accurately, the coder must be familiar with many different reimbursement systems (Table 43–2). In the in-patient setting, codes are a direct link to the hospital's reimbursement for Medicare patients or for any other payer that uses a DRG prospective payment system. Regardless of the payer, the coder must follow basic coding principles. However, the close relationship of coding to reimbursement is something that the coder must be aware of at all times.

In the in-patient setting, the coder must select the principal diagnosis that is listed first. The coder must be careful in reviewing the entire record and determining which of the patient's conditions should be listed as the principal diagnosis. The principal diagnosis is defined by UHDDS as "that condition established after study to be chiefly responsible for occasioning the admission of the patient to the hospital for care." The circumstances of in-patient admissions always govern the selection of the principal diagnosis. For Medicare reimbursement, the DRG assignment is often dependent on the principal diagnosis selected. Next, the coder must be certain that all operating room procedures are identified, as they can affect DRG assignment. Finally, additional diagnoses, particularly complications and certain coexisting conditions that affect DRG assignment, must be identified in order to thoroughly describe each in-patient.

In the ambulatory care setting, diagnosis codes describe the reason for the patient visit; the procedure codes describe what was done to diagnose or treat the condition. Ambulatory surgery patients' services may be reimbursed according to a fee schedule referred to as the ambulatory surgery center list. Providers are paid a set fee based on the CPT-4 procedure code describing the procedure performed. In the near future, hospital outpatient services may be reimbursed by Medicare according to a DRG-like system called the ambulatory patient groups, or **APGs**. This system is likely to be based on ICD-9-CM diagnosis codes and/or CPT-4. Unlike DRGs, in which a patient is assigned to only one group, the ambulatory patient may be assigned to more than one APG. Ambulatory coders must be certain that their coding is accurate and complete to ensure proper reimbursement.

Physician office coding is used in the Medicare system called resource-based relative value scale, or **RBRVS**. Each CPT/HCPCS code is given a rela-

Table 43–2 REIMBURSEMENT SYSTEMS

In-patient/Medicare	Diagnosis related groups (DRG)
Ambulatory surgery	Ambulatory surgery center list (ASC)
Physicians/Medicare	Resource-based relative value scale (RBRVS)

tive value or a number of points that represents three components of that procedure: the physician's work, the physician's practice expense, and the physician's malpractice insurance expense. To compute the physician's payment, the relative value unit is adjusted for the geographic area in which the physician practices and is multiplied by what is called a conversion factor, or a set monetary amount determined annually by the federal government. If the CPT/HCPCS code is incorrect, the physician's payment will be incorrect too.

For patients covered by insurance other than Medicare, the CPT/HCPCS code selected to describe the physician's services will determine the reimbursement, usually according to a fee schedule or pre-established amount based on the services performed.

For the physician services, the assigned ICD-9-CM code is important to justify the services performed, but it is rarely how the reimbursement is determined. The coder in the physician office must be an expert in the CPT-4 coding system and keep up to date with the Medicare, Medicaid, and other insurance companies' policies and procedures concerning coding and billing.

Data Quality

The quality of coded data refers to the reliability, accuracy, completeness, and timeliness of the data (Table 43–3). Reliability is measuring the degree to which something yields the same results in repeated attempts. For example, several different coders using the same record should assign the same code. Accuracy is the degree to which the codes correctly reflect the patient's diagnoses and procedures. Completeness refers to the fact that all the patient's diagnoses and procedures are coded, not just one or two reasons for that individual's health care services. Finally, timeliness means that coding must be done on a daily basis or as frequently as possible to ensure that information about the patient is available for insurance claims processing and for use by the health care provider in determining the types of services performed.

Table 43–3	DATA QUALITY
Reliability	Several different coders using the same record will assign the same code.
Accuracy	The codes assigned accurately describe the diagnoses and procedures.
Completeness	All the patient's diagnoses and procedure are coded.
Timeliness	Coding is performed as soon as possible after the patient's treatment.

Poor data quality usually results from several factors. Frequently, coding errors are made when the coder fails to review the entire record. Other errors may be an incorrect code assignment or the wrong code listed as the principal diagnosis for in-patient stays. Codes for diagnoses and procedures that are not documented in the medical record are considered coding errors. Finally, data quality problems can occur when there is transposition of numbers or the incorrect number of digits in a code. These may be coding errors or data entry errors when code numbers are entered into a computer system.

Improving the Quality of Coded Data

Improving the quality of coded data usually requires several processes. First, coders must be well-trained and knowledgeable. When hiring coders, the employer may want to hire only trained coders, instead of performing on-the-job training. Coders with formal education and/or certification will often assure the employer that quality coding will occur. Second, quality data is dependent on quality information. Even the best coder cannot achieve high quality coding if the patient record is inadequately documented. One way to improve data quality is to work with the physicians to set documentation guidelines. Physicians are usually very willing to provide the details of their patients' conditions once they understand its relationship to the coding of the record and subsequently the physicians' reimbursement. Finally, quality coding requires quality resources. The coder must have current ICD-9-CM and CPT-4 code books. Other resource materials, including medical dictionaries, anatomy and physiology books, pharmacology reference texts as well as insurance company and/or Medicare provider manuals are essential for the coder to achieve a high level of data quality.

Coding Policies and Procedures

It is absolutely essential that coders have established policies and procedures to guide their work. National coding guidelines exist for inpatient and ambulatory care coding. Each facility must develop its own specific policies and procedures that include the national guidelines as well as details unique to that particular facility.

Policies and Procedures

Policies and procedures should describe how the coder performs the clinical coding function. Included in the policies and procedures should be:

- National coding guidelines
- Specific facility guidelines
- Definition of principal and secondary diagnoses and procedures
- How to review and abstract a record
- How to manage conflicting information within a record
- The use of optional codes, such as E-codes and M-codes
- How to use reference/resource materials

Coding policies establish rules and guidelines to be followed. Procedures describe what to do when documentation is incomplete or conflicting; what to do when a code cannot be found; how to review a record; what the UHDDS definitions of principal and additional diagnoses are; the use of optional codes such as E-codes or M-codes; how to review and abstract a record; and how reference materials should be used in the coding process.

Coding managers and coders should work together to develop good-quality coding policies and procedures. These policies and procedures must be continually updated to reflect problems that are encountered in everyday work and as changes occur in national guidelines and payer requirements.

Productivity of Coders

Managers usually set a time standard that states how long it takes to code. The most sophisticated productivity standards are most likely to exist in the in-patient setting. The standard will be the number of minutes that it should take to code a record or the number of records that should be coded within a set period of time, usually an hour. This time standard will vary depending on the type of record, with the in-patient Medicare record usually having the longest time standard. In the ambulatory care or physician office setting, there may be a standard that all records of patients seen in a day are coded the same day or at least within the same business week. Depending on the setting, the standard may be expressed in a time measurement or in a policy statement that says daily coding occurs for patients served in a particular day.

Regardless of the setting, coders must know what is expected of them. Productivity standards will tell the coder how quickly records must be coded or how frequently codes must be communicated to the insurance companies. This is information that the coder needs to meet the productivity standards.

Productivity standards also reflect the degree of accuracy expected of each coder. Regular coding audits are performed by coding supervisors to review the accuracy and completeness of codes assigned by the coding staff members. A quality level of 95 percent or better is usually expected. Staff members who do not meet the quality productivity standard are usually required to complete additional education and be retested. Continually failing the coding quality audits may mean the staff member is released or re-assigned to a different job.

Computer Systems and Support

Computers are often closely tied to the coding process (Table 43–4). Although many coders use the printed ICD-9-CM code books to do their work, more and more coders are using computer products called **encoders.** Encoders are software programs usually run on personal computers to help in the coding process. Encoders exist for ICD-9-CM and CPT-4 coding, and there are two basic types. One is referred to as a branching logic system. After the coder enters the main term for the diagnosis or procedure, a series of questions is returned for the coder to answer in order to make a coding assignment. The second type of encoder is more like an automated code book. The computer screen looks much like a code book page with a point-and-click approach needed to make a coding assignment. Usually, less experienced coders prefer the branching logic system because it provides the rules and direction needed to assign a code. More expert coders find that the automated code book software makes them more productive, as they can use their knowledge and skills to find the correct code quickly. Most encoders include educational material for the coder to consider as well. For example, when a particular diagnosis is entered, the encoder may prompt the coder to look for commonly related conditions or frequently occurring procedures used to treat such a condition. The encoders may also make reference to national coding guidelines for the coder's consideration.

Table 43–4	COMPUTER SUPPORT
Encoder	Software program used to assign codes
Grouper	Software program used to group individual records into DRGs for Medicare reimbursement

Usually included with the encoder software is another form of coding computer support. A **grouper** is a software program used to determine the DRG assigned to a Medicare patient or another patient paid according to a DRG system. In order to use the grouper, ICD-9-CM principal and additional diagnoses as well as the principal and additional procedure codes are entered. Additional demographic characteristics of the patient, including age, gender, and whether discharged alive or expired, are needed in order for the grouper to work. Based on this information, the grouper software tells the coder what the DRG will be as well as how the DRG can change if a different principal diagnosis is selected or if additional diagnoses are entered.

Other computer support used by the coder may be **electronic data interchange (EDI).** EDI is a type of hardware/software configuration that allows for the submission, edit, or payment of health care insurance claims. Instead of completing and mailing paper claim forms to the insurance companies, EDI allows the transmission of data across telephone or dedicated computer lines. The insurance company can also use EDI to directly deposit payments into the provider's bank account and enter claim information into the provider's accounting system. This eliminates the production and mailing (and potential loss) of paper checks and, in general, speeds up the claims processing for all concerned.

Hospitals are most likely to use sophisticated computer support for the coders. Almost every hospital today can afford to buy encoders and groupers and is likely to submit almost 100 percent of its insurance claims via EDI. The use of computers in hospital coding and claims management has become an industry standard.

The ambulatory care facility or physician office is less likely to use coding computer support; however, this too is changing. More and more physician offices are doing their own electronic transmission of insurance claims or using billing companies for that purpose.

Closing Thoughts

The coding process can vary depending on the health care setting. What does not vary is the fact that quality coding depends on the knowledge and skills of the clinical coder and the completeness of the health record. Working together as a team, the clinical coder and the health care provider can ensure that their patient's diagnoses and services are coded accurately, completely, and on a timely basis.

Review Questions

1. Explain the coding process in the in-patient setting.
2. List the various types of ambulatory care settings where the ICD-9-CM classification system would be used.
3. Discuss the importance of coding for reimbursement for healthcare services.
4. List the four measures used to determine the quality of coded data.

Bibliography

Abdelhak M, Grostick S, Hanken M, et al: Health Information Management: Management of a Strategic Resource. Philadelphia, WB Saunders, 1996.

American Psychiatric Association: Diagnostic and Statistical Manual of Mental Disorders, 4th ed. Washington, DC, 1994.

Brown F: ICD-9-CM Coding Handbook with Answers, 1997 Revised edition. Chicago, American Hospital Publishing, 1997.

Bryant G, Prophet S: Growing demand for accurate coded data in new healthcare delivery era. J Am Health Info Mgmt Assoc 1997;69:42–47.

Buck C: Step-by-Step Medical Coding. Philadelphia, WB Saunders, 1996.

Frawley K, Asmonga D: Health Insurance Portability and Accessibility Act addresses healthcare fraud and abuse. J Am Health Info Mgmt Assoc 1996;67:10–11.

Hirschl N: A closer look at ambulatory patient groups. J Am Health Info Mgmt Assoc 1996;67:222–225.

Huffman E: Health Information Management, 10th ed. Berwyn, IL, Physicians Record Co, 1994.

International Classification of Disease, 9th ed. Clinical Modification. Washington, DC, Department of Health and Human Services, 1997.

Nicholas T: Basic ICD-9-CM Coding Handbook. Chicago, American Health Information Management Association, 1997.

Nicholas T: CPT/HCPS Basic Coding Handbook. Chicago, American Health Information Management Association, 1997.

Physicians' Current Procedural Terminology, 4th ed. Chicago, American Medical Association, 1997.

Prophet S: Fraud and abuse implications for the HIM professional. J Am Health Info Mgmt Assoc 1997;68:52–55.

Prophet S: Classification systems: Taking a broader look. J Am Health Info Mgmt Assoc 1997;68:46–50.

Rogers V: Intermediate ICD-9-CM Coding Handbook for Hospitals. Chicago, American Health Information Management Association, 1996.

Rogers V: Ambulatory Surgery Coding. Chicago, American Health Information Management Association, 1996.

Rogers V: Ambulatory patient groups: An outpatient data management tool. J Am Health Info Mgmt Assoc 1996;67:356–359.

44

The Clinical Coder

Lou Ann Schraffenberger

Common Abbreviations

AAPC	American Academy of Procedural Coders
AHIMA	American Health Information Management Association
ART	Accredited record technician
CCS	Certified coding specialist
CCS-P	Certified coding specialist—physician-based
CPC	Certified procedural coder
CPC-H	Certified procedural coder—hospital
HIT	Health information management technology
SCC	Society for Clinical Coding

Objectives

At the completion of this chapter, the reader should be able to:

1. List the six broad areas of coding competency necessary for a clinical coder and give a brief description of each.
2. Name the law that applies to coding that helps combat fraud and abuse and explain why it is important for coders to be aware of it.
3. Describe the steps that a health unit coordinator could take in order to become a clinical coder.
4. Name the two professional organizations for clinical coders.

Education/Knowledge/ Skills Required

The clinical coder (Fig. 44–1) must have a thorough understanding of the content of the medical record in order to locate information to support or provide specificity for coding. Simply transferring diagnoses and procedures to codes without applying clinical knowledge is inadequate. Therefore, the coder must be familiar with the anatomy and physiology of the human body and disease processes in order to understand the etiology, pathology, symptoms, signs, diagnostic studies, treatment modalities, and prognosis of the diseases and procedures to be coded. In addition, knowledge of the coding systems, with their conventions and principles for use, is a basic requirement for a clinical coder.

Both formal education and practical experience are necessary to the development of a clinical coder. Sufficient practice and exposure to patterns of physician documentation enhance the coder's ability to make accurate coding decisions. Clinical coders must also keep up to date on coding guide-

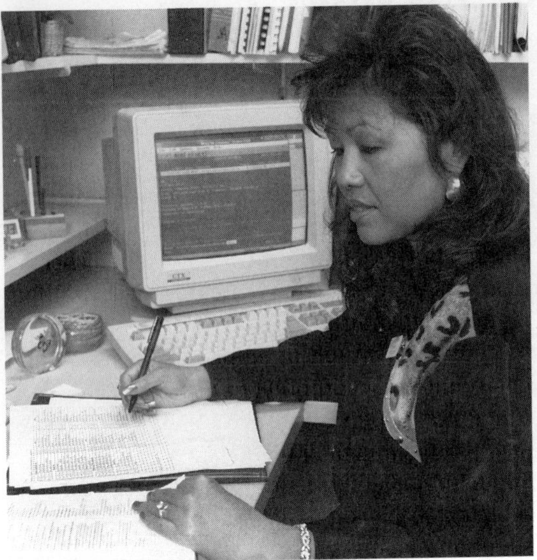

Figure 44–1
The clinical coder.

lines, as new codes and modifications are made in the coding systems annually.

Coding Competencies

The coding competencies for clinical coders working with in-patient records, ambulatory care records, or physician office records are similar. The competencies relate to six broad areas: data identification, coding guidelines, regulatory guidelines, coding, data quality, and computer skills.

Coding Competencies
The skilled clinical coder is knowledgeable in the following clinical coding areas: Data identification Coding guidelines Regulatory guidelines Coding Data quality Computer use

Data Identification

Data identification means that the coder must be able to read and interpret the documentation in the medical record to identify diagnoses and procedures for data capture and billing. This includes all diagnoses, conditions, problems, or other reasons for the care provided as well as all services or procedures performed during that stay. The coder must be capable of assessing the adequacy of medical record documentation to ensure that the documentation will support the codes assigned. Finally, the coder must apply his or her knowledge of disease processes when it is necessary to assign codes to conditions or medical terms that are not indexed in the coding books.

Coding Guidelines

The second area of competency required of all coders relates to the knowledge and use of coding guidelines. The coder must understand the official coding guidelines for the reporting of diseases, as different guidelines apply for in-patient versus outpatient care settings. Knowledge of the guidelines included in the ICD-9-CM and CPT-4 coding books is essential.

Regulatory Guidelines

A third area of competency concerns regulatory guidelines. In-patient coders must be knowledgeable about the DRG system and how it relates to the coding and reporting of diseases and conditions for the in-patient record in the case of Medicare patients and other payers using a similar system. Applying the rules outlined in the Uniform Hospital Discharge Data Set (UHDDS) is essential to define what exactly are the principal diagnosis and procedure and what additional diagnoses and procedures should be reported. For the ambulatory care or physician office coder, knowledge of ambulatory payment groups (APGs) and resource-based relative value system (RBRVS) methodology as it relates to coding must be understood. Using the CPT-4 systems, the coder must understand the concept of the "global surgical package" as it relates to what can and cannot be coded in terms of services rendered to a patient who has a surgical procedure performed. In addition, the ambulatory care and physician office coder must execute policies and procedures related to insurance claims filing and claims appeal.

Coding

Coding is the fourth area of competency for the clinical coder. The coder must apply knowledge of ICD-9-CM instructional notes and conventions to locate and assign the correct diagnosis and procedure codes and sequence them correctly. When using the CPT-4 coding system, the coder must know when to exclude from coding those procedures that are component parts of an already assigned procedure code. The coder using CPT-4 must know how and when to attach modifier codes to a CPT code to adjust the meaning of the codes.

Finally, the coder must know when to assign a level II or level III HCPCS code for services not found in the CPT-4 system. The clinical coder assigning diagnosis and procedure codes must apply knowledge of anatomy, clinical disease processes, and diagnostic and procedural terminology to assign accurate codes.

Data Quality

To maintain data quality, the coder must conduct quality assessment to ensure continuous improvement in ICD-9-CM and CPT-4/HCPCS coding and collection of health care data. Continuous communication with the physicians is essential to gather additional information needed for coding or to clarify conflicting or ambiguous information in the record. Especially true for the ambulatory and physician-based coder is the need to link ICD-9-CM codes to proper CPT-4 codes to ensure accurate insurance claims submission. Finally, the coder must evaluate his or her own educational needs to remain competent. The coder must also determine the educational needs of physicians and staff in terms of coding, reimbursement, and documentation rules as well as penalties and sanction potential for coding fraud and abuse.

Computer Skills

The last area of competency for the clinical coder is computer skills. Knowledge of and ability to work with personal computers is a must for all coders. The in-patient coder works almost exclusively with computer-supported coding systems. He or she must be able to use the computer-based encoders and groupers and have a working knowledge of word processing, spreadsheets, and database software, as all relate to the coding job. The ambulatory and physician-based coder also requires personal computer skills. Although they may not use encoders and groupers as much as in-patient coders do, ambulatory care coders use other software such as scheduling, accounting, and billing programs and electronic claims submission.

Ethical Considerations and Standards

The coder must adhere to ethical principles relating to quality, truth, and accuracy in work performance and productivity. In this era of payment based on diagnosis and procedure codes, the professional ethics of a clinical coder can be challenged. The American Health Information Management Association (AHIMA) established standards for ethical coding. The standards direct the coder to follow established coding guidelines and base the selection of the principal diagnosis and procedures on the definitions in the Uniform Hospital Discharge Data Set. The coder is expected to strive for optimal payment to which the facility or provider is legally entitled, but it is unethical and illegal to maximize payment by means that contradict regulatory guidelines.

In 1996, the Health Insurance Portability and Accountability Act was signed into law. This law establishes a Health Care Fraud and Abuse Control Program, which aims to combat fraud and abuse in Medicare and Medicaid programs as well as in the private health care industry. It is coordinated by the Office of the Inspector General and the Department of Justice. These two federal agencies have been given the power to enforce federal, state, and local laws to control health care fraud and abuse and to conduct investigations and audits pertaining to the delivery of and payment for health care services. According to this Act, criminal penalties are imposed on health care professionals who "knowingly and willfully" attempt to execute a scheme to defraud any health care benefit program (insurance company or payer) or to obtain, by means of false or fraudulent pretense, money or property owned by, or under the custody of, a health care benefit program. Usually this means that the health care institution or physician (whoever is responsible for the delivery of health care in the setting) will be investigated first. This does not mean that the clinical coder will be absolved of wrongdoing if it is found that he or she "knowingly and willfully" performed a job in a manner that would defraud a health care benefit program. The clinical coder must recognize his or her ethical obligations as a professional and refuse to participate in any suspicious or outright fraudulent coding and billing activities.

Resources for the Clinical Coder

Official Sources of Information

The clinical coder must use official sources of information to do the job (Table 44–1). First, this means using the most current edition of the ICD-9-CM and CPT-4 coding books. New books must be purchased yearly to ensure that the most accurate information is being used. Second, the coder must have access to the official coding guidelines for ICD-9-CM. These guidelines are published and regularly updated in a quarterly publication of the American Hospital Association (AHA) entitled *Coding Clinic*. *Coding Clinic* is an absolute necessity for the in-patient coder and is fast becoming essential for all coders. At one time it was written with a hospital focus on coding, but now, as health care has greatly expanded beyond the hospital setting, *Coding Clinic* has followed suit and offers more advice and guidelines pertinent to the ambulatory or physician-based coder.

Another absolute necessity is access to the official American Medical Association (AMA) publication related to CPT-4 coding, which is entitled *CPT Assistant*. This monthly newsletter provides excellent advice and consultation for the CPT-4 coder concerning the use of the codes and other issues related to coding of procedures. The AHA and AMA, in addition to the federal government, are the only sources of information for ICD-9-CM and CPT-4 coding.

Table 44–1	OFFICIAL SOURCES OF INFORMATION
ICD-9-CM	*Coding Clinic*—publication from the American Hospital Association
CPT-4	*CPT Assistant*—publication from the American Medical Association

Publications and Resources

Other publications exist for the clinical coder. The AHIMA, the AHA, and the AMA publish books and educational materials of value to the coder. These books range from basic, how-to-code books to materials developed for the experienced, expert coder. Various other companies produce educational materials for the clinical coder. These materials range from excellent to substandard, so the buyer must be aware of what information is useful.

Insurance companies, in particular Medicare and Medicaid, issue manuals for the coding and submission of claims. Especially important is the monthly Medicare Part B newsletter published by almost every state's Medicare carrier. This newsletter is sent to every physician office and every provider paid under Medicare Part B and is sent by subscription to other interested parties. It contains essential information on Medicare coding and claims submission that cannot be found anywhere else.

Membership Organizations

Clinical coders should also take advantage of resources offered by professional coding organizations, such as the Society for Clinical Coding (SCC) affiliated with the AHIMA and the American Academy of Procedural Coders (**AAPC**). Both organizations sponsor educational programs and newsletters for their members that provide excellent information to support quality coding and competent practice.

Certification

Clinical coders can also become certified or obtain a professional credential by taking examinations offered by the AHIMA and the AAPC.

The AHIMA offers two examinations: one for the hospital-based coder and one for the ambulatory or physician-based coder. Both examinations are intended to demonstrate expert practice. The most successful candidates are usually experienced coders, not entry-level practitioners. Depending on the examination taken, the coder could earn the designation certified coding specialist, or **CCS**, or the designation certified coding specialist—physician-based, or **CCS-P**.

The AAPC offers two similar examinations for the hospital-based coder and the physician-based coder. The designations earned could be certified procedural coder, or **CPC**, or certified procedural coder—hospital, or **CPC-H**.

The Health Unit Coordinator and Coding

The HUC may be doing some coding already in his or her job. There is a natural link between the two careers. The knowledge and skills acquired in the HUC programs, the work experience of interacting with health professionals in medical settings, and the ability to understand the content of the medical record will be beneficial to the HUC who decides to move into a coding position.

Clinical coding is a specialized skill that can be built nicely upon the foundation of the HUC's education and experience. To advance into other dedicated coding positions, however, the HUC might consider additional formal or continuing education opportunities.

One-year coding programs are becoming more available in community colleges and business schools. Typically these coding programs are not accredited by an external agency or group. To select the best programs, the HUC should review the curriculum to see that it contains the necessary information. An outline of the curriculum should include medical record content, medical terminology, anatomy and physiology, disease process or pathophysiology, pharmacology, basic hospital in-patient coding with ICD-9-CM, basic ambulatory care coding with ICD-9-CM, basic CPT-4 coding for ambulatory and physician-based services, reimbursement systems, and possibly advanced ICD-9-CM and CPT-4 coding.

HUCs who desire more advancement opportunities may consider the 2-year health information management technology (**HIT**) programs. About 150 accredited programs exist in the United States in community colleges, business colleges, and vocational/trade schools. Completion of the HIT program allows the graduate to write the national accreditation examination to become an accredited records technician, or **ART**. Many ARTs accept coding positions in hospitals and clinics, but their education, which includes other aspects of information management, allows them to consider more diverse job opportunities, including supervisory positions and research associates.

Other educational opportunities, such as continuing education and independent study, may also be considered by the HUC. Many community colleges offer courses in medical terminology, anatomy and physiology, and pharmacology that can be taken for college credit or for continuing education. These courses may range from 6 to 16 weeks in length. The HUC can examine his or her own strengths and weaknesses, perhaps talk to a health careers academic advisor at the school, and decide which courses will provide an expanded knowledge base without necessitating a formal 1- or 2-year program.

Independent study programs to become a skilled clinical coder are also available. The

AHIMA offers two such programs: one for the ART candidate and one strictly for clinical coding. These programs require the student to complete and return to an instructor the modules and assignments that are mailed to the student. These independent study programs have the same content information as the community college–based programs. Anyone who has ever attempted independent study knows that it requires organization and discipline, because the completion schedule must be determined by the student. There are no classes to attend and no instructor requiring the completion of lessons on a timed basis. However, independent study is invaluable to the working person who cannot take time off from work to go back to school or for the working person who does not have a nearby community college or trade school. Information about the AHIMA independent study programs can be obtained by calling the Chicago office at 312-787-2672. Information is also available on the AHIMA website at www.ahima.org.

Future of Coding

Some people claim that the computer-based patient record will eliminate the job of the clinical coder. There is the potential in the computer-based medical record, through what is known as natural language processing, that the diagnosis and procedure codes will be automatically generated without a human interface. Although this potential exists, the prevalence of the computer-based patient record appears to lie several years in the future.

In the immediate future, the demand for skilled clinical coders is likely to exceed the supply. The greatest expansion of jobs appears to be in non-hospital settings, such as ambulatory centers, physician offices, home health agencies, long-term care facilities, and the like. For many years, payment to these facilities was not determined by coded patient information. This has dramatically changed, and more facilities now appreciate the value of coded data. They rely on the skilled clinical coder to perform that function for them to ensure optimal reimbursement for their services.

The coding systems are likely to change over time. The ICD-9-CM system will probably be replaced by the International Classification of Diseases, 10th edition (ICD-10), between the years 2000 and 2002. ICD-10 will be expanded to six digits for some medical entities and enable more specificity for the coding of certain conditions. A new procedure classification system for hospitals will take effect at the same time. This system, which appears to be radically different from the existing ICD-9-CM procedure system, will be called the I-10 Procedural Classification System. CPT-4 continues to be updated on a yearly basis, and there are no known plans to radically change the system. There have been discussions about the need for one procedure coding system, which would eliminate either the ICD-9 or the CPT-4 procedure system. However, considering the varied and extensive applications of these systems within different sectors of health care, the idea of a single procedure classification does not appear imminent.

Closing Thoughts

Although nothing is absolute, the future seems bright for the clinical coder. Opportunities for employment will continue to exist. Owing to the fact that the coding systems as well as the practice of medicine and its use of technology are likely to change over time, clinical coders will be required to continually update their knowledge and skills to remain competitive in the health care job market. The clinical coder who maintains cutting-edge knowledge of coding systems, medicine, reimbursement systems, and computer technology will be a valuable asset in the health care industry.

Review Questions

1. List the six broad areas of coding competency necessary for a clinical coder and give a brief description of each.

2. Name the law that applies to coding that helps to combat fraud and abuse and explain why it is important for coders to be aware of it.

3. Describe the steps that a health unit coordinator could take in order to become a clinical coder.

4. Name the two professional organizations for clinical coders.

Bibliography

Abdelhak M, Grostick S, Hanken M, et al: Health Information Management: Management of a Strategic Resource. Philadelphia, WB Saunders, 1996.

American Psychiatric Association: Diagnostic and Statistical Manual of Mental Disorders, 4th ed. Washington, DC, 1994.

Brown F: ICD-9-CM Coding Handbook with Answers, 1997 Revised edition. Chicago, American Hospital Publishing, 1997.

Bryant G, Prophet S: Growing demand for accurate coded data in new healthcare delivery era. J Am Health Info Mgmt Assoc 1997; 69:42–47.

Buck C: Step-by-Step Medical Coding. Philadelphia, WB Saunders, 1996.

Frawley K, Asmonga D: Health Insurance Portability and Accessibility Act addresses healthcare fraud and abuse. J Am Health Info Mgmt Assoc 1996; 67:10–11.

Hirschl N: A closer look at ambulatory patient groups. J Am Health Info Mgmt Assoc 1996; 67:22–25.

Huffman E: Health Information Management, 10th ed. Berwyn, IL, Physicians Record Co, 1994.

International Classification of Disease, 9th ed. Clinical Modification. Washington, DC, Department of Health and Human Services, 1997.

Nicholas T: Basic ICD-9-CM Coding Handbook. Chicago, American Health Information Management Association, 1997.

Nicholas T: CPT/HCPS Basic Coding Handbook. Chicago, American Health Information Management Association, 1997.

Physicians' Current Procedural Terminology, 4th ed. Chicago, American Medical Association, 1997.

Prophet S: Fraud and abuse implications for the HIM professional. J Am Health Info Mgmt Assoc 1997; 68:52–55.

Prophet S: Classification systems: Taking a broader look. J Am Health Info Mgmt Assoc 1997; 68:546–550.

Rogers V: Intermediate ICD-9-CM Coding Handbook for Hospitals. Chicago, American Health Information Management Association, 1996.

Rogers V: Ambulatory Surgery Coding. Chicago, American Health Information Management Association, 1996.

Rogers V: Ambulatory patient groups: An outpatient data management tool. J Am Health Info Mgmt Assoc 1996; 67:56–59.

The Professional Organization for Health Unit Coordinators

The National Association of Health Unit Coordinators, Inc. (NAHUC) is the professional association of health unit coordinators. It was established to promote and maintain competent practitioners in the delivery of nonclinical services. NAHUC's mission statement is that the organization is dedicated to promoting health unit coordinating as a profession through education, certification, and complying with the NAHUC Standards of Practice, Standards of Education, and Code of Ethics.

History

In 1977, Myrna LaFleur, an educator from Phoenix, did a national survey to determine the number and kind of unit coordinating educational programs in existence in the United States. She found that not all states had programs but that there were 52 programs located in adult educational centers, community colleges, and vocational/technical schools. Part of the survey asked the participants to indicate if they were interested in the formation of a national association for health unit coordinators. In 1980, Myrna was invited to speak to a group of unit coordinators and unit managers in Minneapolis. She mentioned during her presentation that a state association for health unit coordinators had recently been formed in Arizona. She was delighted to hear that Wisconsin had a local association and that there was a great deal of interest in forming a national association. Myrna was highly motivated by this meeting and contacted those who had responded to her earlier survey and invited these individuals to meet in Phoenix in August 1980. The outcome of the weekend meeting was the development of a constitution and the birth of the National Association of Health Unit Clerks/Coordinators.

It was determined that unit "coordinator" was a term that was not yet universally accepted, so both clerk and coordinator were included in the title. In 1981 the organization was incorporated as a nonprofit professional association.

In 1982 the first national convention was held and the certification board was formed.
In 1983 the first certification examination was given.
In 1984 the Education Board was formed, and the Continuing Education Committee was organized to grant contact hours.
In 1990 the Accreditation Board was formed.
In 1991 "clerk" was officially dropped from the title.
In 1992 the recertification pilot project was begun.
In 1993 the recertification program was initiated.
In 1994 NAHUC became an associate member of the American Hospital Association.
In 1995 the Certification Board developed a plan to form a new corporation in 1998.

General Membership Information

The leadership of NAHUC is vested in a Board of Directors, which consists of a representative from each of nine geographic regions, the directors of the subsidiary boards, and four officers (president, president-elect, secretary, and treasurer). There are several committees to accomplish the duties of the organization.

NAHUC has the following responsibilities to its members:

To conduct the business of the association, through the NAHUC Board of Directors, in the most effective manner available.
To disseminate information to the members regarding the operation of the association and decisions made as well as information that may be useful to increase their knowledge.
To offer and promote educational opportunities on a local, state, regional, and national level.
To support elected officers in conducting the business of the association honestly, diligently, and expediently.
To serve as the official representative of health unit coordinating to allied health professionals, government and educational facilities, and the community.
To certify those who meet the requirements of the NAHUC certification program.
To research and plan for the future needs of the membership and profession.

Active membership is open to health unit coordinators, health unit coordinator educators, and health unit coordinator supervisors. Student membership is open to those currently enrolled in health unit coordinator education programs. Institutional (supporting) membership is open to health care facilities, professional associations, and individual practitioners of other allied health professions. Retired membership is open to those who otherwise qualify for active membership but either have retired or have taken an extended leave of absence from active practice. Honorary membership is awarded to individuals who have rendered outstanding service to health unit coordinating.

Membership in NAHUC grants the individual voting privileges on issues affecting the association, in elections for national offices, for changes in the corporation and its emphasis, for bylaw changes, and in making resolutions at the annual meeting. Membership also offers opportunities for:

Benchmarking
Development of leadership skills through participation at the local, state, regional, and national levels
Serving on committees and boards
Meeting with national leaders
Discounts at NAHUC sponsored events
Continuing education
Networking with peers.

Complimentary member benefit items include:

The NAHUC membership pin
The quarterly newsletter *The Coordinator*
The NAHUC information booklet
The NAHUC national membership directory
Workshop information
Regional newsletter

Members are encouraged to join local chapters and participate in their activities whenever possible.

NAHUC Objectives

Promote recognition of health unit coordinators as professionals with skills and expertise in their chosen field.
Develop and present educational programs that offer continuing education and credit (contact hours) to maintain and increase the coordinator's knowledge and area of expertise.
Increase membership, thereby strengthening our association to accomplish its goals.
Develop accreditation and educational programs.
Promote certification.
Encourage development of health unit coordinating programs in local colleges.
Provide information to prospective health unit coordinating students.
Serve as the official representative of health unit coordinators to allied health professionals, government and educational facilities, and the community.
Encourage the *Dictionary of Occupational Titles* to

accept the name "Health Unit Coordinator" as the title for our profession.

Standards of Practice

A standard of practice is a statement of guidelines serving as a model of performance by which practitioners shall conduct their actions.

These standards are set forth to obtain the best possible service from practitioners for the purpose of providing the organization and competency needed to coordinate the health unit in exemplary fashion, enabling the best care for the patient.

The National Association of Health Unit Coordinators Inc. has formulated standards of practice to encompass all health units. There will be ongoing evaluation and revision in order to keep pace with the advancement of technology and the changes of the objectives and functions of the health units.

Purpose

The purpose of the NAHUC standards is to specify guidelines for health unit coordinators to follow. These standards have as their objectives:

1. Define the realm of the health unit coordinators in the health care system.
2. Specify the primary responsibilities of the health unit coordinator in the nonclinical area of health care.

Basic Assumptions

1. Health unit coordinators provide the nondirect, nonclinical patient care for health services.
2. Standards for these services are established by health unit coordinators, supervisors and educators, and health care agencies.
3. Health unit coordinators accept responsibility for their competency through individual growth, continued education, and certification.
4. Health unit coordinators are responsive to the changing needs and growth of health care.

Criteria for Statements of Standards

A standard is used as a model for the action of practitioners. Criteria used in establishing the NAHUC standards for health unit coordinators are:

1. A standard is established by an authority, in this instance, the National Association of Health Unit Coordinators, Inc.
2. A standard is based upon appropriate knowledge.
3. A standard is broad in scope, relevant, attainable, and definitive.
4. A standard is subject to continued evaluation and revisions.

Standard 1 Education

Health unit coordinator personnel shall be prepared through appropriate education and training programs for their responsibility in the provision of nondirect patient care and nonclinical services.

Guidelines

Education shall be set forth by adopted NAHUC Educational Standards.

Standard 2 Policy and Procedure

Written standards of health unit coordinators' practice and related policies and procedures shall define and describe the scope and conduct of nonclinical services provided by the health unit coordinator. These standards, policies, and procedures shall be reviewed annually and revised as necessary. These revisions will be dated to indicate the last review, signed by the responsible authority, and implemented.

Guidelines

1. Policies shall include criteria based on job description.

2. Personnel policies shall be included.

3. Policies will include the philosophy and objectives of the health care organization.

4. Operational and nonclinical policies and procedures will be included.

Standard 3
Standards of Performance

Written evaluation of health unit coordinators shall be criteria based and related to the standards of performance as defined by the health care organization.

Guidelines

1. Standards of performance shall define functions, responsibilities, qualifications, and accountability, reflecting autonomy of practice.

2. Review shall be on at least an annual basis with evaluation to reflect current job requirements.

3. Standards of performance shall be available to health unit coordinators.

Standard 4
Communication

The health unit coordinator shall appropriately and effectively communicate with nursing and medical staff, all ancillary departments, visitors, guests, and patients.

Guidelines

1. There shall be a written organizational plan that defines authority, accountability, and communication.

2. The organization shall assure that health unit coordinator service functions are fulfilled.

3. Health unit coordinators shall hold meetings no less than six times per year to define problems and propose solutions. A record shall be maintained documenting the content of these meetings for the purpose of monitoring and evaluating their direction.

Standard 5
Professionalism and Ethics

The health unit coordinator shall take all possible measures to assure the optimal quality of nondirect, nonclinical patient care. The optimal professional and ethical conduct and practices of NAHUC members shall be maintained at all times.

Guidelines

1. Health unit coordinators shall participate in staff development.

2. Services shall be provided according to approved policies.

3. All required meetings shall be attended.

4. All current competencies shall be maintained.

Standard 6
Leadership

The health unit coordinator shall be organized to meet and maintain established standards of nonclinical services.

Guidelines

1. Services should be directed by a qualified individual with appropriate education, experience, and knowledge of health unit coordinating services.

2. Leadership and guidance shall be provided to the health unit coordinator.

3. Responsibility and authority shall assure that:

   a. Hospital policy and procedures are followed.

   b. Hospital goals and objectives are met.

   c. Reasonable steps are taken to assure that optimal quality of patient care is provided.

4. It is desirable that the health unit coordinator leader have an associate degree in health service management.

Code of Ethics

This code of ethics is to serve as a guide by which health unit coordinators may evaluate their professional conduct as it relates to patients, colleagues, and other members of the health care professions. This code of ethics shall be subject to monitoring, interpretation, and periodical revision by the association's Board of Directors.

Therefore, in the practice of our profession, we the members of the National Association of Health Unit Coordinators, Inc., accept the following principles:

Principle One

Members shall conduct themselves in such a manner as to gain the respect and confidence of the patients, health care personnel, and community as well as respecting the human dignity of each individual.

Principle Two

Members shall protect the patients' rights, including the right to privacy.

Principle Three

Members shall strive to achieve and maintain a high level of competency.

Principle Four

Members shall strive to improve their knowledge and skills by participating in educational and professional activities and sharing the benefits of their attainments with their colleagues.

Principle Five

Unethical and illegal professional activities shall be reported to the appropriate authorities.

NAHUC National Certification Examination

The national health unit coordinator certification examination is designed to measure knowledge and skill in the areas of health unit coordinator job performance. Review for the examination is recommended. The examination is geared to neither geographic nor specialty areas. The examination is prepared, administered, and graded by a testing agency. The questions for the examination are written by health unit coordinator practitioners and educators.

Certification denotes a process by which the National Association of Health Unit Coordinators, Inc., grants recognition for basic knowledge (or competency) to an individual who has met certain predetermined qualifications specified by NAHUC. Certification is a voluntary process. Certification enhances the personal and professional growth of the health unit coordinator and offers the certificant the right to use the title "Certified Health Unit Coordinator" (CHUC). Certification is another step in the professional ladder that says to the employer, other health professionals, and the consumer that you are actively participating in your professional growth and development.

Requirements

Candidates for certification need not be members of NAHUC. Anyone who is currently a unit coordinator (ward clerk, floor secretary, unit secretary) or who has completed training to become a unit coordinator or anyone who is involved with unit coordinator activities may test for certification.

A 10-question affidavit is answered prior to testing, and identification is required.

The Examination Process

The certification examination is a 120-item (20 pretest items and 100 test items), comprehensive, job-related objective test administered nationally.

While the certification board of NAHUC has overall responsibility for test development and administration, a professional testing agency is contracted to administer the program and provide psychometric guidance for the testing program.

The examination is administered on an electronic testing system known as EXPro. This system eliminates the use of paper and pencil answer sheets. Examination questions and answers are presented on a touch-sensitive screen. A computer memory card records responses and automatically times the examination. EXPro allows you to change answers, skip questions, and mark questions for review. It is not necessary to know typing or computers to use the testing equipment. Examinations are scored immediately. You will leave the test center with your official score in hand. There is a 60-day waiting period for re-examination. There are EXPro centers located throughout the United States. Special testing arrangements may be made in the event that the candidate has a disability that precludes his or her utilizing the conventional examination process.

Recertification

Maintaining certification status is voluntary and the responsibility of the individual CHUC. Recertification is based on a three-year cycle and can be accomplished by either of the following methods:

Provide proof to the NAHUC certification board of having acquired 36 NAHUC contact hours for various education activities during the 3-year period of your certification

OR

Take and pass the certification examination before the expiration date of your present certification.

Upon satisfying either of these requirements, a new card and recertification certificate will be issued. Your original certification date and number will be maintained.

Failure to recertify will result in your no longer being recognized as certified via revocation of the certificate. To become certified after revocation, the examination must be retaken. Upon passing, a new certificate and certification card will be issued.

Continuing Education

Continuing education for the health unit coordinator is essential and a lifelong educational process. The ultimate goal is to be a graduate of an accredited health unit coordinator program or to have health unit coordinator experience combined with continuing education.

In today's rapidly changing health care field, the health unit coordinator risks becoming technically obsolete if his or her knowledge is not current. Continued learning will enhance the health unit coordinator's personal and professional growth. Continuing education is important because it:

Serves as a means of maintaining or improving professional competence.

Is evidence of personal and professional growth to meet changing career demands.

Helps to meet the challenges of a changing labor market by preparing for expanding or new job responsibilities.

Demonstrates a conscious and persistent effort toward personal development.

Serves as documentation of continuing qualifications for recertification.

Continuing education helps to keep you current in your field of expertise. Examples of professional growth courses for the health unit coordinator would be: Current Health Care Changes, Government Regulations, Computer Skills (hardware and software), Communication, Accounting, Office Management, and Interpersonal Skills. These are just a few of the classes available to assist in lateral and vertical career expansion.

Continuing education (and possible education credits) may be acquired in many ways such as:

1. Attendance at educational offerings/workshops/seminars/conventions sponsored by your health care facility. If your facility is not offering continuing education specifically designed for health unit coordinators, encourage it to do so

and to make application for Institutional Providership, which will supply you with the contact hours necessary to maintain your recertification (if you are certified).

2. View a video pertinent to health unit coordinating (which may be obtained from the NAHUC Video Library), complete the post test provided and submit it to the NAHUC Education Board.

3. Write an article for the NAHUC publication *The Coordinator,* for your health care facility newsletter, or for a journal or magazine.

4. Write a book.

As you accumulate continuing education credits, keep a record in your portfolio, in your personnel file at work, and for documents to be submitted for recertification (if you are certified).

Personal and professional growth and development through continuing education should bring satisfaction to the health unit coordinator as well as broadening his or her horizons. Trends in health care are in constant change. We must keep informed and up to date with the changes.

Program Approval Process

Request an application packet for NAHUC contact hours from the NAHUC office. The completed packet with applicable fees is submitted to the NAHUC Continuing Education Committee for approval 60 days prior to the date of the presentation. Upon approval, NAHUC contact hour certificates will be provided to the program coordinator.

The program coordinator is required to return completed program evaluation and attendance report within 30 days after the presentation.

NAHUC Career Ladder

Health Unit Coordinator I

1. Is competent in use of medical terminology.
2. Passes basic human anatomy course.
3. Passes basic pharmacology course.
4. One year clerical/public relations experience.
5. Practices appropriate communication skills.
6. Follows basic job criteria.
7. Graduate of a health unit coordinator training program.

Health Unit Coordinator II

1. Certified by passing the NAHUC certification examination.
2. Practices independent transcription, depending on institution and policies.
3. Precepts other health unit coordinators.
4. Shows the ability to take verbal and phone orders in institutions that allow it.
5. Attends continuing education workshops and in-services.

Health Unit Coordinator III

1. Helps prepare budgets and is responsible for accounting procedures in the unit.
2. Prepares work schedules and monitors productivity for nursing staff/unit.
3. Supervises internal activity and evaluates other health unit coordinators and nonclinical personnel.
4. Plans, teaches, and/or assists with continuing education, workshops, and in-services.

The ultimate goal is to start with graduates of an accredited health unit coordinator program or previous health unit coordinator experience.

Regional and State Associations and Local Chapters

The grassroots of any association is at the local level. The members are able to accomplish that which cannot be done as effectively at the national level. The local chapter and state and regional associations provide a forum for networking with peers in the surrounding area who share the same related issues and common goals. Much more can be accomplished collectively, sharing the expertise of each other.

NAHUC addresses and acts upon issues that are presented by the local affiliates. Participation at the local level is an opportunity to collect ideas and data, problem-solve, and share the information with the national organization. NAHUC can act upon this information for the enrichment of health unit coordinators nationwide.

Many health unit coordinators are not able to travel to the annual national educational conference; therefore, participation at the local level provides many of the same networking and educational opportunities on a smaller scale.

Serving on a committee locally or nationally will help to develop leadership skills that are transferable to a position on the national Boards as well as to enhance career development opportunities.

Forming a Chapter

Five or more NAHUC members in good standing are needed to start a chapter.

Request an application for an affiliation packet from the NAHUC office.
Follow the instructions and step-by-step directions for filling out the application and developing the bylaws.
Submit with fees to the NAHUC office.

The application will be reviewed by the Chapters Committee, and a recommendation will be made to the Board of Directors of NAHUC, who will vote at the winter or summer meeting.

The chapter will be notified of the results within 2 weeks of the respective Board meeting.

Parting Thoughts

The principal authors of this book had the opportunity to serve NAHUC at the national level as well as being chapter members, certified and recertified. It offered us opportunities to meet with other HUCs and share ideas, many of which became items brought before the Board of Directors for vote. It was interesting that many times an idea was brought up by one of us, and by the time it was discussed by others, it became improved (though often barely recognizable). As we reviewed the members' handbook, there are still some bylaws and policies that came about during our terms of service.

We encourage all of the HUCS who read this book to become active members at the local and national level and to become certified. You ***ARE*** *the profession. Your voice needs to be heard.*

Make your institution aware of who you are and what you do. Celebrate HUC Day August 23rd of each year. You can never lose by being proud of who and what you are and educating others to the fact. Use your association to help you get this recognition.

For More Information Contact:
NAHUC*
1211 Locust Street
Philadelphia, PA 19107
1-888-22-NAHUC
FAX 215-545-3310
E-mail 73764.123@compuserve.com

*Address current as of 6/1/98.

Index

Note: Page numbers in *italics* refer to illustrations, page numbers followed by t refer to tables.

D

E

F

G

H

I

Q

R

S

T

HEALTH UNIT COORDINATING

Expanding the Scope of Practice